Principles and Practice of Trauma Nursing

Edited by

Rose Ann O'Shea

RN BN MN DipIMC–RCS(Ed) DPSN PGCE RNT CertMedLaw SRPara

Consultant Nurse, Emergency Care, Redhill, Surrey, UK

Foreword by

Keith Porter

Consultant Trauma and Orthopaedic Surgeon, Selly Oak Hospital, Birmingham, UK

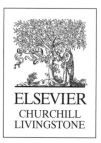

ELSEVIER
CHURCHILL
LIVINGSTONE

EDINBURGH   LONDON   NEW YORK   OXFORD   PHILADELPHIA   ST LOUIS   SYDNEY   TORONTO   2005

ELSEVIER
CHURCHILL
LIVINGSTONE

First published 2005

ISBN 0 443 06405 9

British Library Cataloguing in Publication Data
A catalogue record for this book is available from the British Library

Library of Congress Cataloging in Publication Data
A catalog record for this book is available from the Library of Congress

Notice
Knowledge and best practice in this field are constantly changing. As new research and experience broaden our knowledge, changes in practice, treatment and drug therapy may become necessary or appropriate. Readers are advised to check the most current information provided (i) on procedures featured or (ii) by the manufacturer of each product to be administered, to verify the recommended dose or formula, the method and duration of administration, and contraindications. It is the responsibility of the practitioner, relying on their own experience and knowledge of the patient, to make diagnoses, to determine dosages and the best treatment for each individual patient, and to take all appropriate safety precautions. To the fullest extent of the law, neither the publisher nor the editor assumes any liability for any injury and/or damage.

The Publisher

 your source for books, journals and multimedia in the health sciences

www.elsevierhealth.com

The Publisher's policy is to use paper manufactured from sustainable forests

Printed in China

Contents

Contributors

Peter Bentley BSc(Hons) MSc PGCEA RGN
Lecturer, School of Nursing & Midwifery, City University London, London, UK

John V. Brooke BSc(Hons) MB ChB(Edin) DOOstRCOG DCH MRCGP DipIMC-RCS(Ed)
Member of the emergency service SOS Médecin and General Practitioner, Nice, France

Adam J. Brooks MB ChB FRCS(Gen Surg) DMCC
Fellow in Trauma & Surgical Critical Care, Division of Trauma & Surgical Critical Care, Hospital University of Pennsylvania, Pennsylvania, USA

Helen Burdett MB ChB FRCS
Anaesthetics, Anaesthetic Department, Derriford Hospital, Plymouth, UK

Fiona Churchill RGN CertMinInj
Nurse Practitioner, Minor Injuries Clinic, Western General Hospital, Edinburgh, UK

Elaine Cole BSc MSc PGDipEd RGN ENB199 ENBA86
Lecturer/Practitioner, Accident and Emergency and Trauma, City University School of Nursing and Midwifery, Barts and the London NHS Trust, London, UK

Brenda Cottam DPSN DipIMC-RCS(Ed) RGN
Heartstart UK Regional Co-ordinator (Scotland), British Heart Foundation

Mark Dawes DipHE DipIMC-RCS(Ed) RGN ENB 199,998
Majors Nurse Practitioner, Accident and Emergency Department, Good Hope Hospital, Sutton Coldfield, UK

Bridgit Dimond MA LLB DSA AHSM Barrister-at-Law
Emeritus Professor, University of Glamorgan, Pontypridd, UK

Peter Driscoll BSc(Hons) MD MB ChB FRCS(Ed) FFAEM
Consultant, Accident and Emergency Department, Hope Hospital, Manchester, UK

John Eaton MB BS LRCP MRCS, DipIMC-RCS (Ed), DFFP
General Practitioner, Great Chesterfield, UK

Sharon Edwards MSc DipN(Lond) PGCEA RGN
Senior Lecturer, School of Nursing and Midwifery, University of Hertfordshire, Hatfield, UK

S.M. Gallagher SEN RGN ONC ENB371,998
Clinical Manager, Trauma and Orthopaedics, Worthing and Southlands Hospital NHS Trust, Worthing, UK

Peter L. Gregory MB BS MSc DCH MRCGP PGCAP FFSEM
Director of MSc Sports Medicine, Centre for Sports Medicine, University Hospital, Queens Medical Centre, Nottingham, UK

Teresa A. Griffiths BA(Hons) PMRAFNS
Specialist Nurse Practitioner in Trauma

Barry Hart RN SRPara DipIMC-RCS(Ed) ITU Nursing Cert CCU Nursing Cert
Paramedic, Snetterton Race Circuit, Norwich, UK

John Horton BA Ed(PCA) Dip.IMCRCSEd SRPara
Independent Clinical Practitioner and Training Consultant, Chelmsford, UK

Lesley Jenkins MSc RGN CertB&P CertA&E ATNC(I)
Senior Nurse, Emergency Unit, University Hospital of Wales, Cardiff

Tim Kilner BN(Hons) RGN PGCE SRP DipIMC-RCS(Ed)
Head of Education and Development, Gloucestershire Ambulance Service NHS Trust, Formerly Lecturer in Emergency Nursing, The University of Birmingham, Birmingham, UK

Graham Lethbridge MB BS PGDipSurgAnat
*Critical Care Resident, The Northern Hospital,
Melbourne, Australia*

Nicholas Maartens MB ChB FRACS FRCS(sn)
*Consultant Neurosurgeon, The Royal Melbourne
Hospital, Melbourne, Australia*

Ann McGinley BSc (Hons), MSc RGN ENB100
*Consultant Nurse, Patient at Risk Team, Barts and
the London NHS Trust, London, UK*

Iain McNeil MB ChB FIMCRCS(Ed) MRCGP DRCOG
DFFP EMD
*Associate Director (Ambulance Lead), NHS
Modernisation Agency, Performance Development
Team, Leicester, UK*

Ian Maconochie FFAEM FRCPCH
*Consultant, Department of Paediatrics, St Mary's
Hospital, London, UK*

Janet Marsden BSc MSc MCMI OND RGN
*Senior Lecturer, Department of Health Care Studies,
The Manchester Metropolitan University,
Manchester, UK*

Terry Martin MSc MB BS DAvMed DipIMC FIMC
RCS(Ed) FRCS(Ed) FCARCSI MRCA MRAeS
*Consultant in Anaesthetics, Nuffield Department of
Anaesthetics, John Radcliffe Hospital, Oxford, UK*

Wendy Matthews BSc(Hons) MBBS MRCP FFAEM
*Emergency Medicine Consultant, Chelsea &
Westminster Hospital, London, UK*

Priscilla M. Noble-Mathews BM DipPallMed
FIMC-RCS(Ed) OStJ
Sessional General Practitioner, UK

Rose Ann O'Shea RN BN MN DipIMC-RCS(Ed) DPSN
PGCE RNT CertMedLaw SRPara
*Consultant Nurse, Emergency Care, Surrey and
Sussex Healthcare NHS Trust, Redhill, Surrey, UK*

Lynn J. Parker MSc CertEd ENB329 SRN
*Independent Infection Control Nurse,
Healthcare A2Z, Sheffield, UK*

David R. J. Parkins MBBS FRCS(A&E)Ed FDSRCSEng
FIMC-RCS(Ed) FFAEM
*Consultant in Accident & Emergency Medicine,
Northumbria Healthcare NHS Trust, Wansbeck
General Hospital, Northumberland, UK*

Ann Paynter BSc(Hons) RGN RSCN FETC Cert A&E
ATNC(I)
*Senior Sister/Emergency Nurse Practitioner, Accident
& Emergency Unit, Morriston Hospital, Swansea
NHS Trust, Swansea, UK*

Emyr I. Phillips SBStJ MSc(Dist) MBA BN RGN PGCE
Cert A&E ATNC(I)
*Senior Nurse Manager/Honorary Lecturer,
Emergency Care & Emergency Planning, Accident &
Emergency Unit, Morriston Hospital, Swansea NHS
Trust & University of Wales Swansea, Swansea, UK*

Juergen Rayner-Klein DA(UK) FRCA DipIMC RCS(Ed)
FIMC RCS(Ed)
*Consultant in Anaesthesia and Intensive Care
Medicine, Critical Care Directorate, Derby Hospitals
NHS Foundation Trust, Derby, UK*

Ann Richards BA MSc RGN RNT
*Senior Lecturer, Department of Allied Health
Professions, University of Hertfordshire, Hatfield, UK*

Catherine A. Rowe BSC(Hons) ENB125 RGN
*Nurse Consultant, Critical Care Intensive Care
Units, Derby Hospitals NHS Foundation Trust,
Derby, UK*

Rebecca Salter MBBS BSc MRCPCH
*Specialist Registrar in Paediatric Accident &
Emergency Medicine, St Mary's Hospital, London,
UK*

Tessa Sharpe RGN ENB199 A&E Nursing ENB A86
Trauma Care ALS PALS
*Emergency Department Sister, Accident &
Emergency Department, Addenbrooke's Hospital,
Cambridge, UK*

Howard Sherriff MBChB FRCS Ed FIMC RCS(Ed) MA
(Cantab)
*Consultant, Accident & Emergency Department,
Addenbrooke's Hospital, Cambridge, UK*

Lynda Sibson MSc RGN RSCN ENB901 Asthma Dip
Nurse Practitioner Dip CTHE
*Nurse Consultant, The Modernising Healthcare
Partnership; Managing Director, TIE Europe*

Tony Simcock MB BS FFARCS
*Honorary Consultant Anaesthetist, Royal Cornwall
Hospial, Truro, UK*

Mike Smith MSc PG DipEd RN
*Staff Development Educator, Centre for Nursing,
Evidence-based Practice, Research and Education,
Royal Perth Hospital, Perth, WA, Australia*

Linda Stark BSc(Hons) RGN PSIICertA&E CertMinInj
CertCouns CertHIVN
*Lead Nurse Practitioner, Minor Injuries Clinic,
Western General Hospital, Edinburgh, UK*

Richard S. Steyn MS FRCSEd(C-Th) FIMCRCSEd
MRCGP DRCOG
*Consultant Surgeon, Regional Department of
Thoracic Surgery, Birmingham Heartlands Hospital,
Birmingham, UK*

Karl T. Trimble FRCS (Tr&Orth)
*Squadron Leader; Specialist Registrar in Trauma and
Orthopaedics, Ministry of Defence Hospital Unit,
Derriford Hospital, Plymouth, UK*

Darren Walter MB ChB DipIMC RCS(Ed) FRCS(Ed) FFAEM
*Clinical Director/Consultant in Emergency Medicine,
South Manchester University Hospital, Manchester,
UK*

Stefania Walter BN(Hons) ENB100 EMT-D RGN
*Paralegal, Field Fisher Waterhouse Solicitors
Formerly HEMS Trauma Unit and ITU Staff Nurse,
Royal London Hospital, London*

Matthew K. Wyse FRCA
*Consultant in Anaesthetics & Pre-hospital care,
University Hospitals Coventry & Warwickshire,
Coventry, UK*

Foreword

The development and delivery of trauma care has undergone unprecedented change in the last decade as successive governments have introduced policy and targets affecting both pre-hospital and in-hospital care.

The nursing role is pivotal in many of these changes which are designed to optimise individual performance and collectively enhance patient care. Gone for good is the historical perception of the nurse working in a handmaiden role supporting medical colleagues. In fact many nurses, by virtue of their length of clinical experience and in many cases the possession of a higher degree and extended scope of practice, can offer advice and guidance to doctors, especially Pre-registration House Officers and Senior House Officers, and will continue to do so with the Foundation Year 1 (FY1) and 2 (FY2) practitioners.

The development and advancement of the nursing role has been made possible by the introduction of clinical competency training with underpinning post-registration education. The accredited nurse practitioner, in accepting clinical responsibility and accountability, can deliver appropriate care and function as an autonomous practitioner following clinical guidelines and maintaining high standards of care. In doing so they have the power to make independent decisions and act upon them producing a favourable impact on both the quality of care and the quality of service provided.

In pre-hospital care, ambulance-based clinical practice follows the Joint Royal College Ambulance Liaison Committee (JRCALC) guidelines. With the changes in out of hours general practitioner services, which adds to an increasing workload for ambulance services and Emergency Departments, it is essential that specifically trained paramedics have enhanced assessment skills, broader treatment opportunities, alternative referral patterns and power of discharge from the scene. Whilst this role in some services is being fulfilled by graduate paramedics acting as paramedic practitioners there is an increasingly popular concept of a generic Emergency Care Practitioner (ECP) who can work both in pre-hospital care and in the Emergency Department. Nurses are integral to this development, working for example on an alternating basis between Emergency Departments and the ambulance service or, in some areas, as Immediate Care Practitioners.

In some Emergency Departments, appropriately trained nurses are working as ECPs and are performing triage, assessing and treating patients including requesting and interpreting diagnostics such as x-rays and pathology tests, and undertaking clinical procedures ranging from advanced wound management and fracture management, to more extensive interventions including endotracheal intubation and chest drain insertion. Whilst seen by some to cross professional boundaries, this autonomous role will not compromise junior doctor training; rather it will create more time for junior medical staff, in conjunction with their consultant supervisors, to assess and treat patients with more complex illnesses and injuries.

Nurses who have undergone extended training and education are now working across the interface of primary and secondary care, including working in minor injures units, minor treatment units, primary care centres, walk-in centres and out of hours centres. For the most part nurses remain the key personnel employed by NHS Direct.

Further innovations include the establishment of the role of Consultant Nurses who have the same clinical status as their medical counterparts. These nurses can manage the totality of patient care and have a clearly defined role within the multi-professional team. As nurse leaders, many also have a commitment to research and establishing an evidence base for further developments in practice. Most are involved in producing clinical guidelines and are integral to the development of nurse education programmes, practice development initiatives and ongoing advancement of the nursing role.

A number of hospitals have created the position of Trauma Nurse Co-ordinator, a role which varies between units but which includes co-ordination of the activities of trauma team members including patient assessment and management, and co-ordination of theatre lists and trauma services. In some units this involves data collection for submission to the UK Trauma Audit Research Network (TARN) database.

This book is a timely publication as we increasingly recognise the role of nurses in the care of the ill and injured. Their increased responsibility and the development of autonomous practice reflect a natural development and harnessing of a previously underused resource through competency-based training and postgraduate acquisition of underpinning knowledge. Where necessary the combined nursing and medical authorship of chapters is a reflection of multi-professional co-operation designed to enhance the quality of patient care. As a book specifically dealing with trauma nursing it fulfils its purpose well and provides an evidence-based and contemporary approach to trauma nursing.

Keith Porter
Consultant Trauma Surgeon
Immediate Care Practitioner
University of Birmingham Foundation
NHS Trust

Preface

The incidence of patients who suffer trauma has consistently risen in the United Kingdom over recent years, with many requiring extensive rehabilitation and ongoing care. Those tasked with caring for and managing such patients are all too aware of the need for an effective and efficient team approach to maximise the chance of a successful outcome. Integral to all trauma teams is the trauma nurse, who plays a key role in observing, monitoring and communicating with trauma patients throughout their emergency-care journey. This role is continually expanding, with nurses taking increased responsibility for processes and procedures that were once the exclusive domain of medicine.

To date much of the literature to support the trauma nursing role has come from overseas, with resultant limitations to its usefulness and application by virtue of the different environment in which care is delivered. This book has therefore been produced primarily for nurses practising in Emergency Departments in the United Kingdom who have responsibility for caring for trauma patients. It will also be of use to those nurses who receive patients that have been treated in the Emergency Department into their wards, and to those working in other emergency-care facilities, such as Minor Injuries Units or Walk-in Centres. Additionally, it is hoped that those undergoing further study in emergency, trauma and critical care nursing will find this book a valuable resource and learning tool.

Although comprehensive, this book does not cover aspects of nursing care other than those relevant to the emergency situation. Divided into a number of sections, it examines the biosciences underpinning clinical practice in easily understood terms and adopts a systematic approach to dealing with trauma patients across the lifespan. In doing so, it is hoped that nurses will be able to integrate the theory and practice of trauma nursing and thereby enhance their clinical knowledge and skill.

The first section addresses the epidemiology of trauma, and considers the various contexts in which trauma may occur and its immediate management. Written by experienced clinicians, the mechanisms of injury are explained and considered in relation to single casualty and multiple casualty situations. With the focus on applied biosciences, the second section looks at aspects often overlooked by other texts, concentrating on such areas as the pathophysiology of disease, acid–base balance, the oxygen–dissociation curve and the pathophysiological mechanisms associated with shock. The third section concentrates on resuscitation and stabilisation of the critically ill, incorporates resuscitation guidelines and emphasises the need for appropriate and effective analgesia and anaesthesia. Major trauma and how it affects various anatomical regions is considered in the fourth section, with chapters on burns, blast and gunshot injuries and sports injuries illustrating the range of potentially traumatic circumstances that the trauma nurse may be called upon to deal with. In the penultimate section, attention is given to particular clinical situations and how they may affect the trauma patient, focusing in particular on medical emergencies, paediatric emergencies, the hostile environment and the influence of chemical, biological, radiation and nuclear agents. Finally, the medico-legal aspects of trauma nursing will be considered alongside an analysis of the future of trauma nursing and trauma care delivery in the UK.

Each chapter is supported by details of references or recommendations for further reading which it is hoped the reader will use to further develop their knowledge. It should be noted that the guidelines included are universally agreed and, at the time of going to press, are as up to date as possible. Readers should, however, ensure that they check the latest version of guidelines (such as the European Resuscitation Council Guidelines) before applying their theory to practice. In some sections reference is made to the pre-hospital care of trauma patients as I consider this to be an area where the trauma nurse will have an increasing impact in the future. It is also essential that nurses understand the events that may have transpired before they receive their patients into the controlled environment of the hospital.

Borne out of a need for increased UK-based trauma nursing texts, this book is based on a systematic approach to caring for the trauma patient. The foundation in applied biosciences will, it is hoped, enable clinical pathologies and treatment modalities to be understood and will provide a scientific and evidence-based approach to clinical assessment and patient management. This will reflect developments in the education and preparation of nurses and their need to keep abreast of technological advances in health care. It is envisaged that nurses will use this book to develop their knowledge and underlying expertise required to manage and care for trauma patients, and to support their assessment and diagnostic skills thereby enabling them to contribute more readily to solving patients' problems and meeting their needs.

Written in an authoritative yet easy-to-read style, and prepared by a number of well-known experts in their field, *Principles and Practire of Trauma Nursing* provides the rationale for care through evidence-based practice while maintaining a clinical focus. All chapters have been edited to provide a common approach and format to the book, avoiding duplication where possible, except where it is considered essential to the sense of the topic under discussion. Finally, the last chapter, which discusses some of the potential future directions that trauma nursing may take is, to me, perhaps the most exciting part of this journey. I very much hope that this book will support future generations of trauma nurses, and those responsible for commissioning their research and education, in their quest to develop patient care and their own understanding of trauma and its consequences.

West Sussex, 2004   Rose Ann O'Shea

Acknowledgements

It is not often that one is afforded the opportunity to thank publicly those who have helped and supported them over the years. Although stated simply in a few words, my gratitude is sincere.

In coming up with ideas for this book I have been influenced by a large number of nurses and other clinicians, some of whom are well established and have a recognised and well-deserved reputation, and others who work tirelessly in a quiet, unassuming way unrecognised outwith their own departments and organisations. All are committed to doing their best to ensure that those patients unfortunate enough to fall victim to some form of trauma receive the highest quality of care, and to providing them with the greatest chance of a positive clinical outcome. A wide array of patients, from both hospital and out-of-hospital environments have also influenced my thinking and have shaped my approach to developing the care of the trauma patient through their comments, questions and experiences. To them all I convey my thanks.

In bringing the book to fruition, the contribution of a large number of multi-professional colleagues has been relied upon, each of whom has devoted an enormous amount of personal time and effort to support me in what at times seemed to be an endless project. Too numerous to name, I am proud to be associated with them all and am indebted to them for their unending patience and tolerance, but most of all for their friendship which has not wavered. Thanks are also due to those who gave permission for their illustrations and photographs to be reproduced, which has helped considerably to clarify some areas and thereby facilitate their understanding.

Over the years, I have been encouraged by parents, my family and my husband Iain, who have always supported my efforts and had faith in my endeavours. To them I am also indebted. In closing I would like to thank Keith Porter for his Foreword, and at Elsevier, Alex Mathieson for supporting my initial ideas, and Mairi McCubbin for her patience and unstinting professionalism throughout the long gestation of this publication.

SECTION 1

Trauma care in perspective

Chapter 1

Trauma care in context

Howard Sherriff

INTRODUCTION

The role of nurses in attending to pre-hospital emergencies is relatively new. Community nurses have in the past attended to primary care problems in the community but it has been the traditional role of doctors to attend to those emergencies where patients may require hospitalisation. Trauma care delivery, both within the hospital and in out-of-hospital settings, is traditionally associated with doctors, and emergency physicians in particular. However, in recent years, the unique role of emergency and trauma nurses has begun to be recognised and the ability of nurses to care for patients throughout their continuum of care has been realised. For the most part, such initiatives have focused on in-hospital care. However, the increasing realisation that much of emergency, unscheduled and trauma care can safely be delivered in out-of-hospital settings, has resulted in the realisation that non-traditional nursing roles and the increasing contribution of nurses need to be revisited. This chapter will focus on the potential contribution that nursing has to out-of-hospital emergency care and to pre-hospital trauma care in particular.

PRE-HOSPITAL TRAUMA CARE: THE NURSING CONTRIBUTION

An increasing number of nurses now work in the community and are untapped first-responder resources that may be deployed to patients with critical or life-threatening problems. Fundamental changes within the primary care structure, and the need for time-specific responses when members of the public declare an emergency, have identified the need to look at existing and traditional methods, and to expand these to encompass all health care workers who are appropriately trained and experienced. Until now, nurses attending road traffic accidents or industrial emergencies in the community have been there by virtue of fate or circumstance. Unless members of hospital mobile flying squads, it is unlikely that most will have been specifically called to the scene. Traditionally, ambulance crews encompassing ambulance paramedics and technicians have performed this role. In rural areas in particular, immediate care doctors who are specifically trained in driving techniques and in scene management have responded to accidents, dealing with clinical emergencies in a structured manner. Up to the present, the role of nurses has been a supportive one, mainly as part of hospital flying squads, although some are active members of immediate care schemes.

The future of pre-hospital trauma care for nurses is likely to be one involving nurses responding as part of immediate care teams comprising doctors/nurses or nurses/paramedics, or as independent practitioners. The latter role may be reserved for those attending road accidents, for example, in isolated communities and in rural areas, and may be particularly focused on primary care and community nurses. With increasing leisure activities, the demands on health professional teams to assist in the organisation and running of sports have risen; indeed, many sports, such as horse racing, require nurses with specific pre-hospital care training and expertise to be present. Nurses living in communities can also volunteer for various rescue organizations, which could involve areas of sporting interest, for example, mountain rescue, cave or pothole rescue, and factory or industrial work. This may involve being on call for the community and for rescue work if located near military bases, particularly where there are helicopters, mountain rescue and lifeboat work, or work involving coastguards. For the other services to have confidence in the nurses attending, it is essential that they demonstrate their skills and expertise, their appropriate training, preparation and education, and have a good working knowledge of the equipment supplied by the parent organisation.

With increasing demands on the ambulance service, and the reorganisation and availability of services/systems, such as NHS Direct, criteria dispatching is likely to be the order of the day for ambulance services. A logical result of this is that nurses could respond to emergencies such as myocardial infarctions, acute asthmatic attacks, the assessment of patients following epilepsy or paediatric emergencies in the community, which would require much more than basic first aid or nursing observation. All would demand interventionist treatment. Nurses of the future could expand their role variously, including prescribing and administering intravenous drugs and antibiotics as the first response, for example, to children with suspected meningitis, or administering adrenaline (epinephrine) and other drugs to patients with acute life-threatening asthma or anaphylaxis, in many cases going on to treat them autonomously. Multidisciplinary training courses to support such initiatives are available and are open to nursing, medical and paramedical personnel. By virtue of their existing core training and education, nurses have the requisite skills to enable them to practise in emergency situations both in the community and at the roadside. Not all, however, have experience of applying these – a situation which must be addressed before being exposed to caring for the trauma patient, particularly in the out-of-hospital setting.

> Nurses working in trauma care must be trained in the principles of pre-hospital and in-hospital emergency care

EPIDEMIOLOGY

Trauma remains a significant health problem. The disappointing feature is that it affects the young and active groups of all societies. In the UK, over 14 000 people die from work, domestic and road-related trauma. In 1935, 6000 people are known to have died from road traffic-related deaths in this country. This figure remained static until the 1980s when road improvements, safer cars and some driver improvements progressively occurred. The current figure of 3500 deaths each year in the UK reflects more about the safer roads and active and passive car safety features, than it does driving standards. For example, antilock brakes allow drivers safer cornering, but do not shorten stopping distances. Laws of physics, rather than the types of brakes determine these.

Many children are injured or maimed as pedestrians and cyclists. Prevention is often ignored by so-called responsible and caring adults: head protection is forgotten, seat belts for children are not used, and very young children are still playing on, or near, busy thoroughfares. One of the major reasons for speed limits is to protect pedestrians, particularly children, in residential areas as well as the elderly who may have visual or hearing difficulties or reduced mobility owing to worn and stiff joints. Notably, the home is still the most dangerous place for accidents. The *British Medical Journal* has recently refused to publish articles referring to 'accidents' as all have causes and are, therefore, preventable; most, however, are not actually accidents, which are unpredictable or unexpected events.

Violence is increasing in the UK. This includes assaults in public places as well as domestic violence, including non-accidental injury in children and in the elderly.

With the development of industrial societies, accidents have increased worldwide. Wealth brings with it the consumer society. Industry looks to the vast potential markets in places like China, as car and motor scooter ownership become reality. Untrained and inexperienced populations will suffer health care demands akin to major disasters owing to accidents in the near future. Wars also continue to occur too frequently with devastating injuries to the military and civilian populations involved. The after-effects due to residual weapons like landmines will continue for many decades, making it necessary to ensure that the medical and nursing fraternity does not ignore the principles of war surgery and aftercare.

Trauma is a leading cause of death in all age groups

The trimodal distribution of death

For every trauma death there are two people with disabling injuries

Classically, trauma deaths are described as trimodal and occur at different time intervals (Table 1.1). It is to be remembered that for every trauma death there are two people injured with disabling injuries. The three phases in the trimodal distribution are the immediate, early and late deaths. Immediate deaths are those that occur in the first few seconds or minutes and which are usually due to injuries that cannot be treated, such as brain lacerations, high spinal cord injuries and major damage to the great vessels and the heart. In practical terms, they occur within the first 10 minutes, before trained personnel arrive. A small number in this group are due to obstruction of the airway and account for 50% of trauma deaths. The second group is the early deaths and includes those that die within a few minutes to a few hours after injury. Associated problems include haemothorax, pneumothorax, intracranial bleeding, such as extradural (epidural in USA) and subdural haemorrhages, liver and splenic bleeding, and long bone and pelvic fractures. It is this group that needs to be managed within the first hour after injury, and accounts for 30% of trauma deaths. The late deaths, accounting for up to 20%, occur within days to weeks after the injury. Generally, for audit purposes, these are regarded as the deaths that occur up to 30 days after injury, and are often due to sepsis and multiple organ failure.

Table 1.1	Trimodal distribution of death	
Phase	Time	Causes of death
First	Immediate	Brain lacerations, high spinal cord injuries, major damage to heart or great vessels
Second	Early	Haemothorax, pneumothorax, intracranial bleeding, e.g. extradural and subdural haemorrhages, liver and splenic bleeding, long bone and pelvic fractures
Third	Late	Sepsis, multiple organ failure

Every stage of the patient's management can influence the outcome, so all involved have a part to play. Research has substantiated this, showing that inadequate resuscitation in the first few hours can start a cascade that leads to a downward spiral and death.

> Every stage of the patient's management can influence the outcome

Blunt versus penetrating trauma

The outcome from blunt and penetrating trauma is different. Blunt trauma, with the shearing forces and tearing and splitting of vital organs and structures, is more difficult to treat and the outcome is worse. For this reason, a bimodal timing of death has been suggested for blunt trauma. The two groups are immediate and late deaths owing to complications. Many of the major head injuries that are isolated or that complicate major trauma are not amenable to surgery. Their care is non-surgical occurring within intensive care or intensive therapy units; their victims often becoming the long-term disabled.

Prevention or cure?

Prevention will always be the way to reduce mortality in these late deaths. The thrust of treatment in the first few hours lies in correcting abnormal physiology as it affects the airway, breathing and circulation. Treatment that is given in the first few hours determines the outcome, a finding that gave birth to the concept of *the golden hour*. In pre-hospital care, the *platinum 10 minutes* has also been developed. This is the time that pre-hospital workers have to provide care, unless the patients are trapped. Evidence on outcomes suggests that 'staying and playing' at the scene has a worse outcome than 'scooping and running', where only basic airway, breathing and circulation interventions are provided on scene. The exception to this is advanced airway control, particularly if the hospital is 10 or more minutes away from the scene. In cardiac collapses, the current focus of treatment is in providing defibrillation within minutes. In ventricular fibrillation, the effect of delivery of basic airway care followed by advanced life support and defibrillation within

minutes has been to show improved survival from less than 1% to double figures. As a consequence, community first responders attending patients and initiating basic life support (BLS) with automatic defibrillators present a significant health outcome initiative. This should involve nurses and doctors in the community as well as trained citizens.

SCENE ASSESSMENT

For nurses to be involved in pre-hospital or out-of-hospital care, specific aims and objectives must be met and satisfied. The aims of health professionals in pre-hospital care and trauma care in particular should be to identify actual or potential life threats, to define appropriate and safe management while minimising complications, to carry out any required interventions in a timely and appropriate manner, to arrange early transport of patients to appropriate facilities or to their homes, and to provide support to patients' relatives and to rescue workers involved in their care (Box 1.1).

In order to achieve these aims, pre-hospital trauma team members need to meet specific objectives. They must have a specific reason for being there and should be appropriately trained for the task. Self, scene and patient safety must be paramount at all times, and management of the patient's problems dealt with in an appropriate and recognised manner with evidence-based medicine underpinning specific treatments and interventions. There should be a recognition that the work is hazardous and that, under particular

> **Box 1.1   Aims of health professionals in pre-hospital trauma care**
>
> - To identify actual or potential life threats
> - To define appropriate and safe management minimising complications
> - To carry out required interventions in a timely and appropriate manner
> - To arrange early transport of patients to appropriate facilities or to their homes
> - To provide support to patients' relatives and to rescue workers

circumstances, hazards to individual patients, rescue workers and the community may become apparent and may require appropriate action. There should also be a similar understanding that patients may require extra assistance during their transport to hospital and that appropriate liaison and teamwork between members of the rescue services may be needed while patients are being transferred. Primacy for the patient's care and safety becomes the responsibility of ambulance paramedics and ambulance technicians. However, where there are limitations in the skills of these persons, the more appropriately trained health professionals should remain with the patient until arrival at definitive care.

> Ongoing assessment and monitoring must be continued on route to definitive care

Scene attendance

Work in the pre-hospital environment is inherently dangerous with unknown hazards and problems. One of the outstanding features of work in this environment is the close-knit friendship and teamwork between rescue and emergency personnel. In difficult situations, such as road traffic accidents involving entrapment situations, several different services come together. Although they may have never met before, they work in a coordinated manner acting in the patient's best interests. This is achieved by working to basic principles to which all services adhere. Recognising the command and control structure at the scene, as well as the discipline involved, goes a long way to fostering good teamwork and interpersonal relations. Before attending pre-hospital trauma incidents, particularly road traffic accidents, industrial incidents, sporting accidents or other events, proper planning and preparation must first have taken place.

Firstly, health professionals must be appropriately trained and qualified. Several appropriate courses are available for pre-hospital trauma workers including pre-hospital emergency care courses (PHEC) run by the British Association for Immediate Care (BASICS) and the Faculty of Pre-Hospital Care of the Royal College of Surgeons of Edinburgh (RCSEd), and the Pre-Hospital Trauma Life Support course (PHTLS), which is a sister course to Advanced Trauma Life Support (ATLS) accredited by the American College of Surgeons and which is run as a national faculty by the Royal College of Surgeons of England. Additional courses are now being developed with specific modules focused on generic core skills and specific modules appropriate to particular activities, such as mountain climbing, skiing, lifeboat work, road accident work and different aspects of sports medicine, including crowd medicine at large stadia or concerts. In addition, courses on major incident management are available, which may be an essential part of what may start as seemingly innocuous events.

> Effective multidisciplinary teamwork and cooperation may be achieved by working in a coordinated manner according to basic principles

Arriving at the scene

Where nurses are working independently, they will be expected to arrive at the scene in their own vehicles. The choice of vehicle is important. Many immediate care doctors are looked upon as having high-powered and flamboyant vehicles. However, vehicles that are designed for high performance but which are driven within reasonable limits are inherently safer than small vehicles driven at maximum speed. Secondly, family-sized cars instead of small minis or super minis have more capacity for equipment, and are often better equipped in having built-in features essential for 24 hours a day, all year round, day and night driving.

Most immediate care doctors undergo driver training, often in liaison with the police, with the emphasis on arriving at the incident safely, and not inflicting other casualties on the emergency services. Statistically, immediate care doctors who drive themselves to the accident scene have lower accident rates than professional ambulance and police crews. The use of emergency lighting for emergency workers' vehicles is an area in need of clarification including the issue of on whose behalf and under whose direction the emergency or trauma nurse is responding. There is a fundamental difference between doctors driving to their practice or to hospital emergencies using green lights on their cars, which have not been authorised by callouts from either the police or the ambulance service, to doctors responding to calls authorised by ambulance services. Insurance companies need to be specifically informed that this sort of work will be undertaken, although insurance premiums are rarely increased.

> Vehicle insurance companies need to be specifically informed about the type of emergency work that will be undertaken

Prior to setting out, daily checks of the vehicle should be performed as a regular routine practice, ensuring that there is adequate fuel, oil, windscreen wash fluid and that tyre pressures are satisfactory. Windscreens and mirrors need to be clean, and all medical equipment checked and packed to ensure that it is in date, available and appropriately safeguarded in specialised locked containers where necessary. At the start of the call, protective clothing, usually comprising high-visibility reflective overalls and jackets manufactured to approved specifications, should be worn. This greatly assists emergency services teams in recognising fellow emergency services members. Nowadays, as part of the British Standard, a saturn yellow jacket with green shoulder colours for medical and ambulance personnel is used. The police wear blue shoulder colours and the fire service wear a red variation. Identity badges approved by the parent organisations should be carried at all times. Under certain circumstances, those without official identity will be denied access to the scene.

Responders should be familiar with radio procedures, particularly those of their own controllers or ambulance control. Hands-free communication systems are mandatory both from safety and legal perspectives. Radio use should be kept to a minimum during driving, as full concentration is essential, and mobile telephones must never be used while driving. Safe driving practices should be adopted at all times, including when not responding to emergencies, and should include adherence to speed limits, particularly when cars are marked and the organisation the

health professional represents can be recognised. This is particularly important after an incident, as it sets a good example for road safety to other road users and allows the 'adrenaline rush' to settle.

On approaching the scene, drivers should be aware of the exact location and speed should be reduced. Particular care must be taken, as impatient motorists will frequently 'U-turn' with little or no warning when they come upon traffic tailbacks, and cut directly across the path of emergency vehicles approaching down lines of stationary traffic. Another phenomenon occurs when drivers at the head of queues pull over when they see emergency vehicles in their rear view mirror, but the vehicles behind take an immediate opportunity to overtake without checking their rear view mirrors. This can endanger the immediate care responder.

Slowing down over the last 200 metres or so approaching an incident can reveal some clues regarding the mechanism of injury, enabling an overall assessment of the scene to be made. Where nurses or other health care workers are the first persons on scene, they should park their vehicles safely. On motorways a distance of at least 100 metres back from the incident is recommended.

It should also be recognised that there is a strong possibility of the immediate care provider's vehicle being struck and written off until a police vehicle protects it. Where other emergency vehicles are present, immediate care workers should, if possible, park ahead of the scene, which allows them to leave promptly and accompany patients to hospital where required, but also allows ambulances to park alongside the incident where the injured may be trapped. At the scene, various clues regarding scene safety should be gleaned, including the risk of hazardous chemicals, damaged power lines or leaking gas mains. Fuel spillage is common, but reports of fire caused by burst radiators with steam and antifreeze over the road surface are more common. Overturned vehicles are particularly prone to fuel spillage; the ignition must, therefore, be switched off at an early stage. Night-time portable lighting is also essential. Fully charged torches and mobile searchlights are indispensable and spare batteries are needed.

Safe driving practices should be adopted at all times, including when not responding to an emergency

PATIENT ASSESSMENT

As part of the scene assessment, the mechanism of injury can be established and the patient then approached. Nurses should wear appropriate protective gloves and other protective clothing. It should be recognised that surgical gloves are used as protection against biological hazards, and offer no protection whatsoever against broken glass or metal edges. Leather or synthetic material gloves, which can be washed, however, do provide additional protection.

As part of patient assessment, the fundamentals of pre-hospital care (i.e. airway, breathing and circulation) should be assessed. Recognising the intact or compromised airway, assessing breathing to identify any laboured effort or asymmetry, listening to the pitch of breathing to determine any obstructed airway or narrowing due to bronchospasm, chemicals or burns, are key. Major facial injuries can obstruct the airway and must be managed immediately; a full range of techniques ranging from the basic jaw lift to endotracheal intubation or a surgical airway may be required at the roadside.

Airway compromise in major head injuries is common. One developing area in immediate care is that of rapid sequence induction and intubation using muscle relaxant drugs. Nurses arriving at the scene of incidents are likely to have basic airway skills, although some may not be trained in advanced airway techniques. It is essential that all immediate care providers recognise their limitations and seek help when required at an early stage, emphasising the nature of the assistance required, for example, a compromised airway requiring the attendance of someone able to perform rapid sequence induction and administer relevant medications. Emergency and trauma nurses of the future, particularly those with anaesthetic, critical care or theatre backgrounds, as well as ambulance paramedics may acquire these skills and in so doing perform an even more important role in hospital flying squads. These skills are not easy and should not be undertaken lightly. Where they are practised infrequently, skills are not retained and manual dexterity is lost. Rapid sequence induction or intubation requiring the use of drugs should only be performed by those practising this technique regularly and should not be undertaken by those performing it only occasionally.

Maintaining and updating knowledge and skills is the responsibility of all trauma care providers

Talking to patients on arrival achieves many things not least of which is allaying the many fears and anxieties that patients may have. Human contact tells patients that they are going to be helped and gives a sense of well-being. Some believe that this may be due to endorphin release. These first few calming words are part of the 'care' component of pre-hospital work. Basic observations, such as pulse, respiratory rate, blood pressure and pulse oximetry, are also core components.

Maintaining ongoing communication and establishing rapport with patients is vital

Accident scenes can be extremely noisy. Listening to breath sounds or to the sounds disappearing when trying to measure blood pressure accurately can be difficult. Aggressive or restless patients who are in pain or who are struggling can handicap the measurement of blood pressure using automatic machines. Measurement of the first blood pressure is best done manually and, if necessary, only the systolic pressure recorded. Pulse oximetry is another valuable adjunct in the 'field situation', particularly modern, small pulse oximeters that can be carried in the front pocket of overalls. Oxygen saturation levels of less than 95% are significant. Levels below 90% are indicative of severe hypoxia, the cause of which should be identified. Continued assessment is required throughout. The most immediate life-threatening problem in relation to breathing is a tension pneumothorax. This can be relieved rapidly, one of the most simple techniques being a needle thoracocentesis.

Recognition of shock at the scene is important. It must be assumed that the first cause of shock is hypovolaemia owing to internal or external blood loss. Visible bleeding can be quantified, although it is easy to underestimate the amount of blood loss. Large scalp wounds, for example, can result in the loss of copious amounts of blood. Manual pressure on its own may be inadequate to stem this, and has the disadvantage of taking immediate care workers out of circulation because they have to maintain constant, firm pressure to such wounds. The insertion of large four-way sutures to achieve rapid haemostasis can, however, help to control scalp wounds. The constant concern in shocked patients is that of internal haemorrhage. Only one cure exists for this – the surgeon. Excessive time spent at the scene establishing intravenous infusions and treating shock, but not retrieving the patient to hospital can be self-defeating. Shock can only be treated adequately the first time around; it is much more difficult to resuscitate a patient for the second time. The various classes of shock used in ATLS teachings can provide a rapid and accurate assessment.

> Assume that the first cause of shock is hypovolaemia owing to internal or external blood loss

In high-velocity collisions, overturned vehicles, falls from heights, the risk of spinal injury and spinal cord damage must always be considered. For this reason, many patients are transported to hospital completely immobilised on long boards with semirigid collars and head blocks. This is done as a precaution until cervical spine injuries can be excluded, usually involving appropriate x-rays of the cervical region.

> Assume cervical spine injury until excluded by radiological investigations

Haemorrhage can be reduced by the proper immobilisation of fractures. This also eases pain and reduces the risk of neurovascular compromise or complications. An important observation is the patient's response to rescue workers and whether they speak in the first instance. A rapid assessment of neurological function can be performed by using the AVPU scale to see if the patient is: alert (A), responding verbally (V), responding to pain (P), or is completely unresponsive (U). The next phase involves measuring their neurological status against the Glasgow coma score (GCS) using the three components of eye opening, best verbal response and best motor response.

Once patients have been assessed and resuscitated, they need packaging for transfer to hospital. This should be carried out promptly. In many instances, patients are on scene for far too long with potential detrimental effects on their eventual outcome. A major role of the ambulance crew includes the stabilisation, packaging and transport of patients to places of definitive treatment. The role of emergency, trauma and pre-hospital nurses and immediate care doctors is to assist with this but not to control it. Understanding each other's roles and responsibilities is an essential part of teamwork at the scene. For critically injured trauma patients, there is rarely time to perform a detailed secondary survey other than fracture splintage. However, trauma nurses may be centrally placed to carry out this role and identify injuries present, particularly if they travel with patients to hospital, having first dealt with any life threats.

Part of the preparation of patients for the hospital receiving team is to undress them in line with the exposure (E) component of the primary survey. This enables injuries to be identified that may require treatment at a later stage. Trauma nurses have a key role to play in the care and management of trauma patients, not least being their continuous assessment, reassessment and monitoring particularly with regard to their airway, breathing and circulatory status (ABC), but also in maintaining accurate and comprehensive records.

> Accurate and comprehensive records must be maintained throughout the patient's journey

A structured handover from the pre-hospital trauma team to the in-hospital receiving team is vital and must be heard by all members of the resuscitation team. Additional information given by trauma nurses, such as that relating to patient identification, next of kin and work colleagues, friends or family who need to be contacted, may complement that relating to the scene.

HOLISTIC CARE AT THE ROADSIDE

Part of the scene assessment involves identifying all casualties. Very often in the drama of the situation dealing with critically injured and trapped patients, the attention of all trauma providers is concentrated on them. However, once these patients are stabilised, reassessment and reappraisal of the situation are necessary. Often there may be several other patients involved who have lesser injuries but who still require assessment and examination.

These patients can often be identified sitting at the side of the road or talking to police officers alongside other damaged vehicles and may look pale, drawn and tearful. Commonly, these patients deny that they have any injuries but shortly thereafter may start to develop aching and stiffness in the neck or back, or suffer intense headaches. There is a genuine need for these patients to be seen and examined, and recognition given to the fact that they may wish to release their emotions and cry. For them to do so, professionally trained persons who are prepared to hold their hand and listen can be an effective part of starting the process of rehabilitation. Many individuals try to 'press on' and continue with their journey or activity. Many of these may also suffer symptoms, such as neck-ache, backache or headache, and may become tearful and distressed as a consequence of the incident. The sensible option is for them to return home, ideally having been collected by a partner, friend or relative. In situations involving vehicles, they may sometimes be so badly damaged that they are barely drivable. Talking to patients to determine if they are members of one of the automobile associations that can recover their vehicles and take them home is often forgotten. Trauma nurses can play an important role in ensuring that all those who should be taken to hospital are seen, assessed and transported as appropriate.

> All patients involved in traumatic events should be assessed

Dr Kenneth Easton founded pre-hospital care 25 years ago and is the inspiration behind many immediate care schemes. His model stressed the need to care for patients rather than a total science of treatment. The fact that carers from any of the emergency services, or indeed passing members of the public, take someone's hand and sits with them or puts their arm around them, is remembered long after the event by patients, and very often their family. It is this momentary bond of kindness that makes immediate care worthwhile.

The majority of immediate care schemes in the UK are charities. Traumatic events and memories of them by patients and their friends and communities are often triggers to raise funds to buy the equipment required to keep team members on the road.

At fatalities, which have caused major road disruptions, there are often several witnesses present. Frequently, they have been the first to go to vehicles where there may be deceased persons, or where they have been present during the last moments of life and have heard breathing, leaving them with feelings of self-doubt regarding whether they could have done something more to save a patient's life. In practice, this is extremely unlikely, but for the bystanders they may have witnessed what is to them their worst nightmare without the benefit of previous experience in hospital or medical work. It may be the first time that they have seen anyone deceased who is obviously damaged, and it may be possible that they will suffer unpleasant nightmares and flashbacks. Though physically uninjured, these people are also casualties. They should be taken aside and spoken to by one of the trauma care providers. Benefit may be gained from taking them together in a group because the time available at the scene is limited. However, asking individuals about their fears, warning them of the side effects and encouraging them to talk to each other can be extremely beneficial; indeed, letters of appreciation or telephone calls are not infrequent from people who have been supported in this way at the scene.

Protection of self is an important aspect of immediate and trauma care. One particular area that trauma nurses bring to pre-hospital trauma care is a holistic approach to patient care and understanding of the fact that they may themselves become victims in these stressful situations. For those who attend incidents regularly, seeing several fatalities in the same week can have a detrimental long-term effect and their need for support can be considerable.

> The need for support should not be underestimated

The Fire Service tends to respond with teams of four of five on each vehicle. Scene debriefs followed by a more detailed debrief with their colleagues and officers back at the station are usually commonplace. Police traffic officers often work in single crews or with one partner, and are frequently isolated. More experienced traffic officers, such as accident investigators who spend their lives over a period of several years solely attending fatal accidents, investigating them and carrying out scenes of crime work, fall into this category. Many retire at an early age because they can no longer deal with the stress of seeing and dealing with victims, and in particular with approaching and dealing with their families and experiencing the same emotions. Hospital and mortuary staff as well as hospital chaplaincy staff can also have a major role to play in protecting these individuals, and ambulance and police service teams, both in the pre-hospital trauma phase and in the in-hospital emergency and intensive care phases of treatment.

Finally, it must be remembered that nurses themselves may become victims. If they work in isolation in the community and experience difficult situations, such as dealing with patients with potentially life-threatening illnesses or injuries or fatalities within a relatively short time, they may return to work and try to behave normally when dealing with other patients who are distressed or in need. It is vitally important that these individuals take time for themselves and, if necessary, return to their base or have a break. Talking to other colleagues, and knowing how and where to obtain counselling and support are essential.

One of the attributes of organisations like BASICS is that it is a national network. Many members who have experienced particularly difficult or traumatic experiences contact or are contacted by their BASICS friends and colleagues to seek or to offer help and support, and to talk through their experiences. Such examples range from the Lockerbie bombing to road traffic crashes, such as one in Lincolnshire involving a coach and a people carrier with several children on board. A supportive and long-lasting relationship often results between these professionals. There are many sights that trauma or immediate care providers encounter that they choose not to discuss with their family or friends, and which they will only discuss with or express their concerns to those 'who have been there'. The benefit of such networks in these circumstances cannot be underestimated.

SUMMARY

Pre-hospital trauma care is a challenging, exciting and completely varied activity. The motivation for doing it is something that everyone who participates questions. The strong teamwork and the camaraderie at the scene of incidents, often with black humour and the desire to assist people in distress, have been motivating factors in my own experience over a 25-year period. The involvement of nurses in pre-hospital trauma care will, in many instances, be fraught with difficulties and obstruction. However, nurses have a very specific role to contribute that will complement existing medical and paramedical skills and should be welcomed rather than obstructed.

Further reading

American College of Surgeons Committee on Trauma. *ATLS advanced trauma life support for doctors manual*. Chicago: American College of Surgeons. 1997

Colquhoun MC, Handley AJ, Evans TR. *ABC of resuscitation*. London: BMJ Books, 1995

Driscoll P, Skinner D, Earlam R. *ABC of major trauma*. London: BMJ Books, 2000

Driscoll PA, Gwinnutt CL, LeDuc Jimmerson C, Goodall O. *Trauma resuscitation: a team approach*. London: Macmillan, 1993

Eaton CJ. *Essentials of immediate care.* Edinburgh: Churchill Livingstone, 1999

Emergency Nurses Association. *TNCC Trauma nursing core course manual.* Emergency Nurses Association

Greaves I, Porter K. *Prehospital care*

Chapter 2

Kinetics and mechanisms of injury

John Eaton

INTRODUCTION

In the pre-hospital situation, it is seldom appropriate, or indeed possible, to take a complete and accurate history of the incident and perform a full head to toe examination of the casualty. Casualties may not be capable of giving an accurate history owing to their injuries and the emotional shock of what has happened to them, and may not even be aware of significant and sometimes life-threatening injuries. It is, therefore, important that pre-hospital practitioners are able to make deductions about the casualty's likely injuries by careful observation of the accident scene and then determine the mechanism of injury. To do so they must have an understanding of the physics involved, the way in which impacts occur, how energy is transferred, and the types and patterns of injury that may result.

MECHANICS OF INJURY

Knowledge of the relevant physical principles and laws is essential to fully understand mechanisms of injury (Boxes 2.1 and 2.2). Energy cannot be created or destroyed, but can be changed in form, the main forms of energy being mechanical, thermal, electrical or chemical. When a body stops moving as a result of impacting with another body, some of its energy may be transferred to that other body causing it to move, and some may be changed in form to thermal and chemical energy resulting in deformity or damage to one or both bodies.

Box 2.1   Laws of physics

Newton's first law of motion
- A body will remain at rest and a body will remain in motion unless or until it is acted upon by some other outside force

Newton's second law of motion
- The rate of change of momentum is proportional to the force producing that change and takes place in the same direction as the applied force

Newton's third law of motion
- For every active force there is always an equal and opposite reactive force

---

Box 2.2   Principles of physics

Kinetic energy
- Kinetic energy = $\frac{1}{2}$ mass $\times$ velocity^2

Force
- Force = mass $\times$ acceleration (or deceleration), where mass is the body weight and velocity is the speed of that body

---

From Box 2.2 it can be seen that velocity (speed) increases the production of kinetic energy much more than mass, and the speed of impact is of more importance than the mass (weight) of the impacting objects. The term given to the energy used to deform an object involved in an impact, the effect of which is dependent on the nature of the materials involved, the area of impact and the rate of energy release, is *impact energy*.

Impact energy

The nature of the materials involved, and the way in which energy is dissipated or dispersed through them, is significant. For example, a fall into snow, which is soft, will cause less damage than a fall on to concrete. The body will penetrate the snow and deceleration will be relatively slow as it takes place over a greater distance. If the body was to fall on to concrete, which is hard and non-penetrable, deceleration will be very rapid, as it occurs almost immediately.

The area over which the impact takes place and the energy that is released also have considerable influence on the damage sustained. If the area of impact is small, the amount of energy released per unit area will be greater than if the area of impact is large, thus impact with a sharp instrument will cause more local tissue damage than impact with one that is blunt.

Local tissue damage is greater following impact with sharp objects

---

The release of energy (deceleration) and whether it is gradual or sudden (i.e. the time over which energy is released) have considerable bearing on the damage and injuries sustained. If all the energy is transferred suddenly, more damage will be caused than if it is transferred gradually. For example, before an impact, the driver of a vehicle will be moving at the same speed as the vehicle. If the vehicle stops suddenly owing to an impact, the car and driver will decelerate to a standstill almost simultaneously with most of the considerable decelerative force being transmitted to the driver. If the stopping distance is increased, the deceleration will be less, resulting in proportionately less decelerative force, and less vehicle damage and injury.

Cavitation

In blunt trauma, tissue damage is caused by compression of the tissues under the area of impact, whereas in penetrating trauma, tissue damage is caused by compression and separation of the tissues along the track of the penetrating object. Both blunt and penetrating trauma may result in cavity formation as tissues are forced out of their usual position.

Cavitation occurs as tissues that have collided with the impacting object move away from the point of impact and, in the case of penetrating trauma, the track of the penetrating object as it enters further into the body. The cavities thus created may form and reform several times until all the kinetic energy transferred from the impacting object has been completely dissipated. The amount of cavitation produced and hence the extent of the injury (tissue damage) caused is directly proportional to the amount of impact energy transferred, and will depend on the density of the tissues with which the penetrating object impacts and through which it passes, the size of the frontal area of the penetrating object and the elasticity of the various body tissues involved.

In blunt trauma, there is only temporary cavity formation, whereas in penetrating trauma, especially gunshot injury, there is both permanent and temporary cavity formation. When a fast-moving object with high kinetic energy and a small frontal area impacts with a tissue, it releases its kinetic energy over a small area. If this energy exceeds the tensile strength of the tissue, the object will penetrate that tissue, resulting in permanent cavity formation. At the same time, a temporary cavity will be formed both in front of the object and by the side of its track as it moves through the tissue.

BLUNT TRAUMA

In blunt trauma, injury occurs as a result of the release or transfer of energy produced by tissue compression, a sudden change in velocity such as that which occurs in acceleration or deceleration, or shearing.

Compression injuries

Compression injuries occur when crushing or squeezing of the area under the point of impact causes tissue damage. This may affect both the surface and the underlying internal organs of a body, and is the most common mechanism of injury. Such injuries may be sustained by any part of the body, resulting in a wide range of presentations. *Compression of the head* may, for example, result in scalp laceration and skull fracture, which in turn may cause vascular injury including extradural and subdural haemorrhage, and cerebral contusion. *Compression of the thorax* may result in fractured ribs, including flail chest, pulmonary contusion, pneumothorax and cardiac contusion, as a result of anterior compression of the heart between the sternum and the dorsal spine. *Anterior compression of the abdomen* may result in crushing and rupturing of some of the

underlying internal organs between the anterior abdominal wall and the posterior thoracic cage and lumbar spine; organs thus affected may include the spleen, liver, pancreas and sometimes the liver. Abdominal compression, usually from a frontal impact, may also cause a sudden rise in intra-abdominal pressure, resulting in loss of use of the diaphragm as a respiratory muscle. Herniation of some intra-abdominal organs may also occur, resulting in, for example, herniation of the large bowel into the thoracic cavity causing respiratory impairment and rarely aortic valve rupture as a result of retrograde arterial flow. *Pelvic compression* may cause fractures of the pelvic ring, which (in 10% of cases) may be associated with injury to the bladder, urethra and pelvic blood vessels.

> Damage caused by compression is the most common mechanism of injury

Change of speed (acceleration, deceleration, shear injuries)

Acceleration, deceleration and shearing injuries occur when there is a sudden change in speed (i.e. acceleration or deceleration) of a body composed of two separate but connected parts. If one of the parts stops moving relative to the other, there will be stretching and then tearing of the tissue or material connecting the two parts, or where one part impacts with the other. This tends to occur where a fixed part joins a mobile part (e.g. duodeno-jejunal junction, descending aortic arch or ileocaecal junction). Shearing injuries usually only occur when the acceleration or deceleration is considerable, and are relatively uncommon as mechanisms of injury. Injuries caused in this way are not usually visible and are easy to miss initially if not looked for.

> Shearing injuries are not usually visible and are easily missed

A sudden change in speed of *the head* may, for example, result in cerebral contusion caused by the brain continuing to move inside the cranium at its previous speed until it impacts with the inside of the skull. This may result in vascular shearing injuries with shearing and tearing of blood vessels, temporal or frontal lobe bruising or haematoma formation, subdural haematomas and shearing injury to the spinal cord or brainstem.

Sudden changes in the speed of the casualty's body may result in significant injury to the *cervical spine* and its associated soft-tissue structures, including the spinal cord, similar to that which occurs with shearing injury. In this regard the body may be considered to be similar to two balls, one formed by the thorax and abdomen, which is much larger than the other, and the head, which are connected by a short piece of string (i.e. the neck). If the body suddenly decelerates, the head will continue to move forwards flexing the neck as it does so; this will continue until the head impacts with something or until the neck can flex no further. This may result in a hyperflexion injury of the cervical spine, including anterior wedge fractures, fracture dislocations and ligamentous disruption. If the body suddenly accelerates, the head will tend to be left behind, resulting in neck extension until it can extend no further; the head is then pulled forwards by the body resulting in a possible flexion injury of the cervical spine, a 'whiplash injury', including fracture dislocations and anterior ligament disruption. Sudden sideways acceleration or deceleration will similarly cause lateral flexion to the side opposite to the direction of the movement, a finding often found in association with rotational injuries. The cervical spine has relatively good anterior/posterior stability but is less able to resist lateral and rotational movements, especially when the two are combined. Severe injuries to the cervical spine and its ligaments may result, including injury to the spinal cord sufficient to cause neurological deficit.

The thorax is also at risk of significant injury from these mechanisms. Sudden deceleration as a result of a severe frontal impact, a fall from a considerable height, or acceleration occurring as a result of a severe side (lateral) impact, may result in a shearing injury with rupture (either partial or complete) of the arch of the aorta. This occurs most commonly at the site of the ligamentum arteriosum, as distal to this point the aorta is tethered firmly to the thoracic spine, and proximal to this point the aorta is attached to the heart and is relatively mobile.

Sudden deceleration or, less commonly, sudden acceleration may result in shearing injury to those *abdominal organs* that are not firmly attached close to the abdominal wall. After the initial impact, they will continue to move forward within the abdominal cavity, although the body itself has stopped moving. Shearing injuries usually occur at the site of the attachment of an organ to its mesentery, and result in stretching and then tearing of the mesentery and its blood vessels. Organs that may be affected in this way include the kidneys, spleen, and small and large bowels. In sudden severe deceleration, the liver may also impact with the ligamentum teres as it continues to move forwards and downwards, resulting in severe hepatic laceration.

ROAD TRAFFIC ACCIDENTS: IMPACTS AND INJURIES

In road traffic accidents and other accidents in which there is sudden deceleration, three impacts may occur; the vehicle and the object with which it collides, the casualty with the interior of the vehicle or the pedestrian with the road, and the casualty's brain with the inside of the skull and internal organs with the abdominal wall or thoracic cage (compression injury). There may also be shearing injury as the tissues/materials tethering mobile organs stretch and then tear. In order to assess the injuries that a casualty is likely to be suffering from, knowledge of the mechanism of all three impacts is therefore necessary.

> Three impacts may occur in road traffic accidents and accidents involving sudden deceleration

Vehicular damage

Modern motor cars are designed with impact or crumple zones at the front and rear of the vehicle, which collapse progressively absorbing much of the kinetic energy (impact energy), and a passenger compartment, which is designed to be rigid and minimise any intrusion into it (i.e. 'the passenger safety cell'). The result of this is that less impact energy is transmitted to the passenger compartment, helping to preserve its integrity and there is less intrusion into the passenger compartment with reduced blunt injury to the vehicle occupants caused by intrusion alone. Reduced impact energy is also transmitted to the vehicle occupants when they impact with the interior of the vehicle. Notably, an increasing number of cars also have side impact bars in the doors to prevent side intrusion.

Injuries sustained in road traffic accidents

Vehicle occupants or riders will be subjected to the same direction and type of force as the vehicle in or on which they are travelling. The amount of energy transferred to the vehicle occupant will depend on the impact energy absorbed by the vehicle and whether the deformation of the vehicle has occurred over a relatively long or short time interval. Large vehicles tend to be safer than smaller ones because there is usually more of the vehicle to help absorb the impact energy, more interior space so that the occupants have more room to move in without impacting with the vehicle interior, and more safety features. Where large vehicles impact with smaller ones, the mass of the larger vehicles will affect the movement of the smaller vehicles more than the mass of the smaller vehicles will affect the movement of the larger vehicles.

Injuries sustained by vehicle occupants will depend on the amount and direction of the impact force transferred to them and the nature of the part of the body absorbing the force. Injuries sustained in this way may be subdivided into those caused by compression, shearing and very rarely by penetration.

> Injuries to vehicle occupants depend on the amount and direction of the impact force and the part of the body absorbing the force

TYPES OF IMPACT

Frontal impact (70%)

Frontal impacts occur when the front or front corner of one vehicle impacts with another vehicle or object, causing it to cease forward movement either suddenly or gradually. Rapid deceleration of the vehicle and everything in it may also occur, including its driver and passengers.

Vehicle damage

All or part of the front of the vehicle will be involved in the initial impact, absorbing most of the impact energy and resulting in frontal deformity. This deformity may include exterior damage with shortening of the front of the vehicle and depends upon the impact energy (i.e. the vehicle's kinetic energy and the kinetic energy of the object or vehicle with which it impacts, and the area of impact). For example, impact with another car will cause less intrusion or shortening than impact with a motorcycle with the same kinetic energy, but a much smaller profile or area of impact. The front of the vehicle and its engine compartment are usually designed to absorb most of the impact energy and to collapse progressively without involving the passenger compartment, which only becomes deformed in very severe impacts.

In severe frontal impacts, there will be rearward displacement of the front wing body panels, which may impact with the front of the front doors, making opening them difficult or impossible. The front wheels and the front doors may also be affected, causing buckling of the vehicle's floor pan and roof. Interior damage may include intrusion of a wheel arch, which occurs most often when the impact is offset or oblique, rather than in full-frontal impacts. In full-frontal impacts, the engine helps prevent wheel arch intrusion, rearward displacement of the front fascia (and sometimes the steering wheel), upward displacement and buckling of the floor pan, downwards displacement and buckling of the roof, and sometimes forward movement of insecure seats. In impacts with front seat occupants, deformity to steering wheels may occur pushing them forwards and upwards. Bending or braking off of rear view mirrors, windscreen glass fragmentation and front shelf damage may also occur. When not restrained by seat belts, rear seat occupants may cause damage to the front seats and windscreens.

Vehicle occupant movement

After the impact, unrestrained car occupants continue to move forward relative to the vehicle until they impact with the vehicle interior. It is only then that they experience deceleration and

Box 2.3   Pre-hospital injury assessment protocol

Initial scene assessment
- Safety of self, scene and patient

Primary survey and resuscitation
- Initial triage of patients
- Initial patient assessment, including monitoring and recording of condition, injuries and vital signs
- Simultaneous management of life-threatening medical problems
- Resuscitation

Reassessment of the scene – reading the wreckage
- Re-examination of the accident scene
- Photography

Secondary survey and management
- Reassessment of the patient's condition and injuries
- Identification and management of significant medical problems
- Monitoring and recording of relevant data
- Secondary triage

Overview of the scene
- Reassessment of the scene and mechanism of injury

- Photography of the scene and vehicle wreckage using standard views

Monitoring
- Reassessment of the patient and review of their management:
  - during extrication
  - on the stretcher
  - in the ambulance (with triage)
  - in transit
- Re-examination and collation of patient and scene information
- Transmission of information to the receiving hospital

Handover of the patient
- Briefing of hospital team
- Transfer and replacement of pre-hospital medical and monitoring equipment by hospital medical and monitoring equipment
- Reassessment of the patient with management of those problems requiring immediate attention

Box 2.4   Determining the mechanism of injury

To determine the mechanism of injury these questions need to be answered:
- How was the patient injured?
- What forces were involved?
- What injuries would you expect?

When examining the accident scene a number of factors need to be addressed:
- How did the accident happen?
- What hit what? What happened then?
- What were the road conditions?
- What was the probable speed of impact? Was the airbag deployed?
- What were the forces involved and their direction?
- Why did the accident happen? Was the driver asleep? Has the driver used alcohol, sedating medication or drugs? Is the driver diabetic or epileptic? Did the driver have a myocardial infarction?
- Was excess speed involved? Was there a fault with one of the vehicles? Were there adverse weather conditions?

When examining the vehicle wreckage consider these factors:
- What was the type of impact – frontal, side, rear or rollover?

- Was there deformity of the exterior of the vehicle (the severity of the deformity can give a good idea as to the forces involved and hence the velocity of impact)?
- Was there shortening of the front of the vehicle (rearward displacement of the wheels, doors and body panels, buckling of the vehicle's floor pan or roof)?
- Was there deformity of the interior of the vehicle caused by impact with the occupants? The human body is softer than metal and plastic, and where there is major distortion of metal, it can be predicted that there will be even greater damage to the human body involved, e.g. damage to the windscreen (head), steering wheel (chest), front fascia shelf (knees, etc.), control pedals (feet and ankles)
- Was a seat belt worn and did it lock?
- Were any airbags deployed restricting forward or sideways movement?
- Was there any movement of objects inside the vehicle (e.g. forward movement of seats, unrestrained rear seat passengers, loose luggage)?
- Does the motorcyclist or pedal cyclist's helmet show signs of impact or damage?

Box 2.5   Examining the injury pattern of the casualty – a checklist

- What are the casualty's apparent injuries? (Look for pattern bruising)
- What forces have acted on the casualty, and how did they act?
- How rapid was any deceleration? (The more rapid the deceleration, the more serious the injuries are likely to be)
- Where was the force of the impact transmitted to?
- Was there likely to have been any compression injury? (By cavitation or by secondary collision with internal organs)
- What injury producing movements are likely to have occurred? (Hyperflexion, hyperextension, excessive lateral flexion, etc.)
- What injuries are likely to occur as a result?

the remaining force is transmitted to them, the first significant force being transmitted through the feet in the foot well. If the impact is anticipated and the knees are braced, forward movement may be resisted. At low speeds, knee bracing and arm bracing by drivers may be successful in preventing forward body movement and further body impact with the vehicle; at higher speeds, forward movement is not preventable. Initially, the whole body pivots about the feet until the knees impact with the front fascia. After this the body flexes forward, rotating about the knees and hips until the upper abdomen, thorax and neck impact with the steering wheel (in the case of the driver) and the head impacts with the windscreen, rear view mirror or car roof. Each successive impact occurs with increasing velocity (and, therefore, force), as the body flexes progressively about the last point of impact. Finally, front seat passengers may be ejected through the windscreen, but not usually the driver, whose ejection may be prevented by the steering wheel.

Injury prevention devices
Injury prevention devices are regular features in many modern vehicular designs. These include antisubmarining seats, collapsible steering columns and restraining devices, such as seat belts and airbags, which are designed to prevent or minimise injury.

On impact, occupants may slide forwards in their seats, under the seat belt, if worn, if the seat squabs are too soft, and may suffer severe lower limb injuries as a result. Modern car seats, such as antisubmarining seats, are designed to prevent this. Collapsible steering columns are similarly designed to telescope on impact to prevent the steering wheel intruding further into the passenger compartment in frontal collisions, which may injure the driver's head and chest.

The wearing of seat belts by both front and rear seat passengers is now compulsory with legislation passed to prosecute those who do not comply. Inertia-reel seat belts lock a few milliseconds after a frontal impact, restraining the casualty by reducing forward movement of the pelvis and, to a lesser extent, the thorax and abdomen, thus helping to prevent injuries caused by impact with the front fascia, steering wheel and windscreen. Most new cars are now fitted with seat-belt pre-tensioners, which actively tighten the belt during the first milliseconds of a crash, pulling the occupant back into the seat. During severe deceleration seat belts stretch, increasing the time interval before the body ceases forward movement and reducing the force of deceleration. Seat belts help to prevent forward but not sideways or backwards ejection, and spread the compressive forces over a greater area, thus reducing the force applied per unit area and the severity of injury caused by compression.

Seat belts may, however, actually cause some injuries, which are much less severe than if no seat belt was worn; these may show up as lines of bruising (pattern bruising) or as weals where the seat-belt strap passes over parts of the bony skeleton (e.g. clavicle, iliac crest). Restrained occupants tend to flex their cervical spine more than unrestrained car occupants and may hit the windscreen with their heads. Incorrectly worn seat belts may also cause injuries, especially if the shoulder strap is too high, resulting in neck injury. If the lap strap is loose or too high above the pelvis, there may be compression of the soft intra-abdominal organs between the seat belt and the posterior abdominal wall causing injury to the spleen, liver and pancreas. A sudden rise in intra-abdominal pressure may also occur resulting in diaphragmatic rupture with herniation of intra-abdominal organs into the thoracic cavity, and sometimes an anterior compression wedge fracture of the lumbar spine at the level of T_{12}, L_1, L_2 owing to hyperflexion, similar to that which occurs when the lap belt is worn alone.

Airbags are being fitted to nearly all new cars following their successful use in the USA. They deploy only in medium- and high-speed frontal and oblique frontal impacts, at speeds above 18 mph in European cars where seat belts are worn by more than 95% of front seat occupants, and at 10–12 mph in the USA, where seat belts are not commonly worn. Front airbags are fitted in the steering wheel boss or front fascia in front of the front seat passenger. Their release is triggered by a sensor, resulting in a very rapid chemical reaction, a controlled explosion, which produces a large volume of gas and inflates the bag within a few seconds of a frontal or oblique frontal impact. Vents in the side or top seams allow the bag to deflate almost immediately after inflation, thereby releasing the driver or passenger.

Airbags are effective in spreading the decelerative forces over a large area, reducing forward movement and preventing impact with the front of the interior of the vehicle. They are not, however, effective in preventing secondary injury where there are multiple impacts owing to their rapid deflation after the primary impact. Friction burns are commonly found, usually of the forearms and neck, owing to their rapid inflation, and heat burns, usually of the forearms, owing to the release of very hot gases. Severe, sometimes fatal, hyperextension injuries of the cervical spine may also occur if the driver is short and sitting very close to the steering wheel, or if a baby in a forward-facing child seat is attached to a front seat.

Nowadays, many new cars also have side airbags, which are stored in the seats and are deployed on side impact. Another recent development is the use of side screen airbags, which are stored in the roof side just above the doors, and which are designed to protect the head from excessive sideways flexion, and to prevent it from hitting the side window glass in side impacts.

> Beware of undeployed airbags when attending the scene of a road traffic accident

Vehicle occupant injuries

The range of injuries sustained by vehicle occupants is variable and is dependent on where they are positioned in the vehicle, the type of impact and the use of safety or restraining devices.

Front seat passengers often suffer more severe injuries than drivers as they are usually less prepared for the impact than the drivers, who may anticipate the impact and attempt to prevent forward movement. Unrestrained front seat occupants may suffer compression injuries as they impact successively with the front fascia, resulting in the transmission of impact energy through the knee causing injuries such as patellar fractures, disruption of the patellar ligaments and dislocations with the risk of popliteal artery injury. The impact energy may also be transmitted along the femur to the pelvis resulting in fractures of the femoral shaft, backward displacement (posterior dislocation) of the hip and acetabular fracture.

> Front seat passengers often suffer more severe injuries than drivers

Steering wheels may impact with the upper abdomen resulting in compression of the anterior abdominal wall against the spine and posterior abdominal wall, causing rupture of hollow abdominal organs including the stomach and large and small bowels. Compression injuries of the solid viscera including the liver, spleen, kidneys and rarely the pancreas may also occur. They may also impact with the thorax resulting in compression of the anterior thorax against the spine and posterior thorax, causing anterior chest wall injuries including fractured ribs, anterior flail chest, fractured sternum, and contusion of the heart and lungs; lung tissue is elastic and compressible and is, therefore, not easily damaged. Sometimes, if the casualty anticipates the accident and holds their breath thereby closing the glottis in the process, the lungs may burst, like a paper bag full of air, resulting in a pneumothorax as the thorax is suddenly and forcibly compressed by the impact. Finally, the head may impact with the windscreen glass, frame or side pillars resulting in injury to the forehead including scalp lacerations, skull fracture, cerebral contusion and intracranial haemorrhage. These are now relatively rare since the introduction of seat belts, which have dramatically reduced the severity of this type of injury. The head may also impact with the rear view mirror resulting in, for the person in the right-hand seat, lacerations to the left side of the forehead and injury to the left eye; for occupants in the front left-hand seat this picture is reversed.

Unrestrained drivers and those involved in high-speed frontal impacts may also suffer shearing injuries of the liver and kidneys, with tearing of the vessels and tissues tethering them to the posterior abdominal wall. These injuries are due to the sudden cessation of forward movement as the abdomen impacts with the steering wheel, and result in stretching and tearing of the renal veins and arteries near where they join the inferior vena cava and thoracic aorta, and tearing of the liver caused by impact with the ligamentum teres. They may also suffer from injury to the thoracic aorta where it is tethered to the posterior wall, owing to the sudden cessation of forward movement of the thorax when it impacts with the steering wheel. This can result in transection, or more commonly, a partial tear of the wall of the aorta, resulting in a traumatic aortic aneurysm – a life-threatening event. This type of shearing injury is usually seen in the young as the arteries usually become less easy to tear with increasing age owing to atherosclerosis. Damage to the cervical spine may also occur owing to cervical hyperflexion and hyperextension resulting in severe soft-tissue injury to the neck, fractures of the cervical spine and ligamentous damage.

Unrestrained occupants may be ejected through the windscreen experiencing injuries similar to those sustained by ejected motorcyclists. They may also suffer from severe facial injuries if they impact with hard surfaces, for example, roads, owing to their lack of protective helmets. Front seat car occupants are at risk of being hit by unrestrained rear seat passengers resulting in head, neck and back injuries as a consequence of them hitting the back of the front seats with their knees.

High-speed frontal impacts are associated with an increased incidence of injuries. In particular, they may cause buckling of the roof and the floor of the passenger compartment, resulting in compressive spinal injuries, severe deceleration (shear) injuries (which may not be obvious initially), and fractures of the wrists and forearms as the driver braces the arms in an attempt to prevent forward movement. Offset frontal and oblique frontal impacts present a different clinical picture with injuries such as fractures of the ankles and lower legs caused by front wheel arch intrusion. These are more common and more severe in car drivers as the vehicle's control pedals can injure their feet and ankles, especially the right ankle, which is used for braking.

Seat belt injuries may be sustained by both front and rear seat occupants, with characteristic injury patterns dependent upon their position and location within the vehicle. For those in the right front seat, the chest strap may cause a line of injury extending down across the chest from the right shoulder to the left costal margin and loin. The classic injury pattern associated with this includes subluxation of the acromio-clavicular joint, fracture of the right clavicle, sternum and left lower ribs, and injury to the spleen and left kidney. For those in the left front seat, the line of injury is reversed with liver injury sustained instead of the spleen. Neck injuries may also be sustained due to seat belts that are anchored too high up.

Seat belt injuries to rear seat passengers are usually less severe than those sustained by those in the front seats, as the rear seats are often closer to the back of the front seats than the front seat occupants are to the front fascia. Rear seat passengers usually impact with the back of the front seats, which are usually softer than the front fascia.

Unrestrained rear seat passengers are at particular risk of injury in part owing to the possibility of them being thrown forwards. This may result in them impacting with the back of the front seats and front seat passengers, causing injury to their necks (hyperflexion injuries) and knees. They may also collide with the windscreen and may even be ejected through it, resulting in severe neck and facial injuries. *Restrained rear seat passengers* who are wearing full seat belts may sustain relatively minor facial and knee injuries caused by impact with the back of the front seats. Restrained rear seat passengers using a lap belt alone, usually the central passengers, will flex forward hitting their heads on the seat in front of them. The resultant injury pattern includes head injuries, injuries to the lower abdominal viscera and bladder, potential rupture of the diaphragm owing to the sudden rise in intrathoracic pressure, and knee injuries, especially if they are involved in high-speed frontal impacts. Hyperflexion injuries leading to anterior wedge fractures of the lumbar vertebrae may also occur.

Rear impact

Rear impacts occur when slower-moving or stationary vehicles are hit from behind by faster-moving vehicles (Fig. 2.1). This results in the sudden forward acceleration of the vehicles and their occupants: the greater the difference in speed between the two vehicles, the greater the impact force that is transferred to the vehicle that is hit. If the vehicle then hits another vehicle in front, there will be a secondary frontal impact, and the vehicle and its occupants will experience the effects of the two collisions (i.e. the rear impact followed by the frontal impact).

Vehicle damage
In rear impacts, the rear of the vehicle will absorb most of the impact energy, resulting in shortening and deformity, the severity of which will depend on the force of the impact. The boot is designed to absorb most of the impact and to collapse progressively without involving the passenger compartment, but is less efficient at doing so than the engine compartment, and is relatively shorter. Interior damage includes forward displacement of the contents of the boot and the rear seat, which may impact with any rear seat occupants pushing them forward. They, in turn, impact with and damage the back of the front seats, and with front seat occupants pushing them forward, resulting in damage to the steering wheel, windscreen, rear view mirror and front fascia.

Vehicle occupant movement
Vehicles involved in rear impacts will be accelerated forwards whilst the occupants will appear to move backwards unless they are prevented from doing so by the front of the seat back. The head in particular will move backwards, hyperextending the neck; when the vehicle subsequently stops moving, they will flex forwards. Head restraints may help to reduce the amount of backward movement of the head and minimise the degree of cervical hyperextension. If wrongly positioned, head restraints may be totally ineffective or, if positioned too low, may cause even greater hyperextension of the cervical spine by acting as a pivot around which the head rotates.

Vehicle occupant injuries
Compression injuries, including seat belt injuries, are not uncommon in rear seat impacts. Front seat occupants often suffer posterior chest or spinal injuries as a result of impact with rear seat passengers' knees, whereas rear seat passengers tend to suffer spinal injuries owing to rear intrusion, and knee or femoral injuries owing to impact with the back of the front seat or with the boot contents. Shearing-type injuries may also occur, the most common of which are whiplash (hyperextension) injuries to the cervical spine, with tearing of the anterior cervical ligaments. Other shearing injuries are rare because most intra-abdominal organs are tethered to the posterior abdominal or thoracic wall, which move forward before impacting with the organs, carrying them forward.

Side impact

Side impacts occur when vehicles are hit on one of their sides, with the resultant damage dependent on the speed and force of impact, vehicular design, the use of restraints or protective devices, and the positioning or location of occupants within the vehicles.

Vehicle damage
If the force of impact is insufficient to move the vehicle that is hit sideways, all the force of the impact will be absorbed by the vehicle that is hit, resulting in exterior damage with inward displacement of the doors. This will be less in cars with side impact bars in their doors, but may result in more damage to the vehicle or object impacting with the door. Interior damage may include intrusion into the passenger

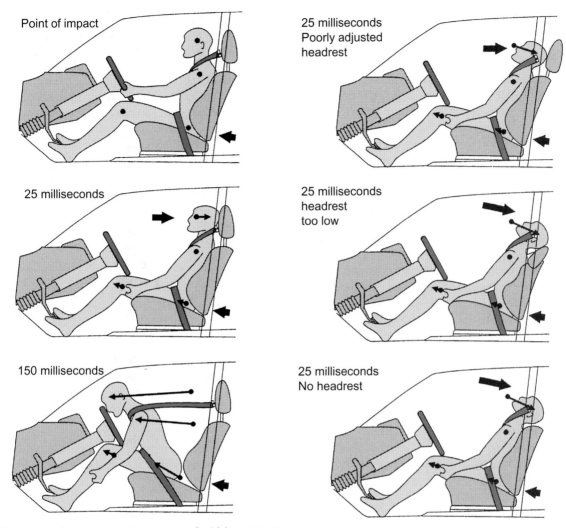

Figure 2.1   Rear impact and movement of vehicle occupant.

compartment. The impact of vehicle occupants with the door on the side opposite to the impact may result in it opening. If the force of impact is sufficient to move the vehicle that is hit, some of the impact energy will be converted to movement energy. In these situations, there may be less damage to the vehicle that is hit.

Vehicle occupant movement

If seat belts are not worn, the body will tend to flex towards the side of the impact, and casualties may hit the side of their heads on the window glass on the same side as the collision. Side intrusions may result in casualties being pushed sideways away from the side of impact. Seat belts, if worn, may prevent sideways movement of the hips and pelvis, but not the thorax and head; classic injury patterns are outlined below. If the impact vehicle pushes the other vehicle sideways, the occupants will be accelerated away from the side of impact after initially moving towards it. When the vehicle stops moving sideways, its occupants will continue to move sideways and may impact with other occupants sitting beside them. Vehicle occupants on the side opposite to that which sustains the impact may be thrown against the door opposite to the impact and, if it opens, may be ejected sideways.

Vehicle occupant injury

In side impacts, vehicle occupants may sustain blunt injury, resulting in lateral compression of the part of the body adjacent to the point of impact. The actual injuries sustained will depend on the side of impact and the level at which it occurs.

On the left side, mid-door intrusion, such as that caused by impact with the front of a car, may result in left lateral flail chest, pulmonary contusion, and rupture to the spleen and left kidney. The casualty's upper arm may rotate posteriorly out of the way protecting it from serious damage, but if the upper arm is pinned between the door and the chest, it may absorb much of the force of the impact transferring some of it to the clavicle and the underlying thoracic wall. This may then result in bony fractures including those of the left humerus, the medial third of the clavicle as it is forced inwards and the outer aspect of the underlying ribs. Right-sided impacts classically cause similar injuries to those on the left side, the only difference being rupture of the liver and right kidney in place of injury to the spleen, left kidney, etc.

Low door intrusion may be caused by impact with the front wheel of a motorcycle. This may result in femoral fractures including impaction fractures where the head of femur is driven into the acetabulum, and pelvic fractures as the ileum is pushed medially, resulting in fractures of the pubic rami anteriorly and the ischium posteriorly. Upper door, window or doorpost intrusion, which may be caused by impact with a lorry bumper, for example, may result in the occupant sustaining head injuries ranging from scalp and facial lacerations to cerebral contusions, skull fractures and cerebral haemorrhage.

Sideways rotation of vehicles involved in collisions will result in occupants sustaining lateral flexion and rotation of the head towards the side of impact. The cervical spine has relatively good anterior/posterior stability, but is less able to resist lateral and rotational movements, especially the two combined. Severe injuries to the cervical spine and its ligaments may result, including injury to the spinal cord sufficient to result in neurological deficit. Seat belts may reduce the direct impact by 'pulling' the casualty away from the point of impact. Vehicle occupants colliding with passengers on the side opposite to the collision may sustain impact injuries to that side of the body. Occupants on the side opposite to the impact may be thrown against the door nearest to them, especially in high-speed impacts, causing it to burst open, sometimes ejecting the casualty sideways. Possible injuries sustained include those to the shoulder, upper arm and chest, the severity of which is dependent on the force of impact, the weight of the casualty and the surface on which they land. Other occupants who may be thrown towards them by the impact may also sustain injuries. Interestingly, if seat belts are worn, there may be greater injury than if the body was free to move out of the way.

> The cervical spine has relatively good anterior/posterior stability, but is less able to resist lateral and rotational movements, especially the two combined

Injury prevention devices

Side impact bars, air bags and impact protection systems are among the most common injury prevention devices in current use. Side impact bars prevent or limit side intrusion into the passenger compartment thereby preventing or reducing the severity of the injury. Some authorities claim that side impact bars may worsen matters as, although they may limit side intrusion when the vehicle occupant comes into contact with the side of the vehicle, there is more energy transfer resulting in more severe chest and pelvic injuries. Side impact bars may also act as a lock in frontal impacts, making it harder for rescue services to force doors open.

Side impact air bags are relatively new developments, which are now being fitted to the seats of some cars to prevent casualties coming into direct contact with doors after side impacts. Their benefits have yet to be fully evaluated. Side Impact Protection System (SIPS) is a system that allows the seats of drivers and front seat passengers to move sideways into a collapsible console in the event of a side impact. Evidence is emerging in relation to their effectiveness.

Rotational impacts

Rotational impacts occur when one corner of a vehicle collides with either an immovable object, or with a vehicle moving more slowly or in the opposite direction. In rotational impacts, the part of the vehicle involved in the impact ceases forward movement while the rest of the vehicle continues to move forwards; this continues until all its kinetic energy is converted to rotational movement, and the vehicle rotates around the point of impact. After the initial frontal impact, the vehicle occupants will continue to move forwards and may impact with the front of the interior of the vehicle before impacting with the side of the vehicle. Vehicular damage and injuries sustained by the occupants are similar to those sustained in frontal and side impacts.

Rollover accidents

Rollover impacts rarely occur in isolation and are often associated with other kinds of impact. The impact is usually spread over a wide area, for example, the whole of the side or roof of the vehicle, and occurs over a relatively large time period as the vehicle rolls over and over. As a result, the amount of damage and injury sustained from the rollover component is usually relatively minor. The vehicle exterior may be deformed with buckling and inward displacement of the roof, owing to its limited strength in resisting direct force, and inward displacement of the doors and floor pan. Unbelted or unrestrained occupants are at significant risk of ejection; front seat occupants are most frequently ejected through side doors, windows or sunroofs, while rear seat occupants are most frequently ejected through the rear window. Injuries sustained by occupants are usually multiple and depend on the points of impact between the car and its occupants. Depression of the vehicle roof may, for example, result in head injuries and injury to the cervical, thoracic and lumbar spine as the force of impact is transmitted down the spinal column. The severity of injury is variable depending on the residual impact energy transferred to the casualty, which is usually small. Fractures of the femur are a relatively frequent occurrence.

Lorries

In large industrial vehicles, such as lorries, the driver's cab usually sits on top of the engine compartment and there is no crumple or impact zone in front of the driver. Should a lorry impact with a car, the interior damage is usually relatively minor, and rarely affects the driver's compartment. However, if the impact is with another lorry, such as in a frontal impact, the entire vehicle front may be damaged, resulting in significant intrusion into the driver's compartment. Rear impacts tend to cause less damage and usually only affect the trailer component. Rollover accidents are relatively common but rarely result in significant injury.

Lorry drivers usually do not wear seat belts nor do lorries have airbags. Consequently, in the event of an impact, occupant movements tend to be similar to those of unrestrained front seat car occupants. From the above it can be seen that frontal or part frontal impacts cause the majority of injuries, the severity of which depend on the forces involved. Steering wheels, which tend to be larger than those in cars, may help to reduce forward driver movement and prevent ejection, which is associated with major secondary injuries. Forward driver movement may result in impact with the steering wheel causing upper and central abdominal injury. Impact with the windscreen may also occur resulting in facial and head injuries, while intrusion of the front of the vehicle may cause severe lower limb injuries. Side impacts involving lorries may result in occupants being ejected sideways if the side door opens.

Motorcycles

Most major injuries involving motorcycles are due to ejection of the motorcyclists on to the road or adjacent surfaces owing to the inherent instability of the motorcycles, and their frequent high speeds. Motorcyclists who lose control on adverse surfaces cause many accidents; inclement weather is usually a contributory factor. Most fatalities in relation to motorcycles and motorcyclists occur as a result of head injuries, despite the wearing of helmets. Lower limb injuries are also particularly common occurring in over 50% of motorcyclists who attend hospital; of these 50% relate to the lower leg.

The wearing of protective clothing and crash helmets have been shown to influence the pattern and type of injuries sustained by motorcyclists, with the severity of injury dependent on the type of impact and protection used. Crash helmets provide protection for the head and face, and can significantly reduce the risk of injury (Fig. 2.2). Indeed, head injuries have been reduced by over 60%, and loss of consciousness by up to 85%. Of particular importance in determining the mechanism of injury are the helmets of pedal cyclists or motorcyclists; these should always be inspected and sent with them to hospital. The main form of protective clothing comes in the form of leather suits. These may help to protect the wearer from dermal injury and friction burns in particular. Tight trousers may also help to reduce blood loss from pelvic and lower limb fractures, through tamponade of the bleeding vessels.

Frontal impact

The impact of the front wheel of motorcycles with other stationary or moving objects may result in the motorcyclist sustaining frontal injuries.

Motorcycle damage Frontal impact with solid objects may result in damage to the front wheel and rearward displacement of the front forks, the amount of displacement dependent on the force involved. After the initial impact, the motorcycle may rotate forwards pivoting about the front wheel as its centre of gravity is above and behind the front axle.

Motorcyclist movement Sudden deceleration will result in the motorcyclist being thrown forwards, impacting with the petrol tank. If the motorcycle decelerates very suddenly and pivots on the front wheel, the rider may be ejected. When the motorcyclist moves forward, the front of the pelvis may impact with the petrol tank resulting in pelvic fracture. In the event that he or she is ejected from the motorcycle, the thighs may impact with the handlebars, especially those having a cow-horn shape, resulting in bilateral femoral fractures.

Motorcyclist injury Injuries sustained by motorcyclists fall into three main categories: those due to ejection, falling over and tailgating. Should motorcyclists be ejected, they will continue to move through the air until they impact with another object or the ground. All the force of the impact will be transmitted through that part of the body that impacts first, resulting in injury at that point; the impact energy will then be transmitted to the rest of the body. The severity of any injuries sustained as a result is dependent on the speed of impact, the trajectory and angle of impact, and the surface on which the motorcyclist lands. Near vertical impacts on to hard surfaces result in the most severe injuries, especially of the head, face, cervical spine, chest and abdomen. Friction burns commonly result from the casualty sliding at speed along the road surface.

Following the initial impact, if the motorcyclist is not ejected, the motorcycle may fall over on to the motorcyclist's legs, crushing them. Secondary injuries of the upper leg, lower leg or ankle are then likely resulting in open or compound fractures of the femoral shafts, tibia, fibula and ankles and dislocations. Collision with the back or side of a vehicle, known as tailgating, may result in hyperextension injury of the cervical spine and head injury, and, in the worst scenario, decapitation.

Side impacts

Side impacts are caused by impact with other moving objects, most often the front bumper or side of cars. Damage to the motorcycle pedals is not uncommon; occasionally damage to the engine and petrol tank are encountered. In side impacts, injuries to motorcyclists are usually caused by direct impact with cars resulting most commonly in fractures of the femur and, less commonly, fractures of the lower leg and ankle. Entrapment of the lower limbs between the motorcycle and the other vehicle or object may also occur. The petrol tank, and less commonly the car wing, usually traps the upper leg with the lower leg trapped between the motorcycle gearbox and the front bumper or corner of the car. Glancing blows may cause tissue rotation resulting in severe soft tissue damage including neurovascular injury. If the motorcyclist is thrown

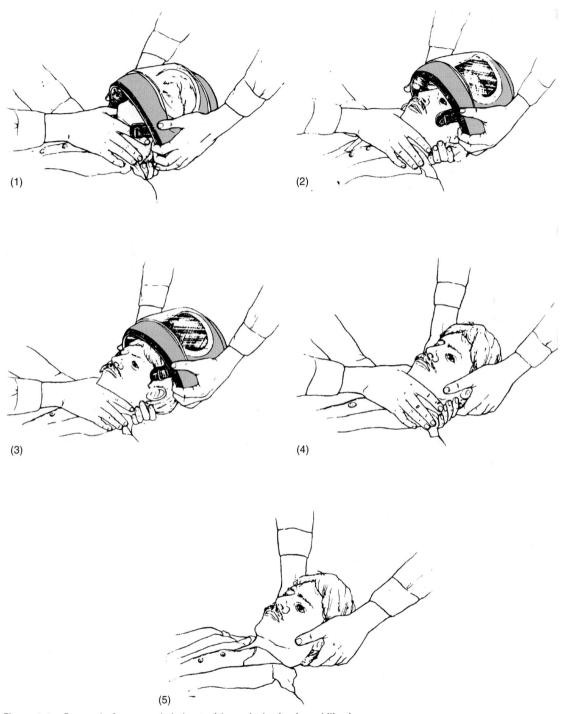

Figure 2.2 Removal of motorcycle helmet with cervical spine immobilisation.

off the motorcycle, he or she may land on the hands or elbows sustaining fractures of the humerus and radius or ulna.

Pedal cyclists

When pedal cyclists collide with stationary objects or slow-moving vehicles, the mechanism of injury is generally similar to that of motorcyclists, but their velocity is usually considerably less and injures are consequently usually less severe. However, if fast-moving cars hit them, the mechanism of injury is similar to that of pedestrians (see later), the difference being that pedal cyclists may be a little higher off the ground sustaining scooping-up injuries. If, on the other hand, lorries hit them, the mechanism of injury is similar to that of pedestrians, with the pedal cyclists sustaining running-over injuries. Rarely, and uniquely, the skin from the lower leg may be stripped (i.e. avulsed, from the lower leg owing to the limb being forced between the wheel spokes). Most child pedal cyclists are injured after losing control and falling from their bicycles. Head injuries are more likely if the incidents occur on hard rather than soft surfaces, and when pedal cyclists have made contact with moving vehicles.

Pedestrians

Pedestrian injuries may be classed as primary or secondary injuries, and usually occur in relation to being hit by moving vehicles, with most pedestrians hit from the side while crossing the road. The type of injuries sustained depends on the age, height and weight of the casualty; adult pedestrians tend to turn away to protect themselves if they anticipate an impact resulting in injuries from lateral or even posterior impacts. Children, on the other hand, tend to turn towards and face the oncoming vehicle.

Primary injury

Primary impacts or injuries are due to the initial collision with the vehicle. Injuries caused depend on the height, weight and age of the casualty, and on the velocity, size and type of vehicle involved.

Adult pedestrians   In primary injuries involving adult pedestrians, the car bumper usually hits them first, knocking their feet from under them. This may result in injuries to the side, if they are facing the vehicle, or injuries to the front of the knee and lower leg, including fractures of the tibia and fibula. The casualties then rotate and flex forwards impacting with the radiator grille, lamps or bonnet causing further primary injury to the thigh or hip, and fractures of the upper femur and pelvis. At low speeds casualties are usually knocked forwards or obliquely sideways, resulting in impact with the front or front corner of the vehicle. At higher speeds, casualties may be thrown into the air on impact. At fairly low speeds, around 20 kph, the body may be thrown violently away to the side of the vehicle but at higher speeds in the region of 60–100 kph, the casualty may be thrown up into the air and may land on the roof of the vehicle. He or she may also travel a considerable distance before hitting the ground or other object, resulting in secondary injuries, which may be more severe than the primary injury.

Scooping-up injuries tend to occur at speeds over 25 kph (cars only) when the casualties have their feet knocked out from under them by car bumpers. This often results in them being thrown up on to the bonnet of the car, resulting in their head impacting with the windscreen (sometimes going through the glass), or windscreen pillar or roof; windscreens deform fairly easily and absorb energy well. Impact with the bonnet may result in fractures of the upper femur, pelvis, ribs and spine, in addition to intra-abdominal and intra-thoracic injuries, whilst impact with the windscreen may result in injuries to the head, face and cervical spine. Once on the bonnet, the casualty assumes the same velocity as the vehicle but seldom stays there long before being thrown sideways on to the road sustaining severe secondary injuries. These include head and cervical spine injury, severe injuries to the side of the body on which they land, and possible injuries from being run over by passing cars. Casualties may also be thrown forwards on to the road, if the driver of the vehicle brakes suddenly, or over the roof of the car, if it is travelling at high speed, causing them to hit the road behind the vehicle and, sometimes the rear window before that. If the vehicle is large, for example, a lorry or bus, the primary injuries may be at a higher level, such as on the chest, arms or head.

Running-over injuries tend to occur when the front part of the vehicle coming into contact with the casualty is relatively high, and the casualty's centre of gravity is relatively low. They are, therefore, more likely to occur in children who are hit by lorries. Running-over injuries are said to occur when a wheel, or the vehicle, pass over the casualty and part of the underside of the vehicle catches on part of the casualty resulting in them being dragged along the road surface. Being run over may result in severe injury to any part of the body, including severe head injuries with gross distortion, serious chest injuries, including flail chest, fractured ribs and sternum, spinal injuries, severe lung contusion and abdominal and pelvic injuries with rupture of the internal organs. Immediate death is also a possibility.

Flaying injuries occur when the wheel, usually of a large vehicle, rotates the body on the ground ripping off the skin and subcutaneous tissue, usually of a leg, arm or the scalp.

Child pedestrians Child pedestrians often sustain serious injuries including head injuries, spinal injuries, especially to the cervical and mid-thoracic regions, and intra-abdominal injuries. As children tend to be shorter and lighter than adults, and have a relatively large and heavy head, any impact usually occurs higher up the body than that which occurs in adults. The first injury caused by impact with the bumper, may result in fractures of the femur and pelvis. The second impact, which occurs almost simultaneously with the first, results in the front of the bonnet impacting massively with the thorax, pushing it backwards. The neck is hyperflexed and the head and face impact with the bonnet. After this, the child may be thrown down and dragged along by the car or knocked to one side. The lower limbs may then be run over by a wheel or knocked backwards, falling under the car where they may be hit by under-car projections and dragged along after getting stuck on part of the car or run over by a wheel.

Secondary injury
Pedestrians impacting with the ground or other object results in skidding, causing secondary injuries. This causes a range of injury presentations including 'brush' abrasions, head injuries (including scalp lacerations, skull and facial fractures with meningeal haemorrhage and cerebral contusions), spinal injuries, especially of the cervical and thoracic regions with spinal cord involvement, chest and pelvic injuries, and fractures of the femur and tibia. The severity of these depends on the weight of the casualty, the surface on which they land or the object with which they collide, their velocity at the time of impact, and the angle of their trajectory.

Elastic recoil
It should be borne in mind that all vehicles, as well as human bodies, exhibit elastic recoil. This means that, although they deform on impact, they are elastic and partially reform afterwards; the deformity seen after an impact is, therefore, not as great as it was at the moment of impact. After an impact, vehicles will tend to spring apart; intrusion into the passenger compartment will be greater than it may appear afterwards, and parts of the body, which may appear not to have impacted with part of a vehicle, may in fact have done so. The tissues and bones of younger bodies are more elastic than those of older bodies, which are more rigid and more inclined to tear and fracture.

> After an impact, intrusion into the passenger compartment will be greater than it may appear

EXAMPLES OF OTHER INJURIES

Falls from heights

In relation to falls, the severity of injury sustained depends on the height of the fall; the greater the height, the greater the velocity achieved by the body and the greater the decelerative force when the casualty impacts with the ground. As a general guide, falls from three times the height of the casualty result in serious injury. The type of surface on which the casualty lands is also of significance; impact with non-compressible surfaces, such as concrete, will result in more severe injuries than impact with relatively compressible surfaces, such as fields, which help to absorb some of the force.

> Falls from three times the height of the casualty result in serious injury

Falls from heights on to the heels or feet result in the whole of the impact force being transmitted through the feet, up the legs and to the spine and head via the pelvis, causing fractured calcaneii and fractured or dislocated hips. After the feet come into contact with the ground and stop moving, the body is forced into flexion as the head, thorax and abdomen continue to move downwards. This results in hyperflexion of the spine at the apex of each of its curves, resulting in compression fractures of the lumbar, thoracic and cervical spine and flexion. Partial relaxation of the ankles, knees and hips prior to the impact may help to absorb part of the decelerative force, or impact energy, and so reduce the severity of the injury. Extension and locking of the ankles, knees and hips prior to impact will, on the other hand, result in the transmission of the decelerative force up the spine and increase the likelihood of significant spinal injury. Falls on to the head with the body in-line, which commonly occurs when diving into shallow water, are also associated with spinal injuries. Here, the whole of the impact force is transmitted through the head and spine, causing a severe hyperextension injury of the cervical spine and, less commonly, severe head injury.

When casualties fall forward on to their outstretched hands to break their fall, they are likely to sustain bilateral Colles fractures and bilateral fractures of the clavicles. The sudden deceleration caused by falls from heights on to hard surfaces may also result in shearing injuries, including rupture of the arch of the aorta. When casualties fall so that another part of their body impacts with the ground, the part of their body that impacts with the ground should be assessed first. The direction in which the resultant force is transmitted through the skeleton should be ascertained and the likely injuries determined.

Sporting injuries

The principles already discussed apply equally to injuries sustained during sporting activities. Injuries may be caused as a result of sudden severe deceleration, excessive compression, twisting, hyperextension and hyperflexion. Other factors involved in their aetiology may include the lack of proper training, inexperience, poor technique, inadequate supervision, poor physical fitness, and lack of adequate protective clothing and equipment. Sports in which relatively high velocities may be achieved include downhill skiing, ski boarding, sledging and tobogganing, water skiing, pedal cycling, skate boarding and horse riding. Should a participant in one of these sports be ejected following an initial collision, the potential injuries are similar to those following ejection from a motor vehicle.

PENETRATING TRAUMA

In penetrating trauma, injury is caused as a result of an object or missile with a small frontal area and high kinetic energy coming into contact with skin and underlying tissues, which it penetrates on entering the body. The object will continue to move through the various tissues in its track, until its progress is either stopped by a tissue that is so dense that it is unable to move forward, ceases forward movement and comes to rest, or it is deflected or exits the body. As it moves through the tissues, it collides with the cells in its track. With each collision there is an exchange of energy resulting in the release of heat and tissue movement, causing the penetrating object to lose some of its kinetic energy. The more kinetic energy the penetrating object/missile loses, the slower it will move. The amount of energy lost or exchanged by the penetrating object depends on the type of target, the density of the tissues through which it passes and its frontal area. A large frontal area will result in a greater number of cells being in the track of the penetrating object resulting in a greater energy exchange, greater tissue damage and larger cavity formation. The frontal area of a penetrating object will depend on its profile; notably, bullets have a small profile, whereas bomb fragments are usually relatively large.

Profile

The shape of the front of the penetrating object or missile, which may be pointed or blunt, is termed its profile. A penetrating object with a sharp point entering a tissue will collide with a smaller number of cells resulting in less energy transfer and less energy loss and will, therefore, cause less tissue damage and cavitation. Alternatively, a penetrating object with a blunt point entering a tissue will collide with a larger number of cells resulting in more energy transfer and greater energy loss, thereby causing greater tissue damage and cavitation. Hollow point bullets have sharp points as they fly through the air losing little kinetic energy as they do so. However, when they penetrate the skin and enter the tissues their points become flattened or blunted, resulting in them colliding with cells, losing kinetic energy and causing tissue damage and cavitation as they penetrate the body further (Fig. 2.3).

Angle of yaw

Most missiles tend to yaw a little from side to side as they fly through the air. This varies during flight and can affect the amount of kinetic energy transferred to tissues by a factor of up to 200, depending on the angle at which the bullet strikes the skin. Thus, the same weapon firing identical rounds may have different effects, and in some circumstances very fast bullets may produce low-energy transfer wounds, whilst slow bullets may produce high-energy transfer wounds.

Tumble

When penetrating missiles or objects, such as bullets, are wedge shaped, their centre of gravity will be nearer their base than their front. When low-energy bullets collide with tissues, they will slow rapidly; however, their centre of gravity will try to continue to move forward, and their bases will try to become their leading points resulting in 'end over end' cartwheel movements or tumbles. As they tumble, the sides of the bullets will become their leading edges, impacting with a greater area than the front or even base of the bullets, thereby causing much greater tissue damage and cavitation.

Fragmentation

When penetrating objects or missiles break apart or separate on impact with the skin or bone, each part or fragment produced may cause significant tissue damage, including multiple exit wounds. The sum of the damage caused by the fragments from one bullet are much greater than that caused by the bullet if it had not fragmented. The multiple pieces of shot or pellets from shotguns produce a similar effect. Bullets with soft or hollow tips or noses, or vertical cuts in the tip (known as *dum-dums*), or the cupronickel coating of fully jacketed rounds fired by high-velocity rifles provide ideal examples of such objects.

Range

Air resistance significantly slows the passage of projectiles: the greater the distance travelled, the greater the reduction in velocity, and the less kinetic energy and injury-causing potential when the projectile penetrates the body. This is of particular significance with regard to shootings, the majority of which take place at close range using handguns; the potential for severe injury is, therefore, high.

Energy levels and tissue damage

The tissue damage likely to be caused by penetrating objects or missiles can be estimated by classifying them according to their kinetic energy and, therefore, the amount of energy likely to be transferred to the tissues. Firearms produce either medium- or high-energy projectiles; the greater the explosive power of the gunpowder in the bullet case or cartridge, the greater the velocity and kinetic energy imparted to the bullet or pellets when the weapon is fired, and the greater the tissue damage caused when those bullets or pellets impact with part of a body.

Low-energy weapons

Low-energy weapons, such as knives, only produce tissue damage at their sharp point or cutting edge. Accordingly, there are usually no

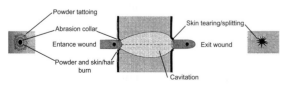

Figure 2.3 Diagrammatic representation of bullet wound.

associated secondary injuries (i.e. there is no energy transfer). Injury only occurs along the penetration track but there is usually some elastic recoil of the tissues after the weapon has been inserted; penetration and tissue damage are, therefore, deeper than they would at first appear. Should the attacker twist the weapon inside the body, extensive tissue damage may be caused.

Almost 25% of penetrating abdominal injuries due to stabbing also involve the thoracic cavity and its contents. This is mainly attributable to the fact that the diaphragm is attached lower down posteriorly than anteriorly, has no bony projection anteriorly and descends during inspiration. Penetrating wounds of the thorax below the nipple line also involve the abdominal cavity.

If the penetrating object has been removed, it is important to ascertain what the object was and, in cases of assault, the gender of the attacker, as men tend to stab with an upward stroke holding the blade on the same side as the thumb, whilst women tend to stab downwards holding the blade on the same side as the little finger.

> If there is one stab wound, there are likely to be others

Medium-energy weapons

The main difference between wounds caused by medium-energy weapons, such as handguns, shotguns and some rifles, and high-energy weapons is the size of the temporary and permanent cavities that are produced when their projectiles penetrate the body tissues. Medium-energy projectiles generally cause damage to tissues on either side of their track as well as to the tissues directly in their track (low-energy transfer wounds), whereas high-energy projectiles cause damage extending far beyond their track.

As the projectiles pass through the tissues, there is a build-up of pressure in front of them, resulting in compression and stretching of the tissues as they move out of their track. As a result,

temporary cavity formation is created, which is usually 3–6 times the size of the projectile's frontal surface area. The amount of tissue damage caused is also dependent on the profile and amount of tumble and fragmentation of the projectiles. The missiles may drag in parts of clothing, etc. as they enter the body; this contamination, however, is confined to the missile track and does not usually result in gross contamination.

High-energy weapons

High-energy weapons, such as hunting rifles and assault weapons, generally cause much greater tissue damage than medium-energy weapons (high-energy transfer wounds) because much larger temporary cavities are produced. These extend far beyond the actual track of the projectiles, resulting in much greater tissue damage and injury than may initially be apparent. The vacuum created behind these projectiles sucks into the wound particles of clothing, bacteria and other debris from the surrounding area, resulting in severe contamination.

CONCLUSION

It is essential that nurses seek an accurate history of the mechanism of injury in all patients who have suffered trauma. Knowledge of the mechanisms of injury should make it possible to predict the injuries that the patient is likely to be suffering from by relating the mechanism of injury to the clinical findings. In interpreting these clinical findings it must be remembered that, in road traffic accidents, three impacts occur: those involving the vehicle(s), the patient(s) and those involving the patient's organs. A good history can lead hospital teams to identify life-threatening injuries more quickly and instigate the necessary treatment. A high level of suspicion must be maintained at all times when the mechanism is suggestive of serious injury. Many lives are saved by staff who maintain this high index of suspicion and act upon it.

Chapter 3

A structured approach to caring for the trauma patient

Elaine Cole and Ann McGinley

INTRODUCTION

From early civilisation to modern day society, the devastating effects of injury have plagued man. This chapter will explore the importance of a systematic approach to trauma management in the UK, its evolution, strengths and limitations, and the developments that may determine subsequent UK trauma care.

THE EVOLUTION OF UK TRAUMA MANAGEMENT

Contemporary trauma management was born out of wartime experience. Triage guidelines, immediate resuscitation and definitive care protocols were created and tested in the battlefield, and the principles later adopted in the civilian situation (Beachley and Snow, 1988; Beachley et al., 1988; Broomfield, 1998; Howell, 1988).

During peacetime, advances in UK trauma management have been sporadic. From the beginning of the National Health Service (NHS) in 1948, casualty units have existed to meet the needs of sick and injured patients. Foremost amongst these has been the Birmingham Accident Centre – a unique facility that was founded by industrialists and health care professionals in 1941, and that has served as a prototype for the development of other UK trauma centres (Sutcliffe, 1990a,b). The 1960s and 1970s saw further refinement of the casualty service with the emergence of accident and emergency (A&E) departments led by specialist consultants (Royal College of Surgeons of England, 1988).

Within the pre-hospital domain, several developments have also occurred. In 1966, a national qualification for ambulance personnel was established, while 1984 saw the widespread introduction of paramedic training. By the early 1990s, the government had pledged to expand this initiative so that, by 1996, each front-line emergency vehicle would be staffed by a fully trained paramedic (Cook, 1991; Lloyd, 1991; Department of Health, 1992).

In addition to the training and preparation of pre-hospital personnel, a number of operational reforms were instigated to optimise the immediate care of the injured patient. These included improvements in communication and dispatch strategies, an increase in the number of rapid-response vehicles and the introduction of national targets for emergency response times (Cook, 1991; Lloyd, 1991; Rouse, 1992; Chadda, 1995; Cross, 1997). Civilian air ambulances were also used to retrieve some of the more seriously injured trauma victims (Caple, 1997).

Despite these achievements, traumatic injury remains a leading cause of death in the under-40-year-old age group and is only surpassed by cancer and ischaemic heart disease in all other age groups (Yates, 1988; Royal College of Surgeons of England and British Orthopaedic Association, 2000).

> Traumatic injury remains a leading cause of death in the under-40-year-old age group

Death, however, is not the only negative performance indicator. In terms of lost revenue, Earlam (1997) reported the societal cost of a premature death to be between £500 000 and £750 000, with those surviving in a debilitated state and who require institutionalised care possibly costing an additional £1000 per week. The human impact of injury in terms of pain, suffering and misery is, however, incalculable, and devastating for all those involved (Yates et al., 1992; Hadfield, 1993).

1988 was pivotal to advancing UK trauma care. Anderson et al. (1988) reviewed a thousand trauma deaths and concluded that 33% were potentially preventable. This finding of sub-optimal trauma care in the UK was confirmed by

the RCS in its report 'Management of Patients with Major Injuries' (RCS, 1988). Together these reports highlighted the enormity of the problem, whilst recognising some of the key contributory factors that accounted for unnecessary premature deaths. Moreover, these findings were consistent with those from the Shock Trauma Institute, Maryland, USA (Davis, 1990; Armstrong, 1995).

West et al. (1979) demonstrated that preventable mortality is partly accounted for by the frequency with which centres treat polytrauma patients. In its report, the RCS (1988) recognised that small units were treating seriously injured patients on an infrequent basis and consequently recommended the development of regional trauma centres in the UK. In response to this, the Advanced Trauma Life Support (ATLS) protocols were adopted (American College of Surgeons, 1997). The RCS (1988) pledged to undertake further research in trauma management and the Major Trauma Outcome Study (MTOS) established in 1990, now superseded by the UK Trauma Audit Research Network (UKTARN).

THE PLIGHT OF UK TRAUMA NURSING

Historically, within the nursing domain, practitioners were equally ill-prepared to care for seriously injured patients. In 1991, Hamilton's survey of 94 emergency nurses found that 46% had no formal training in trauma nursing. Two-thirds of the most junior trained nurses were responsible for caring for the polytrauma patient on a regular basis, whilst their more experienced and senior colleagues rarely practised their skills. Eyre's (1992) survey of 193 A&E departments revealed that only 40% of units surveyed claimed to have had a trauma-trained nurse (Eyre, 1993).

In the early 1990s, trauma training for nurses was restricted to either receiving a single lecture on a post-basic nursing course or attending the medical ATLS course as a non-participant observer (Hadfield, 1993). In practice, the role of the trauma nurse was implicit and often difficult to identify (Lomas and Goodall, 1994). Despite their poor preparation and lack of recognition, nurses remained the one discipline that was strategically placed throughout the trauma continuum (Sutcliffe, 1990b; Hadfield-Law, 1994).

In the USA, it was well established that trauma training was required and that trauma nurses needed to have a specific body of knowledge encompassing resuscitation, stabilisation and rehabilitation (Beachley and Snow, 1988). In November 1990, the Trauma Nurse Core Course (TNCC) was imported in to the UK and the Advanced Trauma Nursing Course (ATNC) followed quickly thereafter. ATNC was an important landmark, as UK nurses began to articulate their philosophical beliefs and values. Central to this philosophy was the acknowledgement that UK trauma victims had the right to be cared for by specifically trained and educated nurses (Hadfield, 1993; ATNC, 1994; Hadfield-Law, 1994). Whilst ATLS principles remained core components of both courses, the role of the trauma nurse, psychosocial aspects of care and the need to initiate change were also included (Hadfield, 1993; Hadfield-Law, 1994). ATNC and TNCC have since become important national and international standards in trauma education for nurses (Bryant, 1989; Zuspan, 1990; Gagnon, 1991; Hadfield, 1993: Inman, 1992; Zimmermann, 1996), both remaining focused on immediate post-injury care and the medical model of trauma management (Hadfield, 1993; Christie, 1994; Hadfield-Law, 1994). Continuous education programmes are clearly required to maintain staff proficiency; and practitioners' needs for training will undoubtedly change over time, as they progress in the specialty and as the specialty itself develops (Zuspan, 1990; Ruth-Sahd, 1993).

Within the USA, the holistic continuum approach to trauma management is well recognized (Beachley and Snow, 1988; Beachley et al., 1988; Beachley, 1989; Scherer, 1989; Daleiden, 1993; Dekeyser et al., 1993; Veise-Berry and Beachley, 1994; Davis and Wood, 1995). This broad approach to trauma care has allowed a number of specialist nursing roles to emerge, such as the pre-hospital nurse, the trauma case manager and the Trauma Nurse Co-ordinator (TNC). The British Association for Immediate Care (BASICS) has also begun to recognise an on-scene role for nurses and the TNC role in UK hospitals is under evaluation (Harrison, 1990; Holleran, 1994; McInulty, 1998).

As trauma care becomes a specialty in its own right, it is important that UK trauma nursing is expanded beyond A&E departments, theatres, intensive care units (ICUs) and orthopaedic nursing. The attributes and preparation of UK trauma nurses requires careful consideration and proactive development. Many of the UK reforms have been imported from the USA and valuable lessons can be learnt from studying the American approach to preparation for practice. Caution must be exercised, however, when translating American nursing into the UK health care culture to ensure that the overall objectives remain congruent with local practice.

INITIAL ASSESSMENT OF THE TRAUMA PATIENT IN THE ACCIDENT AND EMERGENCY DEPARTMENT

When planning the initial assessment, resuscitation and management of the trauma patient, a systematic and collaborative approach is essential to optimise patient outcome. This begins with liaison with pre-hospital care personnel and extends to the interface with definitive care. The aim of the trauma team in emergency departments is to systematically identify and treat those immediately and potentially life-threatening conditions that arise from traumatic injury (Greaves et al., 2001a). Once injuries have been diagnosed, definitive care and patient discharge from the emergency department should be planned.

> A systematic, collaborative team approach is essential to optimise patient outcome

Advanced notification

It is essential that the trauma team in the emergency department have access to accurate information prior to the patient's arrival. The advanced notification given by the pre-hospital team will enable the preparation of equipment and personnel essential to provide the best chance for a successful outcome (Weigelt and Klein, 1994; RCS and British Orthopaedic Association, 2000). In its report into *Better care for the severely injured*, the RCS and the British Orthopaedic Association (2000) recommend the following information as a minimum for advanced notification:

- patient numbers
- age
- gender
- mechanism and type of injury
- heart rate
- blood pressure
- Glasgow coma score (GCS)
- respiratory rate
- oxygen saturation
- treatment given.

Box 3.1   The mnemonic ASHICE

A	Age
S	Sex
H	History
I	Injuries/illness
C	Conscious level
E	Estimated time of arrival

Alternatively, the mnemonic 'ASHICE' (Box 3.1) is useful for gaining pre hospital information.

Once advanced notification has been received, the trauma team should be activated according to hospital protocol (Box 3.2). Activation protocols may vary from hospital to hospital depending on available resources and the type of trauma that is received. It is essential that A&E staff know when to activate the trauma team, and members of the team clearly understand their roles and responsibilities.

The trauma team

The ATLS course is designed such that a doctor can safely look after a multiply injured patient single handedly (American College of Surgeons, 1997). Tasks are performed sequentially, one after the other. This type of approach has been described as vertical organization, and is suggested to be an inefficient method of simultaneous assessment and management of trauma care in terms of timely resuscitation (Driscoll and Vincent, 1992; Adedeji and Driscoll, 1996; American College of Surgeons, 1997). However, within most emergency departments a more defined multi-disciplinary trauma team approach is utilised. Membership of a trauma team is dependent on the institution and available resources as are team

---

Box 3.2   Suggested criteria for activating the trauma team (when requested by the emergency medical services).

Trauma victims with any of the following:
- Actual or potential airway compromise
- Signs of a pneumothorax
- $SpO_2 < 90\%$
- Pulse >100/minute or systolic blood pressure < 100 mmHg (adults)
- A GCS below 14 associated with a head injury
- A penetrating wound anywhere on the torso (including pelvic/perineal regions)
- Any gunshot wound
- Fall from > 25 feet/8 metres

Children with:
- An altered conscious level
- A capillary refill > 3 seconds
- A tachycardia (value dependent on age)
- A pedestrian or cyclist hit by a vehicle

Incidents involving:
- Five or more casualties
- A fatality
- A road traffic accident where the patient was ejected from the vehicle

(Modified from recommendations of the RCS and the British Orthopaedic Association, 2000)

---

roles and responsibilities (Hoff et al., 1997). The trauma team consists of a group of doctors, nurses, technicians and radiographers who each carry out pre-assigned tasks simultaneously to achieve effective, timely, patient management. This horizontal organisation has been shown to lead to significant reductions in resuscitation times (Adedeji and Driscoll, 1996; Hoff et al., 1997). Opinions regarding optimal horizontal team size vary between 4 and 8 with no consensus on team membership or the recommended number of nurses (Weigelt and Klein, 1994; Cudmore, 1996; Deo et al., 1997; Hoff et al., 1997; Greaves et al., 2001a) (Box 3.3).

This more sophisticated method of teamwork requires organisation and an effective team leader to direct individuals. It is recognised that the team leader must have successfully undergone ATLS training, and it is expected that an experienced consultant undertakes the team leader role

(American College of Sugeons, 1997; RCS and British Orthopaedic Association, 2000). This role demands a level of proficiency in team management and excellent communication skills in addition to education and training. Nurses participating in the trauma team, especially those supervising and supporting more junior members of the team, should have completed a trauma nursing course, such as ATNC or TNCC. The development of a common language and an understanding of management goals are essential to maximise patient survival and outcome.

Initial assessment, primary survey and resuscitation

Prior to the patient arriving into the emergency department, all members of the trauma team must take steps to reduce the risk of occupational exposure to blood-borne diseases, such as HIV and hepatitis. In addition to immunisation for all trauma team staff, all blood and body fluids should be assumed to be a potential risk (Greaves et al, 2001a). Each team member should wear gloves, aprons/protective gowns and protective eyewear during the trauma assessment and resuscitation (American College of Surgeons, 1997).

In order to request blood tests, blood products and diagnostic imaging for the trauma patient quickly and safely, a system of pre-arrival registration may be adopted. A&E department staff should be familiar with their local arrangements.

The objectives of the initial assessment, primary survey and resuscitation phase are to rapidly identify and correct any life threatening injuries. Actions by the team may have a potential impact on the patient's later survival, for example, the development of a coagulopathy or an infective process; therefore, an overview of the patient's pathophysiology throughout the trauma continuum is essential.

The assessment is carried out systematically assessing A,B,C,D,E (Box 3.4), using a sequential approach in a vertical trauma team or a simultaneous approach in a horizontal trauma team.

> The assessment is carried out systematically following a sequential approach in a vertical trauma team or a simultaneous approach in a horizontal trauma team

Airway with cervical spine control
The airway must be assessed while the cervical spine is immobilized. The '3Ps' strategy may be adopted in assessing airway (i.e. ensure the airway is patent, protected and, if not, provide it). It is assumed that any patient who has suffered blunt trauma or an injury above the clavicle may

have sustained a cervical spine injury; therefore, manual in-line immobilisation or full immobilisation using a semi-rigid collar, head blocks and tape is essential. The only exception to this is the combative or restless patient where forceful immobilisation may result in further spinal damage. The priority for this type of patient is to identify and treat the cause of restlessness (e.g. hypoxia owing to a tension pneumothorax).

> Assume cervical spine injury in patients who have suffered blunt trauma or injuries above the clavicle

Breathing and ventilation

In addition to providing 100% oxygen via an oxygen mask with a reservoir bag, it is essential to *look, listen and feel* to assess respiratory rate and efficiency, to assist ventilation where necessary and to identify any life-threatening thoracic injuries.

Circulation with haemorrhage control

Priority must be given to arresting haemorrhage. An assessment of circulatory compromise is made and intravenous access should be established ensuring essential blood samples are taken. Fluid resuscitation and blood product administration should be considered and administered dependent upon the patient's status. Contemporary trauma management suggests that the shocked trauma patient may benefit from permissive hypotension (Kreimeier et al., 2000) (i.e. maintaining the systolic blood pressure around 80–90 mmHg, and minimal handling to prevent clot dislodgement). This decision should be made by an experienced trauma clinician. Furthermore, due consideration must be given to maintaining adequate cerebral perfusion pressure where the patient has sustained a concomitant head injury.

Disability

Level of consciousness should be assessed using the Glasgow coma scale and pupillary response recorded as a baseline at this stage. If a neurological injury is identified, an early neurosurgical consultation is essential.

Exposure and environmental control

During the primary survey, examination of the anterior and posterior surfaces may be required to assess for life-threatening conditions. The patient should be fully undressed to facilitate a detailed secondary survey examination, but not left uncovered unnecessarily to avoid hypothermia, and to maintain privacy and dignity.

In addition to the rapid assessment of A,B,C,D,E, a brief history should be obtained. This is most easily recounted using the AMPLE mnemonic (Box 3.5).

Box 3.5   Obtaining an 'AMPLE' history
A   Allergies
M   Medications
P   Past medical history
L   Last food/drink
E   Events/environment related to injury

If the patient is conscious and orientated on arrival, psychological care including explanations of what is going to happen is essential.

Secondary survey

In addition to immediate diagnostic imaging, such as x-rays of the chest, cervical spine and pelvis, a secondary survey may be undertaken after the primary survey is completed and if urgent operative intervention is not required.

This more detailed head-to-toe examination should identify any other injuries and will direct the need for appropriate investigations and management. The patient should be examined starting at the head through thoracic, abdominal, and pelvic regions, bony extremities and soft tissues. Spinal integrity and rectal tone should also be assessed where appropriate. When clinical clearance of the spine cannot be established, spinal imaging must be undertaken. If the skin integrity has been breached with a tetanus-prone wound, then the patient's tetanus status should be reviewed. Analgesia, patient positioning and splinting of extremity injuries should all be addressed as a priority. Urinary catheterisation may be necessary to monitor output. Careful monitoring of the patient must be maintained throughout the secondary survey, in order to closely observe for *any* deterioration in patient status that would warrant a reassessment of A,B,C,D,E. In addition, the patient's response to any intervention, for example, fluid or drug administration should be evaluated to determine its efficacy.

> Careful monitoring of the patient is mandatory throughout the secondary survey

Documentation is crucial throughout the trauma continuum and it is vital that accurate information is recorded during the acute phases of care (Box 3.6). In many emergency departments, a designated trauma sheet or booklet will be used to collate information and avoid the fragmentation of information, which is associated with the use of separate documents (Greaves et al., 2001a).

It is also a nursing responsibility to record the patient's property and valuables, and any interactions with the police, such as handing over of forensic evidence. In addition to caring for the trauma patient, consideration should be given to the patient's family members and close friends. It is suggested that a nurse is designated to liaise with the family members during trauma resuscitation. Resource availability will dictate whether or not this is a trauma team nurse (Hoff et al., 1997).

Witnessed trauma resuscitation

Some relatives *insist* on seeing their relatives during the early stages of their arrival at hospital. This is an area that may provoke strong feelings from members of the trauma team. Arguments for

---

Box 3.6   Documentation

Documentation should include:
- Mechanism of injury
- Haemodynamic, respiratory and neurological monitoring
- Treatment interventions
- Summaries of the patient's status at each stage of the initial assessment and resuscitation
- The name(s) of the nurse looking after the patient and the clinical team(s) taking responsibility for the subsequent patient management.

---

and against the practice of allowing relatives to be present during trauma resuscitation prevail and, whilst rigid guidelines cannot be followed, it is essential that the trauma team have an agreed approach to reaching clinical decisions when faced with this situation (Cole, 2000).

DEFINITIVE MANAGEMENT OF THE TRAUMA PATIENT

Definitive care

The patient may enter definitive care via four routes: diagnostic imaging, the operating theatre, intensive care, or the acute hospital ward. In some instances, admission into definitive care is more complex, as the patient has to be transferred between hospitals for the definitive management of their injuries (e.g. the head-injured patient who requires neurosurgery). Admission to any one of these areas requires clear communication and coordination to ensure appropriate and timely transfer of the patient, and the delivery of expert care. Failure to coordinate and communicate effectively fragments trauma management and delays patient care (Hadfield-Law, 1994; Haire, 1998).

The receiving practitioner should always contrast the injury profile against the mechanism of injury, maintaining a high index of suspicion for missed injury and/or complications that may hamper the individual's recovery. This index of suspicion should be heightened in the immediate post-resuscitation phase when the receiving practitioner should carry out a tertiary survey. An orthopaedic patient, for example, who jumped from a burning building to escape a fire, may have obvious fractures and the inhalation event may not have become manifest in the immediate post-injury phase. The insidious onset of stridor and airway compromise might surprise the unsuspecting carer.

> Always contrast the injury profile against the mechanism of injury

The generic principles that govern immediate trauma management should extend to other parts of the trauma continuum. Collaboration amongst care providers and clinical expertise are pre-requisites to minimising morbidity and mortality (Scherer, 1989).

Hospital personnel caring for trauma victims must be trained and well versed in their role. Zuspan (1990) highlights the need to maintain staff proficiency with continuing education programmes. Scenario training, scavenger hunts, short courses on trauma management and proto-cols have all been advocated in the orientation of new staff (Dunnum and Bailey, 1991; Hamilton, 1991). Virtual reality training using computerised simulation offers a potentially new and exciting way to educate staff on the complexities of trauma care (Rauen, 2001).

In 2000, The RCS and the British Orthopaedic Association reasserted that the provision of optimal trauma care requires:

1. the concentration of trauma services and skills
2. national standards of care for severely injured patients with systematic audit to ensure satisfactory patient outcome is achieved
3. a network strategy between local hospitals to ascertain injured patients receive optimal care, including adequate critical care resources to support the severely injured patient
4. a strategy for rehabilitation
5. trauma life-support training for all paramedics.

It is imperative that at the point of admission to definitive care a consultant should be clearly identified as the clinical lead with overall responsibility for the patient's care. As trauma-tology is not a recognised specialty in the UK, the clinical responsibility of the trauma patient will often come under the auspices of a general sur-geon, neurosurgeon or an orthopaedic surgeon.

> Clinical expertise and collaboration among care providers are prerequisites to minimizing morbidity and mortality

Diagnostic imaging

Within trauma resuscitation, the two plain films advocated by ATLS should be completed (i.e. the chest and pelvic x-rays; American College of Surgeons, 1997). Thereafter, the need for imaging will be determined by the mechanism of injury

and the initial findings in the primary and secondary surveys. All blunt trauma patients who cannot have their spines cleared clinically will require a full set of spinal radiographs (Brooks and Willet, 2001). Trauma centres must have access to computed tomography (CT), a magnetic resonance imager (MRI), and the full range of radiological services (e.g. angiography and ultra-sonography). District general hospitals need to maintain digital links with local tertiary referral centres; those without such facilities need to consider early transfer when appropriate.

Radiography staff are integral to any trauma service and, as such, must be available at all times to perform imaging or diagnostic procedures. Radiologists must be available to interpret findings and consult with their clinical colleagues regarding further diagnostic interventions that may determine treatment. Advanced invasive radiology has allowed the emergence of conser-vative management for solid abdominal organ injury for selected patients who are otherwise cardiovascularly stable (Greaves et al., 2001b).

> All blunt trauma patients who cannot have their spines cleared clinically will need a full set of spinal radiographs

Operative management

Definitive trauma management often incorporates surgical intervention; and immediate access to a fully staffed and well-equipped theatre is mandatory to run an effective trauma service.

Immediate life- or limb-threatening injuries are dealt with in a short 'damage limitation' surgical episode. This procedure is confined to critically injured patients who are shocked and at risk of dying from a triad of hypothermia, acidosis and coagulopathy. If these physiological derangements are established or imminent, the patient should undergo a short damage control procedure aimed at stopping haemorrhage, preventing sepsis and protecting organ function from further harm. Experienced surgeons and anaesthetists should be involved in these procedures. Patients who are metabolically deranged with a lactate debt, hypothermic, hypotensive and coagulopathic, need to return to an intensive care environment for aggressive correction of physiological derangements (Ku et al., 1999; Lewis, 2000). Some centres have well-defined protocols that detail diagnostic work-up and operative courses for specific injuries.

Critical care

For the most seriously injured patients, a period of critical care may be warranted. A tiered approach to critical care provision has now been adopted within the UK, such that critical care personnel may encounter the trauma patient in outreach care (level 1 critical care); high-dependency care (level 2) or intensive care (level 3). The challenge for critical care staff is to escalate or de-escalate trauma patients as appropriate (Department of Health, 2000).

Prior to admission, advanced notification should outline the suspected injury profile, the likely time of arrival and whether the patient will be directly admitted to the intensive care unit or via the operating theatre. Forewarning enables the critical care nurse to be pre-emptive and consider what additional equipment, drugs and monitoring may be required beyond the standard ventilatory and haemodynamic support. For example, the patient with a spinal cord injury with associated chest injuries may require a spinal turning bed that needs to be hired from an external facility. On arrival in ICU, the primary nurse should take a detailed handover noting previous assessments, clinical findings, interventions and specific instructions given to date. The patient will be transferred on to the intensive care equipment ensuring all ventilator and monitor alarms are set (Johnson, 1993). At admission it is also imperative to check the patient is 'labelled' with a hospital identity band – this is particularly important if the patient is unconscious or in the post-anaesthetic phase. Accompanying property must be placed in a bag, labelled and listed as in some instances personal property is required as forensic evidence (McCraken, 2001). Finally, no handover is complete until the next of kin have been identified and updated.

The remit of the critical care team is to support organ function that the patient cannot manage independently and thereby promote homeostatic control. Ventilatory and cardiovascular support is frequently required; thereafter, the nature and degree of injury and the complication sequelae will determine which other organs may be compromised and need support.

Following the patient's initial admission and any surgical episode or major complication, ongoing resuscitation and a period of stabilisation are essential. Invasive monitoring may be required to measure parameters and monitor the patient's progress. During the intensive care phase, specific physiological parameters will be set against which the patient's overall recovery or response to therapy will be judged; for example, mean arterial pressure may be maintained with optimum fluid resuscitation and/or inotropic support. Integrated care pathways or protocols may also be used to guide and enhance care. The critical care practitioner must be discerning, selecting the most appropriate elements of key protocols that may direct the patient's management. For example, a polytrauma patient with head, chest and abdominal injuries may develop acute respiratory distress syndrome (ARDS) in the presence of raised intracranial pressure and abdominal compartment syndrome. Whilst the acute lung injury protocol may advocate nursing the patient in the prone position, their concurrent injuries would prohibit this (Tingle, 1995).

Beyond the high technology surveillance and monitoring, which is integral to the critical care nurse's role, lies the art of caring for the injured patient. The 'art' of nursing is dependent on the individual nurse's competence, background experience and innate intuition. It is not confined to one particular part of the trauma continuum. Benner's (1984) 'Novice to Expert' model depicts how this can change over time as the practitioner not only becomes socialised in the work environment but, more importantly, increases skill acquisition (Ruth-Sahd, 1993). It is the complete experience of caring for multisystem trauma (i.e. the art and the science of nursing), which challenges nurses to meet the physical and psychological needs of the injured patient. Dean (1998) contends that it is the art of nursing that ensures high-technology environments, such as the emergency department or ICU, are humanised and personalised, thus allowing patients and their families to cope and adapt in otherwise stressful situations. Henderson (1960) probably best summarised the art of nursing when she stated that the role of the nurse was to aid the patient in their recovery but, when this was no longer possible, to assist that individual in achieving a peaceful death.

There are seven areas in the care of the critically injured patient that deserve special attention. These are:

1. good pulmonary toilet
2. cardiovascular monitoring and fluid input
3. promotion of skin integrity
4. effective analgesia
5. adequate nutritional intake
6. psychosocial support
7. a peaceful death when recovery is not possible.

Pulmonary toilet

Hypoxia is a real threat that increases the morbidity and mortality of critically injured patients, and is usually associated with the second peak of the trimodal distribution of trauma deaths (Trunkey, 1983). However, long-term problems may ensue beyond the direct pulmonary trauma (e.g. atelectasis and acute lung injury) and may threaten the ventilation perfusion match in patients who may have a greater demand for oxygen. Regular positioning, physiotherapy, suctioning and assisted ventilation may help to redress the balance and ensure that areas of lung remain viable and functioning (Paterson, 1997). Bedside SpO_2 monitoring, serial arterial blood gases and chest x-rays will monitor the progress of events.

> Hypoxia is a real threat that increases the morbidity and mortality of critically injured patients

Cardiovascular monitoring and fluid input

Meticulous attention to fluid intake is essential. Immediately post-injury the nurse, in collaboration with medical colleagues, must ensure that any hypovolaemia that may have compromised organ perfusion has been corrected. It is equally important that overhydration is avoided (Gosling

et al., 1996). Capillary refill, urinary output and haemodynamic parameters of central venous pressure and mean arterial blood pressure should guide ongoing fluid resuscitation. Haemoglobin and haematocrit measurements may reveal late signs of haemorrhage, while ongoing acidosis may be an early indicator for these patients (Ku et al., 1999; Lewis, 2000). Latterly fluid shifts between compartments may occur as oncotic pressure is reduced or the permeability of blood vessels is altered, for example, during a septic episode (Gosling et al., 1996; Metheny, 2000).

Skin integrity

The largest organ of the body is the skin. Although it has many functions, it is an important barrier to external organisms and bacteria. Cutaneous blood flow may also be poor secondary to direct pressure but, more importantly, owing to altered perfusion as seen with gunshot wounds. The autonomic nervous system may preferentially perfuse core organs at the expense of the peripheral circulation. Drugs such as norepinephrine can enhance this autonomic nervous system response as the alpha (α) receptors are stimulated and vasoconstriction occurs (Morrill, 2000). Also, once breached by wounds (traumatic or surgical) and invasive lines, its ability to act as a barrier to infection may be severely diminished. It is imperative, therefore, that invasive monitoring is rationalised and discontinued as soon as possible. Cannulae sited in the field must be removed within the first 24 hours of admission.

Wound management requires strict asepsis. More heavily contaminated wounds require serial surgical debridement. For more complex wounds, Polaroid photographs should be taken serially and incorporated into the wound care plan (Nayduch, 1999). Tissue viability nurses can contribute greatly in advising on wound care and the various pressure relieving devices available for immobile patients who are at risk of developing skin breakdown.

Pain management

Pain is an inevitable symptom that most trauma patients will have to contend with during their recovery. Unrelieved pain will heighten a patient's anxiety level but, more importantly, will increase metabolic demands for oxygen that in an otherwise compromised patient may be deleterious and worsen the pulmonary condition (Cheever, 1999). Consultation with anaesthetic staff or pain nurses should occur early to ensure that the most appropriate drug and mode of analgesia is being used. For example, patients with multiple rib fractures should ideally have epidural analgesia, while other patients may require patient-controlled analgesia (PCA) or regular intramuscular or oral medications. In the context of critical or high-dependency care, the intravenous route may also be used, as patients are more closely monitored and frequently sedated with assisted ventilation.

The choice of opioid is also important. The management of breakthrough pain may require a combination of drugs administered at specific time intervals.

Nutritional intake

Malnutrition is a common phenomenon in hospitalised patients. Delays in establishing an effective feeding regimen are well documented and, for seriously injured patients, may pose a serious threat to their well-being (Riley, 2002). Early enteral feeding is advocated to protect the integrity and immunocompetence of the gut mucosa, as bacterial translocation predisposes the patient to ventilator associated pneumonia with subsequent systemic inflammatory response syndrome and multiorgan failure. Moreover, a hypermetabolic state frequently follows injury, and there is a need for good nutritional intake to allow early tissue repair from traumatic and surgical wounds (Russell, 2001). Resting energy expenditure may increase between 25% and 60%, according to the severity of the trauma and the degree of substrate recycling. The requirements for nutrients alters substrate metabolism, and energy stores are frequently mobilised. Insulin resistance, a negative nitrogen balance and loss of lean body mass are also commonly reported (Say, 1997; Edwards, 2002).

Psychosocial care

The sudden untoward nature of injury may be met with mixed responses from the trauma victims and their family (e.g. disbelief, anger and grief). Fear, anxiety, lack of control and an uncertain prognosis may compound the situation, while flashbacks to the events surrounding the injury are not uncommon. The skilful nurse should try to establish a therapeutic rapport with the patient and their family based on open and honest communication. Enabling the family to develop coping strategies will strengthen the social support network for the patient, which in turn may escalate their recovery.

Additional expert help may be required. Social Workers can ensure that financial burdens and hardship are not additional stressors with which patients have to contend. This is particularly important, as many patients are 'breadwinners' with family commitments. Counsellors also have a unique role to play in helping to minimise long-term psychological disability in patients with post-traumatic stress disorder (Jones and Griffiths, 2002).

The dying patient

Not all patients will survive their injuries. In certain instances, the fight for life is short-lived as the patient's condition never really stabilises. Other patients make some recovery before relapsing and eventually succumbing to the complications of their injuries (Table 3.1).

Achieving a peaceful and dignified death is difficult in a high-technology environment such as an ICU. Families may have little or no time to come to terms with the patient's imminent death. Their anguish may be heightened in situations such as those involving patients who have attempted suicide, or those who are pronounced brain dead where decisions regarding organ donation have to be made. Compassion, understanding and privacy are required. The additional support of religious or bereavement services may be offered, and may be of help to the family.

High dependency care

High-dependency care is an intermediate level of critical care that may be offered to the trauma victim. Dedicated surgical high depencency units (HDUs) are most likely to admit the trauma patient. The main difference in management is

Table 3.1 Complications

Complication	Criteria	Primary event	Secondary events	Monitoring/care required
Abdominal compartment syndrome (ACS) Normal intra-abdominal pressure = 0 mmHg	Raised intra-abdominal pressure Intra-abdominal hypertension: – Mild = 15–20 mmHg – Moderate = 20–25 mmHg – Severe = 25–35 mmHg Additional signs include: – Reduced urine output – Raised airway pressures – Raised CVP	Massive intra-abdominal trauma Pelvic fractures with extensive retroperitoneal haematoma		Measure intra-abdominal pressure via indwelling urinary catheter Laparotomy if intra-abdominal pressure becomes severe
Acute lung injury (ALI)/acute respiratory distress syndrome (ARDS)	ALI – $PaO_2/FIO_2 \leq 300$ mmHg (40 kPa) with bilateral pulmonary infiltrates on CXR and PAOP or ≤ 18 mmHg Identified cause/event ARDS is ALI criteria, but the $PaO_2/FIO_2 \leq 200$ mmHg (27 kPa)	Aspiration Blunt trauma or blast injury Inhalation injury Near-drowning	Burns DIC Fat embolus/pulmonary embolus Massive blood transfusions Multiorgan dysfunction syndrome Neurogenic pulmonary oedema Polytrauma Sepsis SIRS	Assisted ventilation (CPAP; pressure-controlled ventilation with reverse I:E ratios and PEEP; or jet ventilation) Prone positioning, if otherwise not contraindicated Prostacyclin therapy or inhaled nitric oxide Use of steroids controversial Consider ECMO, if conventional respiratory support fails Maximise DO_2 whilst minimizing VO_2
Acute renal failure (ARF)	Urine output ≤ 400 ml/24 hours Urea ≥ 36 mmol/l Creatinine ≥ 310 μmol/l	Burns Hypotension Hypovolaemia	Mismatched blood Nephrotoxic drugs Raised intra-abdominal pressures (> 30 mmHg) Rhabdomyolysis Sepsis SIRS	Treat the underlying cause Careful management of fluids, electrolytes and acid-base balance Daily U and Es Haemodynamic monitoring (CVP; MAP; PAOP) Measure plasma creatinine kinase and myoglobin urinary excretion, if relevant
Compartment syndrome	Signs and symptoms usually occur 6–8 hours post-injury but may be up to 48–96 hours post-injury Intra-compartmental pressure 30–60 mmHg may need treating	Associated with fractures Burns, thermal and electrocution injury Frost and snake bites Soft tissue injury	Casts/traction Hypoperfusion and swelling of muscle Pneumatic antishock garment Prolonged shocked states	Measurement of intra-compartment pressure Fasciotomy threshold varies between 30 and 60 mmHg depending on other clinical signs

Table 3.1 Complications—cont'd

Complication	Criteria	Primary event	Secondary events	Monitoring/care required
Coagulopathy	Abnormal clotting times – thrombocytopaenia; prolonged prothrombin and partial thromboplastin times; elevated D dimers and FDPs; ATIII < 60% normal activity	Burns Hypothermia Hypovolaemic shock Trauma – especially head injury	ALI Mismatched blood Pulmonary/fat embolus Sepsis/SIRS	Management includes treating the cause; transfusing relevant clotting factors. The use of low-dose heparin; ATIII and antifibrinolytic agents remain controversial
Deep vein thrombosis (DVT)	Painful swollen calf; tachycardia; pyrexia Diagnosed on venogram; radioisotope scan; Doppler flow studies or impedance plethysmography	Pelvic or skeletal trauma Spinal cord injury	Altered coagulation Immobility Post-surgery	Inspection of calves and review of D-dimers may increase the index of suspicion for a DVT Anticoagulation (unless contraindicated) Prevention in high-risk patients by using TED stockings or intermittent pneumatic compression boots
Fat embolus	Dyspnoea, tachypnoea, cyanosis, productive of frothy sputum ABG most commonly reveals hypoxia, hypocarbia and metabolic acidosis may be present ECG may reveal right heart strain CXR shows bilateral infiltrates Other signs include: Fever (38–39°C) Hypocalcaemia Abnormal coagulation studies Petechial rash over anterior chest, axillae, neck, conjunctiva and soft palate.	Associated with pelvic and long bone injury Crush injuries Increase adipose tissue disruption	Post-fracture fixation	Early immobilization and fixation of fractures Oxygen therapy ± respiratory support Heparin may be considered
Hypoxia	Headache, confusion, fits or coma PaO_2 < 11 kPa on ≥ 40% FIO_2 Severe if PaO_2 < 8 kPa on ≥ 50% FIO_2 Tidal volumes < 3 ml/kg RR > 30/minute	Airway obstruction Apnoea Hypoventilation due to CNS injury Major thoracic trauma: – flail chest – haemothorax – pneumothorax – diaphragmatic rupture Near-drowning Smoke inhalation and CO poisoning	Anaemia Bronchospasm Respiratory failure – ALI/ARDS – Oversedation – Pre-morbid conditions – V/Q Mismatch Aspiration – Atelectasis – Infection – Pulmonary contusion – Pulmonary oedema	Ensure airway is patent and protected Observe for signs of respiratory failure (increase RR, work of breathing, impaired level of consciousness) Measure FEV_1 ABG CXR – to exclude reversible pathology CVS and SpO_2 monitoring Early respiratory support – oxygen – CPAP – Assisted ventilation

Table 3.1 Complications—cont'd

Complication	Criteria	Primary event	Secondary events	Monitoring/care required
			– Retained secretions Thromboembolic event	Postural drainage and physiotherapy Reduce metabolic demands for the critically injured patient (active cooling and pharmacological paralysis) Consider ECMO, if conventional therapy fails
Ischaemic reperfusion injury	Hypoperfusion leading to anaerobic metabolism and subsequent cellular dysfunction/injury or death	Circulatory shock	Vasospasm Vasoconstriction	Adequate resuscitation Maximise DO_2 Monitor lactic acidosis Specific monitoring for end-organ perfusion, e.g. gastric tonometry Consider antioxidant administration (for oxygen free-radical scavenging)
Multiorgan dysfunction syndrome	Significant failure of two or more critical organ systems	Trauma Burns	Hypoxia Hypoperfusion Infection, including bacterial translocation from the GI tract Rhabdomyolysis SIRS	Cardiovascular and respiratory support Consider goal directed therapy $CI > 4.5$ l/min per m^2 $DO_2 > 600$ mls/min per m^2 Identify and treat infections Early enteral feeding
Pulmonary embolism	Clinical signs of dyspnoea; tachypnoea; anxiety; substernal chest pain; cyanosis; blood stained expectorate ABG – hypoxia and hypocarbia ECG – tachycardia: right ventricular strain, ST depression and T wave inversion in anterior chest leads, ?dysrhythmias, especially AF Raised WBC CXR – normal to evidence of a pulmonary infarction Diagnosed on either a V/Q scan or CT pulmonary angiogram Consider screening for DVT	Arising from DVTs following pelvic and lower limb trauma	Altered coagulation Prolonged bed rest	Analgesia Anticoagulation Monitor APTT, PT and platelets Oxygen ± respiratory and cardiovascular support Consider need for venocaval filter or pulmonary embolectomy

Table 3.1 Complications—cont'd

Complication	Criteria	Primary event	Secondary events	Monitoring/care required
Raised intracranial pressure Normal ICP range 0–10 mmHg	In a head-injured patient, aim is to keep ICP < 20 mmHg with a CPP > 70 mmHg	Direct neurological trauma – fractured skull; intracranial haematomas; cerebral oedema; diffuse axonal injury	Cytotoxic cerebral oedema (hypoxia) Hypercapnia Hypoperfusion Hydrocephalus Loss of autoregulatory function Obstructed venous drainage from the cerebral vasculature Pyrexia Raised intrathoracic or intra-abdominal pressure Seizure activity	Neurosurgical intervention as indicated EEG ICP monitoring (including EVD, if appropriate) Jugular venous bulb oximetry Near infrared spectroscopy Transcranial Doppler ultrasonography Measurement of intracerebral O_2/lactate Close monitoring of temperature; MAP; ICP; CPP and urinary output (observe for DI or response to osmotic diuretics) Monitor ABGs to avoid hypoxia or hypercarbia Ensure sedation level appropriate to reduce basal metabolic demands during critical stage of recovery Nurse head up 15–30° if no other contraindications Maintain head in a neutral position
Sepsis/Systemic inflammatory response syndrome (SIRS)	Core temperature >38°C/ <36°C HR > 90 beats/minute RR > 20/$PaCO_2$ < 4.3 kPa or ventilatory dependent WBC > 12 000 cells/mm³, < 4000 cells/mm³ or > 10% neutrophils in an immature form Sepsis is SIRS criteria plus the presence of a documented infection		High gastric pH Multiple invasive cannulae, drains and wounds Poor nutrition Pre-morbid disease and/or reduced immunocompetence Tracheal intubation	Infection surveillance and treatment of known infections Strict infection control policies, including staff hand hygiene and aseptic management of wounds and lines Active immunization for tetanus and vaccination of splenectomy patients Close monitoring and support of haemodynamic parameters: – adequate fluid resuscitation – vasopressor therapy to maintain MAP > 70 mmHg (> 90 mmHg in neurological patients to maintain adequate CPP) Maximise DO_2 and minimize VO_2 – Ensure adequate cardiac output, Hb and supplemental O_2 – Ventilatory support for severely compromised patients

Table 3.1 Complications—cont'd

Complication	Criteria	Primary event	Secondary events	Monitoring/care required
Shock	Shock is a syndrome that results when metabolic requirements (oxygen and nutrients) of the tissues can not be met by the body	Hypovolaemic – haemorrhage – burns Cardiogenic – cardiac tamponade – tension pneumothorax – severe myocardial contusion Neurogenic – high spinal cord injury – head injury	Hypovolaemic – other fluid losses Cardiogenic – MI – PE/fat embolus Anaphylactic Septic	– Antipyretic therapy ± active cooling Monitor ABGs and serum lactate Early enteral feeding to maintain gut integrity Surgical debridement and drainage of source of infection Treatment of underlying cause Adequate venous access Close monitoring and early support of haemodynamic parameters Consider cardiac output oesophageal Doppler or pulmonary artery flotation catheter to assist with goal-directed therapy Ventilatory support for severely compromised patients

ABG, arterial blood gas; ACS, abdominal compartment syndrome; AF, atrial fibrillation; ALI, acute lung injury; APTT, activated partial thromboplastin time; ARDS, acute respiratory distress syndrome; ARF, acute renal failure; AT III, antithrombin III; CI, cardiac index; CNS, central nervous system; CO, carbon monoxide; CPAP, continuous positive airway pressure; CPP, cerebral perfusion pressure; CT, computerised tomgraphy; CVP, central venous pressure; CVS, cardiovascular system; CXR, chest x-ray; DI, diabetes inspidus; DIC, disseminated intravascular coagulation; DO_2, oxygen delivery; DO_2I, oxygen delivery index; DVT, deep vein thrombosis; ECG, electrocardiogram; ECMO, extracorporeal membrane oxygenation; EEG, electroencephalography; EVD, external ventricular drain; FDP, fibrinogen degradation products; FEV_1, forced expiratory volume at 1 second; FIO_2, fractional inspired oxygen; GI, gastrointestinal; Hb, haemoglobin; HR, heart rate; I:E ratio, inspired:expired ratio; ICP, intracranial pressure; MAP, mean arterial blood pressure; MI, myocardial infarction; O_2, oxygen; PaO_2, partial pressure of oxygen; PAOP, pulmonary artery occlusion pressure; PE, pulmonary embolism; PEEP, positive end-expiratory pressure; PT, prothrombin time; RR, respiratory rate; SIRS, systemic inflammatory response syndrome; SpO_2, peripheral oxygen saturation; TED, thromboembolic deterrent stockings; UＥ, urea and electrolytes; VO_2 consumption; V/Q mismatch, ventilation–perfusion mismatch; WBC, white blood count.

that the patient's acuity is less than ICU: here, the nurse:patient ratio is one nurse to two patients. Full ventilation may not be offered in all HDU areas. For the most part, HDUs will support patients with one system failure providing much of the invasive monitoring associated with the ICU (Department of Health, 2000). The remit of the HDU, however, is akin to that of the ICU (i.e. to support the patient's organ function within the limits of their provision of care). It is, therefore, imperative that HDU personnel recognise when patients' care needs escalate or de-escalate as appropriate. Critically injured patients may, therefore, be admitted to an HDU en route to or on exit from an ICU (Department of Health, 2000).

Ward care

The tenets of good trauma care equally apply to ward and rehabilitation nurses. Ward nurses are often challenged by the nurse:patient ratio such that an acutely ill trauma patient may not receive the appropriate care required.

Astute observation, detection and the interpretation of early insidious signs of deterioration that may herald more serious consequences are mandatory. Early warning systems to identify patients at risk allow early referrals to medical or outreach teams (Department of Health, 2000). Nurses must maintain an index of suspicion until it is proven that all the patient's injuries have become manifest.

Other factors that ward nurses must consider include the provision of effective analgesia, expert wound management and attention to nutritional support, similar to that discussed in the context of the ICU.

The multidisciplinary team approach is of equal importance in the ward environment as that of the higher dependency areas. In addition to medical and paramedical teams, other therapists and social workers have key roles to play in securing patients' recovery in preparation for discharge. Specialist physiotherapists, occupational therapists and speech and language therapists may be required for some patients.

Psychosocial problems usually present themselves in the ward environment, and nurses must be receptive to patients who are expressing difficulties in coming to terms with traumatic events and their injuries. Their critical care stay may have further compounded the problem, as sleep deprivation and additional psychological trauma may have occurred. In recent years, post-traumatic stress disorder has become a well-recognised phenomenon (Jones and Griffiths, 2002) and counselling should be arranged for such patients.

> Astute observation to detect and interpret early signs of deterioration is mandatory

Rehabilitation care

Rehabilitation should start at the point of injury. For the most part, rehabilitation in trauma care in the UK has been largely ignored and under-resourced, with the exception of neurospinal trauma. Investing further resources in rehabilitation care is advocated to improve patient outcome and optimise the use of acute hospital beds (RCS and British Orthopaedic Association, 2000).

> The ultimate outcome of trauma care must be to return the individual patient back to their community in a maximum state of well-being

Systematic approach

Trauma care in the UK is still in its evolutionary phase. A number of units and departments contribute to the overall care and/or recovery of the injured patient. Achieving a unified system is difficult if not impossible when the specialty is largely unrecognised and there is no overview of the patient's journey through the system.

Westaby (1989) contends that trauma care is only as good as its weakest link. Pre-hospital teams and emergency departments have demonstrated that changing the system may have a profound impact on patient care and outcomes, for example, improved pre-hospital communication strategies, emergency department consultants leading trauma teams and the consistent use of ATLS protocols. In these situations, many patients who would have died now survive their immediate resuscitation phase.

With so many disparate entities drawn together to form a trauma system, there is often compromise at the interdepartmental boundaries, where lack of continuity and poor communication negates seamless care (Hadfield-Law, 1994; Beachley and Snow, 1988; Haire, 1998). Definitive care must be revised to reduce the inherent risk of late trauma morbidity and mortality. Ideally, trauma care needs to be delineated as a specialty in its own right; in the interim, two alternative strategies may improve trauma management (i.e. the use of integrated care pathways and the role of the Trauma Nurse Coordinator).

Integrated care pathways

Integrated care pathways (ICPs) are not new, the concept first being introduced in the USA as managed care became established (Laxade and Hale, 1995a). For specific disease pathologies, a care pathway is mapped out with expected time lines against which the patient's recovery is assessed (Latini and Foote, 1992; Hale, 1995; Latini, 1996). Failure of the patient to meet the time lines or deviation from the pathway is recorded as a variance (Hale, 1995; Court et al., 1998). All variances must be examined to determine whether they are patient-specific or system issues that are preventing or delaying care. Outside of trauma care, other UK nurses have used ICPs to good effect, such as those used for cardiothoracic patients undergoing bypass surgery (Laxade and Hale, 1995a). The advantage of using ICPs are multifaceted. They standardise care such that they help the most junior personnel appreciate the care that is required for the patient and thus contribute to the education of staff.

In the case of trauma patients, a relatively unique set of presenting injuries versus their mechanism of injury may be found. Whilst there are key similarities in patterns of injuries, individual trauma patients should never be judged as classical or typical in their presentation. It is, however, possible for ICPs to be devised in relation to specific injuries. With polytrauma patients, due care must be taken in discerning which ICPs should be used and which components of ICPs are contraindicated owing to concomitant injury (Eastes, 1994; Tingle, 1995; Robertson, 1999).

Whilst there are key similarities in patterns of injuries, individual trauma patients should never be judged as classical or typical in their presentation

As a tool, ICPs may enhance communication between disciplines and departments and can map out the clinical course for the patient beyond one specific geographic area (Benton, 1995; Laxade and Hale, 1995b; Latini, 1996; Court et al., 1998). Care can be easily audited, as any variance outside the expected pathway can be explored and system issues that commonly arise formally addressed (Eastes, 1994; Court et al., 1998). The net benefit, therefore, of using ICPs may include reduced length of stay and consequently containment of health care costs (Laxade and Hale, 1995b; Hollingworth-Fridlund et al., 1998; Spain et al., 1998). Finally, the concept of ICPs is congruent with the clinical governance agenda to which all Trusts subscribe.

The Trauma Nurse Coordinator

The Trauma Nurse Coordinator is a specialist practitioner role that was founded in Chicago, Illinois, in 1971, 5 years after the trauma service was established. Over the past 30 years, the role has been widely deployed across the USA, such that trauma centre designation by the American College of Surgeons now dictates that the TNC role is mandatory for level I and II verification (Beachley et al., 1988; Baulch, 1999; Price, 1999).

The remit of the TNC role most closely resembles the UK Nurse Consultant role. The TNC is typically a 'masters' prepared nurse with 5 years post-registration experience in trauma nursing and has four specific subroles (Box 3.7).

The clinical remit of the role ensures that at least one person has an overview of the patient

---

Box 3.7   Role of the trauma nurse coordinator

1. Clinical care
2. Education – delivering both professional and public education programmes
3. Addressing management and quality issues
4. Research and audit

moving through the trauma continuum, that is, from pre-hospital care through rehabilitation (Beachley et al., 1988; Goehring, 1999). Hamric (1989) reports that, where there is a defined patient population, a clinical nurse specialist role is vital. It is this ability to 'know' the patient that allows the TNC to consult and collaborate effectively with other departments and disciplines (Beachley et al., 1988; Tanner et al., 1993). The TNC is frequently considered to be the 'stabilizing force' in a trauma system whose primary purpose is to expedite optimal care for the trauma victim (Daleiden, 1993; Haire, 1998; Price, 1999).

The subsidiary roles of the TNC are critical to ensure that the knowledge and skills trauma nurses are proactively developed; new evidence-based treatment modalities are incorporated into practice, and cost-effective care is provided for the injured patient (Goehring, 1999; Price, 1999). Such has been the impact of the TNCs that their activities have improved patient outcome, shortened length of stay (in both specialist and non-specialist beds), and reduced patient costs by up to $1 million per trauma centre annually in the USA (Dekeyser et al., 1993; Haire, 1988; McInulty, 1998).

Injury prevention

After considering the need for a systematic approach to trauma care, the irony is that traumatic injury is truly the only preventable disease. In addition to the previously stated rates of death and disability caused by traumatic injury, the cost of the devastating effects of trauma on society are incalculable. Seven per cent of the NHS funding is consumed by injury alone (McGinley, 2000).

Despite these figures, there is a fatalistic attitude towards the causation of injuries – 'accidents just happen'. However, they don't! The term 'accident' is a misnomer, traditionally implying an unpredictable event beyond the control of the victim (Hansen, 1998). 'Accidents are not totally random events striking innocent victims like bolts out of the blue...accidents have a natural history in which predisposing factors converge to produce an accidental event' (Bunton et al., 1996).

It is known from experience that injuries occur in specific predictable, often preventable, patterns. A person's environment or behaviour can put him/her at risk so, if unsafe behaviours are modified and precautions taken, injury can be avoided (Martinez, 1996).

Considering that a large number of trauma deaths and disability are preventable, it is notable that, within the field of trauma care, prevention is given less emphasis than resuscitation. Nevertheless, it is acknowledged that the best treatment for a large percentage of trauma-related deaths and injuries is to prevent them happening (Driscoll et al., 1993; Wyatt et al., 1995; Skinner and Whimster, 1999; RCS and British Orthopaedic Association, 2000). A Scottish study comparing the trimodal death distribution of British trauma with the widely acknowledged American statistics revealed that three-quarters of British trauma deaths occur at the time of the injury or shortly afterwards (first peak of death), whilst only half of the American deaths occurred during this period (Trunkey, 1983; Wyatt et al., 1995). This may be attributable to a number of factors, for example, the mechanism of injury (blunt versus penetrating), and the variation in pre-hospital care between the two countries. Nevertheless, one could conclude that, if a large number of people die at the time of the injury and that this is representative throughout Britain, then injury prevention may offer the most effective approach for these patients.

In addition to health professionals recognising the need for injury prevention, the political agenda needs to be considered. Government targets are aimed at reducing injury-related death and disability by 20% in all age groups by 2010 (Department of Health, 1998). Interestingly, less emphasis is placed on individual behavioural change and more on central and local initiatives. It is accepted that successful injury prevention needs a three-pronged approach: education, legislation and engineering (Robertson and Redmond, 1994; Weigelt and Klein, 1994; Gunnels, 1996; Cliff, 1997). Whilst most trauma nurses would regard themselves as experts in care and treatment rather than prevention, there is potential to influence all three areas.

Education, probably the most logical option for trauma nurses, involves raising awareness of risks and how to avoid them by changing behaviour. This can be done on an individual basis by speaking to individual patients about injury prevention and minimisation of risk, highlighting the issue using safety posters, and making literature available in clinical settings. A more structured, collaborative approach could involve trauma nurses participating with community prevention educational programmes. Successful initiatives in the USA have followed this approach (Sheehy et al., 1994; Weigelt and Klein, 1994; Gunnels, 1996; Rush, 1998). One such initiative was conceived by Seattle trauma nurses. Using their specialist trauma knowledge and experience, they are allocated time and given financial support to teach community groups about injury prevention, tailoring the programme to meet the needs of specific groups. Visual images are used to illustrate the consequences of risk and the need for behavioural change. This programme has been received positively with the nurses perceived as credible specialists in their field, and knowledgeable by virtue of their experiences of working in the trauma environment (Sheehy et al., 1994).

Whilst limited in number, UK injury prevention programmes introduced by trauma nurses are said to have had an impact on altering perception and behaviour. These programmes targeted at pre-adolescent schoolchildren, in recognition of a dramatic increase in risk-taking behaviour during teenage years, are taught by health care personnel in collaboration with schoolteachers (Hamilton, 1994; Orzell, 1997), and include causal factors, mechanisms of injury, effects of injury and preventative strategies. Educational strategies for injury prevention may prove challenging to the trauma nurse, not least owing to the lack of importance that is placed on injury prevention within UK trauma courses. By educating others and raising their awareness of injury prevention, it is hoped that nurses will pass on this message to their patients and the general public.

Legislation involving the introduction of legal sanctions against behaviour likely to cause injury or increase the risk of damage from an injury, may be said to have the greatest compliance of all injury prevention strategies, for example, compulsory seat belt wearing (Lane, 1989). However, many trauma nurses and physicians do not consider themselves to be public health experts or social activists. Nevertheless, there are examples (including seatbelt legislation) where physicians have used their knowledge of injury deaths and disability to inform campaigns. One such successful example of legislation involving medical staff collaborating with legal personnel and pressure groups is that aimed at making cycle-helmet wearing compulsory in Australia (Wood and Milne, 1998). Recommendations by professional nursing organisations have also had a positive impact on many areas of injury prevention legislation. Nurses working in collaboration with the government to raise the profile of injury prevention techniques, such as cycle-helmet wearing for children, may help to support future legislation (Emergency Nurses Association, 2000; Lee, 1994).

Engineering involves changing the environment to reduce the risk of injury. Whilst some may adopt a fatalistic approach to such strategies, it is suggested that trauma personnel who are naturally orientated to the front end of care should look even further forward (Lane, 1989). Obvious barriers preventing environmental improvement may exist, for example, cost and the inability of individuals to act alone; recognition is given to the fact that it may be easier for organisations to exact change rather than individuals (Green, 1997). Considering this, trauma nurses could interface with campaigning organisations, develop new relationships outside of the hospital environment to minimise the risk of injury occurring and effect positive environmental change. An example of where environmental strategies could have massive benefits is in road modification and speed restriction. Having witnessed the devastating effects of road traffic accidents, trauma personnel could help to highlight this problem to support and inform speed-restriction campaigns (Stewart and Harlan, 2000). This is reinforced by child health experts who note transport as the single biggest issue in preventative child health, but similarly note a lack of recognition of this by most politicians and medical professionals (Harrabin and Clement, 1999).

Traumatic injury is an epidemic within this country. Given the number of people dying each year, the need for injury prevention is obvious. Despite this, there is an under-reporting of this epidemic within the media. Acknowledgement is given to the plight of those with Creutzvelt–Jacob disease and their families, and the so-called 'economy class syndrome' (deep vein thrombosis; DVT). Calls for changes in legislation and environmental controls in those areas are given a high profile, yet little is said regarding the need for injury prevention. Ten people are killed every day on the roads in the UK – this is the equivalent of one hundred times the Paddington rail crash death toll every year, however, the complacent attitude that 'accidents just happen' and little can be done remains within the public arena (Lee, 1994). Trauma nurses must use their knowledge and expertise to have a positive impact on all aspects of injury prevention supported by appropriately funded injury prevention programmes.

CONCLUSION

Maintaining the momentum of change for the development of UK trauma management is vital. Much has been accomplished since the late 1980s; however, the reform agenda is vast and needs to be strategically implemented, if the desired impact of reducing morbidity and mortality from injury is to be realized.

Appropriate resourcing and preparation of staff is critical to establishing a strong foundation for reform. The continuum ideal must be fostered, whilst trauma care needs to be delineated in its own right so that specialist interdisciplinary practice can be proactively developed. Injury prevention and rehabilitation must assume greater significance.

Finally, nursing must play an integral part in the revision of UK trauma management and thus avoid the stigma of becoming the weakest link in the therapeutic chain of trauma care.

References

Adedeji OA, Driscoll PA. The trauma team – a system of initial trauma care. *Postgraduate Medical Journal* 1996; 72: 587–593

Advanced Trauma Nursing Course. *Advanced trauma nursing course handbook*. Oxford: ATNC, 1994

American College of Surgeons. *Advanced trauma life support course*. (Provider manual) Chicago: American College of Surgeons, 1997

Anderson ID, Woodford M, De Dombal FT, et al. Retrospective study of 1000 trauma deaths from injury in England and Wales. *British Medical Journal* 1988; 296: 1305–1308

Armstrong B, Carpenter J. Shock trauma, Baltimore, USA. *Intensive Critical Care Nursing* 1995; 11: 151–156

Baulch S. The making of a trauma system. In: *Trauma coordinator core course*. (Provider Manual). Maryland: American Trauma Society, 1999

Beachley ML. Trauma nursing is a developing speciality. *Journal of Emergency Nursing* 1989; 15: 372–373

Beachley M, Snow S. Developing trauma care systems: a nursing perspective. *Journal of Nursing Administration* 1988; 18: 22–29

Beachley M, Snow S, Trimble P. Developing trauma care systems: the trauma nurse co-ordinator. *Journal of Nursing Administration* 1988; 18: 34–42

Benner P. *From novice to expert*. Boston: Addison-Wesley, 1984: 1–38

Benton D. The role of managed care in overcoming fragmentation. *Nursing Times* 1995; 91: 25

Brooks RA, Willet KM. Evaluation of the Oxford protocol for total spinal clearance in the unconscious trauma patient. *Journal of Trauma* 2001; 50: 862–867

Broomfield CJ. The preventative treatment of wound shock. In: Greaves I, Ryan JM, Porter KM (eds) *Trauma*. London: Arnold, 1998: 389–397

Bryant KK. ENA's trauma nursing core course: an update. *Journal of Emergency Nursing* 1989; 15: 35A, 36A, 38A, 39A, 40A

Bunton R, Nettleton S, Burrows R. *The sociology of health promotion*. London: Routeledge, 1996

Caple L. Air ambulance operations in England. In: Earlam R (ed.) *Trauma care – helicopter emergency medical service (HEMS)*. Hertfordshire: Saldatore; 1997, 34

Chadda D. State of emergency. *Nursing Management* 1995; 25: 49–51

Cheever KH. Reducing the effects of acute pain in critically ill patients. *Dimensions of Critical Care Nursing* 1999; 18: 14–23

Christie J. Trauma courses. *Surgical Nurse* 1994; 7: 12–14

Cliff KS. Legislation, education and engineering. In: Green J (ed.) *Risk and misfortune: the social construction of accidents*. London: UCL Press, 1997

Cole E. *Witnessed trauma resuscitation – can relatives be present?* Online. available: http://www.trauma.org/nurse/witness.html (8 August 2000)

Cook NB. Prehospital care in the 1990s. *Technic* 1991; 98(Sept): 6–9

Court D, Loupus D, Morrison S. CarePaths: a tool for coping with managed care. *Topics in Spinal Cord Injury Rehabilitation* 1998; 3: 44–52

Cross F. Who owns trauma? The patient. In: Earlam R (ed.) *Trauma care – helicopter emergency medical service (HEMS)*. Hertfordshire: Saldatore, 1997: 174–177

Cudmore JE. Trauma nursing: the team approach. *British Journal of Nursing* 1996; 5: 736–753

Daleiden AL. The CNS as trauma case manager: a new frontier. *Clinical Nurse Specialist* 1993; 7: 295–298

Davis S. Trauma management in Maryland. *Nursing Times* 1990; 86: 58–59, 62

Davis S, Wood I. A trauma centre in the UK: the Stoke experience. *Accident and Emergency Nursing* 1995; 3: 215–218

Dean B. Reflections on technology: increasing the science but diminishing the art of nursing? *Accident and Emergency Nursing* 1998; 6: 200–206

Dekeyser FG, Paratore A, Camp L. Trauma nurse coordinator: three unique roles. *Nursing Management* 1993; 24: 56A, 56D, 56H

Deo SD, Knottenbelt JD, Peden MM. Evaluation of a small trauma team for major resuscitation. *Injury* 1997; 28: 633–637

Department of Health. *The health of the nation strategy: a strategy for health in England*. London: HMSO, 1992

Department of Health. *Comprehensive critical care – a review of adult critical care services*. London: HMSO, 2000

Department of Health. *Saving lives: our healthier nation*. London: HMSO, 1998

Driscoll PA, Gwinnutt CL, LeDuc Jimmerson C, et al. *Trauma resuscitation: the team approach*. Basingstoke: Macmillan Press, 1993: 2

Driscoll PA, Vincent CA. Organising an efficient trauma team. *Injury* 1992; 22: 369–371

Dunnum L, Bailey K. Trauma internship: a success story. *Journal of Neuroscience Nursing* 1991; 23: 253–255

Earlam R. Costs. In: Earlam R (ed.) *Trauma care – helicopter emergency medical service (HEMS)*. Hertfordshire: Saldatore, 1997: 193–196

Eastes LE. Toward continuous quality improvement in trauma care. *Critical Care Nursing Clinics of North America* 1994; 6: 451–461

Edwards S. Physiological insult/injury: pathophysiology and consequences. *British Journal of Nursing* 2002; 11: 263–274

Emergency Nurses Association. *Emergency Nurses CARE: mission, philosophy and objectives*. http://www.ena.org/encare/mission (2000)

Eyre G. Shock treatment. *Nursing Times* 1993; 89: 30–33

Gagnon L. Presidents message: global collegiality in emergency nursing. *Journal of Emergency Nursing* 1991; 17: 3

Goehring M. Role functions of the trauma coordinator. In: *Trauma coordinator core course*. (Provider Manual). Maryland: American Trauma Society, 1999

Gosling P, Bascom JU, Zikria BA. Capillary leak, oedema and organ failure: breaking the triad. *Care of the Critically Ill* 1996; 12: 191–197

Greaves I, Porter K, Ryan J. Patient assessment. In: Greaves I, Porter K, Ryan J (eds) *Trauma care manual*. London: Arnold, 2001a: 18–32

Greaves I, Porter K, Ryan J. Abdominal trauma. In: Greaves I, Porter K, Ryan J (eds) *Trauma care manual*. London: Arnold, 2001b: 87–98

Green J. *Risk and misfortune: the social construction of accidents*. London: UCL Press, 1997

Gunnels MD. Educate, legislate and recreate: making a difference every day through injury prevention. *Journal of Emergency Nursing* 1996; 22: 356–357

Hadfield L. Preparation for the nurse as part of a trauma team. *Accident and Emergency Nursing* 1993; 1: 154–160

Hadfield-Law L. Advanced trauma nursing course (ATNC). *Care of the Critically Ill* 1994; 10: 18–21

Haire J. Communication and trauma management. *Emergency Nursing* 1998; 6: 24–30

Hale C. Key terms in managed care. *Nursing Times* 1995; 91: 29

Hamilton A. Trauma training. *Nursing Times* 1991; 87: 42–44

Hamilton A. The exploratory development of an injury awareness programme for 10–12 year old children in Southampton. Southampton: unpublished MSc dissertation, 1994

Hamric AB. History and overview of the CNS role. In: Hamric AB, Spross JA. (eds) *The clinical nurse specialist in theory and practice*, 2nd edn. Philadelphia: WB Saunders, 1989; 3–18

Hansen KA. Its no accident...it's preventable. *Journal of Emergency Nursing* 1998; 24: 101–103

Harrabin R, Clement B. Speed kills: it's that simple. 20. *The Independent on Sunday*, 28 November 1999

Harrison S. The Heidelberg ten. *Nursing Times* 1990; 86: 39–41

Henderson V. *Basic principles of nursing care*. Geneva: International Council of Nurses, 1960: 7–9

Hoff WS, Reilly PM, Rotondo MF, et al. The importance of the command physician in trauma resuscitation. *Journal of Trauma: Injury, Infection and Critical Care* 1997; 43: 772–777

Holleran RE. Role of nursing in prehospital care. In: Holleran RE (ed.) *Prehospital nursing: a collaborative approach*. St Louis: Mosby, 1994, 3–21

Hollingworth-Fridlund P, Bernal Hall J, Stout P, et al. The nonoperative injury pathway. *Journal of Trauma Nursing* 1998; 5: 75–78

Howell E. The evolution of trauma care. In: Howell E, Widra L, Hill MG (eds) *Comprehensive trauma nursing: theory and practice*. Illinois: Scott Foresman: 1988: 5–33

Inman YO. A look at emergency nursing 'down under': TNCC goes to Australia. *Journal of Emergency Nursing* 1992; 8: 39A–40A

Johnson K. Critical care of the trauma patient. In: Neff JA, Kidd PS (ed.) *Trauma nursing – the art and science*. St Louis: Mosby, 1993: 677–705

Jones C, Griffiths RD. Physical and psychological recovery. In: Griffiths RD, Jones C (eds) *Intensive care aftercare*. Oxford: Butterworth-Heinemann, 2002: 53–65

Kreimeier U, Prueckner S, Peter K. Permissive hypotension. *Schweizerische medizinische Wochenschrift* 2000; 130: 1516–1524

Ku J, Brasel KJ, Baker CC, et al. Triangle of death: hypothermia, acidosis and coagulopathy. *New Horizons* 1999; 7: 61–72

Lane P. Trauma is not a surgical disease. *Archives of Emergency Medicine* 1989; 6: 85–89

Latini EE. Trauma critical pathways: a care delivery system that works. *Critical Care Nursing Quarterly* 1996; 19: 83–87

Latini EE, Foote W. Obtaining consistent quality patient care for the trauma patient by using critical pathway. *Critical Care Nursing Quarterly* 1992; 15: 51–55

Laxade S, Hale CA. Managed care 2: an opportunity for nursing. *British Journal of Nursing* 1995a; 4: 345, 346, 348–350

Laxade S, Hale CA. Managed care 1: an opportunity for nursing. *British Journal of Nursing* 1995b; 4: 290–294

Lee A. Hats off to Angela. *Nursing Standard* 1994; 9: 21–23

Lewis AM. Trauma triad of death – emergency! *Nursing* 2000; 30: 62–64

Lloyd D. Driving force. *Health Service Management* 1991; Dec 261–262

Lomas GA, Goodall O. Trauma teams vs non-trauma teams. *Accident and Emergency Nursing* 1994; 2: 205–210

Martinez R. Creating the future: The emergency nurses role in injury prevention. *Journal of Emergency Nursing* 1996; 22: 265–266

McCraken L. The forensic ABCs of trauma care. *Canadian Nurse* 2001; 97: 30–33

McGinley A. *Accident prevention – does it prevent traumatic injury?* http://www.trauma.org/nurse/accidentprevention.html (2000)

McInulty L. Trauma nurse coordinator – the way forward in trauma care? *A&E Focus* 1998; 8: 3–4

Metheny NM. Fluid volume imbalances. In: Metheny NM. *Fluid and electrolyte balance – Nursing considerations*, 4th edn. Philadelphia: Lippincott; 2000: 40–57

Morrill P. Pharmacotherapeutics of positive inotropes. *AORN* 2000; 71: 173–188

Nayduch DA. Trauma wound management. *Nursing Clinics of North America* 1999; 34: 895–906

Orzell MN. Injury minimisation programme for schools. *Accident and Emergency Nursing* 1997; 4: 139–144

Paterson S. Physiotherapy in intensive care. In: Goldhill DR, Withington PS (eds) *Textbook of intensive care*. London: Chapman & Hall Medical, 1997: 69–77

Price J. *Trauma nurse coordinator benchmarks*. Available online: http://www.trauma.org/archieves/tncbenchmarks.html (5 October 1999)

Rauen CA. Using simulation to teach critical thinking skills. *Critical Care Clinics of North America* 2001; 13: 93–103

Riley ME. Establishing nutritional guidelines for critically ill patients: Part 1. *Professional Nurse* 2002; 17: 580–583

Robertson C, Redmond AD. *The management of major trauma*. Oxford: Oxford University Press, 1994

Robertson K. Trauma nursing – an advanced practice case study. *Canadian Nurse* 1999; 95: 18–22

Rouse A. Emergency ambulance service performance standards. *Health Service Management* 1992; May: 23–25

Royal College of Surgeons of England. *Report of the working party on the management of patients with major injuries*. London: The Royal College of Surgeons of England, 1988

Royal College of Surgeons of England and British Orthopaedic Association. Joint report. *Better care for the severely injured*. London: Royal College of Surgeons of England, 2000

Rush C. Mock drunk driving crash: an exercise in injury prevention. *Accident and Emergency Nursing* 1998; 6: 7–10

Russell L. The importance of patients' nutritional status in wound healing. *British Journal of Nursing* 2001; 10: S42, S44, S49

Ruth-Sahd LA. A modification of Benner's hierarchy of clinical practice: the development of clinical intuition in the novice trauma nurse. *Holistic Nursing Practice* 1993; 7: 8–14

Say J. The metabolic changes associated with trauma and sepsis. *Nursing in Critical Care* 1997; 2: 83–87

Scherer P. Shock trauma. *American Journal of Nursing* 1989; Nov: 1440–1445

Sheehy SB, LeDuc Jimmerson C. *Manual of clinical trauma care*. St Louis: Mosby, 1994

Skinner DV, Whimster F. *Trauma*. London: Arnold, 1999

Spain DA, McIlvoy LH, Fix SE, et al. Effect of a clinical pathway for severe traumatic brain injury on resource utilization. *Journal of Trauma* 1998; 45: 101–104

Stewart RM, Harlan DR. *The problem*. http://rmstewart.uthscsa.edu/Theproblem.html (2000)

Sutcliffe A. The care of the seriously injured patients in the United Kingdom. *Care of the Critically Ill* 1990a; 6: 166

Sutcliffe AJ. A critical appraisal of the RCS working party report on the management of patients with major injuries. *Care of the Critically Ill* 1990b; 6: 176–178

Tanner CA, Benner P, Chesla C, et al. The phenomenology of knowing the patient. *IMAGE: Journal of Nursing Scholarship* 1993; 25: 273–280

Tingle J. Clinical protocols and the law. *Nursing Times* 1995; 91: 27

Trunkey DD. Trauma. *Scientific American* 1983; 249: 28–35

Veise-Berry SW, Beachley M. Evolution of the trauma cycle. In: Cardona VD, Hurn PD, Bastnagel Mason PJ, et al. (eds) *Trauma nursing: from resuscitation through rehabilitation*, 2nd edn. Philadelphia: WB Saunders, 1994: 3–16

Weigelt JA, Klein JD. Mechanism of injury. In: Cardona VD, Hurn PD, Bastnagel Mason PJ, et al. (eds) *Trauma nursing: from resuscitation through rehabilitation*. 2nd edn. Philadelphia: WB Saunders, 1994: 91–113

West JG, Trunkey DD, Lim RC. Systems of trauma care. Study of two counties. *Archives of Surgery* 1979; 114: 455–460

Westaby S. *Trauma: pathogenesis and treatment*. Oxford: Heinemann, 1989

Wood T, Milne P. Head injuries and pedal cyclists and the promotion of helmet use in Victoria, Australia. *Accident, Analysis and Prevention* 1998; 20: 177–185

Wyatt J, Beard D, Gray A, et al. Time of death after trauma. *British Medical Journal* 1995; 310: 1502

Yates D, Woodford M, Hollis S. Preliminary analysis of the care of injured patients in 33 British hospitals: first report of the United Kingdom major trauma outcome study. *British Medical Journal* 1992; 305: 737–740

Yates DW. Action for accident victims. *British Medical Journal* 1988; 297: 1419–1420

Zimmermann PG. Managers ask and answer. *Journal of Emergency Nursing* 1996; 22: 439–442

Zuspan S. Essential trauma nursing knowledge included in a level I trauma center orientation and continuing education programs. *Journal of Emergency Nursing* 1990; 16: 141–144

Chapter 4

Pre-hospital care

Priscilla M. Noble-Mathews

INTRODUCTION

Pre-hospital immediate care is defined as the 'provision of skilled medical help at the scene of an accident, medical or other clinical emergency, and during transport of that patient to hospital'. Evidence exists to show that for every 20 minutes delay in treating patients at the scene of an accident, there is a threefold increase in mortality; the necessity for getting properly trained personnel to such an incident who are able to deliver this care in a rational and disciplined manner can be appreciated. This chapter outlines a brief history of immediate care and summarises the practice of and the problems related to practising medicine in the pre-hospital emergency care environment.

HISTORY OF IMMEDIATE CARE

It was a very far-sighted Senior Medical Officer to the RAF regiment at Catterick, Dr Kenneth Easton, who in the late 1940s was so appalled by the carnage on the A1 and the distance that casualties involved in such road traffic crashes had to travel to hospital, that he obtained permission to go out with colleagues and actually treated the injured on scene before they were removed to hospital. After this, voluntary schemes with doctors from first North Yorkshire, and then from other parts of the country, started to work. From these beginnings was born the necessity for overall coordination, education and international cooperation, and the gold star requirement for cooperation between all the emergency services.

Today the British Association for Immediate Care (BASICS) has over a hundred similar schemes and approximately 2500 doctors under its umbrella, and now incorporates nurses and paramedics as part of its membership. A rigorous accreditation scheme is in existence, run in conjunction with the Royal College of Surgeons of Edinburgh, whereby members of schemes are expected to hold the Pre-Hospital Emergency Care Certificate (PHEC) as the minimum qualification, preferably followed by the Diploma in Immediate Medical Care [Dip IMCRCS(Ed)]. Since the Diploma was opened to nurses and paramedics in 1998, a new qualification for doctors was devised with them now encouraged to apply for a full Fellowship in Immediate Care from the Royal College of Surgeons of Edinburgh.

BASICS is a charity, and all the individual BASICS schemes are charitable organisations. This means that members give their time and services free of charge, and need to raise funds to obtain the necessary equipment, which is becoming increasingly sophisticated as time goes on. Some schemes also provide medical incident officers (MIOs) in addition to their ordinary callouts, who are available on a rotational basis to assist in the event of major incidents. BASICS began as a national organisation and is now internationally recognized. Indeed, BASICS education courses are now delivered to multiprofessional groups internationally and are increasingly sought after. The value of these international links is tremendous and BASICS is increasingly represented globally in many organisations, including the World Association of Emergency and Disaster Medicine.

This international liaison can best be illustrated in the collaborative venture that took place in 1997 between BASICS and Surrey Ambulance Service, where instructor nurses, paramedics and doctors travelled to Romania to train medical and nursing colleagues and firefighters in the fundamentals of pre-hospital emergency care. Here, the baseline level of training and interest in pre-hospital care and in the ambulance service were low, however, the project revealed the potential not only of the nurses but also of the firefighters as emergency technicians. This concept has since been expanded with a similar successful initiative in Malta.

Box 4.1   Features of seamless care

- Smooth initial response
- Clear communication
- Efficient assessment
- Coordinated approach
- Safe and efficient extrication
- Appropriate care and treatment
- Rapid transport to hospital

SEAMLESS CARE

The word 'seamless' is often used to describe the care that should be given to any casualty, from the time of their injury caused by whatever means, until they reach definitive care within the hospital. 'Seamless' is intended to convey the idea of a continuum that has no interruptions, which might break the continuity of care. The concept proposes a totally smooth first response to the incident, efficient assessment of the needs, coordinated handling of the situation, extrication in its broadest sense of removal of the casualty from the environment in which the injury was sustained, and appropriate care and treatment while preparing the casualty for transport as speedily as possible to the correct hospital (Box 4.1). It also, therefore, incorporates the need for effective and efficient communication at all times and the need to ensure that the receiving hospital, the place where the seam is complete, is given as much information about the scene and the casualty as possible.

If integrated care is the seam, then the thread, which must be unbroken and which runs through the whole of this, is undoubtedly communication.

COMMUNICATION

Communication from the scene

Nowadays, particularly with the era of the mobile phone, the first notice of an incident is sent from either casualties themselves or from persons on scene. This provides vital information, such as the description of the type of incident involved with its exact location and, where known, an estimate of the number of casualties (Box 4.2). Having this information may save valuable minutes for the

Box 4.2　Structured message from scene to ambulance control – METHANE

M　Major incident – declared/standby
E　Exact location
T　Type of incident
H　Hazards present
A　Access and egress
N　Number of casualties
E　Emergency services required

emergency services in initiating and coordinating their response. The importance, too, of continually updating this information from ambulance crews to their respective controls, and back to other crews or resource providers cannot be overemphasised. For example, it is by no means unknown for there to be identical place names in different parts of a county and for the emergency services to be sent to the wrong area with a loss of vital time and the potential sequelae for casualty care. Additionally, it is not unknown for an ambulance, helicopter or an immediate care provider to be mobilised to what has been reported as a very serious incident, only for the first crew on scene to find that it is a non-injury situation. This takes valuable resources away from areas where they may be needed more urgently and emphasises the need for information that is passed from the scene by members of the public to be as accurate as possible. Communication must continue, with each unit reporting its arrival on scene, either by voice or by using a predetermined code on the radio. If the incident is likely to be prolonged, it is helpful for ambulance control to know this so that other work can be planned accordingly.

Any requirement for special equipment or specialist personnel must also be clearly stated. In most counties where there is an Immediate Care Scheme in existence, ambulance control will have protocols indicating when members should be used. Hopefully, immediate care providers will be alerted and deployed early on, and not wait for crews to request their assistance. Most immediate care providers prefer to be called early and stood down, if that proves to be the case, rather than be called too late.

Interservice communication throughout any incident is essential to the smooth working of casualty removal. It is extremely helpful when local police, fire, ambulance services and immediate care providers are used to working together and each is aware of the other's role. To be on first name terms, and to be able to discuss and to think through the problems that arise is not only immensely satisfying but also, more importantly, works for the good of the casualties. Where casualties are trapped, the fire service work very closely with the ambulance crew and immediate care providers to assess the best way of extricating the patients, giving due regard to their medical needs. It is vital to know how much time any proposed manoeuvres will take. 'Time critical' patients need to be identified immediately, as this puts a different emphasis on the fire service method of extrication.

Communication with patients

Communication with the casualties themselves is vital. That communication will be by word of mouth initially calling to them, finding out who they are and their recollection of events, and continually giving them reassurance, information, comfort and confidence. Body language is very important; holding a hand or a squeeze of an arm, a pat on the shoulder all communicate a caring situation. It should never be forgotten that hearing is said to be the last sense to go, so great care must be exercised over what is said in front of an apparently unconscious patient.

Communication with hospitals

Communication with the receiving hospitals is essential. Different ambulance services have different arrangements in place for this, although the need is the same throughout the country. Some county ambulance controls provide a direct radio link for ambulance crews to contact emergency department staff members. This would seem to be the most efficient method of communication, as it allows not only for one direct line of communication but also for direct questioning to the crew involved. This also helps to avoid the potential problems associated with misinformation and confusion when information is passed via third parties.

Other services relay messages to the accident and emergency department via ambulance control. The great disadvantage of this method is that it inserts a second link and allows for messages to become distorted. It is easy for clinically untrained members of control staff to mishear and then misreport messages (e.g. 'ketamine' could be confused with 'pethidine'). If the hospital requires further information, they have to request this via control, which has to revert yet again to the crew, who may be busy and unable to respond immediately, and then relay this response back to the hospital. The only reason for following this method is that everything is then logged on tape at control in the event of a later disagreement.

A study by McInerney et al. (2000) found that, when communication between pre-hospital personnel and emergency departments was transmitted via ambulance control, this resulted in information loss during transfer. They also noted that 'suboptimal communication' was a daily occurrence at the pre-hospital and emergency department interface. The Audit Commission's Report 'A life in the fast lane', published in 1998, concluded that, while notification of imminent arrival at hospital of serious cases was good, the information received was not comprehensive enough. This was again put down to the fact that details were relayed through an intermediary link, such as ambulance control. Most ambulance services use a pre-determined structured message, such as the ASHICE message format (Box 4.3). This gives both the sender and receiver of the information a structure upon which to base their report, and can be passed in a few seconds. Information is kept to a minimum but includes the essential details that the emergency department will require to prepare for the patient's arrival.

Box 4.3   Pre-determined message structure to hospital – ASHICE

A   Age
S   Sex
H   History
I   Injuries/illness
C   Current condition and treatment given
E   Estimated time of arrival at hospital

CLINICAL RECORDS

All pre-hospital personnel should complete a patient report form for every patient in their care. This must include detailed information about the casualty/patient, including physiological observations and interventions, and must document changes and trends as time progresses during the incident and during transport. It should also provide notes regarding treatment given and procedures undertaken. Often the first time that this information can be passed to the hospital is when the patient is on the trolley in the emergency department. Sometimes the information is filed in the patient's hospital notes and the admitting staff do not see the details until much later, if at all.

Some hospitals employ an effective and highly focused system, whereby the trauma team is present upon the patient's arrival in the resuscitation room, and all the members of the team listen to the handover by the pre-hospital team member who has been delegated this responsibility. In the case of trauma, the mechanism of injury should be given as well as the injuries found and suspected, as well as details of the clinical observations and treatment given. The earlier the hospital can be given this information, the better prepared they will be for receiving the patient. Telemetry and telemedicine may have a wider role to play in the future, but for the present are likely to be confined to diagnostic interventions, such as electrocardiogram (ECG) interpretation, or for advice about treatment when particularly difficult procedures are required before patients can be extricated.

> All members of the trauma team should receive the patient handover from the pre-hospital team

Photography has a definite part to play in helping to alert emergency department staff to the exact circumstances that the patient – and the pre-hospital staff – has had to endure at the scene. It also gives them a greater understanding of the mechanisms of injury involved. Before Polaroid photography was available, it was difficult for emergency department staff standing under the bright lights of the emergency department with equipment around them at the right level, in a dry and warm environment to visualise what the pre-hospital conditions were like. In particular, they had little understanding of working outside in cold, wet and often muddy conditions, with the only lighting provided by the fire service and with equipment getting wet and slippery. Trying to keep the patient warm and dry with the implications for not exposing an unnecessary amount of the patient's body also poses a challenge. For hospital staff actually to see digital or Polaroid photographs of the wreckage and scene from which the patient has been disentangled (such as those shown in Figures 4.1 and 4.2) does help them to understand the difficulties involved further. It also helps them to have a better picture of what the injuries are or may be.

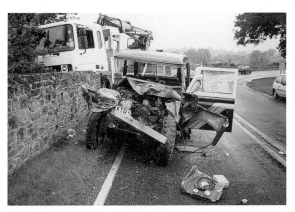

Figure 4.1 Incorrect manoeuvring on a bend caused this crash, resulting in shock for the tanker driver (and owner of the garden behind the wall!), but serious leg injuries for the 4×4 driver.

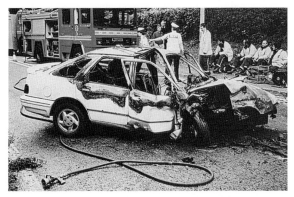

Figure 4.2 Four occupants in this car. What injuries would you predict for the driver?

> Photographic images of the scene can provide information regarding the mechanism of injury and likely injuries sustained

TRANSPORTATION OF CASUALTIES

Transportation to hospital is usually undertaken in an emergency ambulance; however, the increasing availability of air ambulances means that early on in the incident other possible methods of transporting patients should be assessed. Where air ambulances or other aeromedical support is available, consideration needs to be given to the advantages and disadvantages of making use of their facilities. A working knowledge is, therefore, needed of possible landing sites and the presence or absence of landing pads at nearby hospitals. The hospital to which the casualties will be taken must be identified as soon as feasible, to avoid where possible the future need for interhospital transfers. This information should be communicated not only to ambulance control, but also to police officers, who may have the task of informing relatives and who may also need to interview the casualties themselves at a later juncture rather than delay them on scene.

AMBULANCE SERVICE CALL PRIORITISATION

Ambulance services are required to respond to different categories of calls within certain specified times. These are known colloquially as ORCON (operational research consultants) standards or times, and have been laid down by the government as the times within which patients must be attended by the ambulance service for different types of calls.

'Category A' calls must receive an attendance within 8 minutes of the request for help in 75% of cases. Those that are not reached within 8 minutes must be attended to within 14 minutes in urban areas and within 19 minutes in rural areas on 95% of occasions. All 'Category B' and 'Category C' calls must receive an attendance within 14 or 19 minutes of the request for help depending upon the urban or rural categorization of the ambulance service responding. The difficulties of implementing this are self-evident and have led to the use of alternative responses such as paramedic motor-cyclists and rapid response cars, which are 'manned' by experienced paramedics. These are strategically placed or rotated around different areas to enable them to meet the ORCON response time requirements. Paramedic units can assess the situation and may, if safe and appropriate, stand down the ambulance so that it can be deployed elsewhere.

Two 'prioritization' systems are in use that assess the category in to which calls should be placed, Criteria Based Dispatch (CBD) and Advanced Medical Priority Dispatch System (AMPDS). Both are tools devised to assess the category to which the patient's problem will be allocated using specific questions asked in a defined sequence, which the telephone operators must use and follow exactly. From the answers obtained calls will be appropriately categorised by the control dispatcher. Overall, the objectives of the system(s) are to establish critical information from the caller, including telephone number, chief complaint, location, age, sex and conscious level of the patient. The aims of the dispatch systems are listed in Box 4.4.

Criteria Based Dispatch questions are referred to as guidelines rather than the scripted protocols of AMPDS. A study of the two systems by Nicholl et al (1999) concluded that no priority system can be expected to identify life threatening emergency calls and achieve faster response times by focus-ing resources on them without also wrongly identifying some minor calls as life threatening emergencies. Similarly the obverse is true with systems failing to identify some life threatening emergencies. These observations do not obscure the fact that in most cases resources are appropriately deployed.

Box 4.4 Aims of dispatch systems

- Identify a dispatch code
- Decide a priority level of call
- Offer instructions to the caller before the arrival of ambulance personnel
- Provide responders with more detailed information
- Provide medical help to every priority A call within 8 minutes

---

Priority A calls are those where immediate life threatening situations requiring urgent medical assistance are identified, for example, cardiac arrest and uncontrolled haemorrhage. They also include children aged under 2 years and other listed incidents where life-saving skills can be provided through immediate aid and paramedic/clinical intervention. As dispatchers must con-sider utilising the nearest and quickest response to priority A calls, this may mean that 'first responders' may increasingly be used. A number of immediate care schemes also have nurses as integral parts of their team. It is possible and even likely that these nurses will play an increasingly active role in schemes in the future; for some this may develop from their acting as first responders and from being called out to assess Category A incidents within their own geographical areas. For others who have already established confidence and competence in emergency care and interven-tion, both in-hospital and out-of-hospital, their role as full members of the team may be more direct. More experienced pre-hospital nurses may also have a substantive and autonomous role in the future.

Priorities B and C are those categories where serious conditions are identified that are not immediately life threatening, for example, controlled haemorrhage, conscious overdoses or unwell, conscious, diabetic patients.

ON-SCENE TIMES

The length of time that should be spent on scene delivering pre-hospital care remains a subject continually under discussion. The swing of the pendulum from 'scoop and run' to 'stay and stabilise' is, at the current time, returning to a middle balance. Sensibly and logically, if patients are extricated and in the back of ambulances, these should move off as soon as the patients and equipment are secure, and any observations or procedures carried out which cannot be under-taken in moving vehicles have been performed.

There are those who argue that everything can be done in the back of a moving vehicle, and that even cannulation, if not done on scene should be carried out while en route to the hospital. However, most of those who have transported a patient from a scene of trauma will be only too aware of the difficulties associated with this. Obviously, if patients are trapped, the situation will be different and intravenous access and cannulation should be established where appropriate and where possible before they are released.

A study by Mackay et al. in 1997 revealed that paramedics were using their advanced skills selectively. The study showed that paramedics spent longer on scene with cardiac emergency patients, but identified those trauma patients in whom unnecessary delay on scene would be detrimental and transported them to hospital more quickly.

PRE-HOSPITAL CONUNDRUMS

Deakin (1997) published a paper on preventable pre-hospital deaths from trauma in which he discussed a finding by Sampalis in Canada. Sampalis' study examined the detrimental effects of pre-hospital treatment, whereas most other research into this area examined preventable deaths caused by pre-hospital procedures not having been performed. In the Sampalis study, most of the harmful effects noted were caused by endotracheal intubation and by intravenous fluids having been started on scene. The primary reason for the poor outcome was judged to have been the direct result of prolonged time on scene. However, another paper by McDermott et al. (1996) showed that some patients received inadequate airway care and respiratory management, while others had been given inadequate or no fluid resuscitation, thereby implicitly arguing for longer on-scene times. Deakin goes on to point out that head-injured patients in particular receive sub-optimal airway management in the pre-hospital arena. This, he stated, is because realistically only patients with a Glasgow coma scale (GCS) level of three can be successfully intubated without the use of neuromuscular blocking agents.

At present, the use of such neuromuscular blocking drugs is not taught as a standard paramedic skill, so many trauma patients with impaired levels of consciousness who could benefit from endotracheal intubation do not do so. These would typically be patients with a GCS of eight or less who have impaired upper airway reflexes and impaired gas exchange, and who are, therefore, likely to sustain secondary brain injury with the consequential effects on morbidity and mortality. Deakin concludes by emphasizing that most inappropriate care and preventable deaths are related to failure to diagnose and treat basic airway, breathing and circulatory (ABC) problems.

Another linked controversial area in pre-hospital care relates to the amount of fluid and the type of fluid that should be administered. The equilibrium has changed from crystalloids to colloids and now refavours the use of crystalloids. In the past it was held that because, when used, crystalloids were required in a ratio of three to one to replace a given volume of blood (i.e. three times as much crystalloid had to be given compared with the blood loss to achieve haemodynamic stability), and because this would only remain in the intravascular compartment for approximately 30 minutes before diffusing into the interstitial space, that colloids should be used in cases of considerable blood loss – always assuming that blood itself was not available. Colloids, it was believed, remained in the intravascular compartment for at least 60 minutes; therefore, one could give less fluid and thereby reduce the dangers of fluid overload and pulmonary oedema, if these were used. That approach is no longer tenable and crystalloids are back in favour, with the emphasis now on permissive or hypotensive resuscitation. This so-called 'hypotensive resuscitation' has proved to be of greater benefit than trying to match fluid input to estimated blood loss, until surgical control of haemorrhage can be achieved. It has been demonstrated that, if the systolic blood pressure is raised above a level of approximately 90 mmHg, then the risk of further haemorrhage is actually increased. Blood-clotting factors are diluted and any established thrombus may be disturbed with large colloid infusions. In certain circumstances, no fluid given in the pre-hospital phase may prove to be the optimal treatment. The aim, therefore, is to maintain systolic blood pressure at approximately 90 mmHg; this can be achieved even when it is not possible to measure blood pressure physically but where there is access to a radial pulse. (The presence of a radial pulse indicates a systolic blood pressure of 80 mmHg or above.)

> Aim to maintain systolic blood pressure at approximately 90 mmHg

Patients with head injuries need special consideration regarding fluid administration. The method used for assessing cerebral blood flow is best expressed as:

> Cerebral perfusion pressure (CPP) = Mean arterial pressure (MAP) – intracranial pressure (ICP)

Where the ICP is raised, there is an associated risk of greater oedema occurring within the brain with subsequent secondary injury due to compression. Recent thinking advocates the necessity for raising the MAP to ensure adequate cerebral blood flow to ensure that the brain is properly perfused. Therefore, paradoxically, head-injured patients may actually require more fluid and not less. Furthermore, there are also concerns that another of the dogmas of pre-hospital care, namely the application of a hard cervical collar, which is mandatory in all blunt injuries above the clavicle, may actually increase intracerebral pressure. This may be due to impairment of venous drainage to the head and neck; therefore, the hard collar may need to be loosened, but only once the patient is extricated and secured on a long board or vacuum mattress, and the head held by suitable restraints. These are all areas of continuing research.

THE FUTURE FOR PRE-HOSPITAL CARE

Trauma and sudden illness have been described as 'the pandemic of modern society'. Across the European Union (EU) there are 45 000 deaths and 3.5 million casualties per annum whose treatment costs twice the EU budget. Globally, 700 000 people are killed per year and 10–15 million people are injured on the roads at a cost of £300 000 million. These figures have been likened to the equivalent of 1750 airplane crashes a year with nine occurring each year in the UK.

The police force no longer speaks of road traffic accidents (RTAs) but of road traffic crashes (RTCs). Their message is that accidents are truly events that cannot be foreseen (e.g. the Selby rail accident) and so are not directly preventable,

whereas the vast majority of crashes are preventable through better driving, more forethought by drivers and the removal of factors that are known to play a substantial role in them. Alcohol intake, speeding, incorrect manoeuvres, such as overtaking, drugs and lack of due care and attention, for example, owing to the use of mobile phones, are a number of such factors.

Calls and demands on the emergency services to provide pre-hospital care are increasing. Standards of care, education in relation to providing this care and the need for cooperation across the services must rise in parallel. All those engaged in this arena are ever more aware of the demands and expectations for their skills to be honed and updated. The emphasis in pre-hospital care must be to ensure that the right help is given to patients as speedily as possible. The 'right help' is undoubtedly that provided by a team approach. The 'pros and cons' of making nurses part of this team have been discussed in various forums and papers. In 2000, Crouch and Hodgetts examined the actual involvement of nurses within the UK ambulance services. The conclusions were that few ambulance services employed nurses directly. Moreover, a number of people replying to their questionnaire saw as desirable the integration of nurse and paramedic training to develop a 'generic' pre-hospital care worker. One might ask whether the nurses involved would do any 'in-hospital' nursing or how their time would be allocated, and how much 'nursing' would ambulance paramedics undertake and where. Others advocate that, if a nurse is sufficiently interested in pre-hospital care, some sort of conversion course should be designed for them. However, one could argue that this already exists in the form of the standard paramedic course and related examinations.

There are three very active immediate care schemes in the Manchester area. These teams consist of highly trained nursing and medical staff from the emergency department, where they work on a 24-hour rotational basis. All members undergo specific training – both theoretical and practical. Most have completed Advanced Life Support (ALS) and Pre-Hospital Trauma Life Support (PHTLS) courses. If nurses are to be involved as 'nurses' and not as generic pre-hospital workers, then the ambulance service will need to incorporate them into their system. The feasibility of hospital-based nurses working on the same type of callout system as doctors working in the community (GPs) – the system operated by many BASICS doctors – has also been questioned. For this to occur, arrangements will require to be in place whereby they could leave their work, with all the implications raised by this, and respond to calls. Nurses could also be available in their spare time on a voluntary basis, similar to immediate care doctors, or could perhaps be paid like paramedics.

Many nurses do voluntarily attend calls with doctors with whom they already have a working relationship in some of the immediate care schemes. However, if a significant number of nurses were to do this, the logistics and practicalities of callouts would have to be carefully examined. It may well be that one of the most useful roles for most nurses in addition to the care and assistance they can render to patients and to medical and paramedical colleagues on scene, may be to act as first responders as described earlier. This is a concept worthy of further research and scrutiny.

In an editorial in 1998, Matthew Cooke opened the door of immediate care even wider. He reminded us that the care provided by the statutory ambulance services is only one element of immediate care, and refers to mountain rescue teams whose members must be trained and qualified not only in mountaineering but also in survival skills and medicine. This also applies to those who undertake air, sea and cave rescue. Cooke also comments that even mass-gathering medicine is becoming a subspecialty. Innumerable problems are raised by these events, which require skills beyond those needed for the more usual emergency work. All of this emphasises the need for incorporating into the specialty of immediate care all the skills we can utilise. The problem, which must be resolved, is how to match these logistically to the relevant incidents.

There is an argument for clearly defining and delineating the roles of individuals within pre-hospital care. Sometimes there appears to be an almost blind institutional rush to ensure that no one member of the team is less or differently trained than another; hence, the concept of the generic pre-hospital worker. We must ensure that, in our efforts for equality of training, we are not in danger of so blurring the lines that confusion and not care is the ultimate result. Having clearly defined roles does not preclude cooperation, neither does it prevent each person knowing the other's role and in certain circumstances enabling them to undertake it should the need arise. In any team game, each member plays at different individual positions, but the game is only won by the team working as such and moving in a pre-determined way towards the goal. These are exciting times in pre-hospital care and it will be of great interest to see how the specialty evolves in the coming years.

SUMMARY

Pre-hospital care is a vital part of the patient's journey, and must be considered an integral part of the overall resuscitation and stabilisation of patients. The importance of teamwork and of viewing the pre-hospital team as an extension of the trauma team may help to ensure effective communication from the scene to hospitals and other receiving facilities, and ensure that seamless care is delivered where possible, including the use of a structured patient handover. Documentation of findings and interventions in relation to the pre-hospital phase of treatment is essential and, where possible, should include the use of photography.

Having extricated patients from the environment in which they are found, the main aim of the pre-hospital team is to recognise and treat life-threatening problems, and to stabilise and transport patients during their journey to definitive care while optimizing their chances of survival. Of key importance is the ability to recognise and intervene to prevent hypoxia and/or hypovolaemia from developing – the two leading causes of trauma deaths. Although traditionally the majority of pre-hospital care has been provided by ambulance paramedics and, to a lesser extent, doctors, there is little reason why this role could not be undertaken by suitably trained and prepared nurses, who are familiar with the hazards and difficulties of working in the pre-hospital care arena.

References

Audit Commission. *A life in the fast lane*. 2: 42–43. London: Audit Commission, 1998

Cooke M. Editorial. Pre-hospital care – one or several specialties? *Pre-hospital Immediate Care* 1998; 2: 186

Crouch R, Hodgetts T. Involvement of nurse in UK ambulance services: a national survey. *Pre-hospital Immediate Care* 2000; 4: 64–67

Deakin CD. Preventable pre-hospital death from trauma. *Pre-hospital Immediate Care* 1997; 1: 198–203

Mackay CA, Burke DP, Bowden DF. Effect of paramedic scene times on patient outcome. *Pre-hospital Immediate Care* 1997; 1: 4–7

McDermott FT, Cordner SM, Tremayne AB. Evaluation of medical management and preventability of death in 137 road traffic fatalities in Victoria, Australia; an overview. Consultative Committee on Road Traffic Fatalities in Victoria. *Journal of Trauma* 1996; 40: 520–533

McInerney JJ, Ward CT, Hassan TB, et al. Strategies to improve communication at the pre-hospital/accident & emergency interface. *Pre-Hospital Immediate Care* 2000; 4: 176–179

Nicholl J, Coleman P, et al. Emergency priority dispatch systems – a new era in the provision of ambulance services in the UK. *Pre-hospital Immediate Care* 1999; 3: 71–75

Further reading

Eaton CJ. *Essentials of immediate care*. Edinburgh: Churchill Livingstone, 1999

Pre-hospital forum – nurses in pre-hospital care. Forum. *Pre-hospital Immediate Care* 1997; 1: 144–151

Pre-hospital forum – nurses in pre-hospital care. Letters. *Pre-hospital Immediate Care* 1998; 2: 115–119

Nurses in pre-hospital care. Letters. *Pre-hospital Immediate Care* 1998; 2: 53–54

RoSPA. *Care on the road*. 1999; April: 11

Sampalis JS, Boukas S, Lavoie A, et al. Preventable death evaluation of the appropriateness of the on-site trauma care provided by the Urgences Sante physicians. *Journal of Trauma* 1995; 39: 1027–1028

Chapter 5

Stabilisation and transport of the critically ill

Rose Ann O'Shea and Barry Hart

INTRODUCTION

The transportation and management of critically ill patients presents a challenge to all involved in their care. While many nurses and doctors are both experienced and comfortable with managing critically ill patients within their own environments – usually acute hospitals – to be faced with the prospect of working outside of their area in strange surroundings can be daunting.

Things are renowned for going wrong when transferring patients – whether it is in the x-ray department, computed tomography (CT) scanner, magnetic resonance imaging (MRI) department or corridor, or in transit during interhospital or intrahospital transfers. Risks are known to increase when patients are moved, and are affected by numerous factors including staff preparation and training, the availability of and access to safe and effective equipment, environmental factors, the mode of transportation and the ability to react to the unexpected. Although it is hoped that the situation where unprepared staff are suddenly advised of the need for them to escort patients on interhospital or intersite transfers is now a thing of the past, ensuring the stabilisation and safe transport of unstable and critically ill or injured patients must remain paramount. It is essential that all those involved receive adequate preparation and appropriate training in the areas where they are expected to work, and are provided with appropriate and functional equipment as well as personal, protective equipment required for the purpose.

CRITICALLY ILL AND INJURED PATIENTS

From time to time, critically ill and injured patients will require to be moved by staff caring for them. This may include moving the patient from the scene of the accident or incident to hospital, from the emergency department to another location within the hospital for diagnostic purposes (e.g. CT scanning) or from hospital to hospital when specialist treatment is required. The circumstances and possibilities are numerous, and this chapter highlights key factors that must be considered with regard to their mode of transport and the procedures and precautions that must be taken when moving such patients *in extremis*.

It is essential that a structured assessment is undertaken before the patient is moved. This should be repeated after each movement or intervention, with particular attention being given to checking the position and patency of endotracheal tubes, intravenous cannulae and any other clinical or monitoring devices. Should any immediately life-threatening problem be identified during the reassessment process, action must be taken immediately to deal with it promptly.

Patients classed as being critically ill or injured may require to be moved urgently; many are often suffering from conditions that are defined as 'time critical' (Box 5.1). Although there is general agree-ment regarding the parameters that categorise patients as time critical, team members should consult local protocols and guidelines for definitive guidance in their location.

> Trauma is a neglected disease and remains the most common killer of the young

THE PRE-HOSPITAL SETTING

Transportation usually begins with the movement of patients from the scene of the accident or incident to the receiving hospital. This involves various methods of transport and staff with differing levels of ability. While the majority of patients are transported by National Health Service (NHS) ambulance services, other agencies can and do play a vital role. NHS ambulance design and configuration, as well as equipment levels, have improved considerably over recent years. Whereas in the past the role of the ambulance service has been to administer basic treatments and to convey patients to the nearest hospital, this is now evolving into a modern and more sophisticated service providing a high degree of expertise and skill to those who are ill and injured.

Improvements in ambulance design over the years have mainly focused on the addition of extra equipment and the redesign of cabin layouts. This has facilitated access to patients and enabled life-saving interventions to be performed in a more appropriate environment. In UK ambulances, the crew generally consists of two ambulance personnel; typically one drives while the other attends the patient. In more complex situations, additional help may be required to attend the patient; trauma nurses are ideally placed to perform this role and to become an integral part of the transport team accompanying the patient to hospital. In so doing they are also ideally placed to contribute to improving the quality of care provided on route to hospital and to assist in ensuring an effective handover of the patient to the receiving team – an area that is historically associated with difficulty in some areas. Current thinking on the management of trauma and cardiac patients suggests that initial management

---

Box 5.1   Features of time–critical patients

Heart rate > 120 bpm
Systolic blood pressure (BP) < 90 mmHg
Respiratory rate (RR) >30 or <10
Glasgow coma score (GCS) 12 or less
Severe injuries likely to contribute to deterioration in vital signs, e.g.
- severe haemorrhage
- neurovascular compromise
- potential airway burns
- life-threatening asthma
- tension pneumothorax
- massive haemothorax
- unstable coronary syndromes
- more than one long bone fracture
- intrathoracic injury
- intra-abdominal injury
- fulminating infection

of the airway and breathing should take place on scene, but that cannulation should take place in the back of the ambulance en route to hospital.

Managing critically ill and injured patients in the back of an ambulance can be a challenging and daunting experience for experienced ambulance crews, let alone other trauma team members unfamiliar with this environment. To improve safety and to standardise the equipment carried by ambulances, regulations issued by the European Committee for Standardisation have been adopted by UK ambulance services. Known as the CEN guidelines (Committee for European Normalisation), these define the minimum standard for the design and construction of vehicles, the testing and performance of ambulances, and the type and quality of equipment that should be carried and which is used for the transport of sick or injured persons (British Standard, 2000). These guidelines, which are applicable to road ambulances capable of transporting at least one person on a stretcher, however, do not define how ambulances should be laid out and where individual items of equipment should be found. For this reason and to address potential safety concerns, it is imperative that trauma nurses and other immediate care practitioners check their equipment and its location, high-pressure oxygen connections and electrical connections to ensure that they are compatible with those of the transport vehicle in question.

In recent years, the incidence of large-scale transport incidents, such as King's Cross (1987), Clapham Junction (1988), Kegworth (1989), Hatfield (2000) and Potter's Bar (2001), has increased, bringing with it the need to address not only the logistics of transporting the sick and injured to hospital, but also the role of team members caring for them. In such instances, all transport issues and options should be addressed, including the mode and route of transport, environmental hazards and the nature of the injuries involved. Where mass casualty situations or major incidents are involved, decisions regarding patient evacuation and transport to places of definitive treatment are based on the triage sieve and sort (see Ch. 6). Casualty evacuation principles include evacuating patients, usually by emergency ambulance, are based on a system of clinical priorities where those with the greatest level of clinical urgency (i.e. those categorised as priority 1) are transported first. On occasion, the use of ambulance helicopters may be considered appropriate. Those patients allocated priority 2 may need to be removed by emergency ambulance, although those in priority 1 take precedence. Emergency ambulances are not usually required for those designated as priority 3; for these patients, alternative modes of transport such as voluntary aid organisation ambulances, outpatient ambulance vehicles, minibuses, buses, coaches and trains may be used.

In many instances involving single or multiple casualty situations, the need for additional expertise is required en route to hospital. Traditionally, immediate care BASICS doctors or other medical clinicians with an interest in pre-hospital emergency or trauma care have performed this role. Suitably trained and experienced and competent nurses are, however, increasingly demonstrating their ability to perform this role and should be included as integral team members. Identifying the nature of the skills and interventions required rather than professional discipline may work towards achieving this, and to realising the full contribution that nurses can bring to this vital aspect of care.

INTRAHOSPITAL AND INTERHOSPITAL EMERGENCIES

The management of critically ill and injured patients is aimed at recognising and treating life-threatening conditions and emergencies, minimising delays both on scene and en route, effective communication with the receiving staff, and delivering them to the place of definitive treatment in such a condition to optimise their chances of a positive outcome.

In the pre-hospital environment, the decision regarding the hospital to which patients are sent usually rests with the ambulance control manager. Factors influencing this decision include time of day, the environment, risks involved, local arrangements, guidance and the nature of the patient's condition and injuries. Where time-critical injuries have been sustained, the mode of transport is an additional consideration. This is particularly the case in major incidents. In larger urban areas where there is a choice of destination, it is better to select patients for specialist facilities at the scene of the incident. Thus patients who have severe head injuries can be triaged to neurosurgical centres and patients with burns to specialist/regional burns units (Box 5.2). The rarer the condition or circumstance, the more important it becomes to target patients to appropriate specialist centres, even though this may initially appear to be the more difficult course.

Whatever the environment or situation encountered, the importance of teamwork throughout the spectrum of care, including effective, accurate and appropriate communication including pre-alerts and patient handover, should not be underestimated.

Intrahospital emergencies

Moving patients from stretcher to trolley, trolley to bed or from bed to diagnostic imaging facility has the potential for destabilising patients, increasing problems and complications regarding equipment, and for creating unnecessary delays. Where patients are critically ill and injured, it is not unusual for them to require sophisticated observation, monitoring and intervention, which invariably involves the use of cardiac and non-invasive blood pressure monitoring, the administration of intravenous fluids and medications via infusion pumps or devices, and the insertion of various tubes and catheters. Many also are recipients of advanced airway interventions, such as endotracheal tube insertion and mechanical ventilation, and drains, such as chest drains inserted in response to life-threatening emergencies.

Each movement of the patient may exacerbate underlying problems and contribute to haemodynamic or physiological instability, or to equipment problems or failure (Box 5.3). Stabilisation of the patient prior to transfer is, therefore, essential to reduce the impact of such movements, as well as prior planning, preparation and communication between all those concerned.

Patients should be stabilised prior to transfer

Stabilisation is based on securing the patient's airway, providing ventilation and maintaining

---

Box 5.2   Referral to regional burns units (Reproduced with permission from Hodgetts T, McNeil I, Cooke M. *The pre-hospital emergency management master.* London: BMJ Publishing Group, 1995)

Before referring patients to a specialist burns center, be confident that you have excluded and treated any life-threatening associated injuries. Associated injuries are more common than may be at first be anticipated.

Indications for referral to a regional burns unit
1. Full thickness burn > 5% body surface area (children and adults)
2. Partial thickness burn > 10% body surface area in children (< 10 years) and elderly (> 50 years)
3. Partial thickness burn > 20% body surface area in 10–50-year-olds
4. Burns (partial or full thickness) of the face, eyes and genitalia; consider referring burns involving the hands, feet and major joints
5. Electrical burns (the visible skin burn can be deceptively minor)
6. Chemical burns
7. Inhalation injury
8. Less severe burns than those stated in 1–3 if there is coexisting disease
9. Burn + polytrauma, where the burn is the principal injury

Box 5.3   Physiological consequences of transporting the critically ill

Acceleration has a profound effect on normal physiology, which should be anticipated and understood prior to departure. These include:
● Alteration in cardiac output
● Reduction in blood pressure
● Alteration in lung function, even in supine patients
● Alteration in alveolar size
● Increased dead space and resultant underperfusion of alveoli
● Increased shunt, i.e. alveoli are well perfused but underventilated
Reciprocal changes should be anticipated with deceleration

adequate circulation. In addition to meeting the physical and, in a conscious patient, the psychological needs of the patient, the transferring emergency department staff need to arrange a receiving facility, and ensure that they are prepared and ready for the patient's arrival. Locally agreed policies, agreements, transfer forms and specific procedures facilitate this process and enhance communication and the overall quality of care provided to patients. This level of detail should apply to local transfers to diagnostic facilities as well as to transfers to wards, high dependency or critical care areas.

The final step in the process of stabilisation and transportation of patients is deciding the most appropriate mode of transport. With intrahospital transfers, this is relatively straightforward and generally refers to the type of trolley or stretcher most appropriate for the patient's conditions and injuries sustained. With interhospital transfers, this consideration may expand to incorporate the decision on whether to transport via ground or air.

Interhospital emergencies

The transfer of patients between hospitals is generally required to deliver patients to specialist centres or places of definitive treatment. This typically occurs, for example, in remote locations where secondary and tertiary facilities are some distance from the original location, or where the advanced or particular expertise required is provided only at selected locations. Conditions that may warrant such intervention include severe burns requiring treatment at regional or specialist burns units, serious head injuries requiring neurosurgical interventions or significant trauma requiring specialist cardiothoracic review. Access to diagnostic facilities, such as MRI or CT scanning, which may not be available (e.g. at some district general hospitals) may also necessitate this.

As indicated earlier, mode of transport is an important consideration when transferring patients between hospitals. In the majority of cases, the choice is between transfer by ground or air ambulance. The main advantages of ground ambulances include their space and the ability to move in most types of weather. Their disadvantages mainly focus on the length of time

it may take to transport patients, poor road conditions and, in some instances, the lack of available personnel trained in advanced life support. Air ambulance transport offers the advantages of time saved, experienced crews trained in advanced skills and generally a smoother ride for the patient. These are offset by the disadvantages of limited training programmes, weather restrictions and the limited space in which to provide patient care. As with intrahospital transfers, it must be remembered that loading and unloading patients into and out of vehicles, including aircraft, may destabilise the already unstable patient and may produce unnecessary delays.

Where air ambulance or helicopter missions have been selected, it is essential to ensure that both the referring and receiving agencies have spoken with each other and are aware of their roles and responsibilities. Pre-agreed checklists (Boxes 5.4 and 5.5; Figures 5.1 and 5.2) go some

---

Box 5.4 Trauma/helicopter transport checklist (Reproduced with permission from Hodgetts T, McNeil I, Cooke M. *The pre-hospital emergency management master.* London: BMJ Publishing Group, 1995)

Patient precautions
Consider carefully why these patients need helicopter transport and discuss with an expert:
- recent dive (Caisson disease may be precipitated)
- psychiatric disorder
- late pregnancy (risk of supine hypotension)
- critical hypoxia if self-ventilating
- gastrointestinal obstruction
- confusion

Pre-flight checklist
- Is the patient secure and accessible?
- Are there adequate supplies (oxygen, fluid, analgesia) for a long journey?
- Is the electrical equipment compatible with the aircraft electronics?
- Can you use the on-board power supply?
- Have you inserted a chest drain for known/suspected pneumothorax and is it secure?
- Is there water in the endotracheal tube cuff?
- Have you arranged for an ambulance to meet you at the landing site, if needed, for onward transport?

Box 5.5   Pre-transfer checklist

Checks to be made prior to transfer

Airway
- Airway patency
- Placement and stability of endotracheal tube if *in situ*

Breathing
- Adequacy of breathing in the conscious patient
- Consideration of need to sedate and paralyse patient
- Ventilator settings and patient response
- Arterial blood gas levels

Circulation
- Haemodynamic stability
- Vital signs trends
- Control of major haemorrhage
- Adequacy of perfusion
- Intravenous access, and fluid and drug administration, including infusion pumps/syringe drivers
- Review of blood results
- Stability and security of arterial and central venous lines, and urinary catheters, drains, etc.

Neurological/skeletal
- Control of seizures
- Immobilisation of fractures
- Immobilisation of spinal injury patients using appropriate devices, e.g. vacuum mattress

Notes
- Copy of medical records, blood results, scans
- Copies of all relevant documentation
- Patient identification *in situ*
- Samples and documentation labelled appropriately

---

way to avoiding the situation of arriving at hospital where the patient is unexpected and there is no bed or clinician waiting for him/her. Helicopter services must speak to both referring and receiving clinicians, and confirm the clinical status of patients. The time of departure, and estimated time of arrival should also be communicated and all relevant documentation including x-rays, scans and observation charts compiled.

Historically, some groups of patients have been associated with difficulties encountered during transfer/transport. These include those who have sustained spinal injuries. Whereas in the past ambulances tended to travel at significantly low speeds, this practice has been superseded by vehicle redesigns with most ambulances now having a suspension designed to function best at around 30 mph. There is, therefore, now no justification for very slow transfers of patients with actual or suspected cervical spine injuries (Greaves and Porter, 1999).

> Patients requiring specialist centres should be transported to them directly from the scene, where possible

Education, preparation and training

It is essential that those tasked with managing the patient in transit are experienced, trained and equipped for their role. This includes having the ability to react promptly and deal with the unexpected, while maintaining a level head under pressure. Clearly, the novice or junior clinician should not undertake this role. As a minimum, it is strongly recommended that those performing this role are trained in and familiar with advanced trauma life support principles and, ideally, have completed an appropriate training programme such as Trauma Nursing Core Course (TNCC) or Advanced Trauma Nursing Course (ATNC). Where the transfer of children is involved, it is recommended that they have extensive paediatric experience and, where possible, have completed appropriate training programmes. Where the interhospital transfer of ventilated patients is being undertaken, nurses and other clinicians with resuscitation skills and experience of anaesthesiology, intensive care, critical care or emergency care should accompany such patients. Additionally, in the event that aeromedical transportation is required, it is generally advisable that all rescue and retrieval personnel have prior training and experience before undertaking work in the uncomfortable and noisy environment of the helicopter itself, and in the potentially hostile environment of the rescue location.

ANTICIPATION OF POTENTIAL PROBLEMS

The anticipation of potential problems is fundamental to all transfer and pre-hospital work. The

Name

Time of burn...................hrs

Age

Circumstances

☐ enclosed space?

☐ chemical?

☐ electrical?

History of event: ....

....

....

Unconscious at scene:

☐ Yes

☐ No

Signs of inhalational burn?

☐ soot/singeing around nose & mouth

☐ hoarseness

☐ wheeze

Body surface area burn:

Partial thickness..................%

Full thickness.......................%

TOTAL..................................%

Escharotomies:

Site...................   Time...................

Site...................   Time...................

Site...................   Time...................

Oxygen saturation on air = ...%

Saturation on..............% oxygen =..............%

Fluids given:

.... Time ....

.... Time ....

.... Time ....

Associated injuries:

Drugs given:

Pain relief.................   Time...................

Tetanus toxoid   ☐ Y ☐ N

Past medical history:

Other........................   Time...................

FROM A&E

Blood gases:

pH...................

pCO$_2$...................

pO$_2$...................

Intubated? ☐ Y ☐ N

Time..............................

Laryngoscopy..

Size tube...................mm

Length...................cm at teeth

Carboxyhaemoglobin..............%

at...................hrs

☐ Nasogastric tube

☐ Urinary catheter

☐ Chest X-ray

Figure 5.1   Burns/referral checklist. (Reproduced with permission from Hodgetts T, McNeil I, Cooke M. *The pre-hospital emergency management master*. London: BMJ Publishing Group, 1995.)

Tick when completed ✓

Receiving hospital
Name of doctor informed   ☐
Ward name/number informed   ☐

Documentation
All original notes/copies of notes to take   ☐
All original X-rays/copy of X-rays to take   ☐
Cross-matched blood to accompany (clear with transfusion lab)   ☐
Patient preparation
Airway secure
      ET tube size.................mm; length.................cm at the teeth   ☐

Connections secured   ☐
Spine immobilised
      Hard collar ☐   Sandbags and tape ☐   Longboard ☐   KED/RED ☐   Other ....

Chest drains
      Secure ☐   Underwater seal changed for drainage bag ☐   Unclamped ☐
External haemorrhage controlled   Site ....
      Gauge.................Secure

Intravenous lines, preferably two. Note peripheral and central lines.

      Site ....   Gauge ....   Secure ☐
      Site ....   Gauge ....   Secure ☐
      Site ....   Gauge ....   Secure ☐
      Site ....   Gauge ....   Secure ☐

Limbs splinted   ☐
Urinary catheter   ☐
Nasogastric/orogastric tube   ☐

Monitor during transfer
Pulse oximeter   ☐
Non-invasive blood pressure   ☐
ECG   ☐
End-tidal CO_2 ☐
Mean pulmonary artery/invasive blood pressure monitors   ☐
Ensure adequate battery life for these monitors

Equipment preparation
AIRWAY   Spare intubation set   ☐
              Self-inflating bag with reservoir   ☐
              Adequate oxygen supply   ☐
              Suction and suction catheters   ☐

BREATHING   Try patient on portable ventilator and assess for mechanical problems   ☐

CIRCULATION   Supply of colloid/crystalloid/blood   ☐
              Spare intravenous cannulae   ☐

DRUGS   Anaesthetic, muscle relaxant, sedative   ☐
              Analgesic   ☐
              Inotropic   ☐
              Infusion pumps and spare batteries   ☐

Is the patient adequately secured to the stretcher?

Figure 5.2   Trauma/transfer checklist. (Reproduced with permission from Hodgetts T, McNeil I, Cooke M. *The pre-hospital emergency management master.* London: BMJ Publishing Group, 1995.)

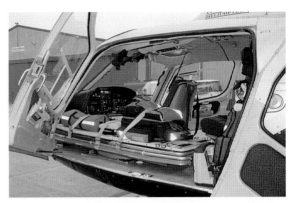

Figure 5.3   Side view of Twin Squirrel helicopter. With this aircraft, both crew are seated behind the pilot, with one person having direct access to the patient.

aim of transport is to transfer patients safely from one point of origin to another and to cause no further harm. Prior preparation and planning are vital to ensure this and to enable potentially life-threatening problems encountered to be managed appropriately (Box 5.6). This relates particularly to the checking of all equipment, including the availability of drugs and devices, the effectiveness and reliability of communication systems, and the availability and accessibility of supplies that may be required for the patient's journey.

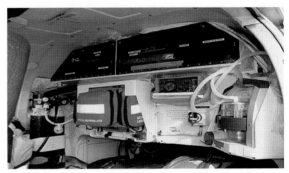

Figure 5.4   Cabin area of Bolkow 105DBS showing layout of equipment and storage.

> Anticipation of potential problems is fundamental to all transfer and pre-hospital work

Where aeromedical transportation is involved, the need for such safety checks and precautions is further heightened. The upper atmosphere (i.e. the air) can be a hostile place. As air pressure declines, less oxygen is available for cellular metabolism and gases trapped within body cavities will expand. Problems associated with motion sickness, such as those encountered in land and sea transfers, may be encountered, as well as those associated with vibration, noise, the cold or humidity, not to mention the psychological terror that may be experienced by those who are afraid of flying. One of the major functional disadvantages of aeromedical care is one of space. Another is that of access to the patient as a whole. In some helicopters, access to the patient's head and airway is all that is possible, whereas others allow greater albeit limited access (Figures 5.3–5.5). Opening boxes or finding equipment may also prove challenging, making some clinical interven-

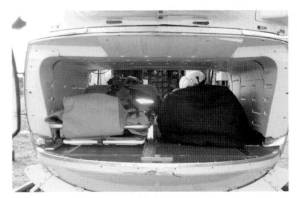

Figure 5.5   Rear view of Bolkow with door open showing the confines of space. In this aircraft, only the patient's chest and abdominal area is easily accessible to the crew.

tions difficult if not impossible. Prior planning and positioning of essential equipment may alleviate some potential problems. Although these problems will never be eradicated, practice and training in delivering care in confined spaces such as aircraft may make such situations more controlled and, therefore, safer.

An essential attribute required of those transferring or transporting critical patients is the ability to know one's limitations and to know when back-up is required. This may relate to equipment or to the need for particular expertise, for example, with reintubation or rapid sequence induction. All need to ensure that adequate medical equipment and medications are available during transit, that they are familiar with them, and that they have the requisite knowledge and skills to deal with both the predictable and the unexpected.

Patient considerations

When considering the effects on patients of long-distance transfer, awareness and anticipation of logistic factors such as the duration of out-of-hospital time, ground transfers, airport formalities, in-flight facilities, equipment and skills available, airborne sector times, time zone changes, stopovers, changes of aircraft, medical facilities at each stage and the actual time of arrival at the destination facility is absolutely vital.

> The aim is to transfer patients safely from one point to another causing no further harm

EQUIPMENT–RELATED PROBLEMS

When planning and preparing equipment for the purposes of patient transfer, it is important to plan for equipment failure and, in particular, for electrical failure. Equipment should ideally be compact, lightweight and rugged enough to withstand the stresses of acceleration, vibration and the possibility of rapid decompression. Electrically powered items must be compatible with ambulance and aircraft supplies, and should be capable of independent battery operation when disconnected from the ambulance/aircraft. Battery life should be adequate for the duration of the entire transit with sufficient reserves for unexpected delays and diversions. Similarly oxygen-powered machines must have reserves sufficient to support the patient's own respiratory requirements.

Equipment is usually categorised according to its purpose and associated specific problems. Diagnostic and therapeutic medical machinery and materials constitute one such category, whereas specific ambulance equipment, such as stretchers, splints, blankets, extrication and immobilisation devices, personal safety and rescue items (helmets, gloves, protective clothing, metal cutters) and communication devices (radio transmitters, mobile telephones), constitute another. The minimum diagnostic and therapeutic equipment specifications for transferring the critically ill and injured are: electrocardiogram (ECG) machine/monitor, defibrillator, pulse oximeter, non-invasive blood pressure monitoring device, suction aspirator, mechanical ventilator, and all equipment necessary to perform safely any of the advanced trauma life support procedures appropriate to the environment in question. Battery-operated suction may be routine but hand-operated suction must also be available. Similarly, duplication of crucial pieces of equipment, such as laryngoscopes and endotracheal tubes, is mandatory. The volume of supplies, such as oxygen and drugs, should be calculated and should include appropriate reserves in case the journey or flight is delayed or diverted or in the event of breakages. Small dependable capnographs, used as a means of detecting misplaced endotracheal tubes (ETTs), and other non-invasive monitoring techniques focusing on cerebral blood flow and cardiac output monitoring are in various stages of development, and may in the future comprise part of the minimum transfer specifications.

In the in-hospital environment, such checks should not be compromised and complacency must be avoided. Frequent checks of resuscitation facilities (at least daily) must be undertaken and immediate access to all essential supplies and materials ensured. Similar checks of ambulance equipment, trolleys, scanning and imaging rooms, and x-ray facilities should be undertaken, and maintenance of elevators and communication devices are mandatory.

Telemetry and telemedicine are increasingly being used to provide treatment as close to the patient as possible in a timely fashion. New and increasingly advanced computerised diagnostic and remote decision support software systems are also being developed to help guide clinicians in the delivery of care with the aim of improving the quality of care provided while maximising the contribution of all team members. Such initiatives have proved to be beneficial, for example, in relation to the delivery of thrombolysis and to pre-hospital thrombolysis in particular. Equipment for these purposes is also increasingly becoming more reliable, affordable and user friendly.

> The minimum diagnostic and therapeutic equipment required to transfer the critically ill and injured must be provided

Some items of equipment are particularly susceptible to gaseous expansion during flight (Box 5.7). These include sphygmomanometer cuffs, glass intravenous fluid bottles, pressure bags, intravenous administration sets, pressurised antishock garments (PASG or MAST), chest drains, nasogastric tubes and other closed drains, endotracheal tube cuffs, catheter balloons and air splints. Special consideration must also be given to selected traction splints, such as the Donway splint. The insertion of water rather than air into endotracheal tube cuffs, for example, will help to minimise problems experienced at altitude and reduce associated complications. Compatibility of

---

Box 5.7   Equipment susceptible to gaseous expansion

Airway and breathing
- Endotracheal tube cuffs

Circulation
- Intravenous administration sets
- Sphygmomanometer cuffs
- Glass intravenous fluid bottles
- Pressure bags
- Chest drains
- Pressurised antishock garments, e.g. military antishock trousers (MAST)

Other
- Nasogastric tubes and other closed drains
- Catheter balloons, e.g. urinary catheters
- Air splints

---

equipment must be ensured prior to departure. In particular, the potential for defibrillation must be considered prior to departure. Regulations issued by the Civil Aviation Authority (CAA) dictate that only those aircraft cleared to use defibrillators in flight may do so; those without such clearance may be required to land in the event that defib-rillation is required. Finally, all equipment must be properly maintained and safely secured in the ambulance, aircraft or trolley prior to departure.

Monitoring and observation

The noise and cramped space of most ambulances and, indeed, helicopters makes the routine work of patient care considerably more difficult in transit. Access to patients is difficult in all but the largest vehicles/helicopters. Listening to the patient's chest with a stethoscope and observing for chest movements may be difficult if not impossible. To compensate for this, patients need to be monitored appropriately with patients being accessible and screens visible where possible. Trends in vital signs measurements rather than absolute values must be noted and prompt action taken where necessary. Endotracheal intubation is difficult in most ambulances, particularly when in transit, and is impossible in most helicopters. Planning ahead and anticipating potential problems and their management is, therefore, essential. Intubated and ventilated patients who have sustained rib fractures are at significant risk of developing a tension pneumothorax, a life threat that requires immediate intervention. Decompression of this by performing a needle thoracocentesis may prevent an impending cardiac arrest but does little to re-expand the lung. A low threshold for tube thoracostomy or chest drain insertion is, therefore, prudent. Attempting to establish an intravenous infusion in the back of an ambulance is a difficult experience at the best of times. This difficulty is exacerbated greatly in the in-flight situation, as there is often limited access and no possibility of pulling into the roadside to have another attempt. It is, therefore, necessary to establish a 'reserve' intravenous line for access in the event of difficulty and in the event that patients require ongoing intravenous therapy.

TRANSPORT/TRANSFER OF THE CRITICALLY ILL

The transport of patients is usually taken to refer to transporting them from the scene of incidents in the pre-hospital phase of their journey to the hospital environment. When considering transport options and issues the transport of staff to the site are of equal importance. To ensure the best possible outcome for patients, the requirements for patient transport/transfer must be understood (Box 5.8).

Patients require to be transported to places of definitive treatment for a range of reasons including where advanced or specialist care not available at the original facility is required, e.g. burns, paediatrics, neurosurgery, cardiac, cardiothoracic, spinal injuries, where the patient has suffered multiple trauma and requires trauma unit intervention, where the specific type of care required by the patient (either nursing or medical) is not available, where additional expertise or diagnostic testing is required, and where conditions that may deteriorate and require care not available at the receiving facility is available. The methods used for making transport decisions are numerous including trauma scoring systems and those based on local protocols, guidelines or national standards. Patients should not be transferred from the resuscitation room or the hospital until stabil-ised and must be fully examined first to ensure that all life-threatening injuries have been identi-fied. This includes stabilisation of the airway, breathing and circulation, monitoring of cardiac rate and rhythm, control of haemorrhage, establishment of intravenous access, assessment of vital signs and any trends in particular, neuro-logical assessment, and cervical spine and injured extremity immobilisation. Prior to transfer, a complete history should be documented, temper-ature control established, interhospital communi-cation initiated and family considerations addressed. The referring hospital must be convinced that the clinical benefits for the patient are better at the receiving facility and the transfer is warranted. Similarly, it must be convinced that the receiving facility is expecting the patient's arrival and has appropriate space and qualified personnel available. It must also be ensured that appropriate staff and equipment are available to perform the transfer. Lastly, the preferred mode of transport should be identified having considered the advantages and disadvantages of each.

Key elements that must be considered when determining the mode of transport and options available in relation to patient needs include the capacity required, the capacity which each vehicle or mode of transport has, their availability and their suitability for the task in hand (Box 5.9). Central to this is an assessment of the speed, safety reliability and level of equipment contained within each.

Land transport/transfer

The prime method of transportation from scene to receiving hospital is by emergency ambulance. Such vehicles are specifically designed to enable safe transport of the seriously ill and injured, and have many facilities for the provision of advanced life support en route (Hodgetts et al., 1995).

Box 5.8   Criteria for successful patient transport

- Familiarity with vehicles used and understanding their limitations
- Understanding of the effects of the mode of transportation on patients and their conditions
- Compatibility between medical equipment used and the mode of transport selected
- Impact of the mode of transport on potential medical interventions
- Understanding the importance of patient packaging, handling and loading
- Impact of the mode of transport on patient/carer communication
- Effective communication between all involved in the patient's care

---

Box 5.9   Criteria for selecting transport

C	Capacity
A	Availability
S	Suitability

Transfer/transport by boat

Transport by water is usually via the use of lifeboats. Medical facilities aboard lifeboats are limited and tend to be dependent on the individuals present. Many have medically trained personnel on board but this is not always the case. Conditions are usually cramped, and the space available and sea conditions often make definitive interventions difficult. Where rescue teams have been called to the sea, the question of winching patients has to be considered. Patients are usually lifted in basket stretchers and must be totally packaged prior to winching, with particular attention paid to preserving their body temperature both in the winching phase and during transport, as helicopters tend to be draughty and cold. Wherever possible, it should be ensured that patients are winched in the horizontal position, as winching in the vertical position can lead to hypotension and collapse, particularly if the patient has been immersed. Large ocean-going passenger liners such as the *QE2* or *Queen Mary II* have extensive medical facilities on board and can cope with significant clinical problems without recourse to land-based facilities.

Aeromedical transport/transfer

The primary reasons for using aircraft for transporting patients are usually clinical (Box 5.10). Those responsible for care should have a firm understanding of the disease process, the rate at which deterioration may occur, the risks that may occur en route and the time which will be required to reach the receiving unit (Box 5.11). Patients at both ends of the trauma or emergency care spectrum may benefit from such a transfer option. For example, those living in remote locations may have to wait several hours until arriving at a place of definitive treatment. This delay carries with it the potential for compromising patient safety and eventual clinical outcome, a delay that could be avoided by aeromedical transportation. Some conditions deteriorate at a rapid rate and require early intervention to optimise the patient's chances of survival. The potential advantages of aeromedical transportation in such examples is evident, including those with severe or life-threatening injuries as a consequence of serious

---

Box 5.10   Aeromedical transportation missions

Primary
- Search and rescue
- Evacuation from incident site to hospital
- Transportation of emergency teams to incident site
- Delivery of medical supplies and equipment to incident site
- Emergency military evacuation

Secondary
- Interhospital transfer
- Military evacuation to next level of care

Tertiary
- Interhospital transfer
- International repatriation
- Transportation of donor organs
- Military strategic evacuation

Box 5.11   Factors to consider when selecting aeromedical transportation

- The disease process
- The likely rate of clinical deterioration
- Potential risks en route to hospital
- Time required to reach receiving facility
- Time of day transport required

---

road traffic crashes, such as tension pneumothorax, massive haemothorax or flail chest. Those who do not die at the scene but who survive to reach a place of definitive treatment, may die days or weeks after the injury, succumbing to problems associated with the third phase of the trimodal distribution of death, such as sepsis or multiple organ failure, all problems which may be related to untreated oxygen or fluid deficits on scene. Minimising the delay to time-critical interventions, such as thoracocentesis or the removal of extra-dural haematoma, is vital and rapid transportation essential.

> The primary reasons for using an aircraft for transporting patients are clinical

The concept that aircraft should transport only specific types of critically ill patients has hindered the wider acceptance of aeromedical transport into health care for many years. Hospital clinicians and purchasers of health care tend to react negatively in response to learning about patients with non-life-threatening problems who have been airlifted. Generally speaking, however, aeromedical transport or transfer does not define a specific type or severity of disease where an aircraft should or should not be used, but rather depends on a number of patient and system-related factors.

As well as the degree of clinical urgency, logistical reasons also influence the choice of transport options. While cost remains an important factor, so too does the issue of time, particularly in relation to secondary transfer roles. Whereas ambulances are often used for the interhospital transfer of patients, this is not uncommonly associated with lengthy transfer times taking a front-line ambulance crew out of action often for periods extending over many hours. The use of aeromedical transport could, in some circumstances, resolve some of these difficulties.

In recent years, the availability and use of helicopters in transporting patients has increased. However, the capacity of those that are specifically designed for patient transport remains small. Other aircraft, such as those that may be provided by the armed forces, are rarely fitted for stretcher use and vary both in capacity and suitability. In general, helicopters are most suitable for use when road networks are disrupted, the terrain is unsuitable for ambulances or the time-critical nature of the patient's injuries gives cause for concern. In some circumstances, however, the disadvantages of helicopter use outweigh their advantages. These range from clinical factors, such as the specific nature of some injuries, e.g. heavily pregnant patients, to practical issues such as the lack of dedicated helicopter landing sites at hospitals, which would necessitate secondary ambulance journeys from distant landing sites, such as school playing fields.

> Helicopters may be considered when road transport is impractical and where air transportation delivers patients to definitive care more quickly

The choice of aircraft used in aeromedical transfers is based on a number of factors, including landing sites, the need for winching capability, the number of patients and crew required, as this may affect aircraft size, aircraft performance in terms of engine size and capability, the environment, wind speed, atmospheric pressure and temperature. The safe weight that can be carried varies from day to day. The weight of medical equipment required, the number of staff and the area the aircraft is required to cover and, therefore, the amount of fuel required, all affect the sort of aircraft used. Civilian helicopters may be hospital based or may be operated by fire, ambulance or police services, for the purpose of transportation directly to and from the accident scene or for urgent secondary transfers of high-dependency patients, or medical supplies or organs for donation. In relation to the accident situation, responsibility for dispatch and control inevitably lies with the ambulance service, which will have local protocol-driven dispatch systems designed to ensure that the helicopter is deployed appropriately.

Repatriation of the ill and injured

Increased commercialism, the affordability of flights and increased tourism have all resulted in an increased number of patients who are ill or injured far from home and who need to be repatriated. International travel is, for many, commonplace nowadays and most people give little thought to their potential health care needs at their destination of travel. Past estimations reveal that 1:500 travellers request some form of help and 1:10 000 requires emergency repatriation (Fairhurst, 1992).

Notably, the aircraft used in repatriation missions are different from those used in the situations referred to earlier. Ambulant patients may travel in conventional passenger aircraft and may only need some form of medical supervision with the provision of emergency drugs and equipment, for the possibility of any untoward problem occurring during the transfer. These patients may require wheelchair transportation but are otherwise treated as normal passengers. Patients with minor disabilities may be offered more seating or legroom. Stretchers take up the space of nine seats on conventional aircraft. Large aircraft dedicated to the air ambulance role, almost exclusively military, are usually converted so that the passenger seats are replaced by frames that can carry multiple stretchers stacked one on top of the other. Critical patients are difficult to manage on conventional passenger-carrying aircraft and airline medical authorities may refuse medical clearance for some types of patient. Privacy and dignity are not secured on these flights, with screening often all that is available. Dedicated air ambulances are used where possible to transfer those in need of 'intensive' care and those who might otherwise be refused carriage by commercial airlines. The repatriation of ill or injured visitors from abroad is an important role of fixed-wing aircraft. A full spectrum of medical care is provided for the patient recovering from a myocardial infarction who returns on a commercial flight with a nurse escort, to the multiply injured anaesthetised and ventilated patient transferred from a remote area in an underdeveloped country. Several UK companies provide such services, but finding suitably trained, experienced and qualified nurses who are able to leave at very short notice and be away for a number of days can be extremely difficult.

For the main part, only those nurses who have opted to work with repatriation organisations or insurance companies have familiarised themselves with the issues associated with alternative means of patient transportation and, in particular, aeromedical transportation. Given the advances in health care technology and the recent developments in emergency care, it would now appear both pertinent and appropriate for emergency and trauma nurses to take up the gauntlet and address this as yet untapped area of trauma nursing care.

SUMMARY

Trauma remains one of the leading causes of death and disability in the young. Advances in trauma, education, training and research, and increased understanding of the identification and treatment of life-threatening problems have contributed to the treatment and stabilisation of such patients, and to improved clinical outcomes. Recognition of the need to minimise delays both on scene and en route to definitive care has encouraged the development of increasingly sophisticated road ambulances, and the availability and use of aeromedical transport appropriate to the patient's needs. An understanding of the risks – both clinical and non-clinical – in the movement of trauma patients has led to an understanding of procedures to minimise related complications and difficulties, and the development of local policies and checklists to ensure effective communication between all those involved in the patient's journey. Advances in medical technology including telemedicine have further enhanced communication, access to appropriate expertise and thereby appropriate clinical decision-making remote from the original location. Through such measures and interventions, intensive trauma care can be brought to patients, instead of patients waiting to be taken to those with the expertise required to care for them. Trauma and pre-hospital nurses have a vital contribution to make to this arena.

References

British Standard BS EN 1789:2000 *Medical vehicles and their equipment – road ambulances.*

Fairhurst RJ. Health insurance for international travel. In: Dawood R (ed.) *Travellers' health*, 3rd edn. Oxford: Oxford University Press, 1992: 317–325.

Greaves I, Porter K. *Pre-hospital medicine: the principles and practice of immediate care.* London: Arnold, 1999

Hodgetts T, Mackway-Jones K. *Major incident medical management and support.* London: BMJ Publishing Group, 1995

Hodgetts T, McNeil I, Cooke M. *The pre-hospital emergency management master.* London: BMJ Publishing Group, 1995

Further reading

Advanced Life Support Group. *Pre-hospital paediatric life support*. London: BMJ Publishing Group, 1999

Advanced Life Support Group. *Advanced paediatric life support – the practical approach*. London: BMJ Publishing Group, 2000

American Academy of Pediatrics. *Pediatric education for pre-hospital providers*. Sudbury, MA: Jones and Bartlett, 2000

American College of Surgeons Committee on Trauma. *ATLS advanced trauma life support for doctors manual*. American College of Surgeons, 1997

Browner BD, Pollack AN, Gupton CL (eds). *American Academy of Orthopaedic Surgeons emergency care and transportation of the sick and injured*, 8th edn. Rosemont, IL: American Academy of Orthopaedic Surgeons, 2002

Caroline NL. *Emergency care in the streets*, Boston: Little Brown & Co., 1995

Driscoll PA, Gwinutt CL, LeDuc Jimmerson C, Goodall O. *Trauma resuscitation – the team approach*. London: Macmillan, 1993

Emergency Nurses Association. *TNCC Trauma nursing care course manual*. Park Ridge, IL: Emergency Nurses Association

Greaves I, Porter K. *Pre-hospital medicine: the principles and practice of immediate care*. London: Arnold, 1999

Harding RM, Mills FJ. *Aviation medicine*. London: BMJ Publishing Group, 1993

Hodgetts TJ, Porter C. *Major incident management system*. London: BMJ Books, 2002

Hodgetts T, McNeil I, Cooke M. *The pre-hospital emergency management master*. London: BMJ Publishing Group, 1995

Hodgetts T, Mackway-Jones K. *Major incident medical management and support*. London: BMJ Publishing Group, 1995

Holleran RS. *Emergency and flight nursing review*. St Louis: Mosby, 1996

Nicholson PJ. The helicopter in the immediate care environment. *Journal of the British Association of Immediate Care* 1988; 11: 54–57

Pre-Hospital Trauma Life Support Committee of the National Association of Emergency Medical Technicians in co-operation with the Committee on Trauma of the American College of Surgeons. *PHTLS basic and advanced pre-hospital trauma life support*. St Louis: Mosby Lifeline, 1990

Ramage C, Kee S, Bristow A. Interhospital transfer of the critically ill by helicopter. *British Journal of Hospital Medicine* 1990; 43: 147

Trunkey D. Towards optimal trauma care. *Archives of Emergency Medicine* 1985; 2: 181–195

Chapter 6

The management of major incidents and mass casualty situations

Iain McNeil and C. John Eaton

CHAPTER CONTENTS

INTRODUCTION

Major incidents and mass casualty situations have in recent years taken on a high profile within the UK. The rights and expectations of patients, and intense media attention and scrutiny of incidents, such as the 9–11 attact on New York, mean that the health response to large-scale incidents must be impeccable. We must be fully prepared to meet the difficult challenges of patient care in very hostile conditions under the spotlight of the world's media – not just after the event but from the very moment it happens. This chapter is aimed at addressing some of the issues about the management of the health service response to major incidents and mass casualty situations with the emphasis on the pre-hospital phase.

A BRIEF HISTORICAL PERSPECTIVE

The recorded origins of pre-hospital care date back to Roman times (Hines, 1998) when the Roman army organised medical care on the battlefield. This concept was later copied by the armies of Napoleon, where troops were triaged with a view to identifying those who would be most likely to return to the battlefield after treatment. Many of the current practices in major incident management were developed and refined during war. The Great War of 1914–1918, the Second World War and the war in Vietnam all saw major advances in mass casualty treatment.

In civilian spheres, there are many recorded major incidents in history that show that nothing changes. These include, for example, an incident in 1867 when the Royal Humane Society dealt with an incident where 200 people fell through ice on an ornamental lake in Regents Park (Neal, 1997). A train crash in 1857 on the North Kent Line illustrated that specialist equipment was required when rescuers had to extricate injured patients with the use of a single jack (*The Times*, 1857). In Sunderland during 1883, 183 children were killed following a crush in a theatre (Lambert, 1883), and in 1917 an explosives factory in Silverstone blew up, killing 73 and injuring 1000 (Morris, 1917). In 1884, Scotland Yard was bombed by the Fenians.

As transport systems become more complex, history shows that the incidence of disasters continues unabated: large aircraft are blown from the skies in terrorist attacks, such as in the Lockerbie crash, and an aircraft crashes on landing as at Kegworth. Terrorists continue their activities by blowing up civilian targets, and the rail system continues to fail and cause death as evidenced by crashes at Clapham, Purley, Hatfield and Berkshire. Nature also plays its tricks with floods and earthquakes occurring frequently. The list could go on, but it is clear that there are many parallels and similarities with disasters that have occurred in the past few years. It is sad to note that many of the lessons in public and transport safety have not really been heeded, and society continues to make the same mistakes.

During the latter half of the 20th century, many clinicians campaigned tirelessly to ensure that the health response to major incidents became more organised. In 1977, The British Association for Immediate Care Schemes (BASICS) was born after a 10-year struggle by Dr Ken Easton OBE and a number of other dedicated supporters; this organisation supports a network of volunteer doctors who assist the statutory emergency services at serious accidents and major incidents. Hospitals began to take more notice of their responsibilities in responding to serious incidents and developed the concept of mobile medical teams. Regrettably, there was no formal links between the National Health Service (NHS) and the volunteers working in BASICS across the UK, and the provision of support was piecemeal. There was no official guidance for those responding to major incidents and, in 1985, BASICS published the first edition of *Guide to major incident management*. It was not until 1990, when the Department of Health published its first comprehensive guidance for major incidents that there was clear advice available to those tasked with dealing with such problems. This advice has since been regularly updated.

Training for major incidents has also been rather haphazard with individual emergency services following their own internal training programmes; occasional interservice exercises improved the situation, but in health terms there was no way of training staff. BASICS ran a number of courses in conjunction with the Hammersmith Hospital and continues to do so, but these courses were infrequent and could not support the numbers wishing to be trained. In 1995, the Advanced Life Support Group (ALSG) developed the multidisciplinary Major Incident Medical Management and Support Course (MIMMS). This course has proved very successful and personnel from all areas of the emergency and military services have undertaken the training, which focuses specifically on those areas of interest to the health service.

DEFINITIONS

Major incidents are defined as those unexpected events, which overwhelm the normal resources available. In health terms, a major incident

> is said to exist when any occurrence presents a serious threat to the health community or the health service is disrupted or there are, or are likely to be, so many living casualties that special arrangements are necessary to deal with them. (MIMMS, 1995)

It should be noted that a major incident for one service is not necessarily a major incident for the others. For example, a large fire may be a major incident for the fire service but the health service could be unaffected. Additionally, a plane crash in which there are no survivors would not be regarded as a major incident for the hospitals, whilst the other emergency services may be overstretched.

Mass casualty situations are those situations, normally declared as a major incident, where the number and severity of the casualties overwhelms the ambulance and medical resources available for their treatment (Eaton, 1998).

Major incidents and mass casualty situations can be further classified into simple or compound incidents and compensated or uncompensated.

A *simple incident* is one in which the infrastructure surrounding the incident remains intact. Thus roads, rail links, hospitals and communication systems remain unaffected, and can be used in the response to the incident.

A *compound incident* is one in which the infrastructure is damaged. This is most often seen in natural disasters, such as earthquakes, when there is significant disruption to the inflow of resources, the outflow of the injured and the resources available within the area affected.

A *compensated incident* occurs when the problems caused by the incident can be dealt with using available resources that can be brought easily to the scene.

An *uncompensated incident* occurs when the resources available are inadequate to deal with the situation. This happens most often in mass casualty situations and in incidents occurring in remote areas.

Most major incidents in the UK are 'simple and compensated'.

Types of major incident

Major incidents can also be classified according to their cause, as either natural or man-made.

Natural disasters are the result of, for example, drought, famine, flooding, earthquake, forest fire or earthquakes. There are many of these that have been recorded in history with perhaps the worst occurring in China in 1887, when the Yellow River burst its banks killing 900 000 people with a further 1 million dying as a result of the famine and disease that ensued (MIMMS, 1995). In more recent times, the two earthquakes in Turkey in 1999 led to the deaths of approximately 18 000 people and in 2003 in Iran an earthquake took 50 000 lives (Figure 6.1).

Man-made disasters are very diverse in their aetiology. They may be deliberate, as in terrorist activity, or accidental, as in a train crash. They occur when large numbers of people are present

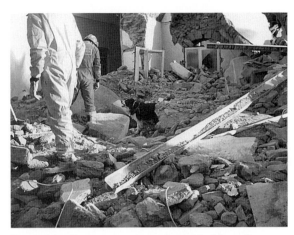

Figure 6.1   Rescuers search a collapsed building after an earthquake in Iran, 2003.

for any given activity, such as leisure, sports, work or travel.

Large leisure and sports venues, most of which are classed as mass gatherings, have resulted in many deaths in recent decades. The fire at Bradford City football ground (1989), a crush at a football match in South Africa (2000), echoing similar disasters in Ibrox, Glasgow (1971), Brussels (1985) and Hillsborough (1989), show the potential for pleasure to turn to disaster in moments.

Transport disasters resulting in large numbers of deaths happen approximately three to four times a year in the UK. Most are the result of train or aircraft crashes, although coach crashes also feature in the statistics. No matter what mode of transport is used, there is scope for disaster – disasters that are repeated through history. The 'safest ship ever designed', the *Titanic*, sank in 1912, the *Herald of Free Enterprise* sank in 1987, whilst the passengers were on a shopping day trip, and in 1994, a ferry sank killing 852, whilst travelling the short distance between Sweden and Finland. Aircraft continue to fall from the sky, either through accident as in the Kegworth crash of 1989, in the Concorde crash in Paris of 2000, or terrorist activity as in the bombing of a fully laden Boeing 747 over Lockerbie in 1988. Trains, despite much work on passenger and system safety measures, continue to cause significant numbers of deaths.

Industrial incidents are usually the result of a foreseeable risk. These include as examples explosions in chemical plants (Bhopal 1984), fires on oilrigs (Piper Alpha 1988), explosions in fireworks factories (China and Holland 2000). Nuclear plants also pose a significant risk as evidenced by the Chernobyl disaster in Russia in 1986 when 40 000 residents were exposed to very high levels of radiation, the effects of which will be felt for at least two generations.

Terrorist activity in the UK is not a new phenomenon; with the first IRA bombing in the UK occurring in 1867 and the most recent being in Ealing in August 2001, the risk is well known to most in the country.

PREPARATION FOR A MAJOR INCIDENT RESPONSE

Adequate preparation is one of the most important elements of major incident management. There are three main areas of preparation: planning, training and equipment.

Planning

Every agency involved in major incidents should have plans for such eventualities. These plans should be regularly tested and reviewed. The Department of Health appoints health emergency planning advisers, who are responsible for ensuring that the health services in their area are ready to respond. Additionally the Department of Health has published a series of guidelines. These include HC (90) 25, HSG (92) 35 and 'Emergency planning in the NHS: health service arrangements for dealing with major incidents' [EL (96) 79].

It is important that any planning is undertaken in conjunction with all the other services and providers that might potentially respond alongside your own so that there is a fully integrated plan and response. Plans should build on everyday processes so that those involved work in an area in which they are familiar rather than thrusting them suddenly into new and unfamiliar roles in a crisis.

> To fail to plan is to plan to fail.
> Planning and preparation prevent particularly poor performance

All hospitals equipped to receive casualties must be capable of providing a mobile medical team and must have plans that detail the required actions of key individuals within the hospital. Ambulance services must also have detailed plans with clear guidance for all involved.

Training

It is essential that all those involved in the provision of major incident responses be appropriately trained to fulfil their roles either in hospital or at the scene. This should include theoretical instruction as provided by the ALSG with their MIMMS course or BASICS. Practical training should also be undertaken. This may consist of tabletop exercises, a paper exercise or fully integrated simulations of major incidents (Figure 6.2).

All hospitals are expected to test their plans on an annual basis. Many high-risk sites are expected to test their plans routinely, alongside the statutory emergency and health services. Major airports are required to have a full interservice simulation every 2 years; this is observed by the licensing authorities of the airfield and, if performance is not satisfactory, the airport could be shut down until the services expected are in place.

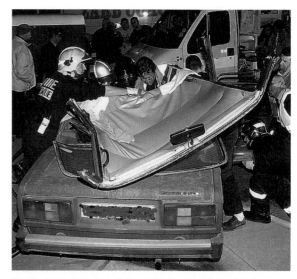

Figure 6.2 Exercises. It is normally possible to become involved in individual small-scale exercises run by the various emergency services; this is invaluable preparation for a full-scale incident.

Box 6.1   Equipment required at major incidents

- Personal protective equipment
- Communications equipment
- Medical equipment
- Reference equipment
- Recording equipment
- Personal supplies, e.g. food/drink

Equipment

It is essential that any team deployed to the scene of a major incident be properly equipped. The equipment that should be provided is listed in Box 6.1.

Personal protective equipment should include a high-visibility jacket and overtrousers, a safety helmet, protective footwear and gloves

Communications equipment should be in the form of a hand-held radio. Any radio must be capable of communicating with the local ambulance service on normal 'domestic channels' and on the 'emergency reserve channel' (ERC). This will ensure that communications are carried out on a common network and that all messages will be recorded. Mobile phones may be of limited use; however, it is unlikely that they will be used, as they pose a number of problems: all conversations are unrecorded as are radio messages and thus you will have no record of the call; it is quite possible that no lines will be available as the cells are often blocked by the press; and also communications may become uncoordinated if a large number of people are using phones to contact others.

Medical equipment should be appropriate to the needs of the casualties and the nature of the incident. All equipment should be compatible with the local ambulance service and should augment rather than duplicate the equipment carried by ambulances.

Reference equipment should include maps of the local area and any identified high-risk sites, such as airports or chemical plants. It would also be useful to have available the location and contact details of specialist centres and specialist advisors (such as the radiation advisor).

Recording equipment should include a means of keeping a log of your actions and messages –

a large notebook would suffice. In addition, a camera may be of use to photograph the scene or entrapped patients. Dictaphones can also be used, but there can be problems with ambient noise levels at an incident and they are therefore not always useful. Adequate numbers of patient report forms and triage cards are also required. You should remember that all records you make, even if written on the back of a scrap of an old envelope, are legal documents and must be kept in their original form for the enquiry.

Personal supplies should include some food and drink, some money, and spare and warm clothing. Additional items might include torches, light sticks, spare pens and spare batteries for electrical equipment. You will not be able to rely on others to provide such items and you should have them with you.

All equipment to be used at a major incident should be routinely checked. It is essential that all the equipment brought to the scene is serviceable and safe, and that all the drugs are within their shelf life.

THE ROLE OF THE STATUTORY EMERGENCY SERVICES

At any major incident, the statutory emergency services, which have responsibilities to respond that are laid down in law, will be in attendance. These include the police, fire service and ambulance service. It is essential that anyone involved in providing pre-hospital medical care is fully conversant with the roles and responsibilities of these services. Additionally, they must ensure that they are fully integrated within the teams attending.

Depending upon the nature and location of the incident, other agencies may be involved; these include the coastguard, local authorities, voluntary services, hospital teams and immediate care schemes. Additionally, the military may be on scene. Other services, such as railway companies, gas and electricity, airports authorities and the environment agency may also have a vital role to play in the management of any major incident. All these organisations must work closely with the statutory services.

In general, the police are responsible for the overall command of the scene and will often treat the incident site as a scene of crime. It is thus important that any health workers appreciate this fact and act accordingly to protect forensic evidence when possible. The police have specific responsibilities to protect property and safeguard life, and they must uphold the law. Additionally, they must facilitate the working of the other statutory services and manage a coordinated group of senior officers from the services on scene. They will work with the coroner and, in the early stages, will provide the role of coroner's officer. The police will set up a casualty bureau, which provides information to relatives and the public. They are also responsible for the safe custody of the dead at mortuary facilities. The police are responsible for liaising with the media.

The fire service leads the rescue and extrication processes as well as dealing with any inherent hazards, such as chemicals or fire. They are also expected to provide specialist rescue equipment, such as lifting gear, lighting and decontamination equipment. They are expected to ensure the safety of all other services within the incident area and deal with any hazards present. They also provide access to specialist advice for chemical and radiation incidents.

The ambulance service has a duty to provide clinical care to casualties and to transport them to a suitable care facility. They are also expected to decide upon the need for medical support from hospital teams, the need for a medical incident officer and to transport them to the scene, if required. They are also expected to provide inter-hospital transfers as required. Additionally, they must provide the logistical support and communication systems for the health care resources at the scene.

THE ROLE OF THE MEDICAL SERVICES IN THE PRE-HOSPITAL ARENA

Medical services will only be called to the scene of an incident if the ambulance service requires assistance at the scene. This decision is usually determined by the number, severity and type of the expected injuries. Their role is to support the ambulance incident officer (AIO) in the command and control of the incident, and to provide triage and treatment for the casualties. The source if this

help can be from a pre-hospital medical team or from a mobile medical team from a hospital.

Whatever the source of the teams on scene, the responsibilities are the same. The senior doctor on scene assumes legal responsibility for the medical treatment of the injured. The teams will primarily provide triage and treatment, but may also provide confirmation of death. They will work closely with the ambulance service and will liaise with receiving hospitals. They may also be expected to provide medical care to the other rescuers on scene and, if required, may advise the police on forensic matters.

Pre-hospital medical teams are usually part of BASICS. They are in the main made up of doctors but, increasingly, nurses are developing an independent operational role within such schemes. The members of the schemes are all specially trained and experienced in pre-hospital emergency care, and regularly work with the other services at 'routine' incidents. It is likely that, where they are available, they will provide the primary medical support in the event of a major incident.

Mobile medical teams (MMTs) are teams sent from hospitals to support the ambulance service at the scene. They are not commonly dispatched in areas where BASICS schemes are present and tend to provide support where either BASICS is unavailable or is overwhelmed by the size of the incident.

It is essential that MMTs are not sent from a hospital that is likely to receive casualties from the incident. To do so would compromise the working of that hospital. It is, therefore, likely that the MMT will be required to travel some distance and their attendance is often delayed. There are other problems associated with MMTs. These include lack of experience in the pre-hospital environment and the lack of a cohesive team used to working together, as there is no guarantee of who will be available at any time. Generally MMTs will have a surgeon, an anaesthetist and a number of nurses. They are, however, very useful when specific tasks, such as surgical procedures, are required.

Mobile medical teams should not be deployed from a hospital receiving casualties from the incident

Some hospitals provide a routine response to pre-determined needs, for example, Frimley Park Hospital in Surrey will provide a team of doctors and nurses to give care and support in the survivor reception centre for Gatwick Airport. This process is regularly exercised.

DECLARING A MAJOR INCIDENT

In health terms, anyone can declare a major incident. In other services, it is often only a senior officer who can do so. When declaring a major incident, it should be done via ambulance control. They will require information about the incident and this is best given by following the mnemonic 'METHANE' (Box 6.2).

The police and fire service may use another mnemonic 'CHALET', which imparts the same information in a different order.

It should be remembered that a major incident might be declared for reasons other than a mass casualty disaster. For example, flooding, as happened in the winter of 2000/2001, caused widespread disruption to ambulance services and many declared major incidents because of the extraordinary arrangements that they had to put in place to deal with the problems.

MAJOR INCIDENT MANAGEMENT

The management of any major incident should be carried out according to a few basic principles. These principles, first propounded on early MIMMS courses, and later developed and expanded by ALSG, have become international standards for major incident management and have been adopted by NATO and a number of foreign countries. The principles (Box 6.3) can be regarded as being as important as the 'ABC' of resuscitation. The CSCATTT of major incident management should be adhered to whenever you are involved. It provides a clear structure upon which to base your decisions and will help you through a difficult situation.

COMMAND AND CONTROL

The successful management of a major incident relies totally on proper command and control by those who know their own role and that of the teams working with them. Command and control must be established early in the incident and strict discipline must be applied. There is no place for those who will not carry out instructions without argument, or those who will not adhere to the command structure and process.

Interservice coordination is essential, and it is important that the senior officers on scene cooperate and communicate at all times. The relationship between the key senior officers, the police incident officer (PIO), the fire incident officer (FIO), the ambulance incident officer (AIO) and the medical incident officer (MIO), is shown in Figure 6.3.

The hierarchy of command and control

A common system of nomenclature for senior officers involved in the management of major incidents has been devised to help identify the status, role and service of those people speaking over radio systems, or delivering command and control at the scene.

Box 6.2 Information required when declaring a major incident

M	Major incident declared (or stand by), with time and your name
E	Exact location of the incident
T	Type of incident
H	Hazards on scene
A	Access to incident, i.e. route/road/rendezvous point
N	Number of possible casualties
E	Emergency services on scene and required

Box 6.3 The principles of major incident management

- Command and control
- Safety
- Communication
- Assessment
- Triage
- Treatment
- Transport

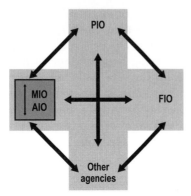

Figure 6.3 Key incident officer relationships. PIO, police incident officer; FIO, fire incident officer; AIO, ambulance incident officer; MIO, medical incident officer.

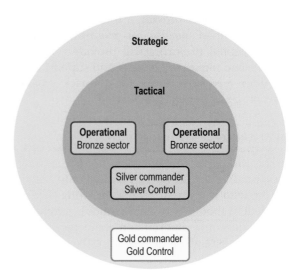

Figure 6.4 The tiers of command.

In each service there are officers with designations of 'gold', 'silver' and 'bronze'. The status can be used as a prefix to the role to identify an individual at a major incident scene (e.g. bronze triage officer would be the triage officer in the forward area of the incident). These tiers of command are depicted in Figure 6.4.

'*Gold*' denotes the most senior level of command. This function is often carried out from a location remote from the incident site at 'gold control', at which the senior 'gold commanders' congregate. The functions are in the main strategic and advisory.

'*Silver*' denotes the most senior commanders/incident officers present at the scene. These people have the responsibility for tactical management of the whole scene of the incident. The ambulance incident officer will be denoted as 'silver medic' and will operate a silver control from the site. The medical incident officer is denoted as 'silver doctor'.

'*Bronze*' officers are those with specific operational roles within the scene of the incident, for example, 'bronze loading' is the ambulance service officer with responsibility for loading ambulances with patients and despatching them to hospitals.

It is essential that those personnel tasked with management roles do not get involved in treating patients, as they will be unable to carry out their key function, if distracted by other matters.

The chain of command

Each service will appoint officers to key functions depending upon their role. Each service will have a clearly identified chain of command from the appointed incident officer, down through the various operational officers to the staff at the scene of the incident. All interservice liaison should be carried out through the proper chain of command. Thus, should firefighters need help with a patient, they should pass that request up to their own senior officer, who will in turn discuss the priorities with the AIO. The AIO may then deploy personnel to assist and advise them to do so through his or her own chain of command. This process may seem cumbersome to many used to working in hospitals; however, it is designed to ensure that scarce resources and manpower are deployed to the best effect for the greatest number of casualties, rather than concentrating significant resources on a single specific individual. Additionally, it ensures that the senior officer knows exactly who is doing what and where. If staff were to be redeployed without going through this process, chaos would soon reign.

The ambulance service will, when resources allow, appoint the following 'point' officers:

● gold commander – often the chief ambulance officer

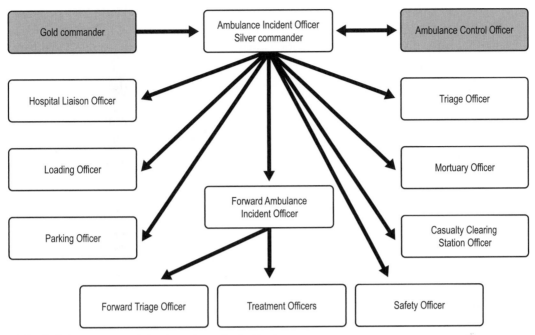

Figure 6.5 Ambulance command structure at a major incident.

- silver commander – the ambulance incident officer and the medical incident officer
- bronze officers to the following key positions:
  - forward ambulance incident officer
  - forward (primary) triage
  - triage
  - casualty clearing station
  - parking point
  - loading point
  - safety
  - hospital liaison officer.

These positions, outlined in Figure 6.5, may be replicated by medical staff attending the scene or, more likely, when resources are scarce, medical staff may be appointed in the clinical areas of triage and treatment instead of ambulance staff.

Responsibilities of senior officers in the medical services at a major incident scene

The ambulance incident officer has the overall responsibility for the work of the ambulances service at the scene. In the very early stages, this role will be carried out by the attendant of the first ambulance that arrives on the scene. He or she is responsible for establishing liaison with the other services on scene and ensuring that the ambulance service is responding appropriately. As more senior and appropriately trained personnel arrive, the responsibility will be passed up the chain of command. It is likely that an officer of middle or senior rank will ultimately fulfil the role.

The AIO will liaise very closely with his medical counterpart, the medical incident officer, at all times. Indeed, they should be almost inseparable throughout the duration of the incident. All decisions should be made in consultation with their counterparts.

The forward ambulance incident officer (FAIO) is responsible for the command of personnel within the scene or a designated bronze sector. He will liaise closely with the Forward Medical Incident Officer (FMIO) should one be appointed. The FAIO and FMIO are essentially the eyes and ears of the incident officers right up at the sharp end of the incident. These officers do not have a treatment role.

The (primary) triage officer is either an ambulance service officer or paramedic or a doctor. His or her role is to carry out the triage sieve (see later) on all casualties before they are treated in the casualty clearing (or treatment) station (CCS). This role will be carried out either within the scene itself or at the front entrance to the CCS, the aim of which is to establish the early treatment priorities of casualties; occasionally, it is carried out at both locations.

The casualty clearing station officer (CCSO) is responsible for the smooth running of the CCS. He or she may be a member of ambulance staff initially but is likely to be replaced by a doctor once enough resources are available. The CCSO is responsible for overseeing the treatment of all casualties and for retriaging them using the triage sort (see later) with a view to establishing evacuation priorities. He or she will liaise with the AIO/MIO and loading officer.

The ambulance loading officer (ALO) is responsible for ensuring that casualties are dispatched to the most appropriate hospital in as short a time as possible. The ALO will liaise with the AIO and CCSO.

The ambulance parking officer (APO) is responsible for marshalling all the transport at a predetermined parking point and ensuring that the ALO has a steady supply of vehicles to take casualties to hospital.

The ambulance safety officer (ASO) is responsible for overseeing, on behalf of the AIO, all aspects of safety relating to the health care response. This will include liaison with the fire service safety officer and all the senior incident officers. The ASO is responsible for ensuring that the safety of the working environment is as good as it can be, and for making sure all health care rescuers are suitably clothed with personal protective equipment.

A number of *treatment officers/doctors* will be appointed to carry out the hands-on treatment of casualties at the CCS. Occasionally, they will be sent forward into the scene to deal with entrapped casualties that have been identified to need additional clinical skills or advice in their management.

The ambulance control officer (ACO) is the communication officer in charge of providing the communications at the scene. He or she will do this in liaison with the ambulance control (usually at headquarters), the other emergency services and the AIO. The ACO is also responsible for ensuring that a log of all messages passed to and from those at the incident is kept.

All of the above 'point officers' are responsible for maintaining a log of their key decisions and actions and all messages that they pass to others.

Organisation at the scene

The overall organisation of the scene, especially in the early stages, is of paramount importance if the incident is to be effectively managed. Therefore, it is important that everyone addresses the issues using the same concepts about how the site should be organised.

The incident site may spread over a considerable area, especially in rail and aircraft accidents, and it may be necessary to set up a number of 'bronze operational sectors', each with its own bronze command structure that in turn report to a single silver command.

There are a number of basic organisational entities of which all staff responding to an incident must be aware. These are listed below.

- *Rendezvous point* – this is the area, often manned by the police and remote from the actual incident, where all emergency personnel and their vehicles are assembled, logged and briefed prior to their being sent forward to the scene itself. Large high-risk sites, such as airports, will have a number of pre-determined rendezvous points.
- *Outer cordon* – this is a cordon, set up by the police, around the whole of the incident. Its purpose is to prevent unauthorised persons gaining access to the incident and to optimise the free movement of the emergency services in the area.
- *Inner cordon* – this is a cordon that surrounds the immediate vicinity of the incident; it is often manned by the fire service. Its purpose is to prevent unauthorised entry to the site. It acts as an additional safety measure, as all emergency personnel are logged in and out of the site. Thus, the authorities know exactly how many people are working within the scene.
- *Incident control point* – this is the central area where all the control vehicles are usually situated. The incident officers are also in this area. It is often some distance from the actual incident.

- *Ambulance control point* – this is the ambulance control vehicle. In the early stages, it may be a single ambulance but, in time, it will be replaced by a purpose-built control unit. It is usually based at the incident control point.
- *Ambulance parking point* – this is the place where all the available ambulances are parked prior to loading patients.
- *Triage point* – this is a single point at which all triage is carried out. All casualties must pass through this point.
- *Casualty clearing station* – this is an area set up specifically for the treatment of the casualties. It may be a building or a tent, but may also just be a patch of ground where casualties can be conveniently brought.
- *Loading point* – the point at which all casualties are loaded on to an ambulance. It is situated beside the casualty clearing station.
- *Body holding area* – this is a place where those bodies that are inadvertently removed from the scene, or those who die prior to transportation, are taken for temporary safekeeping. Those who are found dead within the scene should not be removed from their resting place.
- *Temporary mortuary* – this is a building, which is adapted for use as a temporary mortuary. Most counties have a number of pre-determined sites that will be used; however, in some situations, a building near the incident may be used. It is here where the forensic examinations will take place.
- *Survivor reception centre* – this is a place, usually well away from the scene, where survivors are taken for minor first aid, documentation and interview by the police. This is often a leisure centre or sports centre where suitable facilities are available. Some airports have specific lounge areas that will be used for this purpose.
- *Hospital liaison* – this takes place continually between relevant incident officers at the scene, but if manpower permits, ambulance services will send a liaison officer direct to accident and emergency (A&E) departments to act as a go-between and to ensure communication is maintained.

The schematic diagram in Figure 6.6 shows how the various points are linked with an ambulance transport circuit.

SAFETY AT THE SCENE

The safety of the personnel and the scene itself should be considered in the following order – self, scene, then the casualties. No rescuers should ever be exposed to unnecessary risk and become casualties themselves.

Safety is the overall responsibility of the fire service. It is they who will set up the inner safety cordon and control access to the site. The fire service will liaise closely with the individual who is designated by the AIO as safety officer for the ambulance and medical services.

The ambulance and medical incident officers are responsible for overseeing the welfare of their staff and must be aware of the potential for exhaustion, environmental hazards, scene hazards, the need for rest and recuperation, and food and drink.

It is essential that all staff attending a major incident are provided with appropriate personal protective equipment (PPE). The essential items have been highlighted above. PPE should include high-visibility jacket, helmet and protective footwear. Appointed officers should wear suitable identification denoting their role at the scene. The safety officer will deny access to anyone not wearing adequate clothing.

> Personal protective equipment must be worn at all times

Anyone entering the scene of the incident must be briefed as to the hazards they might expect to encounter. These could include chemicals, sewerage, glass, jagged metal, hot surfaces and fluids. It is unlikely that they will encounter fire, as the fire service will not allow access to the site whilst there is still a significant risk.

Falling masonry and unstable structures are of considerable concern, as rescuers may be required to enter such structures to get to casualties, especially in earthquake situations. Aftershocks or the heavy lifting equipment used in the rescue process may dislodge unstable structures and bring them down on rescuers.

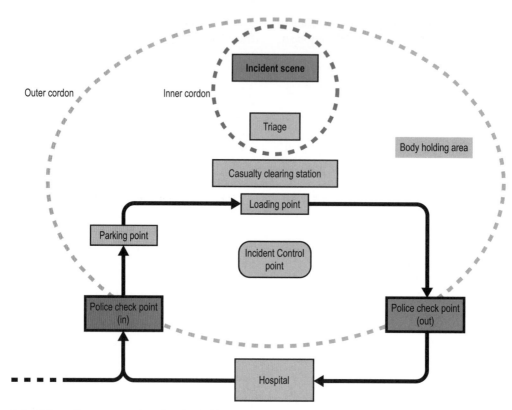

Figure 6.6   Schematic representation of major incident scene.

On railway lines, rescuers should be aware of the high voltage 'third rail' or overhead cables. No one should approach an electrified railway line until it is confirmed that the power has been turned off, and even then great care should be taken not to touch any electrical parts, as the charge can be stored for some time. Remember also that electric charges can arc a considerable distance, especially in a wet environment. Additional hazards on railway lines include 'coasting locomotives', whose power has been cut but which take a considerable distance to stop, and diesels on an electric line!

In suspected terrorist incidents, where bombs have been placed, rescuers should be aware of the potential for a 'secondary device'. A secondary device is often placed at a point where rescuers and survivors might congregate after an initial blast, thus nobody should approach a scene of a bomb blast until the police have given permission. Additionally, rescuers should not use radio and mobile phones within the vicinity of a bomb lest the signals set off the bomb.

On the roads and railways, there are huge numbers of chemical tankers and mixed chemical loads. Potential rescuers should be familiar with the various types of hazard warning signs on such vehicles, such as the 'HAZCHEM' sign or the 'KEMLER CODE' signs. These signs will provide enough information to the emergency services to tell whether it is safe to approach or not. If in doubt, stay clear.

All those who enter the scene of an incident must be aware of the evacuation signal. This is often a whistle blown repeatedly. If the evacuation signal is heard, all rescuers must immediately leave the scene even if this means leaving live casualties behind.

All personnel likely to attend an incident in the pre-hospital setting should make themselves familiar with the risks they face. This can best be done by reading the book *Safety at scene* (Calland, 2000).

COMMUNICATIONS

The key to effective command and control of a major incident is good communications. The ambulance service will usually provide communications for the medical services, but where that is not the case, all communications provided by the medical teams must be compatible with those of the ambulance service. There are a number of means of communications that might be used at a major incident (Box 6.4).

It is essential that the emergency services are able to communicate within their own organisation, with other services on scene and with agencies remote from the scene. Thus, the AIO on scene may need to communicate with, for example:

- the gold command centre
- the police
- the fire service
- all its personnel on site
- immediate care schemes
- the receiving hospitals
- the survivor reception centre
- the local authority
- specialist centres
- other ambulance services
- the health authority.

It can be seen, therefore, that the communications systems can be very complex. They need to be robust, regularly tested and strict discipline in their use must be maintained at all times.

Radio communications are the most often used method; however, problems arise as each statutory service is not normally able to communicate

on the other's channels. There is a nationally agreed radio channel, channel 69, which can be used by all services; however, the infrastructure for this is extremely expensive and there are few places in the UK where it is available. The ambulance service does have one common channel that is used by all other ambulance services, the emergency reserve channel. This is often used in the early stages of an incident, but it soon becomes overloaded with radio traffic, thus other channels are brought into play.

Mobile phones are in theory very useful, but this is not borne out in practice. Firstly, reception is variable and cannot be relied upon and, secondly, it is unlikely that you will be able to get a line, as the media often swamp the systems as soon as they know a major incident has occurred. It is possible to use a system known as access overload control (ACCOLC) on the Vodaphone network. This blocks out all but those authorised by the Home Office. It is rarely used, as it is very expensive and cannot block out those who are already on the network in the process of making a call. Additionally, it is difficult to maintain discipline in the chain of command, if communications do not go through the ambulance control unit.

> All communications must go via the ambulance control point

Radio networks get very busy at major incidents. It is, therefore, very important that only essential messages are passed over the air, and those messages should be short, succinct and to the point. Radio discipline is important: only one person can speak at a time and it is possible that whilst you are speaking you are preventing a more important message being passed.

In the event that radio communications are not available, 'runners' can be used to pass messages between services or officers. Any message passed via a runner should be written down – word of mouth is notoriously unreliable. Any reply to a message should similarly be written down.

ASSESSMENT OF THE SCENE

Assessment of the scene is a vital part of the command and control function. It begins as soon as the first responders arrive on the scene and should go on throughout the time the incident is running.

The key elements of assessment include the element of the 'METHANE' report, as detailed earlier. As the incident unfolds, the incident officers will continually reassess the needs of the rescuers and casualties. Of particular importance is the assessment of the need for additional support and specialist facilities. This is often a role of the gold commanders, who may be required to arrange for access to specialist facilities many miles away. Incident officers must be constantly aware of the changing needs of the casualties and the rescuers, and any changes in environmental conditions.

From the medical point of view, the key areas that require constant monitoring are the triage, treatment and transport requirements.

TRIAGE AT THE SCENE

Triage, from the French word 'triager' (to sort), is the process carried out at the scene to identify casualty's needs for treatment and evacuation to hospital. The overriding principle of triage in a major incident or mass casualty situation is 'that the needs of the many outweigh the needs of the few'. Additionally, it is a process aimed at ensuring that the casualties reach the right hospital in an appropriate time frame for definitive care.

> Triage is a dynamic process – casualties should be frequently retriaged and constantly reassessed

Triage begins at the incident scene where *primary triage* is carried out. This is done by any of the rescuers present within the incident site, and on occasions a 'primary triage officer' may be appointed specifically to carry out this role. This activity is carried out before any treatment is commenced. Primary triage may also be carried out at the entrance to the casualty clearing station. Primary triage is often referred to as the *triage sieve* and consists of a rapid assessment of airway, breathing and circulation. The primary aim of the sieve is to allocate a triage category and thus a treatment priority to casualties.

Table 6.1 Triage categories

Priority	Triage label colour	Sieve treatment priority	Sort TRTS
P1	Red	Immediate	1–10
P2	Yellow	Urgent	11
P3	Green	Delayed	12
P4	White	Dead	0
P3E	Green with red corners	Expectant	1–10

TRTS, triage revised trauma score.

A more selective assessment of the casualties is carried out within the casualty clearing station. This is often known as *secondary triage* or the *triage sort,* and is based upon the triage revised trauma score (TRTS). Its purpose is to identify those in most need of evacuation.

The triage categories of the sieve and sort are shown in Table 6.1, and listed below.

- *Immediate priority casualties (P1)* are those requiring immediate life-saving procedures.
- *Urgent priority casualties (P2)* are those who require definitive treatment (often surgical) within 4–6 hours.
- *Delayed priority casualties (P3)* are those whose injuries do not require urgent treatment, or those who are involved in an incident but are uninjured.
- *Dead casualties (P4)* are those who die at the scene.
- *Expectant casualties (P3E)* are those whose injuries are so severe that they are expected to die no matter how much treatment they receive. This category is rarely used and should usually be reserved for incidents that are both compound and uncompensated. In the event that there is a need to use the P3E category, all incident officers at gold and silver level should be involved in making the decision.

It is essential that all casualties are regularly reassessed as their condition may deteriorate or improve depending upon their injuries. For example, a patient with internal haemorrhage may initially present as walking and be categorised as P3, but as the bleeding progresses and

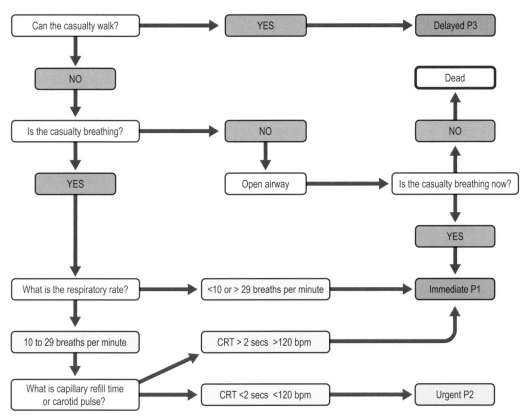

Figure 6.7 The triage sieve.

they become shocked, they may collapse and be retriaged as P1.

The triage sieve is outlined in Figure 6.7.

Triage labelling

Once casualties have been triaged, they will be labelled with a coloured label or marker as denoted in Table 6.1 and Figure 6.7. This allows rescuers to identify the casualties' needs at a glance. Triage labels also have space for recording treatment and observations, and are part of the clinical record of each casualty. There are a number of different systems in use within the UK, but all adhere to the principles of colouring and categorisation as detailed above.

The dead

Where possible, the bodies of the dead should be left *in situ*, to aid the police in any forensic investigation. Where possible, a doctor will be allocated to identify the dead and label them accordingly within the scene. This must be done in the presence of a police officer whose identification number must be put on the triage label along with the date, time and name of the doctor confirming death. This is a vital role, as it is important that the dead are quickly identified, so that non-medical rescuers do not waste valuable resources trying to obtain treatment for casualties who are already known to be dead.

> The dead should in left *in situ* whenever possible

Paediatric triage variations

It will be seen that the triage sieve outlined above will triage paediatric casualties into a high level of category even when their vital signs are in fact normal. This problem can be dealt with by using a number of commercially available triage tapes (akin to the Broslow Tape©), which are available for use in paediatric resuscitation.

TREATMENT AT THE SCENE

The medical and ambulance services at the scene have the primary responsibility for the treatment of the casualties. It is true, however, that many others will become involved in treating patients, especially in the early stages when medical resources are scarce.

Initially, treatment will be provided by bystanders and survivors of the incident, and with first aid treatment being provided by the early arrivals from the emergency services. As the resources build up, the treatment available will grow in capacity and complexity until such time as a casualty clearing station is established and evacuation to hospital is possible.

Treatment can be carried out within the area of the incident, especially if casualties are trapped and also at the casualty clearing station. Only personnel tasked with the specific responsibility of treatment should become involved; thus, the triage officer or a forward medical incident officer should not actually lay hands on a patient, as they will compromise their ability to carry out their command role if they do.

It must be emphasised that the primary aim of any treatment at the scene is to allow the patient to reach the most appropriate hospital safely; it is not to restore the patient to full health. The treatment given will initially depend on the triage priority allocated to the casualty and the nature of the problem presented. A patient with airway problems will require much faster and intensive treatment than someone with, say, a fractured tibia.

A schematic representation of a casualty clearing station is shown in Figure 6.8.

It will be noted that *all* casualties brought from the incident site *must* go through the primary triage sieve process and then a triage sort at the CCS. It is likely that those with minor injuries or no injuries at all will be transported away from the scene very quickly, whereas those with injuries may require 'stabilisation' within the CCS.

Casualties must not be loaded direct from the scene on to transport

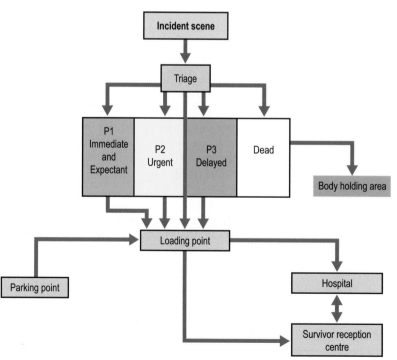

Figure 6.8 Schematic diagram of a casualty clearing station and patient flows.

The scope of treatment is usually confined to ensuring adequacy of the airway, breathing and circulation. The procedures may include basic life support manoeuvres and advanced life support interventions, such as intubation, cannulation and infusion and drug administration, and from time to time advanced interventions, such as needle thoracocentesis, needle cricothyrotomy and intra-osseous infusions, may be required. Additionally, as part of the transport process, casualties will be 'packaged' for transport, if their injuries demand it; thus, a cervical collar and full spine immobi-lisation may be applied, or splintage of fractures. Very occasionally, advanced surgical interventions, such as amputation, are required at the scene.

TRANSPORT

Transport is the responsibility of the ambulance service. Close attention must be paid to the transport needs of patients so that they are taken to the most appropriate hospital in a timely fashion. The structure of the transportation process has been shown in Figures 6.6 and 6.8 above.

The order in which casualties are evacuated should, where possible, be determined by the triage priority following the triage sieve in the CCS. The availability and capacity of vehicles suitable for transport may lead the officer in charge of the CCS and the loading officer to evacuate less severe casualties in, say, a minibus, before more serious casualties are taken in a traditional ambulance. Additionally, the avail-ability of suitably qualified staff to accompany seriously ill casualties may affect the timing of evacuation.

The destination hospital is in the main chosen by the loading officer, although he or she will be in constant contact with the AIO and MIO to determine the capacity of receiving hospitals. If possible, the loading officer will ensure that those casualties requiring specialist treatment (e.g. burns or neurosurgery) are taken directly to hospitals with those facilities. If this is not possible, then the casualties should be taken to a general hospital and the potential need for secondary transport logged with ambulance control so that it can be included in their plans.

The loading officer will, where possible, ensure that the distribution of casualties is spread across a number of hospitals, ensuring that no given A&E department is swamped with more patients that it can cope with. This requires considerable skill and constant liaison with the incident officers and the receiving hospitals.

Types of transportation

There are a number of transport modes available to the emergency services. These are listed in Box 6.5.

The best mode of transport for casualties is an emergency ambulance, as these vehicles are specifically designed and equipped for the safe transport of seriously ill patients. However, in a major incident, the number of casualties will usually outnumber the available ambulances and so other methods may need to be used. These may include patient transport ambulances, which are of a lower specification than emergency ambulances, cars and minibuses.

It may be possible to use public transport vehicles, such as coaches, buses and taxis; these are of particular value in taking uninjured casualties to a survivor reception centre or those with very minor injuries to a hospital some distance from the incident, thus ensuring that more local hospitals are kept clear for the more seriously injured. In the event that an incident occurs in an area that is not well served with hospitals, it is possible that the rail network could be used to distribute large numbers to hospitals many miles away.

Public transport is often chosen by survivors of major incidents; they have been known to self-evacuate to hospital even before the emergency services have arrived on scene, as occurred at the now infamous Clapham rail crash.

Box 6.5   Types of transport in a major incident

- Emergency ambulance
- Patient transport ambulance
- Car
- Minibus
- Public transport – bus/taxi/railway
- Helicopter – air ambulance, military, civilian

Helicopters, especially air ambulances, are becoming increasingly available. Air ambulance helicopters can, however, only transport one casualty at a time, so their use may be limited in mass casualty situations. They are, however, invaluable when access to the site is difficult owing to road problems or difficult terrain. Military helicopters are capable of carrying more than one casualty, but they are not designed for medical evacuation and so pose problems in securing casualties on stretchers and keeping them warm. The best use of helicopters is perhaps in providing direct transport to a distant specialist centre and in due course for secondary transfers between hospitals.

Civilian helicopters are not recommended as a suitable method of transporting casualties, although they could be used to allow senior officers to gain a bird's-eye view of the incident site.

THE HOSPITAL ROLE IN MAJOR INCIDENTS

A major incident is not just a problem for the services deployed to the scene, it is also a significant problem for the hospitals receiving casualties from the incident. Hospitals must, therefore, be prepared to handle such an eventuality and have robust plans in place that are exercised regularly.

The hospital response is normally under the command and control of a *hospital coordination team*. This consists of a medical coordinator (often the medical director), the senior nurse, a senior manager and the hospital triage officer.

The hospital coordinator is, in effect, the silver commander and is responsible for the overall response by the hospital. The triage officer is responsible for performing retriage as casualties arrive at the hospital and determines the location in which casualties will be treated. The senior nurse is responsible for ensuring that the clinical areas required are made available. These include A&E, theatres, intensive care and the wards. The senior manager is responsible for ensuring that administrative needs are met. These include staff resourcing, hospital information centre, documentation, care of relatives, media liaison and laboratory facilities (including blood transfusion).

It is possible that additional staff may be called into the hospital. This is usually done via the hospital switchboard personnel, who use a cascade system to reach as many people as possible.

Declaration of major incident within the hospital

It is unusual for a hospital to declare a major incident without first hearing from the ambulance service. It is essential, however, that a hospital be prepared to do so if casualties begin to arrive in large numbers, whether the ambulance service has declared a major incident or not.

The key alert messages that will be passed are:

- major incident stand by
- major incident declared
- major incident stand down.

These will be passed to the hospital switchboard by ambulance control. On receiving any of these calls, the switchboard operators will instigate an action plan putting in motion the response that is required.

Action after incident declared

Once a major incident is declared, all staff should report to their predetermined reporting point for instructions. Action cards will be distributed to those who will be expected to fulfil key roles in the response. The action cards briefly describe the duties of that individual and ensure that the role is carried out to the full, even when someone who has not performed that role in the past is appointed.

Treatment at hospital

Treatment will be prioritised according to the patient's needs, as identified by the hospital triage officer. Casualties may be categorised into two groups – those with medical and those with surgical needs. Senior physicians and surgeons will then liaise with all those required to ensure that definitive treatment is carried out within the hospital and theatres. This entails considerable juggling with the needs of both the existing patients of the hospital as well as those from the major incident. It is vital that the treatment given to all patients is fully documented within the case notes.

THE MEDIA AT A MAJOR INCIDENT

A major incident is of considerable interest to the media. Their hunger for an exclusive story is immense and many will go to extreme lengths to get one. It is likely that there will be both national and international interest, and it is not uncommon to see the incident and its aftermath being played out in real time and relayed across the world on television. This places considerable pressure on the casualties, their relatives and the rescuers alike. It is, therefore, essential that good relationships be established with the media at an early stage so that an effective media handling process can be instigated.

The key points to consider are that the police are, in the main, responsible for dealing with the media at the scene and will establish a media rendezvous point. They will also provide a media liaison officer who will provide regular updates to the media. It is possible that the police will also allow a small number of journalists restricted access to the scene on the understanding that any information and film footage is shared with other media representatives. It is possible that, in protracted incidents, a media centre will be established, providing a focal point for journalists and members of the emergency services media liaison teams.

At the hospital, similar arrangements will be made to ensure that the media response is controlled.

If you are asked to give an interview, it is essential that you clear the content of your interview with the police and other incident officers. Any interview should fulfil the criteria in Box 6.6.

Box 6.6   Giving a statement to the media

- Content should be agreed with the police and other incident officers.
- Statements should avoid contradiction and conflict.
- Statements should be factual and brief.
- Do not give an opinion as to the cause.
- Do not apportion blame.
- Do not give details of individual casualties.
- Do not give estimates of numbers of casualties or dead unless these have been confirmed.

CLOSING A MAJOR INCIDENT

Once all the live casualties have been removed from the scene and all the dead have been identified and labelled, the ambulance incident officer, in collaboration with the other incident officers, will 'declare the incident closed'. This message will be relayed to the receiving hospital and all those at the scene.

The senior officers should make sure that arrangements are made to ensure that medical cover is retained, where required, for those working within the wreckage of the scene. This requirement may go on for some days, as happened when the cruiser the *Marchioness* sank in the Thames, when a medical presence was maintained for 3 days.

Incident officers should ensure that all the records from the incident are kept and not destroyed, as they will become part of the legal documentation for the inevitable inquiry. All those involved in a major incident would be well advised to write down as much as they can remember about their own involvement at the incident as soon as possible. This will help considerably when they are later required to submit formal reports.

DEBRIEFING

It is essential that debriefs take place to ensure that all the facts about the incident are collated. Of equal importance is to provide an opportunity for rescuers to have a 'psychological debrief'.

A very short debrief should be arranged as the incident is closed to ensure that all staff are safe and well, and to congratulate them on their efforts. A formal debrief should be arranged within the next 48 hours. This will allow staff to share their initial thoughts and worries. Another debrief should be arranged approximately 1–2 weeks after the incident to allow staff to further explore their feelings in a place of safety and report back. A formal multiagency debrief will be arranged some weeks after the incident to give the senior officers the opportunity of sharing their experiences and to learn from the incident.

Senior officers should be aware of the need to watch out for signs of *post-traumatic stress disorder*

Box 6.7   Symptoms of post–traumatic stress disorder

- Anxiety
- Apathy
- Withdrawal
- Depression
- Poor concentration
- Marital problems
- Irritability
- Misplaced outbursts of anger
- Palpitations
- Exhaustion
- Increased use of alcohol or use of drugs

(PTSD) in their staff. It is increasingly recognised that rescuers can suffer severe emotional and psychological disorders after exposure to a major incident. It should be recognised that PTSD is a normal reaction to an abnormal situation. The onset of PTSD can be delayed for many months and on occasion many years. Potential symptoms are detailed in Box 6.7.

Counselling is the mainstay of treatment; however, it must be emphasised that many will only accept such treatment from those who have a true insight into the problems they faced at the incident. Occasionally psychiatric treatment and drug therapy are required.

CONCLUSION

It can be concluded, therefore, that the successful management of a major incident, of whatever type, is wholly dependent on a cohesive team approach. Good command, control and communication will ensure that the various services involved in the response work in concert with each other. A sound understanding of the roles and responsibilities of all the organisations and their tiers and chains of command are essential to this. A thorough understanding of the principles of triage and emergency medical care in a hostile environment is also vital. Above all, discipline and a willingness to serve as part of a large team will ensure that a major incident is managed with the minimum of error. Planning, training and multi-service exercises will help organisations and individuals prepare for the eventuality. It will happen again, for certain, and you must be ready to respond.

References

BASICS. *Guide to major incident management.* 1985
Calland V. *Safety at scene.* London: Mosby, 2000
Department of Health. *Emergency planning in the NHS: health service arrangements for dealing with major incidents.* HC (90) 25. London: HMSO, 1990
Eaton J. *The medical aspects of major incident management.* Ipswich: BASICS, 1998

Lambert, BMJ June 23 1883
MIMMS, ALSG. London: BMJ Books 1995
Morris EW. *1917 House Governors Log London Hospital*
Neal W. *Trauma care HEMS.* Saldatore Ltd, 1997
The Times, June 28, 1857

Further reading

Advanced Life Support Group. *Major incident management and support – the practical approach.* London: BMJ Publishing Group, 1995.
Calland V. *Safety at scene.* London: Mosby, 2000
Cooke M. *Churchills pocketbook of pre-hospital care.* Edinburgh: Churchill Livingstone, 1999
Eaton J. *The essentials of immediate care.* Edinburgh: Churchill Livingstone, 1999
Eaton J. *The medical aspects of major incident management.* BASICS, 1998

Hines K. *BASICS comes of age.* Ipswich: BASICS, 1998.
Hodgetts T, McNeil I, Cooke M. *Major incident management master.* London: BMJ Publishing Group, 1995
Joint Royal Colleges Ambulance Liaison Committee (JRCALC). *Pre-hospital clinical guidelines*, Issue 3, 2004. London: JRCALC, 2004.
Kuehl AE. *National Association of EMS Physicians pre-hospital systems and medical oversight,* 2nd edn. St Louis: Mosby Lifeline, 1994

SECTION 2

Applied biosciences in trauma care

Chapter 7

Homeostasis

Peter Bentley and Wendy Matthews

INTRODUCTION

Little in life is constant: our body's activity levels vary throughout the day depending on what we do. Our activities may range from eating a large meal to vigorous exercise or, when time allows, resting. To enable the body to undertake these activities effectively, internal adjustments in the body's systems need to be made. Throughout our lives, the body makes these continuous adjustments to prevent imbalances occurring. They range from the regulation of fluids and electrolytes ingested in our diets to maintaining normal body temperature. These processes are collectively referred to as homeostasis.

> Homeostasis is the maintenance by an organism of a constant internal environment; the process involves self-adjusting mechanisms in which maintenance of a particular level is initiated by the substance to be regulated (Hale et al., 1995)

HOMEOSTATIC MECHANISMS

Homeostatic systems have at least three interdependent components that enable the careful regulation of numerous body functions. Firstly, a control centre acts to determine what is called the 'set point' or normal range in a variable. The hypothalamus of the brain contains a temperature control centre, which monitors changes in the body temperature. Normal body temperature is between 36–37° C, which is the optimum temperature for the different body systems to work at. Alterations in our body temperature affect the body systems, with sustained hyperpyrexia leading to death owing to our proteins denaturing at high temperatures. Periods of hypothermia may similarly lead to death. The control centre functions by analysing variables, such as body temperature, and initiates appropriate responses to try to return the variable to a normal level. The information about a change in a variable, such as increased body temperature, is detected by sensors or receptors. These second components direct the information to the control centre. Examples of such receptors are the small sensory or afferent neurons found in the skin, which detect increased temperature and direct this information to the control centre. The final component of the homeostatic system relates to the effectors. These provide the response initiated by the control centre via motor or efferent neurons. This response may be vasodilation of blood vessels or increasing sweating. These three components function to regulate a wide range of processes, such as levels of electrolytes in the blood and the control of blood glucose levels within normal ranges for the needs of the different body systems (Figure 7.1).

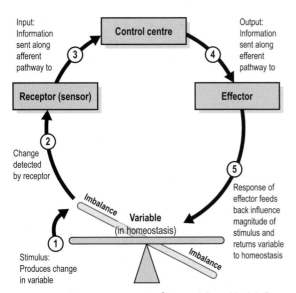

Figure 7.1 The control system. (Adapted from Marieb E. *Human anatomy and physiology*, 5th edn. Boston: Benjamin Cummings, 2000: 11.)

Feedback mechanisms

In order to maintain mechanisms, such as normal blood glucose levels, feedback systems aid homeostatic processes. Most feedback mechanisms operate by negative feedback, where changes in the variable cause changes in the opposite direction. When blood glucose levels rise above normal, insulin production is stimulated; however, when the glucose levels return to normal, the stimuli for insulin are reduced and insulin production ceases. In contrast, positive feedback sees the output from the system being increased: during labour, the stimulation of the uterus to contract owing to the pressure of the baby's head increases the levels of the hormone oxytocin, increasing the contraction of the uterus. When the baby is born, the oxytocin production ceases. Positive feedback mechanisms tend to regulate more infrequent events, with blood clotting a further example of a homeostatic mechanism that is regulated by this process.

Feedback mechanisms aid homeostatic processes

The role of two of our body's systems has been briefly mentioned in relation to homeostatic feedback mechanisms. The nervous system's role occurs very rapidly by producing electrical signals, which are conveyed by neurons in feedback systems. However, whilst the nervous system acts rapidly, the endocrine system, in contrast, acts more slowly producing chemical messages called hormones. Hormones are derived from either amino acids or are described as being steroids, which are made from the lipid cholesterol. Most hormones are produced by the organs of the endocrine system, namely endocrine glands. Examples of these are the thyroid gland and the pituitary gland. Some hormones, however, are produced by organs that have other functions, for example, as well as secreting the hormone insulin, the pancreas also secretes enzymes used for digestion. Hormones are secreted into the blood and travel to particular sites in the body. Although many hormones are synthesised in a complete form, some hormones, such as testosterone, are inactive and are modified to become active after being secreted by their endocrine gland.

Some hormones are very specific and target only a particular site. For example, thyroid stimulating hormone (TSH) only targets the thyroid gland. In contrast, the hormone thyroxine acts on a wide variety of different sites in the body stimulating increased metabolism. Hormones create their effect by interacting with targets on cell surfaces called receptors; this then alters the activity of the target cell. The changed activity inside the cell may lead to actions, such as the production of an enzyme or other regulatory substances, which aid homeostatic mechanisms. The endocrine and nervous systems work together in maintaining homeostasis by ensuring that changes in the body's internal environment are carefully regulated to prevent large alterations that could be detrimental. The production of hormones acts to aid homeostasis but the secretion of hormones is carefully regulated. There are three different forms of stimuli that regulate the production of hormones; these are neural, hormonal and humoral stimuli (Marieb, 2000).

REGULATION OF HORMONES

Neural stimuli

'Neural control' refers to nerve fibres stimulating the production of hormones. Secretion of the hormone adrenaline increases when the sympathetic nervous system stimulates the adrenal glands. Similarly, the release of oxytocin and antidiuretic hormone by the posterior pituitary glands is also stimulated by neural stimuli from the hypothalamus.

Hormonal stimuli

'Hormonal stimuli' refers to the process by which hormones stimulate other glands to produce their own hormones. The action of TSH on the thyroid gland stimulating the production of thyroxine is a good example of this form of stimulus. Hormones, such as TSH, which act in stimulating the production of hormones by other glands, are called tropic hormones.

Humoral stimuli

The stimulus for this form of hormone production comes from altered levels of substances in the blood affecting the level of hormones. Increasing blood glucose levels, for example, stimulate the action of insulin. Insulin facilitates cells to take up glucose and converts excess glucose to glycogen, which will be stored in the liver. Thus, the actions of this hormone aid the return of normal levels of blood glucose and are an important homeostatic mechanism in this process.

Although the regulation of the production of several different hormones has been described, some endocrine glands may be regulated by more than one of the different control processes. The duration of the hormonal effects varies: some have a short action that may last seconds, whilst the effects of others can last for several days. Once hormones have exerted their effects, they are degraded and excreted by the liver or kidneys.

FLUID COMPARTMENTS

Fluid balance is an important homeostatic mechanism. An average 70 kg male consists of around 40 litres of fluid, which constitutes 60% of his body weight. At younger ages, there is a greater proportion of body water, with an infant's body weight consisting of over 70% water. By adulthood there is some differences between the sexes, with females having slightly less body water than males owing to lower amounts of skeletal muscle, but greater amounts of fat. With the ageing process, the amount of body water diminishes in both sexes. Dissolved in body fluids are essential electrolytes, such as sodium and potassium, non-electrolytes, such as glucose, urea and creatinine, and various proteins.

> Fluid balance is an important homeostatic mechanism

The different areas of the body where fluids and electrolytes are found are referred to as fluid compartments (Figure 7.2). The first fluid compartment relates to fluids found inside of the cells and is known as the intracellular fluid (ICF) compartment. This compartment accounts for two-thirds of the body's fluids. Outside of the cells, the remaining one-third of fluids is found in the extracellular fluid (ECF) compartment. This compartment is further divided into the region

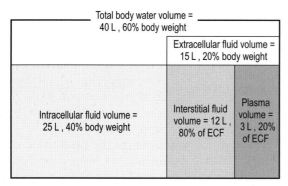

Figure 7.2 The major fluid compartments of the body. (Adapted from Marieb E. *Human anatomy and physiology*, 5th edn. Boston: Benjamin Cummings, 2000: 11.)

that surrounds the cells (i.e. the tissues or interstitial fluids), which contains around 80% of the fluids, and the remaining 20%, which is found in the blood vessels (i.e. plasma). Extracellular fluids are also found between serous membranes, such as the pleura and peritoneum, around synovial joints and also in the cerebrospinal fluid of the central nervous system. There are much greater levels of potassium and magnesium in the intracellular compartment compared with levels in the extracellular compartment. This, however, contrasts with higher levels of sodium, chloride and bicarbonate ions in the extracellular compartment.

Before consideration is given to homeostatic mechanisms relating to fluid and electrolyte transport between these compartments, each of the compartments components will be discussed.

INTRACELLULAR FLUID COMPARTMENT

Knowledge of the structure and function of cells has come a long way since the discovery of cells by Robert Hooke around 1665. An understanding of the important role of cells in animals and plants led to the development of the 'cell theory'. This theory describes five basic concepts (listed below) that are relevant to the normal function of the human body.

1. Cells are the building blocks of all plants and animals.
2. New cells are produced by the division of pre-existing cells.

3. Cells are the smallest units that perform all vital physiological functions.
4. Each cell maintains homeostasis at the cellular level.
5. Homeostasis at the tissue, organ, organ system and organism levels reflects the combined and coordinated actions of many cells.

Humans have trillions of cells, which display enormous variation both in their size and in their appearance (Figure 7.3). Cell sizes vary from being several micrometers long to the much larger smooth muscle cells, which can be up to 30 cm in length (Marieb, 2000). Diagrams of cells often depict them as having an organised circular appearance, but this can be contrasted with cells that are more irregular with a more branching appearance such as neurons. There are several distinct components of human cells that are important in their normal function.

Surrounding human cells is the cell membrane. This structure protects the internal contents of the cell and regulates transportation of substances entering and leaving it. Membranes comprise a complex arrangement of lipids including cholesterol, proteins and a lesser amount of carbohydrates. The carbohydrate component is present on the external surface of the cell membrane and is known as the glycocalyx. The glycocalyx is important in cellular recognition processes. The presence of these components on a cell membrane acts to enable interactions with some cells in the same group, but they also act as receptors on the cell surface to which drugs and hormones can interact. The glycocalyx on the surface of erythrocytes has the important role in determining ABO blood groups.

Located inside human cells is a watery fluid known as the cytoplasm where various cellular activities occur. Many of these activities occur inside structures known as cellular organelles. The main function of some of the organelles is worthy of discussion.

Mitochondria are elongated oval-shaped organelles that function in the production of a stored form of energy, adenosine triphosphate (ATP). The generation of ATP in mitochondria is oxygen dependent; this process is often, therefore, referred to as aerobic metabolism. The ATP is then

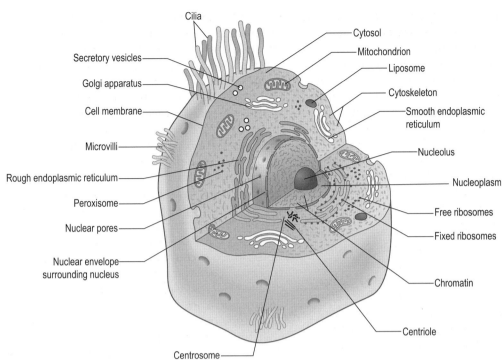

Figure 7.3 The anatomy of a representative cell. (Adapted from Martini F. *Fundamentals of anatomy and physiology*, 4th edn. London: Prentice Hall International, 1998: 67.)

Labels: Cilia; Secretory vesicles; Golgi apparatus; Cell membrane; Microvilli; Rough endoplasmic reticulum; Peroxisome; Nuclear pores; Nuclear envelope surrounding nucleus; Centrosome; Cytosol; Mitochondrion; Liposome; Cytoskeleton; Smooth endoplasmic reticulum; Nucleolus; Nucleoplasm; Free ribosomes; Fixed ribosomes; Chromatin; Centriole

released from the mitochondria for cellular processes that require energy. Cells that have high energy needs, such as those in the liver and muscle, are rich in mitochondria. Mitochondria have a small circular copy of DNA; mutation of genes in this DNA can lead to rare genetic disorders.

The endoplasmic reticulum (ER) forms a complex network of passageways where the synthesis and storage of various cellular substances occurs. The ER forms an important transportation route throughout cells. ER also removes drugs and toxins that are rendered harmless. The ER is divided into one of two types: the rough ER has ribosomes present on its surface where proteins are synthesized, whereas the smooth ER lacks ribosomes but appears to be more important in the production of hormones.

Golgi apparatus form flattened sacs that interact with the cells' nuclei. They function in synthesising enzymes and hormones, which they package and transport around the cell; some are exported from the cell for use in other areas of the body.

Lysosomes are small sacs containing enzymes, which digest cellular debris including bacteria.

Central to the control of cells is the nucleus, which is present in all human cells except for erythrocytes. The nucleus is surrounded by its own nuclear membrane, which regulates the movement of substances entering and leaving the nucleus. The main component of the nucleus is deoxyribonucleic acid (DNA), which carries the code for over 100 000 proteins. This code is converted and conveyed to the ribosomes by messenger ribonucleic acid (mRNA), where proteins ranging from important enzymes to components of blood are synthesised. Damage to the DNA, known as mutations, can lead to abnormal protein production, which can cause severe imbalances in some cells leading to genetic diseases ranging from cystic fibrosis to various cancers.

EXTRACELLULAR COMPARTMENT

Interstitial fluids

Surrounding the cells is the interstitial fluid, which contains water, electrolytes and substances such as glucose and urea. Surrounding the interstitial fluid is a network of blood and lymphatic vessels. Whilst the blood vessels transport important nutrients and oxygen to the cells, both lymphatic and blood vessels function to remove fluid and waste from the interstitial fluid, some of which are products of metabolism from the cells. There are small differences in the concentrations of the different components between the interstitial fluid and the plasma components of the extracellular compartment. These are minor when compared with the differences between the ICF and ECF (Martini, 1998). The main difference is that there are higher concentrations of proteins in the plasma than in the interstitial fluid.

Plasma

Plasma is an important component of blood, accounting for around 55% of its total volume. The remaining 45% is referred to as formed elements and contains the blood cells. Plasma has a straw-coloured appearance and is predominantly formed of water, which accounts for over 90% of its contents. Plasma proteins form an important group of substances present in the plasma, with three of these being particularly important.

Albumin accounts for 60% of the plasma protein population and have an important role in regulating the movement of fluids between the capillaries and the tissues. When albumin is present in reduced levels in the blood, there is increased loss of fluid from the capillaries into the tissues leading to oedema. Globulins are important proteins that form hormones and antibodies, whilst fibrinogen is an important plasma protein that contributes to blood clotting.

The remaining components of plasma include electrolytes, nutrients, respiratory gases and wastes.

The formed elements can be divided into three main groups of cells. Erythrocytes or red blood cells form over 99% of the formed elements. The remainder is made up of the leucocytes or white blood cells and the thrombocytes, which are known as the platelets. These cells are derived from stem cells in the bone marrow, which undergo a process known as haemopoiesis to develop into the members of each cell group.

Erythrocytes

Adults have approximately 5 million erythrocytes per microlitre of blood. Their distinctly round appearance is described as a biconcave disc. Erythrocytes contain the pigment haemoglobin, which has a key function in oxygen carriage. When combined with oxygen, it forms oxyhaemoglobin, which enables oxygen to be transported to the tissues for the cell's activities. Haemoglobin is also responsible for carriage of approximately one-quarter of carbon dioxide with which it combines to form carbaminohaemoglobin, thereby aiding the excretion of carbon dioxide. The haemoglobin is formed of four units of the iron-rich haem to which oxygen binds and four protein chains formed by the globin to which the carbon dioxide binds. Erythrocytes are very flexible and are able to change shape, which enables them to squeeze into narrow capillaries due to the protein spectrin. Erythrocytes lack a nucleus, so are unable to divide like many other cells. They are withdrawn from the circulation as they begin to wear out, a process that usually occurs after approximately 120 days. Erythrocytes are degraded in the liver and spleen; much of the iron is reused for new erythrocytes whilst other components are eventually excreted in the urine and faeces. The production of erythrocytes is a carefully regulated homeostatic mechanism, where hypoxia acts as a driver to stimulate increased erythrocyte production owing to the actions of the hormone erythropoietin. This hormone is mainly produced by the kidneys and acts to stimulate the bone marrow to increase erythrocyte production. However, when the erythrocytes are functioning successfully in gas carriage, fewer new erythrocytes are produced.

BLOOD GROUPS

Although there are over 20 different blood groups in humans (Tortora and Grabowski, 2000), the two main groups that tend to be of most clinical significance are the ABO and rhesus groups.

ABO blood groups

Erythrocytes have very specific glycoproteins, known as antigens, on their cell surface on the glycocalyx. It is these antigens that aid the determination of which ABO blood group someone belongs to. There are only two types of these antigens: antigen A and antigen B. Located in the plasma around the erythrocytes are antibodies, which are also of two types, referred to as anti-A and anti-B. These antibodies form an important immune response when incompatible blood is transfused to patients, often with devastating affects.

An individual with type A antigens belongs to blood group A but has the opposite antibodies, anti-B, in their plasma. Those with type B antigens belong to blood group B, but also have opposite antibodies, anti-A, in their plasma. Members of the population with both type A and type B antigens on their erythrocytes belong to blood group AB, but have no antibodies in their plasma.

Those who lack any antigens on their erythrocytes belong to blood group O, but will have both anti-A and anti-B antibodies in their plasma. Variations in the UK and Western European population for ABO blood groups are shown in Table 7.1.

Two terms are used in relation to blood transfusion. The recipient is the person who receives the blood; this contrasts with the person donating the blood, the donor. Transfusion reactions owing to incompatible blood groups tend to occur when donated blood has the same antigens as the recipient's antibodies. Thus, if a patient who is blood group A receives transfused blood from a donor of blood group B, the recipients anti-B antibodies will attack the donor's type B antigens.

Rhesus blood groups

Rhesus is an antigen present on the cell surface of erythrocytes. Over 85% of the UK population have this antigen and are known as rhesus positive.

Table 7.1 ABO blood groups. (Adapted from Hinchliff S, Montague S and Watson R. *Physiology for nursing practice*, 2nd edn. London: Baillière Tindall, 1996)

Blood group	Antigens	Antibodies	Percentage of UK and Western Europe population
A	A	b	42
B	B	a	9
AB	A + B	None	3
O	None	a + b	46

Situations can occur in pregnancy when women who are rhesus negative may develop antibodies to their rhesus-positive fetuses. Good antenatal screening can detect this situation, which can be treated by the administration of antirhesus gamma globulin, thus preventing this complication from occurring.

Leucocytes

These cells are crucial to the body's defences at times of infection. Many leucocytes are able to migrate out of blood vessels by a process called diapedesis enabling them to travel to the tissues and other regions of the body. Neutrophils are the main population group, which can account for between 40% and 70% of leucocytes. They destroy pathogens by phagocytosis, where they surround and digest their prey. In contrast, basophils and eosinophils provide the body's immune response at times of allergy. Lymphocytes are divided into one of two types: B lymphocytes, which eventually divide and form antibodies that act as specific targets against microbial antigens; and T lymphocytes. The T lymphocytes act by secreting toxic chemicals called cytokines and also have a regulatory role in the body's immune responses. Feedback systems also regulate the immune system, with hormones and an array of other substances stimulating the recruitment of immune cells when the body is under attack by pathogens. Immune responses can also be reduced, preventing unnecessary production of leucocytes and antibodies. This process may be imbalanced in autoimmune disease, where antibodies damage healthy tissues.

Thrombocytes

Thrombocytes are also referred to as platelets and have an essential role in blood clotting. Structurally they have the appearance of flattened discs and contain granules that are rich in chemicals that aid blood clotting. Platelets form plugs in damaged blood vessel walls, which act to slow blood loss. The production of platelets also occurs in the bone marrow and is regulated by the hormone thrombopoietin. Normal levels of platelets in the blood range from between 150 000 and 400 000 platelets per microlitre of blood

(Tortora and Grabowski, 2000). Organs such as the spleen act as sites where platelets can be stored and easily released at a time of haemorrhage.

FLUID BALANCE

Maintenance of the composition of fluids and electrolytes in the different fluid compartments is largely dependent on dietary intake. Water is an essential nutrient. A healthy adult should have a water intake of approximately 2500 ml per day. Most of this intake is from drinking fluids; however, many foods contain water, with nearly one-third of daily water intake obtained from moist foods. The remaining water input is produced as a result of metabolism, mostly owing to the production of ATP in the mitochondria with water produced as a byproduct. In order to maintain fluid balance, water gains have to be balanced by water losses. Urinary losses account for 60% of water output. The remaining losses are harder to quantify and are referred to as insensible losses. The majority of insensible losses of water occur as a result of respiration and sweating; less than 5% occurs in the faeces. These forms of insensible losses can increase in some patients who may be at risk of developing dehydration owing to hyperpyrexia, tachypnoea or diarrhoea.

Water and electrolytes present in food and drinks are absorbed across the wall of the intestines into the blood (Figure 7.4). Movement of substances out of blood vessels occurs owing to hydrostatic pressure, which pushes fluids out of capillaries at the arterial end into the tissues, although most proteins and the erythrocytes remain in the capillaries. Some of the fluids and electrolytes that enter the tissues will pass across cell membranes and enter the cells. Homeostasis of fluid and electrolyte balance is maintained by movement of substances either back into the venous end of the capillaries or into the lymphatic system, which returns some of the tissue fluids back to the blood.

In order to maintain sufficient levels of water in the plasma, important feedback mechanisms involving a number of different hormones act to minimise the effects of dehydration or fluid overload. The term osmolarity describes a measurement to describe the concentration of substances

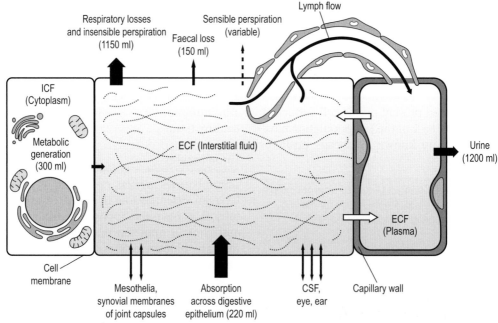

Figure 7.4 Fluid exchanges. (Reprinted from Hinchliff S, Montague S, Watson R. *Physiology for nursing practice*, 2nd edn. London: Baillière Tindall, 1996.)

present in the blood. When the body fluid is depleted, the osmolarity increases and this is detected by structures called osmoreceptors. The osmoreceptors present in the hypothalamus act to stimulate drinking and the release of antidiuretic hormone (ADH) from the pituitary gland. ADH acts on the nephrons of the kidneys promoting water reabsorption back into the blood. As a result of this, losses of water in the urine are reduced, with the urine appearing darker and more concentrated. The adrenal glands secrete a hormone called aldosterone; this also acts on the nephron to increase water reabsorption. The action of both these hormones is reduced when osmolarity decreases, when water levels in the plasma return to normal levels. Alcohol is known to block the action of ADH, promoting a diuresis. Large quantities of alcohol are associated with heavy losses of water that can lead to dehydration and the phenomenon described as a hangover.

Fluid balance is often discussed with electrolytes. The actions of major electrolytes and the imbalances seen in the trauma patient will be discussed in the next chapter.

CONCLUSION

Homeostatic mechanisms, such as fluid and electrolyte balance, blood glucose and temperature control are important processes, which need to be understood by those involved in caring for trauma patients. An understanding of these processes will improve patient care, especially in the critically ill patient whose limited capacity to maintain these homeostatic mechanisms may often be impaired.

References

Hale W, Marghan J, Saunders V. *Collins dictionary: biology.* London: Collins, 1995

Marieb E. *Human anatomy and physiology,* 5th edn. Boston: Benjamin Cummings, 2000

Martini F. *Fundamentals of anatomy and physiology,* 4th edn. London: Prentice Hall International, 1988

Tortora G, Grabowski S. *Principles of anatomy and physiology,* 9th edn. New York: J Wiley, 2000

Chapter **8**

Applied biochemistry pertaining to the trauma patient

Wendy Matthews and Peter Bentley

INTRODUCTION

A series of biochemical tests is carried out on a patient's blood and urine on admission to hospital. This biochemical profile is used to evaluate any pre-existing abnormalities, aid diagnosis, and monitor and guide appropriate therapy to restore the optimum physiological environment. Samples are taken of venous blood, arterial blood and, when possible, urine. The following is a brief description of these standard measurements and their use when caring for the trauma patient.

BIOCHEMICAL INDICES

Urea and electrolytes

Urea and electrolytes (U&Es) are routinely measured from venous blood samples and give an indication of the patient's electrolyte balance, renal function and level of hydration. They include sodium (Na), potassium (K), urea, creatinine and sometimes chloride (Cl) and bicarbonate (HCO_3).

Liver function tests

Liver function tests (LFTs) reflect the level of liver enzymes that are released from hepatocytes, and are raised in liver disease and trauma. These include alkaline phosphatase (alk ph), alanine aminotransferase (ALT), aspartate aminotransferase (AST) and albumin, which may be used as an indicator of nutritional status and synthetic function of the liver. Bilirubin, a product of the breakdown of red blood cells that is conjugated by liver cells, is also included. When the bilirubin level is raised, it is important to know if it is conjugated or unconjugated. If it is unconjugated, this is indicative of a pre-hepatic cause, such as increased breakdown of red blood cells in haemolysis. If it is conjugated, then the problem relates to obstruction of the common bile duct. If the result reflects mixed conjugated and unconjugated bilirubin, this is suggestive of liver disease.

Glucose

The blood glucose level is measured within the biochemical profile, and is raised in diabetes and as a consequence of the stress response.

Amylase

Amylase is a pancreatic enzyme that is raised in pancreatic damage and pancreatitis.

Bone profile

The bone profile is a useful measure that reflects calcium and phosphate levels. The ionised calcium level is reported and is corrected in relation to the albumin level. This is also dependent on the pH of the body with more calcium ionised in the presence of acidosis. The blood level does not reflect the total body calcium accurately because of the large reservoir in bone. Bone metabolism is altered in patients with bony metastases from cancer, osteomalacia, Paget's disease, renal disease and myeloma.

Osmolality/osmolarity

Osmolality refers to the number of solute particles per unit weight of water (mmol/kg of water), and can be measured directly or calculated. Osmolarity refers to the number of particles of solute per litre of solution (mmol/l). A solute is the substance that is dissolved in a solvent. These measurements indicate the 'tonicity', which determines the osmotic pressure exerted by a solution across a membrane. If a solution is isotonic, this indicates that it has the same osmotic pressure. If the osmolarity of a solution goes up, a cell within that solution will lose water to the solution and the cell will shrink. If the osmolarity of a solution goes down, the cell will absorb water

and will swell and burst. This effect demonstrates the need to maintain a stable equilibrium throughout the body tissues to prevent cell death.

Creatine kinase

Creatinine kinase (CK) is an enzyme that catalyses a reaction in muscle producing creatine and ATP (adenosine triphosphate) (energy). The CK level rises as a result of strenuous muscle activity and muscle damage, such as myocardial infarction or crush injury. It is released from cells when they break down or necrose (rhabdomyolysis). A very high CK level is a predictor of renal damage, as it reflects a large degree of cell breakdown and release of cellular components such as myoglobin (a muscle protein). If the patient is not adequately hydrated, these cell breakdown products block the renal tubules causing acute tubular necrosis and renal failure.

Arterial blood gas samples

Arterial blood gas measurements are obtained from a sample of arterial blood usually taken from the femoral or radial artery. They are taken in a specially prepared syringe containing heparin and are placed in a blood gas analyser producing results for pH, pCO_2, pO_2, HCO_3^-, base excess and oxygen saturation. The significance of these results will be discussed in the next chapter.

Urine

Urine can be tested for osmolarity, and to assess sodium and potassium excretion. If urine osmolarity is high, i.e. the body is producing concentrated urine, this is suggestive of the body conserving water and of fluid depletion.

This is under the influence of the renin–angiotensin system and the production of anti-diuretic hormone (ADH) and is a normal response to 'stress'. This response also conserves sodium in order to conserve water and the urinary sodium level is usually low. The volume of urine output is extremely important in the assessment of fluid balance.

It is important that each sample is placed in the appropriate bottle (usually a heparinised sample for arterial blood) and that the venous blood sample is not taken from a site near an intravenous line. Results will not be accurate if the sample has haemolysed, as intracellular components will be included in the analysis.

Trauma can result in direct organ or tissue damage and haemorrhage. Significant haemorrhage, which reduces the body's circulating volume, triggers responses to preserve perfusion of vital organs. Any tissue that is not adequately perfused will experience hypoxia and resultant cell death. The aim of resuscitation is to reverse this pathological process by trying to maintain a normal physiological environment. The biochemical analysis will guide and evaluate the resuscitation.

NORMAL BIOCHEMICAL VALUES

The range of normal biochemical values can vary slightly between laboratories. Box 8.1 provides an outline of one such range.

Box 8.1 Range of normal biochemical values	
Blood plasma	
Sodium (Na)	135–145 mmol/l
Potassium (K)	3.5–5.0 mmol/l
Urea	2.5–6.7 mmol/l
Creatinine	70–150 mmol/l
Glucose	4–6 mmol/l
Chloride (Cl)	95–105 mmol/l
Bicarbonate (HCO_3)	24–30 mmol/l
ALT/AST	5–35 iu/l
Alk ph	30–300 iu/l
Bilirubin	3–17 mmol/l
Amylase	0–180 iu/l
Albumin	35–50 g/l
Calcium (total; Ca)	2.12–2.65 mmol/l
Phosphate (PO_4)	0.8–1.45 mmol/l
Creatine kinase (CK)	25–180 iu/l (variable depending on ethnicity and sex)
Osmolality	278–305 mosmol/kg
Urine	
Osmolality	350–1000 mosmol/kg

ELECTROLYTES AND THEIR CLINICAL SIGNIFICANCE

Sodium (Na) and potassium (K) exist as electrolytes (positively charged ions) in solution throughout the body and are vital for cell function.

Total body sodium is approximately 4200 mmol/l and is roughly divided into: 50% in extracellular fluid, which is divided between the interstitial and vascular compartments (135–145 mmol/l); 10% in intracellular fluid (10 mmol/l); and 40% in bone. The total amount is a balance between intake in the diet and excretion by the kidneys. The regulation between intracellular and extracellular fluid is dependent on the energy driven sodium/potassium pump (Na^+/K^+ pump) in the cell membrane, which pumps the sodium against the concentration gradient from inside the cell to outside the cell. In conditions of hypoxia, the cell ceases to produce sufficient energy, the sodium pump fails and the concentration gradient cannot be maintained.

Potassium is the main intracellular cation. Total body potassium is approximately 2500 mmol: 98% is intracellular (140 mmol/l) and 2% is extracellular (3.5–5.0 mmol/l). Potassium is exchanged for sodium in the Na^+/K^+ pump, and moves into cells in conditions of alkalosis and with insulin (which is used as treatment for hyperkalaemia).

The volume of the extracellular fluid is determined by the amount of sodium. Water moves between compartments and is reabsorbed or excreted in the kidneys to maintain a balanced osmolality in response to changes in sodium concentration. From this it can be understood that the figure obtained in the venous sample biochemical analysis reflects the extracellular sodium concentration (i.e. the relative amount of sodium to water in that compartment), but does not directly reflect the absolute amount or volume of either, or the total body situation.

> The volume of the extracellular fluid is determined by the amount of sodium

Haemorrhage

In the patient who has had a significant haemorrhage there will be a total loss of electrolytes and volume in a normal amount relative to each other. Therefore, before the body's compensatory mechanisms begin, the biochemistry results will be unchanged. The initial compensatory change will be for the kidneys to preserve sodium so that the water will follow, thus restoring circulating volume. A later biochemistry sample may show a higher sodium level. This does not indicate increased body sodium but low total body water. After a further period of time, the relative values will have been restored by further reabsorption of water or rather the decreased excretion of water. If the body does not have enough total body water or enough intake of water to replenish the loss, the sodium level will remain high and the patient is dehydrated. The aim of resuscitation is to avoid this situation and to replenish lost fluid volume with isotonic fluids, such as Hartmann's solution, normal saline 0.9% or blood so that the kidneys can continue to control normal homeostasis with adequate total body fluid.

The electrolyte components of some intravenous fluids

The electrolyte components of some intravenous fluids are shown in Table 8.1.

Diabetic ketoacidosis

Other medical conditions may also cause deranged results prior to the onset of trauma. For example, an insulin-dependent diabetic patient may lapse into a ketoacidotic coma whilst driving his car. His pre-trauma biochemistry will show hyperglycaemia and acidosis, resulting in hyperkalaemia. The high potassium level is not a reflection of increased body potassium but of depleted intracellular potassium with potassium in the extracellular compartment whilst the total body potassium is low. On treatment with insulin

and fluids, the plasma potassium level will fall as the potassium is transported into the cells, requiring potassium to be added to the intravenous fluids to maintain equilibrium.

Acute renal failure will cause a raised potassium level, which is important to note at the onset of rhabdomyolysis or acute tubular necrosis after a period of hypovolaemia. Chronic cardiac failure is often reflected as a low plasma sodium level as a result of high total body water with normal or high total body sodium.

These examples demonstrate the need to interpret biochemical results within the context of pre-existing conditions, the acute history and therapeutic interventions undertaken.

> Biochemical results must be interpreted within the context of pre-existing conditions, the acute history and therapeutic interventions undertaken

Urea

Urea is the end product of the breakdown of amino acids by the liver and is excreted by the kidneys. A low dietary intake of protein will result in a low plasma level of urea. A high level on plasma sampling can reflect several things, such as a high-protein diet. A pathological example of this is gastrointestinal haemorrhage. High urea may be an indication of dehydration but, in conjunction with a raised creatinine, is suggestive of renal failure.

Creatinine

Creatinine is also an end product of muscle breakdown excreted by the kidneys. It is formed from creatine by the loss of a water molecule. A total of 1–2% of total body muscle creatine is lost in this way, thus the figure is directly dependent

Table 8.1 The electrolyte components of some intravenous fluids

	Na (mmol/l)	K (mmol/l)	Cl (mmol/l)	Ca (mmol/l)	HCO$_3$ (mmol/l)
Normal plasma	142	4.5	103	2.5	26
Normal saline (NaCl; 0.9%)	150	–	150	–	–
Glucose 5%	–	–	–	–	–
Hartmann's	131	5	111	2	29

on muscle bulk. Creatine is part of the reversible reaction in which a phosphate ion is donated from creatine phosphate to yield energy for muscle contraction. The significance of creatinine is that the kidneys do not reabsorb it so the urinary excretion in relation to the blood level indicates renal function.

THE EFFECT OF TRAUMA ON BIOCHEMICAL INDICATORS

The effect of trauma can be direct, causing tissue or organ damage such as cardiac, respiratory, renal or brain injury. Alternatively, it may be indirect as a result of failure of body systems after haemorrhage or secondary sepsis. On a cellular level, injury can result from direct cell trauma or disruption of the normal physiological environment, such as a period of hypoxia secondary to hypoperfusion after haemorrhage at a distant site in the body. A normal cell with an adequate supply of oxygen maintains a complex intracellular environment requiring a constant source of energy. Cellular respiration provides this free energy by the breakdown (oxidation) of foodstuffs. There are three main stages in cellular respiration: glycolysis, the Krebs cycle and oxidative phosphorylation.

> There are three main stages in cellular respiration: glycolysis, the Krebs cycle and oxidative phosphorylation

CELLULAR RESPIRATION

Energy within the body is obtained by the breakdown of food. Initially, the food is broken down into smaller molecules. Proteins are broken down to amino acids, polysaccharides into simple sugars such as glucose, and fats into fatty acids and glycerol. These simpler molecules are then broken down, or reduced, to carbon and hydrogen atoms within the cell in small steps, each step controlled by a specific enzyme releasing the energy stored in the molecular bonds. Finally, the carbon and hydrogen atoms are oxidised to carbon dioxide and water, which is the most energetically stable form of carbon and hydrogen atoms.

In the bloodstream, oxygen dissociates from haemoglobin and diffuses down the concentration gradient into the cell. Amino acids, glucose and free fatty acids also enter the cell. The first step, *glycolysis*, takes place in the cytosol. It does not require oxygen and, under anaerobic conditions, will continue providing some energy. Glycolysis is the process in which glucose, a molecule with six carbon atoms, is converted to two molecules of pyruvate (three carbon) by nine separate steps. During this process, adenosine triphosphate (ATP) and nicotinamide adenine dinucleotide (NAD$^+$) are formed. Both these molecules function as a store of energy. When ATP is hydrolysed, it converts to adenosine diphosphate (ADP) and an inorganic phosphate (P$_i$), releasing energy that was present in the bond. NAD is important for its ability to transfer electrons. It is able to accept H$^+$ ions (i.e. two electrons with a proton) to form NADH. In this structure, the hydride ion can be readily transferred to other molecules.

The overall reaction of glycolysis is:

Glucose + 8ADP + 8P$_i$ + 2O$_2$ → 2 Pyruvate + 8ATP + 4H$_2$O (aerobic)

Glucose + 2ADP + 2P$_i$ → 2 Lactate + 2ATP + 2H$_2$O (anaerobic)

Without oxygen, lactate is produced as the end product. With ongoing hypoxia this builds up resulting in lactic acidosis.

The next step in cellular respiration is the citric acid cycle, also known as the *Krebs cycle* or *tricarboxylic acid cycle* (TCA cycle; Figure 8.1). This takes place in the mitochondria and is oxygen dependent (i.e. it can only occur aerobically). Pyruvate and fatty acids (breakdown products from fats) are selectively transported from the cytosol into the mitochondria. Pyruvate is broken down by the enzyme pyruvate dehydrogenase and fatty acids are broken down by the fatty acid oxidation cycle to acetyl coenzyme A (acetyl CoA). Acetyl CoA then enters the citric acid cycle. At the beginning of the cycle, acetyl CoA reacts with oxaloacetate and forms citric acid. Then follow seven reactions all catalysed by different enzymes, resulting in the regeneration of oxaloacetate (hence the cycle) and two molecules of CO$_2$. The energy that is released in the cycle when the C-H and C-C bonds are oxidised is transformed into a

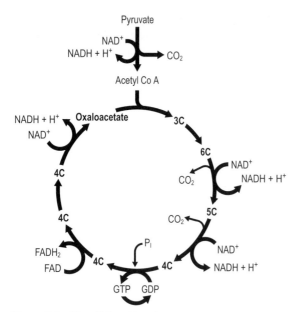

Figure 8.1 The citric acid cycle.

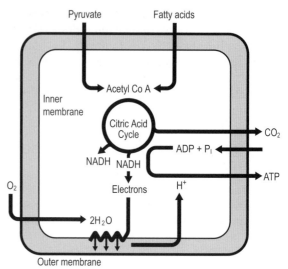

Figure 8.2 Aerobic cell respiration.

high-energy phosphate bond and the readily transferred electrons on the carrier molecules NADH and $FADH_2$. That is, through each turn of the cycle, three molecules of NAD^+ are converted to NADH and one flavine adenine nucleotide (FAD) is converted to $FADH_2$.

The next step is *oxidative phosphorylation*. Electrons from NADH and $FADH_2$ pass down the *electron transport chain* (Fig. 8.2). This takes place on the inner membrane of the mitochondrion where all the electron carrier molecules are embedded. At each step of the chain the electron falls to a lower energy state. At the end of the chain the electrons are transferred to oxygen molecules to form water. Oxygen molecules have a high affinity for electrons and so they are at a low-energy state. With the energy released, protons (H^+) are pumped from the inner to the outer mitochondrial membrane. This creates an electrochemical proton gradient. The H^+ then travels back into the inner membrane down its gradient via an enzyme complex involving ATP synthase, which catalyses the production of ATP from ADP + P_i. The ATP is then pumped out to the rest of the cell to be used as energy. After the ATP has been used in the cytosol and has been hydrolysed to ADP, it is transported back for

recharging. The complete oxidation of glucose yields $6CO_2$ + $6H_2O$ + 38ATP.

The electrochemical gradient is used to transport many other molecules across the membrane (e.g. phosphate, calcium ions, pyruvate, Na/K pump). It is easy to see that, without this process of cell respiration carrying on in a continuous fashion, the cell will quickly run out of ATP. Without ATP the cell cannot maintain the concentration gradients that allow the cell to continue to function.

The immediate intervention following trauma is to control and treat any compromise to the airway, breathing and circulation whilst ensuring no major disruption to the cervical spine. This approach is aimed at preventing the effects of hypoxia on the body systems. A safe airway and effective ventilation ensures that oxygen is getting into the lungs. Optimising the circulation ensures that the oxygen is being transported around the body to tissues and vital organs, thus preventing the onset of shock. Shock is defined as inadequate tissue perfusion. The body has many mechanisms that can compensate to prevent the onset of shock. In acute haemorrhage there is a decreased circulating blood volume. The sympathetic nervous system response will increase the heart rate, improve the contractility of the heart and constrict the peripheral blood vessels. With adequate resuscitation at this point, oxygenated blood flow will return and the effects of transient hypoxia can be reversed. Without resuscitation, the condition will progress to prolonged shock. The arterial vasoconstriction relaxes whilst the venular vasoconstriction continues leading to a raised oncotic pressure and oedema with leakage of fluid from capillaries to surrounding tissues. After 30–40 minutes the extravascular interstitial fluid replenishes the plasma volume through the capillaries in a volume equal to the volume of blood lost. This is the stage of compensated shock. If this progresses further, worsening circulation and metabolic imbalances make the situation irreversible despite any efforts of resuscitation because the oxygen debt is too large.

Shock is defined as inadequate tissue perfusion.

In the lungs, the initial decrease in circulating blood volume causes an increased dead space as less of the lung tissue is being perfused. The muscular work increases to compensate but, with decreased perfusion, the muscles begin to fail. Initially there is hypoxia and hypocarbia because of the increased respiratory effort but, as shock progresses, carbon dioxide rises and lactic acid rises from increasing anaerobic respiration resulting in a respiratory and metabolic acidosis.

In the kidneys, decreased perfusion initiates vasoconstriction and sodium and water retention. Continued hypoperfusion causes ischaemic cell damage and direct renal tubular damage from cell breakdown products and stasis. Failing renal function causes a metabolic acidosis and decreasing urine output.

On a cellular level, hypoxia results from hypoperfusion. Lack of oxygen halts aerobic respiration. Anaerobic glycolysis takes over, producing lactate and insufficient ATP. Intracellular pH falls owing to the production and build-up of lactic acid and an increase in inorganic phosphate. The sodium pump cannot function without ATP resulting in a rise in intracellular sodium and diffusion of potassium out of the cell. These effects can be seen in changes in morphology of the cell with clumping of the nuclear chromatin, loss of granules in the mitochondrion and dilation of the endoplasmic reticulum. Water follows the net gain of sodium causing the cell to swell. Continued

---

Box 8.2   Pathophysiology of hypoxia

Reversible
- ↓ Oxidative phosphorylation
- ↑ Lactic acid
- ↑ P_i
- ↓ ATP
- ↓ Na/K pump
- ↓ pH
- Ca influx
- ↓ Protein production
- ↑ Intracellular water and Na
- Efflux of K

Irreversible
- Membrane injury
- Calcium influx
- Mitochondrial dysfunction
- Release of lysosomal enzymes
- Leakage of cell enzymes
- Influx of extracellular molecules

---

hypoxia decreases protein production further, reduces mitochondrial function and increases membrane permeability. This stage is still reversible if oxygen is restored but, if not, the process progresses with marked swelling of the mitochondria, damage to the plasma membrane, leakage of enzymes and other cell constituents, and a massive influx of calcium. Lysosomal membranes are damaged with release of hydrolytic proteases, lipases and phosphatases into the cell resulting in cell autolysis.

The effects of hypoxia (Box 8.2) vary between the type of cell and the environment. Brain cells cannot survive a few minutes of hypoxia whereas skeletal muscle cells can recover after 30 minutes. Hypothermia prolongs the time to irreversible cell injury.

Hypothermia prolongs the time to irreversible cell injury

The aim of active resuscitation is to prevent the stepwise deterioration to cell and organ failure by preventing cellular hypoxia. Supplementary oxygen is given via a facemask or endotracheal intubation to maximise alveolar oxygen concentration. Intravenous fluids are infused to maintain intravascular volume and optimise tissue and organ perfusion. In mild shock the intravenous fluid recommended is Hartmann's solution. Three times the volume of Hartmann's must be infused for the equivalent volume of blood lost because this solution does not remain in the intravascular compartment but is also distributed to the interstitial fluid. More significant haemorrhage should be replenished by blood to improve oxygen carriage.

After initial resuscitation, the patient will go on to definitive care for sustained injuries such as laparotomy or orthopaedic care for fractures. There is a group of patients with major trauma who, despite adequate early resuscitation and definitive treatment, are at risk of later onset multiorgan dysfunction syndrome (MODS) and death. Respiratory problems are usually the first sign and may begin at 24 hours after injury. The most severe form of this is the acute respiratory distress syndrome (ARDS). Despite intensive organ support, the condition progresses, leading to coagulation problems, in particular disseminated intravascular coagulation (DIC), renal problems, such as acute tubular necrosis (ATN) and liver failure with decreased cardiac output and intractable shock. The pathogenesis of this syndrome is not fully evaluated but is thought to involve occult hypoperfusion, particularly in the splanchnic area and the release of inflammatory mediators. The inflammatory response leads to decreased systemic vascular resistance and a high cardiac output state. The body is already in a highly catabolic state following trauma and, despite adequate resuscitation at this stage, the process progresses with failure of utilisation of oxygen in the microcirculation owing to interstitial oedema, uncoupling of oxidative phosphorylation and malfunctioning of the mitochondria. The inflammatory mediators involved include cytokines, tumour necrosis factor, nitric oxide and interleukins. Current therapeutic advances have been aimed at intervention to modify the inflammatory response. Death from MODS usually occurs at 1–6 weeks following injury.

CONCLUSION

Biochemical tests are essential adjuncts to assessing and monitoring the care of the trauma patient. Although of intrinsic value in themselves, all biochemical results must always be interpreted within the context of any pre-existing conditions, the acute history and therapeutic interventions undertaken. Actions must then be based on an understanding of the underlying physiological processes with monitoring continued against which to gauge progress.

CASE STUDIES

Case study 8.1

A young motorcyclist is brought into the accident and emergency (A&E) department having been involved in a road traffic accident (RTA). He has been trapped under a car involved by his legs for one hour. He is found to have bilateral tibial and fibular fractures. Biochemistry results from initial blood test on arrival are normal. His urine dipstick test is positive for blood. Microscopy of his urine shows no red blood cells. Imaging shows no renal damage. He undergoes fixation for his fractures but the following day his urine output drops to 10 ml/hour and repeat biochemistry is: Na 137, K 6.7, urea 22, creatinine 420, CK 4300.

The patient has sustained severe crush injuries and rhabdomyolysis. This is shown by the high CK and the presence of myoglobin in the urine. Urine myoglobin gives a false-positive test for blood on testing when no red blood cells are in the urine. Red blood cells would be present if there had been renal trauma hence the significance of the normal renal imaging and normal urine microscopy. He has developed acute renal failure most likely from acute renal tubular damage from muscle breakdown products. Treatment involves vigorous fluid resuscitation at the time of injury but once renal failure has developed renal dialysis may be necessary.

Case study 8.2

An elderly gentleman is pulled from his burning car. He suffers extensive burns (30%). On arrival he is intubated and cared for on the intensive care unit (ITU). His initial arterial blood gas measurement shows a carboxyhaemaglobin level of 15%.

The patient has been in an enclosed area inhaling carbon monoxide. The formation of carboxyhaemoglobin instead of oxyhaemoglobin causes decreased oxygen delivery to organs and tissues as carboxyhaemoglobin has a high affinity for oxygen and does not readily give it up to the tissues. A usual level in the blood is approximately 1% for a non-smoker and up to 5% for a smoker. A level of more than 10% is significant and requires a high concentration of inspiratory oxygen to displace the carbon monoxide. A level of more than 40% or with other signs, such as confusion or coma, requires hyperbaric oxygen treatment at a specialist centre. The following day his biochemistry results show: Na 148, K 5.2, urea 24, creatinine 200.

The patient is dehydrated. Burns require aggressive fluid resuscitation as a large amount of fluid is lost from the burn area. Set formulae are used to calculate fluid requirements and the aim is to maintain a urine output of 30–50 ml/hour in the adult. In the immediate management it is important to keep the area covered and to keep the patient warm. Any patient with extensive burns is in a highly catabolic state and often requires parenteral nutrition to aid healing.

Case study 8.3

A 19-year-old man is brought to casualty following a fight. He has sustained a stab wound to his upper abdomen. He has a heart rate of 160 beats/minute and is anxious and uncooperative. Resuscitation is commenced with oxygen and intravenous Hartmann's solution. He remains cardiovascularly unstable with suspected peritonitis and is taken for laparotomy. Whilst in theatre, the A&E house officer pursues the biochemistry results, which are reported with an amylase of 1200. In theatre, a laceration to the pancreas is found.

Case study 8.4

A 40-year-old woman is brought into the A&E department from the scene of a road traffic accident at 8 am. She was the driver of a car

that was witnessed to mount the pavement and drive into a shop window. Bystanders thought that the driver had been 'fitting' at the wheel. On arrival, she is 'thrashing' around with no obvious sign of injury. Glucose 'stick' testing reads 'low'. She is given 50 ml of 50% glucose and calms down and begins to talk normally. She reveals that she is an insulin-dependent diabetic who had given herself her morning dose of insulin and was going to have something to eat at work for breakfast. Unfortunately, her insulin had begun to bring her blood sugar down before she had eaten. Laboratory results confirm a blood glucose reading of 1.2 mmol/l. Low blood glucose caused the fitting.

Case study 8.5

An elderly gentleman is found wandering near the supermarket at 2 am. He is disorientated in time and place. On examination he has a large haematoma on the occipital area of his head, which appears to be a few days old. His biochemistry results are: Na 122, K 3.6, urea 8. His urine osmolality is 800 mosmol/kg, with plasma osmolality 270 mosmol/kg.

He has the syndrome of inappropriate antidiuretic hormone release (SIADH) as a result of his recent head injury. Antidiuretic hormone is being 'inappropriately' released causing the retention of body water. Increased body water 'dilutes' the plasma sodium even though the body total sodium remains the same or increased. The urine is 'inappropriately' concentrated compared to the plasma osmolality. The low Na level causes confusion and, if it continues, fitting.

Case study 8.6

A middle-aged lady has undergone a splenectomy after being involved as a passenger in a high-speed road traffic accident. Three days postoperatively she is noted to be oedematous. Biochemistry results show: Na 129, K 4.7, urea 4.7 and creatinine 95. On review of her fluid chart, she has been given 5 litres of fluid per day postoperatively two-thirds of which was 5% dextrose.

She has developed interstitial oedema from a combination of overzealous treatment with intravenous fluid and 5% dextrose and the after effects of the 'stress' hormone response, which leads to retention of salt and water.

Case study 8.7

A middle-aged known alcoholic gentleman is brought into the A&E department having been found at the bottom of a stairwell. He is breathing spontaneously but has obvious rib fractures on the right side with pain on breathing. He has a significant head laceration and boggy swelling on the right side of his head and his Glasgow Coma Score (GCS) is calculated to be 11. His temperature is 34°C. He has a mid-shaft femoral fracture with gross deformity and swelling. He is initially treated with high-flow oxygen by mask, intravenous fluids, reduction and splintage of his femoral fracture, and active warming. Initial blood gases were pH 7.28, pCO_2 7.1, pO_2 8.2. It was decided to commence intubation and mechanical ventilation, which was performed successfully. A chest x-ray post-intubation showed a haemothorax and a chest drain was inserted. His arterial blood gases improved slightly.

His biochemistry results were: Na 136, K 4.8, urea 10.2, creatinine 190, bilirubin 35, ALT 120, alk ph 260, albumin 33, corrected Ca 2.4. The following day on the intensive care unit his oxygenation could not be maintained and his arterial blood gases deteriorated: pH 7.14, pCO_2 7.6, pO_2 7.2. His haemoglobin dropped and his clotting became deranged despite treatment with clotting factors. Repeat biochemistry showed Na 140, K 6.1, urea 23, creatinine 280, bilirubin 45, ALT 563, alk ph 410, albumin 28. His urine output dropped to less than 10 ml/hour and it was decided to commence renal dialysis on the third day. Oxygenation was still poor and a worsening acidosis was developing. By the third day his clotting worsened and he developed disseminated intravascular coagulation. He suffered a massive pulmonary haemorrhage and died.

This is an example of multiple trauma with coexistent renal and liver impairment. The lung contusion led to respiratory failure, which could not be reversed by mechanical ventilation. There followed a cascade of renal, liver and coagulation failure, which, despite organ support, led to irreversible decline and death.

Further reading

Alberts B, et al. *Molecular biology of the cell*, 3rd edn. New York: Garland, 1994

Devlin T (ed.) *Textbook of biochemistry with clinical correlation*, 4th edn. New York: Wiley-Liss, 1997

Gutierrez G. Cellular energy metabolism during hypoxia. *Critical Care Medicine* 1991; 19: 619–626

Kumar V, Cotran RS, Robbins SL. *Basic pathology*, 6th edn. Philadelphia: WB Saunders, 1997

Pastores SM, et al. Posttraumatic multiple-organ dysfunction syndrome: role of mediators in systemic inflammation and subsequent organ failure. *Academic Emergency Medicine* 1996; 3: 611–622

Stene JK, Grande CM. *Trauma anaesthesia*. Philadelphia: Williams and Wilkins, 1991

Stoner HB. Interpretation of the metabolic effects of trauma and sepsis. *Journal of Clinical Pathology* 1987; 40: 1108–1117

Chapter 9

Acid–base balance

Peter Driscoll

INTRODUCTION

Acid–base balance is a potentially complex and difficult subject. It is, however, based upon a number of simple concepts. This chapter is intended to outline these concepts. The chapter will cover the meaning of the commonly used terms in acid–base balance, and will outline how the body removes carbon dioxide and acid, and will also cover the interpretation of an arterial blood gas result from a trauma patient.

TERMINOLOGY

It is important that the terms commonly used, when discussing acid–base balance, are clearly understood. These are detailed below.

Acids and bases

Originally the word 'acid' was used to describe the sour taste of unripe fruit but subsequently many different meanings have been attributed to it. This led to considerable confusion and misunderstanding, which was not resolved until 1923, when the following definition was proposed:

> An acid is any substance that is capable of providing hydrogen ions (H^+)

A strong acid is a substance that will readily provide hydrogen ions and, conversely, a weak acid provides only a few. The body mainly deals with weak acids, such as carbonic acid and lactic acid.

The opposite of an acid is a *base* which is defined as any substance that 'accepts' hydrogen ions. One of the commonest bases found in the body is bicarbonate (HCO_3^-).

The pH scale, acidosis and alkalosis

The concentration of hydrogen ions in solution is usually *very* small, even with strong acids. This is particularly true when dealing with the acids found in the body, where the hydrogen ion concentrations are in the order of 40 nanomoles/litre (nmol/l).

---

1 nanomole = 1 billionth of a mole

To gain a perspective on how tiny this is, it is interesting to compare it with the concentration of other commonly measured electrolytes. For example, the plasma concentration of sodium is around 135 mmol/l (i.e. three million times greater).

Dealing with such very small numbers is obviously difficult and so, in 1909, the pH scale was developed. This scale has the advantage of being able to express any hydrogen ion concentration as a number between 1 and 14 inclusively. The pH of a normal arterial blood sample lies between 7.36 and 7.44, and is equivalent to a hydrogen ion concentration of 44–36 nmol/l, respectively.

Crucially, though the pH value *increases*, the concentration of hydrogen ions *decreases*. This is a consequence of the mathematical process that was used to develop the scale. Therefore, an arterial blood pH below 7.36 indicates that the concentration of hydrogen ions has increased from normal. This condition is called an *acidaemia*. Conversely, a pH above 7.44 would result from a reduction in the concentration of hydrogen ions. This condition is called an *alkalaemia*.

Another important consequence of the derivation of the pH scale is the fact that *small changes in pH mean relatively large changes in hydrogen ion concentration*. For example, a fall in the pH from 7.40 to 7.10 means the hydrogen ion concentration has risen from 40 to 80 nmol/l (i.e. it has doubled).

Buffers

Many of the complex chemical reactions occurring at a cellular level are controlled by special proteins

---

Box 9.1   Key points: pH scale, acidosis and alkalosis

- Hydrogen ions are only present in the body in very low concentrations
- As the hydrogen ion concentration increases, the pH falls
- As the hydrogen ion concentration falls, the pH rises
- An acidaemia occurs when the pH falls below 7.36 and an alkalaemia when it rises above 7.44
- Small changes in the pH scale represent large changes in the concentration of hydrogen ions

---

called enzymes. These substances can only function effectively at very narrow ranges of pH (7.36–7.44). However, during normal activity, the body produces massive amounts of hydrogen ions, which, if left unchecked, would lead to significant falls in pH. Clearly a system is required to prevent these hydrogen ions causing large changes in pH before they are eliminated from the body. This is achieved by the 'buffers': they 'take up' the free hydrogen ions in the cells and in the bloodstream, thereby preventing a change in pH.

There are a variety of buffers in the body. Intracellularly the main ones are proteins, phosphate and haemoglobin. Extracellularly there are also plasma proteins and bicarbonate. Proteins 'soak up' the hydrogen ions like a sponge and transport them to their place of elimination from the body. In the majority of cases, this is through the kidneys. In contrast, the bicarbonate reacts with the hydrogen ions to produce water and carbon dioxide. The latter is subsequently removed by the lungs (see later).

With these common terms defined, we can now consider why trauma victims can become acidotic and how the body tries to correct it.

ACID PRODUCTION AND ITS REMOVAL

The body, whether healthy or injured, produces large amounts of water, acid and carbon dioxide each day. A healthy adult will normally produce 15 000 000 nmol of hydrogen ions each day as part of the waste products of food metabolised to release energy. As this process occurs at a cellular

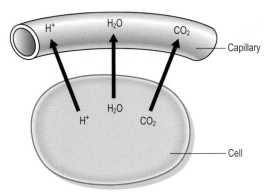

Figure 9.1 Removal of waste products from cells.

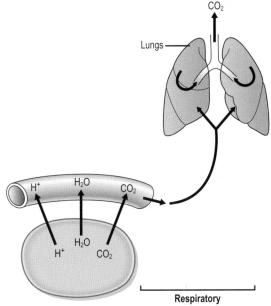

Figure 9.2 Removal of carbon dioxide by the lungs.

level, it is here that these products initially accumulate. Irreparable cellular damage occurs if this is left unchecked.

The first acute compensatory mechanism is the intracellular buffering system. As described previously, this provides the cell with a temporary way of minimising the fluctuations in acidity. Subsequently, these waste products (i.e. carbon dioxide and hydrogen ions) are excreted into the bloodstream where they are taken up by the extracellular buffers (Figure 9.1).

However, this is only a temporary solution because there is only a limited amount of buffer. If this was the sum total of the body's defence to acids and carbon dioxide, then the buffers would soon be exhausted, thereby allowing the products of metabolism to accumulate in the bloodstream. A system is therefore needed to remove these harmful substances from the body so that they do not reach toxic levels and, at the same time, regenerate the buffers. Fortunately, the body can eliminate these waste products by the lungs and the kidneys.

Carbon dioxide removal (the respiratory component)

Carbon dioxide (CO_2) released from cells is transported in the blood to the lungs, diffuses into the alveoli, and is ultimately removed from the body during expiration (Figure 9.2). If CO_2 is produced faster than it can be eliminated, or there is a blockage to its elimination, then it will accumulate in the bloodstream. Here it reacts with

Table 9.1 Results from an arterial blood sample taken during respiratory acidosis

	Normal	Respiratory acidosis
pH	7.36–7.44	↓↓
$PaCO_2$	36–40 mmHg	↑↑
	4.8–5.3 kPa	
HCO_3^-	21–27 mmol/l	21–27 mmol/l

water in the plasma with the result that hydrogen ions (H^+) are produced along with bicarbonate:

$$CO_2 + H_2O \rightleftharpoons H^+ + HCO_3^-$$

The greater the amount of CO_2, the more H^+ is produced. If this increase in plasma concentration of hydrogen ions causes the pH to fall below 7.36, then an *acidaemia* will occur. As the cause of the acidaemia in this case is a problem in the respiratory system, it is known as a *respiratory acidosis*. If a sample of arterial blood were taken immediately this occurred, then the result shown in Table 9.1 would be obtained.

As a byproduct of the reaction between CO_2 and water, the bicarbonate concentration also increases by the same amount as the hydrogen ions. However, this increase is usually in the order of several nanomoles. As the normal concentration is 21–27 mmol (i.e. 21–27 *million* nanomoles) the net increase in bicarbonate is very small. Consequently, these changes in concentration are enough to change the pH scale but are not large enough to alter significantly the plasma bicarbonate concentration.

In an injured patient, the respiratory component needs to excrete over 12 000 000 nmol of H^+ per day. It is, therefore, easy to see that there can be a rapid onset of acidosis during episodes of hypoventilation.

ACID REMOVAL (THE METABOLIC COMPONENT)

As already described, acids are continually produced as a result of cellular metabolism. The amount produced from normal metabolism is approximately 3 000 000 nmol/day. This acid load is soaked up by buffers in the bloodstream in order that they can be transported safely to their point of elimination (Figure 9.3). One of these buffers is bicarbonate (HCO_3^-), which is generated by the kidneys and released into the bloodstream, where it reacts with free hydrogen (Figure 9.4).

In certain circumstances, so much acid is produced by the cells that it exceeds the capacity of both the protein buffers and bicarbonate. If this results in an accumulation of free hydrogen ions

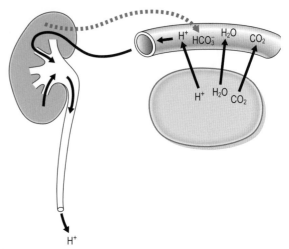

Figure 9.4 Restoration of bicarbonate by the kidney.

Table 9.2 Results from an arterial blood sample taken during metabolic acidosis

	Normal	Metabolic acidosis
pH	7.36–7.44	↓↓
$PaCO_2$	36–40 mmHg	36–40 mmHg
	4.8–5.3 kPa	4.8–5.3 kPa
HCO_3^-	21–27 mmol/l	↓↓

in the plasma such that the pH falls below 7.36, then an acidaemia has been produced. As this is a result of a defect in the metabolic system, it is termed a *metabolic acidosis*. If an arterial blood gas sample were taken when this occurred, then the result shown in Table 9.2 would be obtained. The bicarbonate level has fallen as a consequence of reacting with the free hydrogen ions to produce carbon dioxide and water.

> Carbon dioxide and acids are being produced continually by cellular metabolism
> The removal of CO_2 by the lungs is termed the respiratory component
> The removal of acid by the kidneys is termed the metabolic component

The respiratory–metabolic link

It can be seen from the above that the body has two distinct methods of preventing the accumulation of hydrogen ions and the subsequent

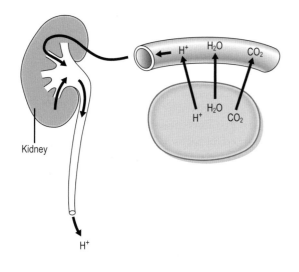

Metabolic

Figure 9.3 Removal of hydrogen ions by the kidneys.

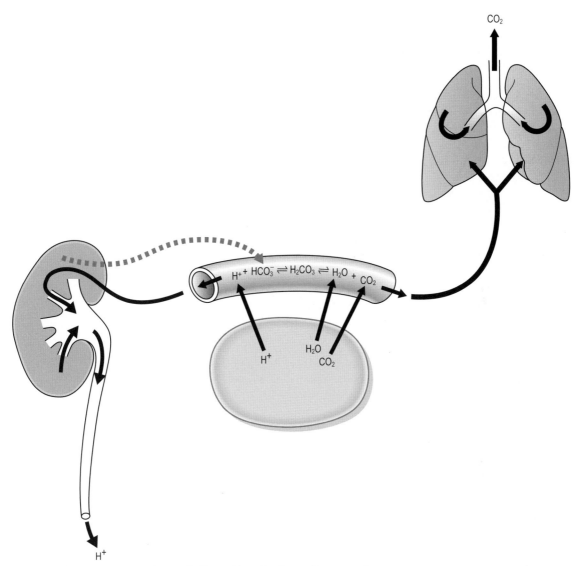

Figure 9.5 Carbonic acid–bicarbonate buffer: acid production and its removal.

development of an acidaemia. As a further protection, these two components are in balance (or equilibrium) so that each can *compensate* for a derangement in the other. This link between the respiratory and metabolic systems is due to the presence of *carbonic acid* (H_2CO_3; Figure 9.5).

The ability for each system to compensate for the other becomes more marked when the initial disturbance in one system is prolonged. The production of carbonic acid is dependent upon an enzyme called carbonic anhydrase, which is present in abundance in the red cells and the

kidneys. It is, therefore, ideally placed to facilitate the link between the respiratory and the metabolic systems. The following examples consider how this link can help the body respond to an excess of either carbon dioxide or acid.

Example 1

In a head-injured patient with inadequate alveolar ventilation, carbon dioxide accumulates. As we have seen, this will tend to cause a respiratory acidosis. Rather than the

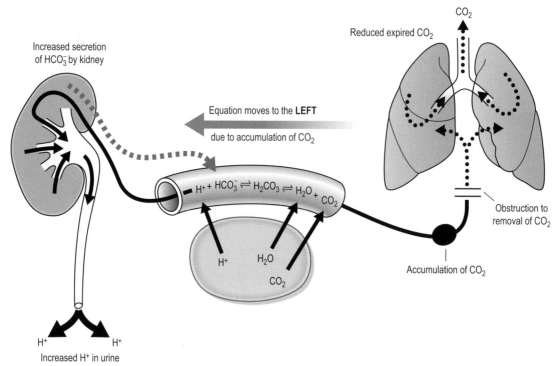

Figure 9.6 Metabolic compensation to respiratory acidosis (i.e. the metabolic system is compensating for the respiratory system).

body existing in a chronic state of acidosis, the metabolic system can help compensate by increasing bicarbonate production by the kidneys (Figure 9.6). Utilising the carbonic acid link, this enables the removal of some of the excess carbon dioxide. However, this compensation takes over 24 hours to become effective, as it is dependent upon the increased production of enzymes in the kidney.

It is important to realise that, in the acute situation, *the body does not fully compensate.* Consequently, if an arterial blood sample is taken early on, it will demonstrate that there is still a persistent but slight underlying acidaemia (Table 9.3).

Example 2

Shocked trauma patients sometimes develop a state of excess acid production known as *lactic acidosis*. The excess cellular acid is released into the plasma to be transported to the kidney for excretion. However, the kidneys are only able to excrete the additional acid load

Table 9.3 Results from an arterial blood sample taken during early metabolic compensation

	Normal	Respiratory acidosis	Metabolic compensation
pH	7.36–7.44	↓↓	↓
$PaCO_2$	36–40 mmHg	↑↑	↑↑
	4.8–5.3 kPa		
HCO_3^-	21–27 mmol/l	21–27 mmol/l	↑

slowly and a metabolic acidosis develops. The kidneys are slowly stimulated into increasing bicarbonate production to counteract this but it takes 24 hours. In the meantime, owing to the carbonic acid link, some of the excess acid can be converted to carbon dioxide and eliminated by the respiratory system (Figure 9.7).

This compensation is facilitated by the fact that the excess hydrogen ions are detected by special receptors in the brainstem, which, in turn, increase the respiratory rate and depth within minutes. (Compare this with the slow

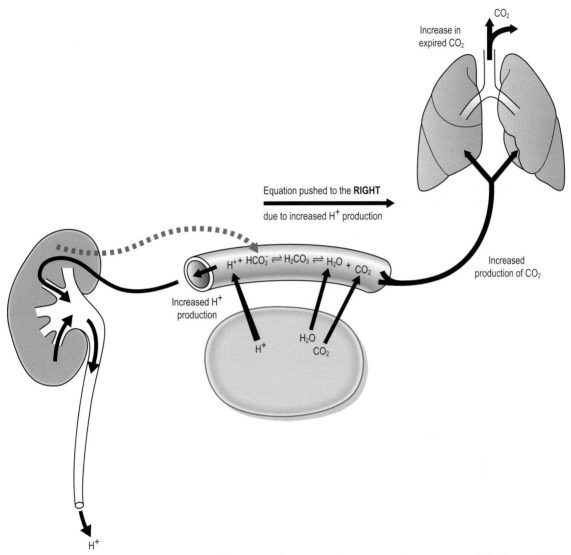

CO$_2$

Increase in
expired CO$_2$

Equation pushed to the **RIGHT**

due to increased H$^+$ production

$$H^+ + HCO_3^- \rightleftharpoons H_2CO_3 \rightleftharpoons H_2O + CO_2$$

Increased H$^+$
production

Increased
production of CO$_2$

H$^+$

H$_2$O
CO$_2$

H$^+$

Figure 9.7   Respiratory compensation to metabolic acidosis (i.e. the respiratory system has compensated for the metabolic system).

response of the kidneys.) This process enables the body to eliminate the extra carbon dioxide providing there is no obstruction to ventilation. The lowering of the carbon dioxide levels in the blood encourages further free acid to be converted into carbonic acid and eventually carbon dioxide. However, the body does not fully compensate in the acute situation. Therefore even after several hours, respiratory compensation will only be partial and the patient will still be slightly acidaemic (Table 9.4).

The body does not fully compensate in the acute situation

It must also be remembered that the degree to which the respiratory system can compensate is dependent upon the work involved in breathing and the systemic effects of a low arterial concentration of carbon dioxide. The compensatory mechanisms can thus be summarised as in Box 9.2.

Table 9.4 Results from an arterial blood sample taken after several hours of respiratory compensation

	Normal	Metabolic acidosis	Respiratory compensation
pH	7.36–7.44	↓↓	↓
PaCO$_2$	36–40 mmHg	36–40 mmHg	↓
	4.8–5.3 kPa	4.8–5.3 kPa	
HCO$_3^-$	21–27 mmol/l	↓↓	↓↓

Box 9.2   Summary of compensatory mechanisms

- The metabolic component of the body's acid elimination mechanism can compensate for a respiratory acidosis by increasing the production of bicarbonate by the kidneys
- Compensation by the metabolic component usually takes over 24 hours to achieve
- The respiratory component of the body's acid elimination mechanism can compensate for a metabolic acidosis by increasing ventilation of the lungs and eliminating carbon dioxide
- Compensation by the respiratory component usually takes place within minutes
- In the acute situation, the body does not fully compensate, therefore the underlying acidaemia will remain

---

A SYSTEMATIC APPROACH TO ANALYSING AN ARTERIAL BLOOD GAS (ABG) SAMPLE

Before analysing a blood gas result, it is important to assess the patient first and to be aware of the clinical history and current medications. A review of the other laboratory investigations is also helpful. In the emergency situation, however, these data may not be immediately available. Consequently, the initial results must be interpreted with caution and trends followed, whilst the rest of the information is being obtained (Box 9.3).

Data interpretation

Is there an acidaemia or alkalaemia?
In most cases, the patient will have an acute single acid–base disturbance. In these circumstances, the body rarely has the opportunity to compensate completely for the alteration in hydrogen ion

---

Box 9.3   Systematic approach to analysing an ABG sample

History
- Are there any symptoms of conditions likely to cause an acid–base disturbance?
- Are there any symptoms resulting from an acid–base disturbance?

Data interpretation
- Is there an acidaemia or alkalaemia?
- Is there evidence of a disturbance in the respiratory component of the body's acid–base balance?
- Is there evidence of a disturbance in the metabolic component of the body's acid–base balance?
- Is there a single or multiple acid–base disturbance?
- Is there any defect in oxygen uptake?

Integration of history and data
- Do the conclusions from the history agree with the data analysis?

---

concentration. Consequently, the pH will remain outside the normal range and thereby indicate the underlying acid base disturbance.

> pH less than 7.36 = Underlying acidaemia
> pH greater than 7.36 = Underlying alkalaemia

In acute, single acid–base disturbances the body usually does not have time to compensate fully. The pH will, therefore, indicate the primary acid–base problem

Nevertheless, a normal pH does not necessarily mean the patient is free of an acid–base disturbance. In fact, there are three reasons for a patient having a pH within the normal range as listed below.

- There is no underlying acid–base disturbance.
- The body has fully compensated for a single acid–base disturbance.
- There is more than one acid–base disturbance with equal but opposite effects on the pH.

Using the knowledge gained from the patient's clinical history and examination, it is possible to have a good idea which of these options is the true answer. However, to confirm or refute early suspicions, it is necessary to see if there is any evidence of alterations in the respiratory and metabolic components of the body's acid–base balance.

Is the abnormality due to a defect in the respiratory component?

Checking the $PaCO_2$ gives a good indication of ventilatory adequacy because it is inversely proportional to alveolar ventilation. When combined with pH, it can be used to determine if there is either a problem with the respiratory system or if the respiratory component is simply compensating for a problem in the metabolic component.

Take, for example, an arterial sample with a pH of 7.2 and a $PaCO_2$ of 60 mmHg (8.0 kPa). A pH of 7.2 indicates that there is an acidaemia. As the $PaCO_2$ is raised, this indicates that there is a *respiratory acidosis*. Consider now a patient with a similar pH but a $PaCO_2$ of 25 mmHg (3.3 kPa). There is still an acidaemia but, as the $PaCO_2$ is lowered, it would imply there is *respiratory compensation to a metabolic acidosis*. To confirm this, the metabolic component would need to be assessed.

Is the abnormality due to a defect in the metabolic component?

To determine the metabolic component, the concentration of bicarbonate is measured. In a similar situation to that described above, when the bicarbonate concentration is combined with pH, it can be determined if there is either a primary metabolic or compensatory metabolic problem.

Using the second example above, the bicarbonate was found to be 9.5 mmol/l. This is below the normal range (22–27 mmol/l). Consequently with a pH of 7.2 and a $PaCO_2$ of 25 mmHg (3.3 kPa), it is in keeping with the idea that this patient has a *metabolic acidosis with partial respiratory compensation*.

In addition to bicarbonate, the base excess is also often provided in the ABG result. This provides a better assessment of the metabolic component of the body's acid–base status because it takes into account all the buffers in the blood not just bicarbonate. Base excess is defined as the number of moles of *bicarbonate* which must be added to the equivalent of 1 litre of the patient's blood, so that a pH of 7.4 is produced. Respiratory influences are eliminated by keeping the partial pressure of carbon dioxide constant at 40 mmHg (5.3 kPa). The value should be zero but a normal range is from –2 to +2 mmol/l. For example, an arterial blood sample with a pH of 7.25, a $PaCO_2$ of 25 mmHg (3.3 kPa) and a base deficit of –15 indicate that there is a metabolic acidosis with partial respiratory compensation.

Is there a single or multiple acid–base disturbance?

To narrow down the diagnosis even further, you need to consider how much the $PaCO_2$ and bicarbonate (base excess) concentration has changed. If these changes fall within certain limits, then there is usually only a single acid–base disturbance. Alternatively, if they are outside this range, then it is likely that the patient has more than one acid–base disturbance.

There are two methods of assessing these changes. Both are equally effective; one uses a graphical method and the other relies upon arithmetical calculations. However, in using these methods, be aware that they only provide an initial approximation. The results need to be interpreted in light of clinical findings. The ABG should then be repeated after approximately 15 minutes of therapy. Re-analysis will help to refute or confirm the initial conclusions.

> Trends in ABG results are a more accurate way of detecting multiple acid–base disturbances than a single reading

Graphical method

In order to understand the graphical method, it is necessary to be familiar with the layout of 'Flenley's graph', as shown in Figure 9.8. In particular, the following points should be noted.

- The graph is showing how the pH alters with changes in $PaCO_2$.
- Cutting diagonally across the graph are lines that indicate the concentration of bicarbonate. These are known as *isopleths*.
- As the concentration of bicarbonate increases, the gradient of the isopleths falls.
- The square box indicates the normal range for pH, $PaCO_2$ and bicarbonate concentration.

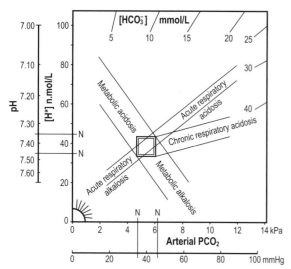

Figure 9.8 Flenley's graph.

- Fanning out from this box are the possible ranges of normal responses you could expect with single acid–base disturbances.
- The bands representing the acute respiratory disturbances run approximately parallel to the isopleths. This is because the pH and $PaCO_2$ are altered but there is little effect on the bicarbonate concentration. These bands do not include patients who have had long enough to develop metabolic compensation and so have altered their bicarbonate concentrations. Instead, these patients are represented in the chronic respiratory acidosis group.
- The band representing the metabolic disturbances runs across the isopleths. Therefore, metabolic acidosis and alkalosis will alter the bicarbonate concentration as well as the pH and $PaCO_2$. These bands include patients who are using respiratory compensation to counteract the pH changes. However, it does not include those patients who have had long enough to develop metabolic compensation (i.e. those who have a chronic metabolic disturbance).

Using this graph, one can plot the results from the blood gas analysis. If it lies within one of these bands, then there is likely to be only one acid–base disturbance. Conversely, if the results lie outside these normal ranges, then there is likely to be more than one acid–base disturbance.

Box 9.4 Expected changes

Acute respiratory acidosis
A 1.0 mmHg rise in $PaCO_2$ produces a 0.1 mmol/l rise in HCO_3

Chronic respiratory acidosis
A 1.0 mmHg rise in $PaCO_2$ produces a 0.4 mmol/l rise in HCO_3

Acute respiratory alkalosis
A 1.0 mmHg fall in $PaCO_2$ produces a 0.2 mmol/l fall in HCO_3

Chronic respiratory alkalosis
A 1.0 mmHg fall in $PaCO_2$ produces a 0.5 mmol/l fall in HCO_3

Metabolic acidosis
A 1.0 mmol/l fall in HCO_3 produces a 1.0 mmHg fall in $PaCO_2$

Metabolic alkalosis
A 1 mmol/l rise in HCO_3 produces a 0.6 mmHg rise in $PaCO_2$

All these values are taken from the middle of the normal ranges.

Arithmetic method
This system has the disadvantage of using the older units for $PaCO_2$ (i.e. millimeters of mercury – mmHg). Nevertheless, by applying the numbers listed in Box 9.4, it is possible to determine if the changes in $PaCO_2$ and bicarbonate are appropriate for a single acid–base disturbance. If there is any inconsistency between the actual results and those derived by calculation, then it is likely that the patient has more than one acid–base disturbance.

Having now finished the interpretation of the parameters in the blood gas analysis, which provide information on the patient's acid–base balance, it is then necessary to assess one more important value in an arterial sample – the partial pressure of oxygen. This is important because a failure to take up oxygen can lead to many adverse conditions, including hypoxia. With regard to the acid–base balance, hypoxia can give rise to metabolic acidosis because it causes the cells to change to anaerobic metabolism and so produce excessive quantities of lactic acid.

Is there a defect in oxygen uptake?

In knowing the inspired oxygen concentration (FiO$_2$), it is possible to predict what the PaO$_2$ would be if the patient was ventilating normally. Since atmospheric pressure is 760 mmHg (approximately 100 kPa), 1% is 7.6 mmHg (about 1 kPa). This would mean inspiring 30% O$_2$ from a facemask would produce an inspired partial pressure of oxygen of 30 kPa (228 mmHg). This should lead to an arterial concentration of around 20–25 kPa (152–257.6 mmHg) because there is a normal drop of about 7.5 kPa (57 mmHg) between the partial pressure of oxygen inspired at the mouth and that in the alveoli. A drop significantly greater than 10 kPa (76 mmHg) would imply there is a mismatch in the lungs between ventilation of the alveoli and their perfusion with blood.

For example, an arterial PaO$_2$ of 33 kPa (approximately 250 mmHg) in a patient breathing 40% oxygen is within normal limits. In contrast, an arterial PaO$_2$ of 24 kPa (approximately 180 mmHg) in a patient breathing 50% oxygen indicates that there is a defect in the take up of oxygen because the expected value is at least 40 kPa. (An inspired oxygen of 50% will have a partial pressure of approximately 50 kPa. This would mean the expected PaO$_2$ would be at least 50–10 = 40 kPa.)

The following case study illustrates how blood gases should be interpreted using the system outlined above.

Case study

A previously well 23-year-old man is brought to the emergency department with a head injury having fallen off a 3-metre wall. In the department, he became increasingly drowsy.

RESULTS

Whilst receiving 85% oxygen by a non-rebreathing mask with reservoir, an arterial sample was taken for blood gas analysis. The results were as shown in Table 9.5.

ANALYSIS OF HISTORY AND RESULTS

History
Are there any symptoms of conditions likely to cause an acid–base disturbance?
Answer: Yes.

Table 9.5   Results from an arterial blood sample taken from a patient with a head injury receiving 85% oxygen

	Normal	Patient
pH	7.36–7.44	7.05
PaCO$_2$	35–45 mmHg	80.4 mmHg
	4.7–6.0 kPa	28.5 kPa
HCO$_3^-$	21–28 mmol/l	15.5 mmol/l
Base excess	±2 mmol/l	−7.5 mmol/l
PaO$_2$	Over 90 mmHg*	119.9 mmHg
	Over 12.0 kPa	15.8 kPa

*On room air.

Respiratory depression will lead to carbon dioxide retention and, therefore, a respiratory acidosis. In view of the acuteness of the history, it is unlikely that there would be any measurable metabolic compensation. It is also possible the person may have sustained other injuries in the fall, which could cause internal haemorrhage. As a result, the patient may have developed a lactic acidosis owing to inadequate tissue oxygenation. Impaired ventilation can also lead to poor oxygen uptake by the lungs. This can be compounded by any associated chest injuries that could be present.

Are there any symptoms resulting from an acid–base disturbance?
Answer: None from the information provided.

Data
Is there an acidaemia or alkalaemia?
Answer: Yes
The pH is reduced, therefore, there is an acidaemia.

Is there evidence of a disturbance in the respiratory component of the body's acid–base balance?
Answer: Yes.
The carbon dioxide level is raised, which is in keeping with a respiratory acidosis.

Is there evidence of a disturbance in the metabolic component of the body's acid–base balance?
Answer: Yes
The bicarbonate (base excess) is low. This is in keeping with a metabolic acidosis.

Is there a single or multiple acid–base disturbance?
Answer: There is a multiple acid–base disturbance

There is both a respiratory and metabolic acidosis. The Flenley graph shows that the results lie outside the normal bands for acute respiratory acidosis and metabolic acidosis. This implies there is more than one acid–base disturbance. By using the arithmetic model, if the patient only had a respiratory acidosis the expected bicarbonate would be:

$$24.5 + [0.1 \times (80.4 - 40)] = 28.5 \text{ mmol/l}$$

This is well above the actual figure of 15.5 mmol/l. Again, this implies there is more than just a respiratory acidosis.

Is there any defect in oxygen uptake?
Answer: Yes.

The expected PaO_2 should be at least 570 mmHg (75 kPa). The actual result is much lower, indicating there is a defect in patient's ability to take up oxygen.

Integration
Do the suspicions from the history agree with the data analysis?
Answer: Yes.

This patient has a combined respiratory and metabolic acidosis as well as a defect in the oxygen uptake.

SUMMARY

The body's system for removing the carbon dioxide and acid produced by metabolism has both a respiratory and metabolic component. These are linked by carbonic acid, which enables one component to compensate for a defect in the other. Following trauma both components can be affected. In addition, there can be defects in the oxygen uptake. It is, therefore, important that a systematic way of interpreting the arterial blood gas results is adopted, so that all the available information can be acquired.

Chapter **10**

The oxygen dissociation curve

Terry Martin

INTRODUCTION

Oxygen is well known as the first 'drug' of choice for trauma patients. It is vital for normal cellular metabolism and a continuous supply of adequate oxygen molecules is essential to prevent damage from cerebral hypoxia. A long-term impairment of oxygen uptake, carriage or delivery will also result in other end-organ dysfunction and damage. Oxygen in the body can be measured in a number of ways, and it is necessary to understand exactly what each measurement means and how it is related to oxygen carriage and delivery in the blood.

PARTIAL PRESSURE OF OXYGEN

Oxygen *partial pressure* (PO_2), otherwise known as *tension*, is the fraction of the total pressure of a mixture of gases that is exerted by oxygen alone. Dalton's law of partial pressures states that each gas in a mixture exerts the same pressure as if it were present, alone, in the same volume occupied by the mixture. The PO_2 difference between two areas determines the direction and rate of flow of oxygen molecules, even when the oxygen is in solution. Henry's law states that the amount of gas dissolved in a given volume is proportional to the partial pressure of the gas at the gas–liquid interface. Therefore, in terms of partial pressure of oxygen, a gradient exists in which flow occurs 'downhill' from alveolar air to arterial blood and then to the tissues (Figure 10.1).

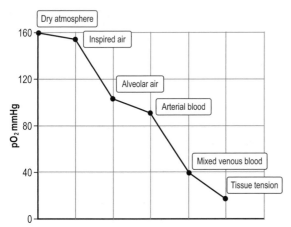

Figure 10.1   The partial pressure gradient for oxygen.

OXYGEN CONTENT OF BLOOD

The amount of oxygen transported to the tissues would be grossly inadequate if it were simply dissolved in physical solution in plasma. The actual amount of oxygen carried in the blood is determined predominantly by the amount in reversible chemical combination with the red blood cell pigment, haemoglobin. This oxygen-carrying protein increases the oxygen capacity of the blood 70-fold.

The total oxygen content of the blood (i.e. that quantity of oxygen contained in the red cells plus the quantity dissolved in solution) is defined as the volume of oxygen in millilitres per decilitre of blood. It can be calculated using:

$$CaO_2 = Hb \times 1.34 \times SaO_2 + 0.023 \times PaO_2 \text{ kPa}$$

or

$$CaO_2 = Hb \times 1.34 \times SaO_2 + 0.0034 \times PaO_2 \text{ mmHg}$$

where:

CaO_2 is the arterial oxygen content (in ml/dl) of blood;

Hb is the haemoglobin concentration (in g/dl) of blood;

1:34 is the volume of oxygen (in ml) carried by 1 g of fully saturated haemoglobin;

SaO_2 is equal to the fractional haemoglobin saturation;

0.023 is the solubility coefficient of oxygen in plasma (in ml of oxygen/dl, for PaO_2 in kPa);

0.0034 is the solubility coefficient of oxygen in plasma (in ml of oxygen/dl, for PaO_2 in mmHg);

PaO_2 is the arterial oxygen tension (measured in kPa or mmHg).

Approximately 99% of the oxygen in blood combines with haemoglobin. Without this special protein, the amount of oxygen carried would be so small that the cardiac output would need to be increased enormously to give an adequate oxygen flux. This would require a considerable increase in blood volume. The physiological significance of haemoglobin is clearly immense.

OXYGEN SATURATION OF HAEMOGLOBIN

Haemoglobin saturation depends on the partial pressure of oxygen and the position on the curve that describes the relationship between PaO_2 and SaO_2 (i.e. the oxygen dissociation curve) and not on the amount of haemoglobin present. This latter point causes confusion but can be better understood by this hypothetical question:

> If a trauma patient receiving 100% oxygen has lost almost all his blood and it is replaced by crystalloid leaving only one red blood cell, and the haemoglobin in that cell is fully saturated, every time that cell passes the pulse oximeter probe, the measurement would be SaO_2 100%. But does this tell us anything about the patient's oxygenation?

Clearly, the answer is 'no'. This is further illustrated in the discussion on anaemia below.

Saturation can be expressed in two ways, depending on the degree of accuracy required.

Fractional saturation is defined as the ratio of oxygen haemoglobin to total haemoglobin:

Fractional saturation = SaO_2 = $HbO_2/(HbO_2 + Hb + metHb + COHb)$

where:

HbO_2 is the oxyhaemoglobin concentration;

metHb is the methaemoglobin concentration;

COHb is the carboxyhaemoglobin concentration.

More frequently, the *functional saturation* is used because it ignores the presence of non-oxygen-carrying methaemoglobin and carboxyhaemoglobin. This is the measure provided by blood gas analysers, which estimate saturation from PaO_2 and the oxygen dissociation curve:

Functional saturation = SaO_2 =
$HbO_2/(HbO_2 + Hb)$

HAEMOGLOBIN

Haemoglobin is a globular oxygen-binding protein with a molecular weight of 64 458 Daltons. It is the principal soluble protein in erythrocytes and gives the cells their red colour. Its main function is to pick up oxygen as the cells pass through the pulmonary capillaries and to release it in the capillaries of other tissues, where it is consumed during cellular metabolism.

The structure of haemoglobin was elucidated using x-ray crystallography techniques by Perutz and fellow workers in Cambridge during the 1960s. A knowledge of its molecular structure provides an understanding of its remarkable properties. The haemoglobin molecule consists of four protein chains, each of which carries a haem group (a tetrapyrrole ring with a central iron atom; Figure 10.2). The commonest type of adult human haemoglobin (HbA) has two types of polypeptide chains, two of each occurring in each molecule, i.e., two alpha (α) chains, each with 141 amino acid residues, and two beta (β) chains, each with 146 amino acid residues. In both types, the haem group is attached to a histidine residue. The HbA molecule is designated $\alpha_2\beta_2$ and, although the four chains lie 'crumpled' together in a ball, the actual shape (the quaternary structure) is of critical importance and determines the nature of the reaction with oxygen.

There are a number of alternative amino acid sequences in the haemoglobin molecule, and the normally occurring alternative chains are described as gamma (γ) and delta (δ). Fetal haemoglobin (HbF) comprises a combination of two gamma chains with two alpha chains ($\alpha_2\gamma_2$), whereas A2 haemoglobin (HbA2) is comprised of two alpha and two delta chains ($\alpha_2\delta_2$). HbA2 forms 2–3% of the total haemoglobin in normal adults.

In comparison with the beta chains of adult haemoglobin, the gamma chains in fetal haemoglobin possess fewer positive charges in the space where a product of glucose metabolism called

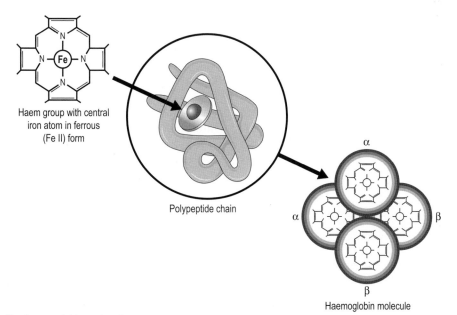

Haem group with central iron atom in ferrous (Fe II) form

Polypeptide chain

α

α β

β

Haemoglobin molecule

Figure 10.2   The haemoglobin molecule.

2,3-diphosphoglycerate (see 'Factors affecting the affinity of haemoglobin for oxygen') is bound. This feature allows oxygen to be bound more tightly (i.e. with greater affinity) than with adult haemoglobin and facilitates the movement of oxygen from the mother to the fetus. HbF is gradually replaced by adult haemoglobin over the first few months of life.

Other variations in the amino acid chains are considered to be abnormal, and many are associated with disordered oxygen carriage or impaired solubility.

BINDING OF HAEMOGLOBIN AND OXYGEN

The haemoglobin molecule comprises four haem complexes made up of a porphyrin (tetrapyrrole ring) and an atom of ferrous (II) iron. Each of the four iron atoms can bind reversibly to one oxygen molecule. Since it contains four haem units, the haemoglobin molecule (Hb_4) reacts with four molecules of oxygen to form Hb_4O_8 (Box 10.1). The reaction is very rapid, requiring less than 0.01 second, as is the deoxygenation (reduction) of Hb_4O_8 back to Hb_4.

The quaternary structure of haemoglobin determines its affinity for oxygen. The shape is maintained by loose bonds between neighbouring amino acids on the same and different chains. The resulting looped structure places the haem group in a crevice, which limits and controls the ease of access for oxygen molecules.

When haemoglobin takes up oxygen, the two beta chains move closer together, whereas they move further apart when oxygen is given up. The movement of the chains is associated with a change in the position of the haem groups, which assume a relaxed (R) state that favours oxygen binding, or a tense (T) state that decreases

---

oxygen binding. The transition from one state to another occurs about 10^8 times in the life of a red blood cell.

The unique ability of haemoglobin to accept oxygen in the presence of high oxygen partial pressure, and yet release it when the partial pressure is low, results from the specific characteristics of haem–haem interactions within the haemoglobin molecule. These interactions allow the oxygenation of one subunit to alter the oxygen affinity of the other subunits. The recruitment of more subunits in the molecule will occur at a lower partial pressure of oxygen than otherwise would be required. The rapidity with which the fourth subunit combines with oxygen is approximately 300 times faster than the first subunit. This is called an *allosteric* effect, that is, when a bound substance (ligand) changes the affinity of another part of the protein for the same ligand (in this case, oxygen). Perhaps more importantly, in the presence of low oxygen tensions, oxygen release from haemoglobin will occur in a similar manner (i.e. the release of oxygen from the first haemoglobin subunit facilitates release of further oxygen).

This enhancement of oxygen uptake and release is the cause of the sigmoid shape of the oxygen dissociation curve and defines the percentage saturation of haemoglobin at any partial pressure of oxygen.

OXYGEN–COMBINING CAPACITY OF HAEMOGLOBIN

When blood is equilibrated with 100% oxygen (PO_2 = 101 kPa or 760 mmHg), normal haemoglobin becomes 100% saturated. When fully saturated, each gram of haemoglobin contains approximately 1.34 ml of oxygen. The haemoglobin concentration in normal blood is about 15 g/dl (14 g/dl in women and 16 g/dl in men). Therefore, 1 dl of blood contains 20.1 ml (1.34 ml × 15) of oxygen bound to haemoglobin when the haemoglobin is 100% saturated. The amount of dissolved oxygen is a linear function of the PO_2 (0.023 ml/dl blood per kPa PO_2).

Under normal circumstances, the haemoglobin in blood at the ends of the pulmonary capillaries is about 97.5% saturated with oxygen (PaO_2 = 97 mmHg or 12.9 kPa). Because of a small amount

---

> **Box 10.1   The reaction of oxygen with haemoglobin**
>
> $Hb_4 + oxygen \equiv Hb_4O_2$
> $Hb_4O_2 + oxygen \equiv Hb_4O_4$
> $Hb_4O_4 + oxygen \equiv Hb_4O_6$
> $Hb_4O_6 + oxygen \equiv Hb_4O_8$

of mixing with venous blood that bypasses lung capillaries, haemoglobin in systemic arterial blood is only 97% saturated. The arterial blood, therefore, contains a total of about 19.8 ml of oxygen per dl (19.5 ml bound to haemoglobin and 0.29 ml in solution).

Because of the lower saturation whilst breathing atmospheric air, the oxygen-combining capacity of adult haemoglobin is approximately 1.31 ml/g. Haemoglobin concentrations are based on iron content, not on oxygen-combining capacity and, since some of the iron is in the form of methaemoglobin and carboxyhaemoglobin, the observed oxygen-combining capacity is less than the theoretical values above.

THE OXYGEN DISSOCIATION CURVE

The characteristic sigmoid-shaped oxygen (or, more correctly, oxyhaemoglobin) dissociation curve relates percentage saturation of the oxygen-carrying power of haemoglobin to the PO_2 (Figure 10.3). When haemoglobin takes up a small amount of oxygen, the R state is favoured and additional uptake of oxygen is facilitated. As previously described, combination of the first haem group in the haemoglobin molecule with oxygen increases the affinity of the second haem for oxygen, and oxygenation of the second increases the affinity of the third, and so on, so that the

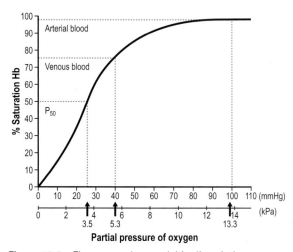

Figure 10.3   The oxygen–haemoglobin dissociation curve.

affinity of haemoglobin for the fourth oxygen molecule is many times that for the first.

The standard oxygen dissociation curve is useful for predicting haemoglobin saturation under a number of conditions, since many factors are known to shift the curve and hence will affect uptake and release of oxygen. The conventional method for quantifying a shift of the dissociation curve is to measure the PO_2 required for 50% saturation (the P_{50}).

Under standard conditions (Box 10.2), the P_{50} is 3.5 kPa (26.3 mmHg). The other important points on the standard curve are:

- arterial blood, which normally corresponds to 97% saturation at a PO_2 of 13.7 kPa (103 mmHg);
- venous blood, which normally corresponds to 75% saturation at a PO_2 of 5.3 kPa (40 mmHg).

A small drop in PO_2 from normal arterial levels causes only minimal decrease in saturation because the curve is almost at a plateau. However, if PO_2 is already low (for pathological or environmental reasons), the same small decrement in PO_2 will cause significant desaturation because of the steep part of the curve.

The steep part of the curve lies within the normal physiological range of extrapulmonary PO_2 levels and explains the unloading of oxygen to the tissues. In effect, a small fall in tissue PO_2 results in a large dissociation and liberation of oxygen from haemoglobin.

FACTORS AFFECTING THE AFFINITY OF HAEMOGLOBIN FOR OXYGEN

The structure of haemoglobin is altered by factors that influence the strength of the loose bonds between the polypeptide chains. Alteration of these bonds affects the accessibility of the haem

Box 10.2   Standard conditions for the oxygen dissociation curve

Blood temperature	33.7° C
Blood pH	7.08
Blood base excess	−7 mmol/l

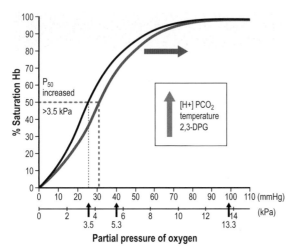

Figure 10.4 Right shift of the oxygen–haemoglobin dissociation curve.

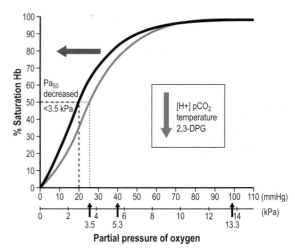

Figure 10.5 Left shift of the oxygen–haemoglobin dissociation curve.

groups to oxygen (and hence its affinity). In general, four important factors can shift the oxygen dissociation curve: pH, PCO_2, temperature and the concentration of 2,3-diphosphoglycerate (2,3-DPG). A rise in temperature, hydrogen ion concentration (i.e. a fall in pH), PCO_2 or concentration of 2,3-DPG will all shift the curve to the right and increase the P_{50} (Figure 10.4). When the curve is shifted in this direction, a higher PO_2 is required for haemoglobin to bind a given amount of oxygen. In other words, saturation is *lower* for any given PO_2. Oxygen is bound *less avidly* and unloading in the tissues is favoured.

Conversely, a decrease in any of these parameters shifts the curve to the left and decreases the P_{50} (Figure 10.5). Under these circumstances, a lower PO_2 is required to bind a given amount of oxygen. In other words, saturation is *greater* for any given PO_2. Oxygen is bound *more avidly* but results in less liberation in the tissues.

The Bohr effect: pH and CO_2

The decrease in oxygen affinity of haemoglobin when the pH of blood falls is called the Bohr effect and occurs because, in a reversal of the normal allosteric effect, deoxyhaemoglobin binds hydrogen ions more avidly than does oxyhaemoglobin. This reaction helps to liberate oxygen in metabolising tissues that are not only consuming oxygen, but are also producing hydrogen ions

(H^+) and CO_2. A fall in pH by 0.2 (e.g. from 7.43 to 7.23) can increase oxygen release by 25%.

According to carbon dioxide metabolism (CO_2 + H_2O ≡ H_2CO_3 ≡ HCO_3^- + H^+), the pH of blood falls as its PCO_2 content increases, so hypercarbia will shift the curve to the right and the P_{50} rises. The negative effect of CO_2 on oxygen binding is mainly due to this tendency for pH to become more acidic (i.e. hydrogen ion concentration increases) as PCO_2 climbs. However, CO_2 in the form of bicarbonate ions (HCO_3^-) also binds preferentially to deoxyhaemoglobin to form carbamino-Hb (the *Haldane effect*) and promotes release of oxygen. In effect, most of the desaturation of haemoglobin that occurs in the tissues is secondary to the decline in the PO_2, but an extra 1–2% desaturation is due to the rise in PCO_2 and local shift of the curve to the right.

Temperature

An increase in temperature dissociates oxygen from haemoglobin and the curve is shifted to the right. Blood bathing in warm metabolising tissue will, therefore, release more oxygen than blood flowing in cold tissues. Conversely, cold air in the lungs shifts the curve to the left, thereby increasing the haemoglobin avidity for oxygen (i.e. more is picked up) and, similarly blood liberates oxygen less readily in peripheral cold tissues (the cold 'red nose' phenomenon).

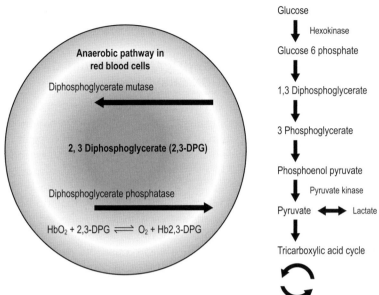

Glucose

Hexokinase

Glucose 6 phosphate

1,3 Diphosphoglycerate

3 Phosphoglycerate

Phosphoenol pyruvate

Pyruvate kinase

Pyruvate ⟷ Lactate

Tricarboxylic acid cycle

Anaerobic pathway in red blood cells

Diphosphoglycerate mutase

2, 3 Diphosphoglycerate (2,3-DPG)

Diphosphoglycerate phosphatase

$HbO_2 + 2,3\text{-DPG} \rightleftharpoons O_2 + Hb2,3\text{-DPG}$

Figure 10.6   Formation of 2,3-diphosphoglycerate in the glycolytic pathway.

2,3–Diphosphoglycerate

The presence of some organic phosphates in erythrocytes can also have a significant effect on the P_{50}. The most important of these compounds is 2,3-DPG, a highly negatively charged molecule, which is plentiful in red blood cells. In essence, 2,3-DPG reacts with haemoglobin to release oxygen and, therefore, moves the dissociation curve to the right. It is formed from 3-phosphoglyceraldehyde as a product of the breakdown of glucose (glycolysis) in the absence of oxygen. This is called the Embden–Meyerhof pathway (Figure 10.6). 2,3-DPG binds to positive charges on the beta chains of deoxyhaemoglobin, resulting in a conformational change that reduces oxygen affinity. One mole of deoxyhaemoglobin binds 1 mol of 2,3-DPG and an increase in the concentration of 2,3-DPG causes more oxygen to be liberated. On the other hand, as haemoglobin binds more oxygen, the protein shape changes to allow the beta chains to move closer together and compress the sites where 2,3-DPG would otherwise be bound.

The level of pH affects the concentration of 2,3-DPG by its actions on the enzymes used in red cell glycolysis. At high pH (decreased H^+ concentration, i.e. alkalosis), activity of the enzyme DPG mutase is enhanced, whereas DPG phosphatase activity is reduced, both of which favour an increase in the level of 2,3-DPG. Similarly, 2,3-DPG concentration falls when the pH is low (increased H^+ concentration, i.e. acidosis). Hence changes in pH have direct and indirect effects, which have opposing actions on the oxygen dissociation curve. For instance, an increase in H^+ ion concentration tends to shift the curve to the right (via the Bohr phenomenon), whereas a tendency towards left shift will also occur because the acid pH results in a lower concentration of 2,3-DPG. In effect, the decrease in 2,3-DPG occurs after several hours of acidosis and helps push a right shift back towards the left.

Changes in the level of 2,3-DPG are also responsible for curve shifts due to chronic hypoxia, chronic anaemia, prolonged exercise, some abnormal haemoglobins and erythrocyte enzyme abnormalities, abnormal hormone activity (thyroid hormones, growth hormone, and androgens), and in stored blood.

Exercise

Exercise causes elevation of temperature, CO_2 and metabolites in active tissues, and a lowering of pH. The net result is an increase in 2,3-DPG with subsequent rise in the P_{50} with right shift. In addition, as more oxygen is removed from blood flowing through active tissues, the tissue PO_2 declines. At low PO_2 values, the oxygen dissociation curve is steep and large amounts of oxygen are liberated per unit drop in PO_2.

Abnormal haemoglobins

2,3-Diphosphoglycerate is also implicated in the differences in oxygen affinity associated with amino acid substitutions in haemoglobin chains. For instance, the greater affinity of fetal haemoglobin for oxygen facilitates the movement of oxygen from the mother to the fetus. The cause of this greater affinity is the poor binding of 2,3-DPG by the gamma polypeptide chains that replace beta chains in fetal haemoglobin. Some abnormal haemoglobins, which do not adequately bind 2,3-DPG, have low P_{50} values and the resulting high oxygen affinity of the haemoglobin causes enough tissue hypoxia to stimulate increased red cell formation with resulting polycythaemia.

In summary, the oxygen dissociation curve is shifted to the right (P_{50} raised) by an increase in hydrogen ion concentration, PCO_2, temperature, and 2,3-DPG, whereas a decrease in any of these parameters will cause a shift to the left (Table 10.1).

CLINICAL SIGNIFICANCE OF SHIFT OF THE DISSOCIATION CURVE

When the oxygen dissociation curve shifts to the right (for instance, in acidosis) oxygenation of haemoglobin is impaired but release of oxygen in the tissues is increased. If arterial PO_2 is assumed to be 13.7 kPa (103 mmHg) and arterial saturation is decreased by a reduction of pH, the effect is small. However, in the venous circulation, the oxygen tensions are very markedly affected. Over a wide range of conditions, a shift of the curve to the right will always raise the venous PO_2 provided other factors remain constant.

The seriously injured patient is likely to have derangements of the oxygen dissociation curve, predominantly because of the pathophysiology of the trauma (such as blood loss, i.e. reduced haemoglobin concentration). Additionally, dissociation may be affected by treatment (such as blood transfusion) and possibly also because of a pre-existing condition (such as sickle cell disease). Knowledge of these factors will help optimise oxygen carriage and subsequent oxygen delivery to hypoxic tissues.

Table 10.1   Causes of shift of the oxygen dissociation curve

P_{50} decreased < 3.5 kPa (left shift)	P_{50} increased > 3.5 kPa (right shift)
Saturation is *greater* for any given PO_2. Oxygen is bound *more avidly*, but results in less liberation in the tissues	Saturation is *lower* for any given PO_2. Oxygen is bound *less avidly*, and unloading in the tissues is favoured
By direct action Decreased [H^+] Decreased PCO_2 Decreased temperature Fetal Hb Carboxyhaemoglobin Methaemoglobin	**By direct action** Increased [H^+] Increased PCO_2 Increased temperature
By decreasing 2,3-DPG Increased [H^+] Decreased thyroid hormone Hyperoxia Panhypopituitarism Blood storage	**By increasing 2,3-DPG** Decreased [H^+] Thyroid hormone Hypoxaemia Congestive heart failure Hepatic cirrhosis

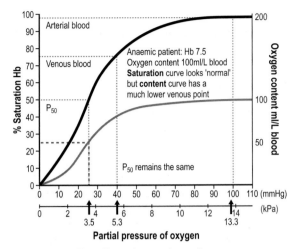

Figure 10.7 The effect of anaemia on the oxygen dissociation curve.

Anaemia

In anaemia there is decreased haemoglobin content, therefore, *ipso facto*, less oxygen content. A decrease in PO_2 has a more profound effect because less oxygen is available for the tissues and there is a smaller gradient to drive it. The effect is best seen in an alternative oxygen dissociation curve, one that describes the relationship between PO_2 and oxygen *content*, CaO_2 (Figure 10.7).

Chronic anaemia results in chronic hypoxia. Red cell 2,3-DPG concentration is increased in a variety of diseases in which chronic hypoxia exists. The curve is shifted to the right and increases the P_{50} in the order of 0.5 kPa (3.8 mmHg) higher than control levels. This facilitates the delivery of oxygen to the tissues by raising the PO_2 at which oxygen is released in peripheral capillaries.

Blood transfusion

Storage of bank blood with acid-citrate-dextrose (ACD) preservative results in depletion of 2,3-DPG within 3 weeks and P_{50} is reduced to about 2 kPa (15 mmHg). In effect, the ability of this blood to release oxygen to the tissues is reduced. This decrease limits the benefit of the transfusion when given to a hypoxic patient. A massive transfusion of old blood shifts the dissociation curve to the left but restoration occurs within a few hours. Storage of blood with citrate-phosphate-dextrose (CPD) substantially reduces the rate of 2,3-DPG depletion.

Abnormal forms of haemoglobin

Sickle cell anaemia (HbS) is a hereditary condition in which glutamic acid is replaced by valine in position 6 on the two beta chains. This single substitution is sufficient to cause insolubility of the haemoglobin molecule in the reduced state, leading to impaired oxygen carriage, red cell deformity and microemboli.

Thalassaemia, another hereditary disorder, consists of a suppression of HbA formation with persistent compensatory production of HbF. In this condition, the oxygen dissociation curve is shifted to the left.

Iron in the haem group may combine with other abnormal ligands (i.e. other inorganic molecules in competition with oxygen). The reaction products are often more stable than oxyhaemoglobin and, therefore, block the uptake of oxygen. Clinically, the most important of these compounds is carboxyhaemoglobin, but reaction products may also be formed with nitric oxide, cyanide and ammonia. Along with the loss of oxygen-carrying power, there is a left shift of the dissociation curve so that the remaining oxygen is only released at lower tensions of oxygen. This may cause tissue hypoxia despite the fact that the arterial PO_2 and oxygen content appear to be in the normal range.

Methaemoglobin (metHb) is haemoglobin in which the iron atom is in the trivalent ferric (Fe III) form. It may be hereditary (deficiency of the enzyme metHb reductase), or acquired (prilocaine, phenacetin and sulphonamide toxicity, etc.). Although it is unable to combine with oxygen, metHb is slowly reconverted to haemoglobin in normal patients. Reducing agents such as ascorbic acid or methylene blue may be used to convert the iron from the ferric to ferrous states when oxygenation is significantly impaired.

Effect of anaesthetics

Although it has long been known that some anaesthetics (e.g. halothane, methoxyflurane and diethyl ether and cyclopropane) bind to haemoglobin, there is no evidence for any significant change in P_{50} and no discernible detrimental effect with modern anaesthetic agents.

Respiratory failure

Respiratory failure does not appear to cause any significant change in either 2,3-DPG levels or the P_{50}.

Shock

Hypovolaemic and septic shock do not appear to be associated with any significant changes of 2,3-DPG or changes in P_{50}.

ALTITUDE AND AEROMEDICAL TRANSPORT OF TRAUMA PATIENTS

On climbing through the atmosphere, although the relative composition of air remains constant, both pressure and density decline. Effectively this means that fewer oxygen molecules are available for physiological use. Beyond 10 000 ft, the paucity of oxygen becomes physiologically problematic. The deficiency of oxygen is called *hypoxia*. At the same time, gases trapped within body cavities will expand in obeyance of Boyle's law (i.e. volume is inversely proportional to pressure when temperature remains constant).

The effects on normal respiratory physiology

Alveolar gas is air saturated with water at body temperature and contains carbon dioxide. Since CO_2 is soluble and diffuses readily, its partial pressure in blood leaving the pulmonary capillaries ($PaCO_2$) is almost in equilibrium with that of alveolar gas (P_ACO_2). Pulmonary ventilation (the volume and rate of breathing) is automatically regulated to keep pace with CO_2 production and, under normal circumstances, the P_ACO_2 and $PaCO_2$ are constant, at about 5.3 kPa (40 mmHg). In contrast, because of normal physiological shunting and the shape of the oxygen dissociation curve, the arterial partial pressure of oxygen (PaO_2) is lower than that of alveolar gas (P_AO_2). The partial pressures of the components of the alveolar gas mixture at sea level are shown in Box 10.3.

Box 10.3 Partial pressures of the components of alveolar gas at sea level	
Nitrogen	75.8 kPa (570 mmHg)
Oxygen	13.7 kPa (103 mmHg)
Carbon dioxide	5.3 kPa (40 mmHg)
Water	6.2 kPa (47 mmHg)
Total (ambient pressure)	101.0 kPa (760 mmHg)

Box 10.4 Partial pressures of the components of alveolar gas at 2440 m (8000 ft)	
Nitrogen	56.4 kPa (424 mmHg)
Oxygen	7.4 kPa (56 mmHg)
Carbon dioxide	5.0 kPa (38 mmHg)
Water	6.2 kPa (47 mmHg)
Total (ambient pressure)	75.0 kPa (565 mmHg)

The total ambient pressure at the maximum equivalent altitude in a pressurised aircraft, 2440 m (8000 ft), is 75.1 kPa (565 mmHg). The partial pressure of oxygen in dry air would, therefore, be 21% of 75.1, that is, 15.8 kPa (119 mmHg). However, within the alveoli, the partial pressures are as shown in Box 10.4.

Since alveolar gas is fully saturated, the vapour pressure of water remains constant at 6.25 kPa (47 mmHg) at all altitudes. The partial pressure of CO_2, however, is reduced because of the hypoxic drive to increase pulmonary ventilation, effectively washing CO_2 out of the lungs.

The PO_2 axis of the dissociation curve can be changed to represent altitude and it becomes clear that ascent through lower ambient pressure is reflected in a reduction of PaO_2. Figure 10.8 shows the relationship between altitude, pressure and saturation, and demonstrates that the onset of hypoxic symptoms occurs at around 3050 m (10 000 ft), where the dissociation curve steepens and haemoglobin is less avid for oxygen. Below 3050 m (where PaO_2 is of the order of 7 kPa or 52.5 mmHg), the rightward shift of the dissociation curve is less advantageous, since oxygenation in the lung is impaired and the gain of improved off-loading in the tissues gives negligible net benefit.

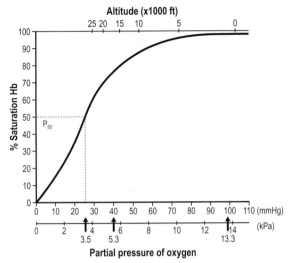

Figure 10.8 The relationship between altitude, pressure and oxygen saturation.

Hypoxia

Hypoxia is defined as oxygen deficiency sufficient to cause impairment of physiological function. The most relevant type of hypoxia in the flight environment is *hypobaric (hypoxic) hypoxia*, which becomes apparent above 3050 m (10 000 ft) in normal individuals. Without supplemental oxygen, SaO_2 at sea level of 98% will decline to about 90% at 3050 m (10 000 ft) and 65% at 6100 m (20 000 ft). Although hypoxic hypoxia is caused by an inadequate partial pressure of oxygen in inspired air (and inadequate gas exchange at the alveolar-capillary membrane), it is also experienced by those with a ventilation–perfusion defect or with an airway obstruction. Since these patients are hypoxic at sea level, they will clearly be at increased risk of hypoxic damage during flight.

Other forms of hypoxia will also exacerbate the complications of hypobaric hypoxia. *Hypaemic (anaemic) hypoxia* is caused by a reduction in the oxygen carrying capacity of the blood. This may be due to anaemia, hypovolaemia, carbon monoxide poisoning, heavy smoking, or congenital or drug-induced methaemoglobinaemia. *Stagnant (circulatory) hypoxia* is oxygen deficiency due to reduction in tissue perfusion. It occurs when cardiac output fails to satisfy tissue requirements (cardiogenic shock), after long periods of positive pressure breathing or from venous pooling,

arterial spasm or occlusion of blood vessels. *Histotoxic hypoxia* is the inability of the body tissues to utilise available oxygen, for instance, in cyanide poisoning, which uncouples oxidative phosphorylation, the final cascade in the release of energy-rich phosphates in cell mitochondria.

SUMMARY

Although some oxygen is dissolved within the plasma, most is carried in combination with haemoglobin in erythrocytes.

The oxygen saturation is:

$$SaO_2 = \frac{\text{Amount of oxygen combined with Hb}}{\text{Oxygen-carrying capacity}} \times 100\%$$

The relationship between oxygen saturation and oxygen tension (partial pressure of oxygen in the blood) is described by the sigmoid-shaped oxygen dissociation curve. This characteristic shape is of great importance. The flat upper portion ensures that moderate variations of alveolar oxygen tension around the norm at 13.7 kPa (103 mmHg) at sea level have little effect on the amount of oxygen combined with haemoglobin in arterial blood (i.e. its saturation). The steep portion at lower oxygen tensions ensures optimal dissociation of oxygen from haemoglobin into the tissues. A large drop in saturation (as a large quantity of oxygen is given up to the tissues) results in only a small fall in tension. This is important in maintaining oxygen tension at tissue level.

The shape is not influenced by the concentration of haemoglobin, but the position of the curve may be shifted left or right by disturbances in acidity (pH), arterial CO_2 tension ($PaCO_2$), temperature and concentrations of 2,3-DPG. Tissue that works hard will produce hydrogen ions, CO_2 and heat. A fall, therefore, in pH, and/or a rise in $PaCO_2$, temperature and 2,3-DPG levels will shift the curve to the right and thereby increase the amount of oxygen given up by the blood at a given oxygen tension. The net effect is improved oxygen delivery to the tissues.

CONCLUSION

A knowledge of the uptake, carriage and delivery of oxygen is essential to appreciate the necessity for high inspired oxygen and adequate circulating fresh haemoglobin in seriously ill and injured patients. Therapy can be directed according to anticipated changes in the oxygen dissociation curve. For instance, warm fresh blood is inevitably more efficacious than cold stored blood, and the correction of ventilation impairment will improve the respiratory component of acidosis. Furthermore, problems during transportation can also be predicted and prevented. For instance, in an aeromedical transfer, raising the aircraft cabin pressure will prevent the already hypoxic patient from slipping down to the steep part of the dissociation curve. Clearly, there is a theoretical advantage to a right shift of the dissociation curve in that a greater delivery of oxygen to the tissues is likely at a PO_2 around 50 mmHg and the likely effects of 2,3-DPG mediated changes in P_{50} appear to be of minimal significance in comparison with changes in arterial PO_2 and tissue perfusion. Unfortunately, there is little evidence that a shift in the curve makes any significant difference to critically ill patients and the optimum curve for these patients remains unclear. Similarly, there is no evidence that drug-induced shifts of the dissociation curve have any therapeutic role.

Further reading

Fishman AP, Farhi LE, Tenney SM, Geiger SR. *Handbook of physiology*, Section 3: *The respiratory system*, Vol. 4: *Gas exchange*. Baltimore: Waverly Press, 1987

Ganong WF. *Review of medical physiology*, 19th edn. Connecticut: Appleton and Lange, 1999

Healey TEJ, Cohen PJ. *A practice of anaesthesia*. London: Edward Arnold, 1995

Lumb A JF. *Nunn's applied respiratory physiology*. London: Butterworth-Heinemann, 1999

Martin T, Rodenberg HD. *Aeromedical transportation: a clinical guide*. Farnham: Avebury, 1996

West J. *Respiratory physiology*. London: Lippincott Williams and Wilkins, 1999

Widdicombe J, Davies A. *Respiratory physiology*. London Edward Arnold, 1991

Zubay GL, Parson WW, Vance DE. *Principles of biochemistry*. Dubuque: WCB, 1995

Chapter **11**

Applied physiology pertaining to the trauma patient

John V. Brooke

INTRODUCTION

For life to be sustained, oxygen must flow from the atmosphere in which we live to each of the body's cells. The oxygen present in the air must be able to pass freely through the *airway*, the anatomical space between the lips and the nose and the alveoli in the lung, moved by the mechanism of *breathing*, and then be transported from the lung to each of the body's cells by the *circulation*.

This chapter sets out the route by which oxygen passes from the atmosphere to each of the body's cells, and then describes how an interference at some point along this route leads to loss of homeostasis, shock and death in those who are seriously ill or injured.

The atmosphere is the mixture of gases overlying the surface of the earth. It is made up of: nitrogen 78%, oxygen 20.93%, argon 0.9%, carbon dioxide 0.03%, a variable amount of water vapour, and trace amounts of hydrogen, ozone, methane, carbon monoxide, helium, neon, krypton and xenon (Figure 11.1).

At sea level, atmospheric pressure is approximately 760 mm mercury (Hg), or 101 kilopascals (kPa). One kilopascal is approximately equal to 7.5 mmHg. The partial pressure of a gas in a mixture of gases (such as the atmosphere) is the pressure which that gas would exert if it alone occupied the volume occupied by the mixture of gases. Thus, at sea level, the partial pressure of oxygen in dry air is:

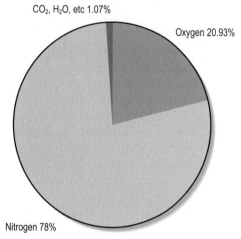

Figure 11.1   The composition of the atmosphere.

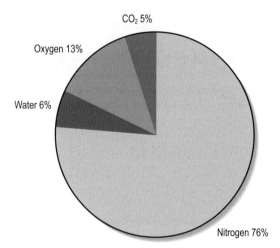

Figure 11.2   Alveolar gas composition.

$$\frac{20.93}{100} \times 760 = 159 \text{ mmHg } (21.2 \text{ kPa})$$

CHANGES THAT OCCUR IN INSPIRED AIR DURING ITS PASSAGE THROUGH THE AIRWAY

In the upper airway, air is warmed and humidified with water vapour. The partial pressure of the water vapour in the humidified air in the airway is approximately 47 mmHg (6.2 kPa). The addition of water vapour to the gases in the airway will, by definition, lower the partial pressure of the other gases in the airway. The partial pressure of the dry gases of the atmosphere is, therefore, reduced to:

760 – 47 = 713 mmHg (95 kPa)

Oxygen continues to constitute 20.93% of the dry gas of the atmosphere and, therefore, the partial pressure (PO_2) in the upper airway following humidification is reduced to:

$$\frac{20.93}{100} \times 713 = 149 \text{ mmHg } (19.9 \text{ kPa})$$

As the warmed and humidified air enters the lower airway, the partial pressure of oxygen is further reduced as it mixes with gases, which have diffused from the pulmonary capillaries across the alveolar membrane into the alveolar space. The mixture of gases that will diffuse from the

pulmonary artery capillary into the alveolar space will reflect the gas content of mixed venous blood (Figure 11.2). Mixed venous blood has a partial pressure of oxygen (PO_2) of 40 mmHg (5.3 kPa) and a partial pressure of carbon dioxide (PCO_2) of 45 mmHg (6 kPa). Thus, the mixture of gases present in the alveolar space will differ considerably from the atmosphere by having a lower PO_2 and a higher PCO_2.

There is a significant difference in the composition of the alveolar gases between the apices and bases of the lung. The highest PO_2 is to be found in the alveoli present in the apices of the lung and the lowest at the bases. The PCO_2 is at its highest value at the lung bases and at its lowest value at the lung apices.

An average value for the PO_2 in the lung alveolar space would be of the order of 100 mmHg (13.3 kPa). The PCO_2 in the alveolar space is approximately 40 mmHg (5.3 kPa).

THE AIRWAY IN THE ADULT AND THE CHILD

The airway starts at the mouth and nose, and becomes the space within the pharynx, larynx, trachea and bronchi. In the adult, the volume of the airway is approximately 150 ml.

There are significant and important differences between the airway of a child and an adult; these differences are summarised in Box 11.1.

Box 11.1   The paediatric airway

- The tongue of the child is relatively large and is attached to a relatively small mandible.
- The adenoidal and tonsillar tissues attain their greatest size between the ages of 3 and 8 years, and even in health may significantly reduce the size of the airway.
- The epiglottis of the child projects more posteriorly than in the adult, at an angle of about 45° to the vertical plain. It is horseshoe-shaped compared to the leaf-like shape of the adult.
- The child's neck is shorter than the adult's and, therefore, the relationship between the various parts of the airway and the cervical spine are also different.
- Thus the child's larynx is at the level of the second and third cervical vertebrae, whereas in the adult it is lower, at about the level of C5.
- The larynx is the narrowest part of the adult upper airway. In the child, the narrowest part of the upper airway is at the level of the cricoid cartilage.
- Compared to an adult, the child's trachea is short, soft and easily compressible.

Table 11.1   Respiratory rate according to age

Age (years)	Respiratory rate (breaths/minute)
12 to adult	12–16
5–12	15–20
2–5	20–30
Under 2	30–40

BREATHING – ITS MECHANISM AND CONTROL

Breathing is the mechanism that brings the air from the atmosphere into contact with the alveolar membrane. The number of breaths per minute, i.e. the respiratory rate, decreases with age between infancy and puberty (Table 11.1).

The respiratory rate decreases with age between infancy and puberty

The mechanism of breathing

During the inspiratory phase of respiration, air is drawn through the airway and into the lungs by a reduction in intrathoracic pressure. Intrathoracic pressure is reduced by increasing the intrathoracic volume. The volume of the thorax is increased by increasing the internal dimensions of the intrathoracic space (as descibed below).

- The inferior–superior dimension is increased by contracting the diaphragm, which results in its descent.
- The anterior posterior dimension of the thorax is increased through the action of the intercostal muscles. These muscles act to raise the ribs, therefore, making them more horizontal. (The anterior end of each rib is normally situated at a lower level than the rib's posterior articulations at the costovertebral joints.) Thus, as a result of a contraction of the intercostal muscles, the anterior end of each rib is displaced forwards and upwards, and the anterior–posterior dimension of the thorax is thereby increased.

In an adult, a reduction in the intrathoracic pressure to –5 mmHg (–0.6 kPa) will result in a normal resting breath, the volume of which will be in the order of 500 ml. The volume of air taken through the airway during a single breath is termed the *tidal volume* (VT). *Ventilation* (VE) is the product of tidal volume and respiratory frequency (*f*). Thus

$$VE = VT \times f$$

Minute ventilation is the volume of air that passes into the airway during one minute.

The work of breathing

The work of breathing depends on the rate of breathing and the amount of energy required to move air through the airway, which in turn depends upon the resistance to airflow within the airway.

The pressure flow characteristics of tubes were first described by the French physician, Poiseuille. His work demonstrated that in a tube of length *l* and radius *r* through which a substance of viscosity *n* was passing, the resistance to flow *R* could be calculated from the equation:

$$R = \frac{8nl}{pr^4}$$

From this equation, it may be seen that the resistance to airflow is inversely proportional to the fourth power of the radius of the airway. Thus, if the radius of the airway is halved, the resistance will increase by a factor of 16.

The control of breathing

Breathing is controlled by the respiratory centre, which is situated in the pons and upper medulla. The afferent input to the respiratory centre is from the central receptors in the medulla and from the peripheral receptors situated in the carotid bodies and the aortic bodies. These receptors are sensitive to changes in the PCO_2, change in the hydrogen ion concentration (pH) and, to a lesser extent, to changes in the PO_2.

Situated within the part of the respiratory center that is located in the pons is the *pneumotaxic centre*. This area regulates the efferent discharges from the respiratory centre in such a manner that the stimulation of the muscles responsible for respiration is intermittent and reciprocal, thereby establishing a regular pattern of inspiration and expiration – normal breathing.

In a healthy subject, small changes in PCO_2 or pH will affect the respiratory drive from the respiratory centre.

CIRCULATION: ITS COMPONENTS AND REGULATION

Breathing delivers atmospheric oxygen to the alveolar membrane. From this site within the lung, it must be absorbed and delivered to every cell in the body.

The components of the circulatory system

The system that manages the delivery of oxygen is the circulatory system. This has three components:

1. A fluid with oxygen carrying capability – the blood.
2. A system of conduits in which the blood may circulate – the arteries and veins.
3. A pump to circulate the blood – the heart.

The regulation of the circulatory system

Regulation of the circulation is under the control of the suprapontine region of the brainstem, which receives its afferent input from both the sensory and autonomic nervous systems.

Baroreceptors and *chemoreceptors* monitor blood pressure and blood chemistry. Changes in blood pressure and blood chemistry are detected and transmitted to the brainstem, which coordinates the circulatory response with the aim of achieving homeostasis (see Chapter 7). The systemic arterial baroreceptors, which monitor blood pressure, lie in the adventitia of the arterial wall at the locations detailed in Box 11.2 below.

The carotid sinus is innervated by the glosso-pharyngeal nerve, with the remainder of the baroreceptors supplied by branches of the vagus nerve. Both the glossopharyngeal nerve and the vagus enter the brainstem at the level of the medulla.

The chemoreceptors that transmit information regarding PO_2, PCO_2 and pH are situated in the carotid body, which lies at the bifurcation of the common carotid artery, and in the aortic bodies which are found in two main sites: at the root of the right subclavian artery, and around the transverse part of the aortic arch. The carotid body is innervated by the glossopharyngeal nerve and the aortic bodies by branches of the vagus nerve.

> The rate of flow and the pressure within the systemic arterial system is a function of the output of the heart and the resistance offered to the circulating blood by the blood vessels through which the blood is flowing

The efferent fibres of the sympathetic nervous system innervate the heart, the arterioles and the adrenal glands. Activation of the sympathetic nervous system increases the rate of the heart and constricts the arterioles, and, as *blood pressure* is a function of cardiac output and the resistance

---

Box 11.2   The location of arterial baroreceptors

- Within the carotid sinus, i.e. the dilatation at the origin of the internal carotid artery
- Within the transverse part of the aortic arch
- At the root of the right subclavian artery
- Scattered along the course of the common carotid artery

offered to that output by the systemic arterial system, this will have the effect of increasing blood pressure. This effect will be enhanced by the increase in output of norepinephrine from the adrenal glands, which follows upon sympathetic stimulation of these structures.

Fibres present within the vagus nerve represent the main contribution of the parasympathetic nervous system to the circulatory system. The vagus nerve supplies parasympathetic fibres to the heart, the lungs and the abdominal viscera. The cardiac effect of parasympathetic stimulation is to induce a slowing of the heart. The para-sympathetic nerves that supply the abdominal viscera are primarily concerned with mechanisms of emptying those viscera and hence the para-sympathetic activity, which induces a bradycardia may at the same time result in nausea and vomiting.

The normal parameters of the circulatory system

The blood within the circulatory system represents about 8% of body weight. *Blood volume* may, therefore, be calculated as approximately 80 ml/kg of body weight. Total blood volume, thus, varies with age (Table 11.2).

In an adult with a blood volume of approximately 5 litres, the distribution of this volume will be approximately as follows:

- heart – 0.6 litres;
- lungs (pulmonary arteries, capillaries and veins) – 0.9 litres;
- the systemic circulation – 3.5 litres;
- of the 3.5 litres of blood in the systemic circulation, approximately 60% of this volume will be present in the veins.

Blood pressure increases through childhood, achieving adult levels in the early teens (Table 11.3).

The output of the heart, the *cardiac output*, is measured in litres per minute. It is the product of the amount of blood ejected by each contraction of the heart – the *stroke volume* and the number of times the heart beats each minute.

As described earlier, the volume of blood in an adult heart is approximately 0.6 litres, the left ventricular *end diastolic volume* is about 140 ml and the stroke volume approximately 90 ml. At the

Table 11.2 Variation of blood volume with age

Age (years)	Approximate weight (kg)	Blood volume (ml)
Adult	70	5600
12	40	3200
5	20	1600
1	10	800

Table 11.3 Variation of blood pressure with age

Age (years)	Systolic blood pressure (mmHg)
12 and over	100–120
5–12	90–110
2–5	80–100
Less than 2	70–90

completion of systole, approximately 50 ml of blood remains in the left ventricle, i.e. the *end systolic volume*. The percentage of the end diastolic volume which is ejected at each contraction of the heart, is termed the *ejection fraction*. Thus:

$$\text{Ejection fraction } (\%) = \frac{\text{Stroke volume}}{\text{End diastolic volume}} \times \frac{100}{1}$$

The *cardiac index* defines cardiac output in terms of body size and is the cardiac output in litres per minute per square metre of body surface area. Therefore:

$$\text{Cardiac index (litres/minute per m}^2） = \frac{\text{Cardiac output (litres/minute)}}{\text{Body surface area (m}^2)}$$

A mean cardiac index in the resting state would be of the order of 3.5 litres/minute per m², with a normal range of between 2 and 5 litres/minute per m².

The cardiac index may also be defined in terms of cardiac output per kilogram of body weight; this may be the most convenient calculation for children. If it is calculated in this way, the following normal values will be obtained:

- birth – 300 ml/kg;
- adolescence – 100 ml/kg;
- adult – 70–80 ml/kg.

Using these values, it may be calculated that the cardiac output of an adult weighing 70 kg will be of the order of 5–5.5 litres/minute.

The cardiac index is at its greatest value at birth and declines thereafter

A high cardiac index at birth, when the stroke volume at birth is low must, by definition, require a rapid heart rate. Thus, the heart rate is at its highest values at birth and declines until adulthood (Table 11.4).

The transport of oxygen by the circulation

At rest, the tissues of a healthy adult require approximately 300 ml of oxygen every minute. This oxygen passes from the alveolar space in the lung to the capillaries in the alveolar wall by diffusion. Oxygen diffuses in accordance with the laws of diffusion of gases (Graham's and Fick's laws).

Graham's law states that 'the rates of efflux of different gases through a porous membrane under given conditions are inversely proportional to the square roots of their molecular weights'. *Fick's law* states that 'the volume of a gas which diffuses across a membrane in unit time (V) depends upon the permeability coefficient of the membrane (D), its area (A), its thickness (T), and the partial pressure of the gas on either side of the membrane ($P1$ and $P2$)'. Fick's law is represented by the following equation:

$$V = D(A/T) \times (P1 - P2)$$

In health, the alveolar membrane is 0.0003 mm in thickness and, in an adult, has an area of between 50 and 100 m^2. An average value for the PO_2 within the alveoli is 100 mmHg (13.3 kPa) and the PO_2 of the blood entering the alveolar capillary from the right side of the heart (mixed venous blood) is approximately 40 mmHg (5.3 kPa).

The time taken for a particular red cell to pass through the alveolar capillary is approximately 0.75 seconds at rest but may be reduced to less

than 0.25 seconds during exercise. During this time, the PO_2 on either side of the alveolar membrane will have equilibrated; therefore, the PO_2 of the blood, which has passed through the alveolar capillary and is destined for the systemic circulation, will be 100 mmHg (13.3 kPa). This blood will have dissolved within it 0.3 ml of oxygen per 100 ml and, therefore, with a cardiac output of 5 litres/minute about 15 ml of oxygen dissolved in the blood, will be distributed by the circulation each minute. This is about 1/20th of the body's requirement at rest.

Haemoglobin

The fact that the volume of blood ejected from the heart each minute, the cardiac output, can contain within it sufficient oxygen to provide for the body's needs in a wide variety of circumstances is due to the presence within the circulation of a substance that is able to combine reversibly with oxygen, uplifting oxygen from the alveolar capillary and releasing it to the cells of the body. The substance with this remarkable quality is *haemoglobin*.

Haemoglobin (Hb) in man and vertebrates is a protein molecule with a molecular weight of 64 585 Daltons. It is made up of two pairs of polypeptide chains; alpha chains, each consisting of 141 amino acids; and beta chains, consisting of 146 amino acids joined to one another by peptide links. At one end of the chain is an alpha amino group, at the other end a free carboxyl group. A haem group is attached to a histidine residue on each chain and each haem group contains one atom of ferrous iron. The molecule of haemoglobin, therefore, consists of the four polypeptide chains, four haem groups and four atoms of ferrous iron.

The haem group is common to all species, but differences in the amino acid sequence of the polypeptide chain account for the different characteristics of haemoglobin noted in different species. Variants on the polypeptide chain amino-acid sequence of adult haemoglobin account for the human haemoglobinopathies.

Haemoglobin is able to act as a carrier for oxygen owing to the ability of the ferrous iron of the haem group to combine reversibly with molecular oxygen, yet always remaining in the

Table 11.4	Heart rates according to age
Age (years)	Heart rate (beats/minute)
12 and over	60–100
5–12	80–120
2–5	95–140
Less than 2	110–160

ferrous state. Each molecule of haemoglobin is oxygenated in four steps. At each step, one of the four subunits combines with oxygen.

The four steps are from deoxygenated haemoglobin (deoxyhaemoglobin), via two intermediaries, to fully oxygenated haemoglobin (oxyhaemoglobin). As each haem subunit is oxygenated, it facilitates the oxygenation of a further haem subunit so that, as oxygenation proceeds, combination with further molecules of oxygen is made easier. This is described as 'cooperative interaction' between the binding sites of the haemoglobin molecule. Thus, the affinity of haemoglobin for oxygen depends on the amount of oxygen that is bound to it.

> The affinity of haemoglobin for oxygen depends on the amount of oxygen bound to it

Haemoglobin that has been oxygenated (oxyhaemoglobin) has a higher affinity for oxygen than haemoglobin, which has not combined with oxygen (deoxyhaemoglobin). This characteristic explains the efficiency of haemoglobin as a carrier of oxygen (Figure 11.3). Thus haemoglobin returning to the lungs as mixed venous blood, which has released a proportion of its bound oxygen to the tissues, will have a lower affinity for oxygen than fully oxygenated haemoglobin. It will, however, be entering an environment, the alveolar capillary, where the PO_2 is high (100 mmHg; 13.3 kPa) and, at this high PO_2, the low-affinity deoxyhaemoglobin will be rapidly fully oxygenated.

The fully oxygenated oxyhaemoglobin, with its high oxygen affinity, will only release a significant percentage of its bound oxygen when it enters an environment with a relatively low PO_2; the organs and tissues of the body. The dissociation curve for oxyhaemoglobin depicts the manner in which oxyhaemoglobin releases the oxygen that is bound to it (Chapter 10). The high affinity of oxyhaemoglobin for oxygen results in a comparatively small percentage release of oxygen during the early phase of PO_2 reduction.

Thus, in a well person with normal physiological values, it is not until the haemoglobin with its bound oxygen (oxyhaemoglobin) has entered an environment with a PO_2 of 60 mmHg (8 kPa)

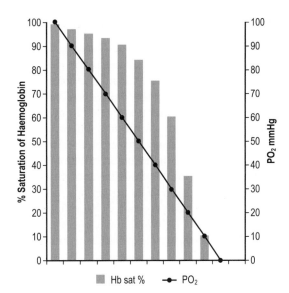

Figure 11.3 Relationship between the percentage saturation of haemoglobin (Hb sat %) and the partial pressure of oxygen (PO_2).

or less that significant unbinding of oxygen takes place. Average tissue PO_2 is approximately 40 mmHg (5.3 kPa) (although actively metabolising tissue such as heart muscle, or exercising skeletal muscle will have a PO_2 which is considerably lower than this) and thus, at a PO_2 of 40 mmHg (5.3 kPa), oxyhaemoglobin will have released only 25% of its bound oxygen.

Therefore, in health, blood returning from the tissues to the right side of the heart as mixed venous blood still contains 75% of the oxygen that it contained when it left the alveolar capillary to return to the left side of the heart and from thence to enter the systemic circulation.

The quantity of oxygen carried by haemoglobin

The quantity of oxygen being carried by the circulation at any one time does, of course, depend on the concentration of haemoglobin in the blood. One gram of haemoglobin has the ability to combine with approximately 1.36 ml of oxygen; thus, in a person with a haemoglobin of 15 g/100 ml of blood, the amount of oxygen carried in the blood, if the haemoglobin is 100% saturated with oxygen, will be:

$$1.5 \times 1.36 = 20.4 \text{ ml (oxygen)}$$

Assessment of the percentage oxygen saturation of haemoglobin

The normal range for oxygen saturation is 97–100%. Oxygen saturation may most conveniently be assessed by using a pulse oximeter. This instrument passes light, generated by two light-emitting diodes, through an extremity which is being perfused by blood, and measures the absorption of light energy by the structures through which the light is passing. Each diode emits light of a different wavelength. The absorption spectra of oxygenated and deoxygenated haemoglobin are different, and the light-emitting diodes emit light at those frequencies at which the absorption spectra of oxygenated and deoxygenated haemoglobin show the greatest difference. By computing the relative concentrations of oxygenated and deoxygenated haemoglobin that is passing between the light-emitting diodes and the photodetector, the instrument will give direct readings of the percentage of haemoglobin, which is oxygenated.

Pulse oximeters have an accuracy of 2–3% in the range 70–100% saturation but, as the instrument measures light energy absorption, inaccuracies may result from pigmentation or contamination of the skin. The most potentially dangerous inaccuracy arises from the fact that the pulse oximeter will interpret carboxyhaemoglobin, produced by the combination of carbon monoxide with haemoglobin, as being fully oxygenated haemoglobin.

Factors that affect the binding of oxygen to haemoglobin

The affinity of haemoglobin for oxygen and, therefore, the amount of oxygen that remains bound to haemoglobin at any particular PO_2 value is affected by changes in partial pressure of carbon dioxide (PCO_2), changes in hydrogen ion concentration (pH) and changes in temperature. In health, there is a significant variation in these values in the different tissues of the body and, following illness or injury, there may be further very significant change.

The elimination of carbon dioxide

The oxidative processes from which cells obtain their energy result in the generation of 'acidic products'. The word 'oxygen' means 'generator of acid'. Of these 'acidic products', carbon dioxide is quantitatively the most important. In an adult, approximately 300 litres of carbon dioxide is expelled from the lungs each day; in terms of its acidic effect, this is the equivalent of 15 litres of normal hydrochloric acid.

Carbon dioxide is transported from the metabolic sites in the cells to the lung in the following three ways.

1. As dissolved carbon dioxide. Carbon dioxide is approximately 20 times more soluble than oxygen; dissolved carbon dioxide accounts for 10% of the total carbon dioxide transported to the lungs.
2. In combination with haemoglobin. Carbon dioxide combines reversibly the alpha-amino group of haemoglobin to form a carbamino compound plus hydrogen ions:

$$Alpha\text{-}NH_2 + CO_2 \rightarrow Alpha\text{-}NHCOO^- + H^+$$

   About 30% of carbon dioxide is transported in this manner.
3. As bicarbonate, formed by the reaction of carbon dioxide with water:

$$CO_2 + H_2O \xrightarrow{\text{Carbonic anhydrase}} H_2CO_3 \leftrightarrow HCO_3 + H^+$$

   60% of carbon dioxide is transported in this manner. The enzyme *carbonic anhydrase* which catalyses this reaction is abundantly present in the erythrocyte, and represents about 4% of total red cell protein. It is one of the most efficient catalysts known, one molecule of carbonic anhydrase catalysing the hydration of more than one million molecules of carbon dioxide every second.

Once H_2CO_3 reaches equilibrium with CO_2, the rate of hydration of CO_2 within the cell becomes entirely dependent on the rate of movement of HCO_3^- out of the cells. HCO_3^- diffuses out of the cell in exchange for chloride ions (Cl^-), which move in the opposite direction to maintain electrochemical equilibrium.

Reduced (deoxygenated) haemoglobin is less acidic than oxyhaemoglobin and is, therefore, able to accept more hydrogen ions than oxyhaemoglobin, as it is a better proton acceptor. The hydrogen ions produced by these two reactions involved in the transport of carbon dioxide are accepted by the reduced haemoglobin, thus enabling both reactions to move in a rightwards direction, and facilitate the transport of carbon dioxide by these mechanisms. It is, of course, in those tissues where carbon dioxide concentrations are high that deoxygenated haemoglobin will be most abundant.

In a healthy person, the PCO_2 of arterial blood is 40 mmHg (5.3 kPa) and the PCO_2 of resting tissues approximately 46 mmHg (6.1 kPa).

THE PHYSIOLOGICAL RESPONSE TO THE DEMANDS OF EXERCISE

Exercise, by definition, is an increase in muscular activity. The oxygen requirement of the muscle cells is increased, and this demand is met by an increase in the flow of air into the alveoli and an increase in cardiac output.

The heart muscle (myocardium) contracts with greater force if it is stretched, and thus, according to the Frank-Starling law, an increase in the volume of blood returning to the heart (preload), by filling the chambers and stretching the sarcomeres, will increase cardiac contractility and cardiac output. This response is an intrinsic characteristic of heart muscle. Interestingly, the subepicardial myocardium and subendocardial myocardium respond to different ranges of stretch to produce, in the healthy heart, i.e. normal physiological response to exercise – an increase in cardiac output, which may be 5–6 times the resting value.

THE PHYSIOLOGICAL BASIS OF THE TREATMENT OF TRAUMA

Trauma is life threatening when it impedes the transport of oxygen to the vital organs of the body to such an extent that homeostasis cannot be maintained. This loss of homeostasis presents itself clinically as the syndrome known as shock. The treatment of shock is the treatment of its cause, which is always the treatment of a problem that is interfering with the flow of oxygen from the atmosphere to the tissues, and particularly to the vital organs of the body. Logically, therefore,

shock may result from an interference with the flow of oxygen from the atmosphere to each of the body's cells at any point along the route that has already been considered in the earlier part of this chapter.

Shock related to the respiratory system

Problems that can be classified as being related to the respiratory system can occur even before air enters the upper airway. If a gas that is not a normal component of the atmosphere is present in significant quantity, it will, according to the law of partial pressure, reduce the percentage of oxygen in the air inspired and, therefore, reduce the amount of oxygen that may be transported to each cell. One such gas that can interfere very seriously with the transport of oxygen, even if it is present in the air that we breathe in only very small quantities, is carbon monoxide. This gas has an affinity for haemoglobin that is 210 times greater than the affinity of oxygen for haemoglobin. Once haemoglobin has combined with carbon monoxide, it is no longer available as a transporter of oxygen. Importantly, it must be stated that the assessment of such a patient is rendered difficult by the fact that the pulse oximeter cannot recognise the difference between haemoglobin that has combined with oxygen and haemoglobin to which carbon monoxide is attached.

Interference with the flow of oxygen from the atmosphere may next occur, as a result of any physical obstruction to the airway either by the physical presence of material within the airway or by external compression of the airway. Spasm of the airway that produces an effective block may result from the inhalation of water or other liquid, or the inhalation of an irritant gas. An increase in the temperature of inhaled air, particularly associated with the inhalation of irritant or toxic gases following combustion, will produce spasm in the airway and also oedema of the wall of the airway. Certain gases will also damage the alveolar membrane.

Interference with the mechanisms of breathing can occur with chest wall trauma, which prevents the normal movement of the thorax or prevents the formation of a negative pressure within the thorax, as occurs with a flail chest injury. The presence of air (pneumothorax) or blood (haemo-thorax), or blood and air (haemo-pneumothorax) in the potential space between the lung and the chest wall effectively diminishes the volume of the thorax that the lungs are able to occupy, and thereby interferes seriously and, in the case of a tension pneumothorax, progressively, with respiration.

Shock as a result of interference with the pumping action of the heart

Clearly, if the heart is unable to act as an effective pump to the circulatory system, blood and, therefore, oxygen cannot be supplied to the cells of the body. Direct physical trauma may affect the pumping ability of the heart either by directly traumatising the heart muscle or, as in the case of a cardiac tamponade, by restricting heart function by the compressing effect of blood or fluid in the potential space between the pericardium and the heart. Trauma may also interfere directly with heart function by provoking abnormal heart rhythms.

Shock as a result of obstruction to the circulation

Major blood vessels can be obstructed by compression, as the result of trauma or by obstruction within the blood vessel due to blockage by a blood clot, as in the case of pulmonary embolus, by bubbles of gas such as that which occurs in 'the bends', or by amniotic fluid emboli, which can occur during labour.

Shock related to the distribution of blood by the blood vessels

In health, the body regulates the circulation in a manner appropriate to the body's needs. This correct distribution of blood is possible only if the autonomic nervous system is able to function normally and the blood vessels that this system controls are able to respond in a normal manner. Trauma, such as head injury, may directly damage the function of the autonomic nervous system.

It has already been noted that blood pressure is a function of the output of the heart and the resistance of the circulatory system to that output.

This resistance is maintained by the muscular tone of each artery and arteriole, and it is this muscular tone that the autonomic nervous system modifies continually throughout life. Loss of this tone results in dilatation of the blood vessels of the arterial system, a reduction in the resistance of the circulatory system and, therefore, a reduction of the blood pressure. The ability of the blood vessels to maintain the normal tone can be affected by direct trauma, by poisoning and the inhalation of toxic gases, by the toxic effects of infection on the blood vessels such as in septi-caemia, or by the excessive production by the body of histamine and other substances with vasodilator capability, such as in anaphylaxis.

Shock related to loss of fluid from the circulatory system

For the circulation to be maintained, an adequate volume of fluid must occupy the circulatory system. As noted earlier, in health approximately 5600 ml of blood occupies the space within the circulatory system of an adult.

Fluid may be lost from the circulation as whole blood, as a result of haemorrhage, but fluid may also effectively be lost from the circulation owing to the loss of fluid from other organs, e.g. from the gastrointestinal system as a consequence of vomiting or diarrhoea, or from the skin, as may occur particularly in hot climates when patients are incapable of hydrating themselves as a result of trauma or illness.

Fluid may also be lost from the circulatory system as a result of trauma to the blood vessels and tissues; this situation is seen particularly in burn trauma. The permeability of the blood vessels can also be affected by the toxic effects of an infection that has progressed to a septicaemia, permitting leakage of fluid from the circulation. In the case of meningococcal septicaemia, the toxic damage to the blood vessels is so severe that whole blood may be lost from the circulation, presenting as petechial haemorrhages. The mediators released during the process of anaphylaxis also increase the permeability of the blood vessels, permitting fluid loss from the circulation.

Clearly, the treatment of shock related to the loss of fluid from the circulatory system is, in the first instance, to take whatever measures are necessary to prevent further fluid loss and to replace the fluid that has been lost in order to maintain a volume of fluid within the circulatory system that is sufficient to permit that system to function. For the shocked patient, the fluid will need to be replaced as soon as possible by intravenous infusion, ideally, with the fluid best adapted to the loss that has taken place. In the emergency situation of the traumatised patient, however, the necessity is first to restore within the circulatory system a volume of fluid that will permit that system to function and, therefore, permit the uninterrupted flow of oxygen by way of the circulation from the atmosphere to the vital organs of the body.

Without an adequate circulation these vital organs will be unable to perform their function. The physiology and the biochemistry of the body will deviate progressively from the normal values and, as the situation deteriorates to the point beyond which the restoration of homeostasis is no longer possible, a state of irreversible shock will be reached followed by death; a death which has occurred essentially because it has not been possible to maintain the vital flow of oxygen from the atmosphere to the cells of the body.

CONCLUSION

It can be seen that the prime driving force of the physiological process is to deliver oxygen to the tissues and to remove waste products. Any derangement of this process in the trauma patient whether due to a reduced oxygen supply from obstruction of the airway or impaired breathing, or circulatory failure due to blood loss will quickly lead to significant physiological problems. These problems in turn manifest themselves as shock and will, if uncorrected, lead to death. The aim of all clinical interventions must, therefore, be to prevent further insult and restore physiological normality as quickly as possible by the maintenance of adequate tissue oxygenation. It is from this basic principle that the underlying basis of the ABC approach to the trauma patient is derived.

Further reading

Advanced Life Support Group. *Advanced paediatric life support*. London: BMJ Publishing Group, 1995

4th Alfred Benzon Symposium. *Oxygen affinity of haemoglobin and red cell acid base status*. Copenhagen: Royal Danish Academy of Science and Letters, 1971

Baldwin J. A model of co-operative oxygen binding of haemoglobin. *British Medical Bulletin* 1976; 32: 213–218

Brooke J. *The physiological basis of immediate care medicine*. Edinburgh: Scottish Academic Press, 1999

Eaton J. *Essentials of immediate medical care*. Edinburgh: Churchill Livingstone, 1993

Haljamae H. Does pre-hospital hypertonic infusion therapy improve the survival of trauma patients. *Lakartidningen* 1999; 96: 1014–1017

Jamieson E. *A companion to manuals of practical anatomy*. Oxford: Oxford University Press, 1950

Kroll W. Hypertonic-hyperoncotic solution: possibilities and limits. *Schweizerische Rundschau fur Medizin Praxis* 1998; 87: 683–689

Remy B. Red blood cell substitutes: fluorocarbon emulsions and haemoglobin solutions. *British Medical Bulletin* 1999; 55: 277–298

Standl T. Artificial oxygen carries as red blood cell substitutes – perfluorocarbons and cell-free haemoglobin. *Infusionstherapie und Transfusionsmedizin* 2000; 27: 128–137

Chapter 12

Haemodynamic disturbances

Sharon Edwards

INTRODUCTION

Haemodynamic changes following trauma are common and may alert the nurse to the deterioration in a patient's condition. The detection of these changes is, therefore, vitally important so that early therapeutic interventions can occur. An understanding of the underlying physiological principles of haemodynamic changes that occur during trauma is imperative.

This chapter provides a comprehensive review of the haemodynamic changes that occur following trauma and before any form of shock is detected, and the mechanisms by which the body maintains homeostasis through its compensatory mechanisms. Some of these mechanisms are so effective that the patient's condition may not change until shock is well established.

It is important that those caring for the trauma patient have an understanding of the response to injury and the practical application of this knowledge to treatment in order to avoid death, not only from the immediate effects of the injury but also from later multiple organ failure.

PHYSIOLOGICAL RESPONSES TO TRAUMA

There is now a sophisticated understanding of the complex metabolic response of the human body to traumatic injury. Following trauma, the initial physiological responses that occur are: neuroendocrine responses; changes in oxygen supply and demand; alterations in metabolism; inflammatory/immune response (IIR); and post-trauma capillary leak. These physiological responses are initiated to protect the body from cell, tissue and organ damage.

Neuroendocrine response to injury

One of the earliest responses to injury is neuroendocrine activation. This occurs in response to cytokine release from the site of injury and stimulates the sympathetic nervous system, hypothalamus, pituitary and adrenal glands (Tan, 1998; Edwards, 2002). The nervous system generates biochemical agents such as hormones and the endocrine system produces substances that mediate activity within the central nervous system.

Following an insult, activation of the neuroendocrine system stimulates the release of numerous substances into the circulation, including the following:

- Catecholamines (adrenaline and noradrenaline). These are released via the sympathetic nervous system and the adrenal cortex causing tachycardia, increased cardiac output, blood pressure, rate and depth of respirations, blood flow redistribution, glycogenolysis, gluconeogenesis and lipolysis.
- Glucocorticoids. These are produced via the hypothalamus which releases corticotropin-releasing hormone (CRH) and the anterior pituitary gland which secretes adrenocorticotrophic hormone (ACTH). The adrenal cortex then releases cortisol, a glucocorticoid that results in gluconeogenesis, proteolysis and lipolysis, and anti-inflammatory and cell-protective effects to prevent damage from excessive activation of the metabolic response.

The stimulation of the sympathetic nervous system occurs almost immediately with the autonomic nervous centres of the brain stimulating almost all the sympathetic nerves at once, effecting change in target organs with extreme rapidity and intensity. Heart rate can double in 3–5 seconds, cardiac output can increase fourfold, while selective vasoconstriction and vasodilatation occurs to redistribute circulating volume to the vital organs (heart and brain) (Huddleston, 1992).

The neuroendocrine response to injury is to protect the body from the effects of injury. However, it causes an increase in oxygen consumption and myocardial work. The redistribution of blood flow away from the 'non-vital' gut reduces the integrity of the gut lining and may result in translocation of bacteria and endotoxins into the circulation resulting in septic shock (Hoffman and Natanson, 1993) and the high catecholamine level can lead to arrhythmias causing a compromised heart to arrest (Tan, 1998). Therefore, if this response is prolonged, it is believed to contribute to lactic acid production and may contribute to multisystem organ failure and a reduced mortality.

Oxygen supply and demand

An imbalance between oxygen supply and tissue demands is fundamental to the nature of trauma. Under normal circumstances, whole-body oxygen consumption (VO_2) is maintained over a wide range of oxygen delivery (DO_2) by varying oxygen extraction (Skowronski, 1998). For example, as VO_2 increases, so too does DO_2, and is presented as a positive correlation. When VO_2/DO_2 increases (e.g. owing to the excess demands of trauma, stress, blood loss and hypermetabolism), and if DO_2 falls below a critical level, the DO_2/VO_2 relationship becomes linear. This supply-dependent state gives rise to an oxygen debt and hypoxia occurs.

The most important effect of hypoxia is that the cell has to resort to anaerobic metabolism. This causes a reduction in adenosine triphosphate (ATP) concentrations in the mitochondria of the cell, which fall within 15 minutes following hypoxia (Gosling, 1999). Mitochondria activity is thus diminished owing to a lack of oxygen and ATP from glycolysis. The end product is lactic acid, which rapidly builds up in the cell and in the blood, lowering the pH. The net result of anaerobic metabolism is the production of lactic acid and a decrease in the energy available for cell work, consequently leading to metabolic acidosis, and tissue and organ dysfunction.

If cellular acidaemia becomes extreme, cellular dysfunction becomes worse, the hypoxic cell swells and becomes distorted and finally ruptures, causing disintegration of the mitochondrial matrix. If hypoxia is allowed to continue, the process becomes irreversible (see Ch. 13).

It is clear that an adequate oxygen supply is essential for mitochondrial function and avoidance of an intracellular energy deficit. However, delivering high-concentration oxygen alone to patients with trauma does not always lead to the prevention or recovery from cellular hypoxia, and aerobic respiration is not always fully restored (Gosling, 1999).

Alterations in metabolism

With the stimulation of the neuroendocrine system, there is a substantial increase in metabolic rate, oxygen consumption, and the production of carbon dioxide and heat. This amplification of energy production is accomplished at the expense of lean body mass. The loss of lean body mass in trauma is different from that observed during starvation. The body preferentially uses fat sources for fuel during starvation in an attempt to preserve lean body mass, with protein being protected until the final stages of malnutrition (Edwards, 2000). However, patients with profound multiple trauma who hypermetabolise usually use mixed fuel sources as an energy supply.

Energy requirements are amplified to supply nutrients and oxygen to tissues and organs involved in the defence against the results of injury. Inflammation, immune function and tissue repair all require an increase in energy substrates to support their functions. The increased demand is sensed by the hypothalamus, pituitary and adrenal glands, which quickly mobilise regulatory hormones, including glucagon, catecholamines and glucocorticoids, which have synergistic effects on each other (Lehmann, 1993).

All potential sources of glucose are mobilised as sources of fuel. Amino acids and glycerol are converted into glucose via gluconeogenesis, and glycogen stores are converted via glycogenolysis. The result is hyperglycaemia. The beta cells in the pancreas continue to secrete increased amounts of insulin, but cellular insulin resistance also develops, resulting in high levels of circulating insulin and hyperglycaemia.

The release of catecholamines causes decreased deposition of fat stores, or lipogenesis, and increased breakdown of fat, or lipolysis. The liver degrades fatty acids for use as fuel, and fat deposits may accumulate in the liver leading to signs and symptoms of liver failure. These include hyperbilirubinaemia, elevated levels of liver enzymes and hepatic encephalopathy (Cheevers, 1999). Zinc, distributed via the liver, becomes deficient and this contributes to impaired wound healing (Tan, 1998).

As protein continues to be broken down and used for energy, serum levels of protein are reduced (Cheevers, 1999). Circulating proteins are responsible for maintaining the stability of the colloid oncotic pressure of the vascular bed. A decreased level of these proteins (e.g. albumin) results in decreased colloid oncotic pressure and hypoalbuminaemia, which causes pooling of fluid in the interstitial space and leads to oedema. Protein loss is accompanied by potassium, magnesium and phosphate loss (Tan, 1998).

All energy sources are utilised following trauma, as a result of the increase in metabolism. Fats, stored glucose and protein are all broken down. This causes a reduction in energy stores and sources, and deprives cells of nutrients, thus reducing their function. In addition, the increase in cellular metabolism increases oxygen consumption, cardiac work and carbon dioxide production, which can become detrimental rather than protective.

Inflammatory/immune response

The wound or injury site plays a role in the systemic response that has become the focus of recent questions and investigation (Edwards, 2003). The wound produces extensive inflammation by attracting nutrients, fluids, clotting factors, and large numbers of neutrophils and macrophages to the damaged site. These are activated to protect the host from invading microorganisms, to limit the extent of blood loss and injury, and to promote rapid healing of involved tissues. This activation is known as the *inflammatory/immune response* (IIR) and represents a major physiological event in the body.

To attract nutrients, fluids, clotting factors and further white blood cells to the site of injury, the damaged tissue and mast cells release mediators such as cytokines [e.g. interleukins, interferon and tumour necrosis factor (TNF), histamine and prostaglandin], oxygen-derived free radicals and prostaglandins. This in turn leads to increased capillary permeability causing the swelling, redness, pain and oedema often observed in inflammation.

Other enzymes and other blood components, such as complement, will also play a role in inflammation and in assisting the immune system in preventing microorganism invasion (Figure 12.1). These include opsonisation of foreign particles, activation of phagocytic cells and lysis, haemostasis (the mechanism of coagulation and fibrinolysis), kinins (which stimulate neutrophil chemotaxis, phagocytosis and microvascular permeability) and mast cells (which release bradykinin, histamine and chemotactic factors that may cause systemic or localised disturbances, such as anaphylaxis or asthma).

The mechanism of coagulation and fibrinolysis is closely linked to the IIR. Activation of haemostatic mechanisms normally accompany injury, localised inflammation and damage to endothelium as they are necessary to prevent excessive blood loss and isolate the injured site (Huddleston 1992). Several circulating components play a role in both processes: kallikrein/kinin cascade, complement, Hageman factor, and platelets. Activation of the IIR often leads to concomitant activation of coagulation processes or alterations in the haemostatic balance causing systemic thrombosis or gross haemorrhage. When these develop simultaneously in one patient it is known as *disseminated intravascular coagulation* (DIC).

The IIR mediators are numerous and the process is initiated to protect the host, but a lack of appropriate regulation, via the hypothalamic-pituitary-adrenal axis, can lead to an uncontrolled intravascular inflammation that ultimately harms the host. The mediators run wild and become toxic to other cells, damaging tissues, vessels and organs distant from the initial injury (Huddleston, 1992). These effects often develop as *adult respiratory distress syndrome* (ARDS), *systemic immune response syndrome* (SIRS) or *multiple system organ failure*.

A vicious, self-activating cycle can occur, and a previously protective mechanism actually contributes to widespread maldistribution of volume, imbalance of oxygen supply and demand, and alterations in metabolism (Huddleston, 1992). If these pathophysiologic changes cannot be reversed or slowed, organ dysfunction and failure ensue.

Post–traumatic capillary leak (fluid shifts)

Following injury, there is a rapid and proportional increase in capillary permeability caused by the mediators discussed earlier. This evolves at a local level as a beneficial response to allow the macromolecules of the innate immune system (complement, kinins and neutrophils) and clotting factors to reach the site of injury. The localised swelling is caused by extravasation of plasma proteins and accompanying water. This causes the localised interstitial oedema necessary for effective healing, repair and prevention of infection. However, if the inflammatory mediators get into the systemic circulation, capillary permeability and severe interstitial oedema can be detected in capillary beds remote from the site of injury, and this can have negative effects on tissue oxygen delivery. As overfilling of the 'third space' becomes critical, oxygen diffusion from capillary to cell is impaired, producing hypoxic damage to organs.

This process may predispose a major trauma victim to excessive stimulation of inflammatory pathways leading to severe and prolonged increase in vascular permeability. The result of this is hypovolaemia and, in the presence of inflammatory mediators, it may lead to further interstitial oedema. This condition is the result of intense inflammatory stimulation and is associated with SIRS (Reilly and Yucha, 1994).

Factors affecting the physiological responses to trauma

Not only do trauma patients experience direct injury, they may also be suffering from other concomitant diseases, such as diabetes or hypertension, and are exposed to stress, fluid replacement therapies (e.g. blood transfusions), surgery/anaesthesia and starvation, all of which will affect their physiological response to trauma.

Pre-existing clinical conditions directly affect the patient's physiological response to trauma

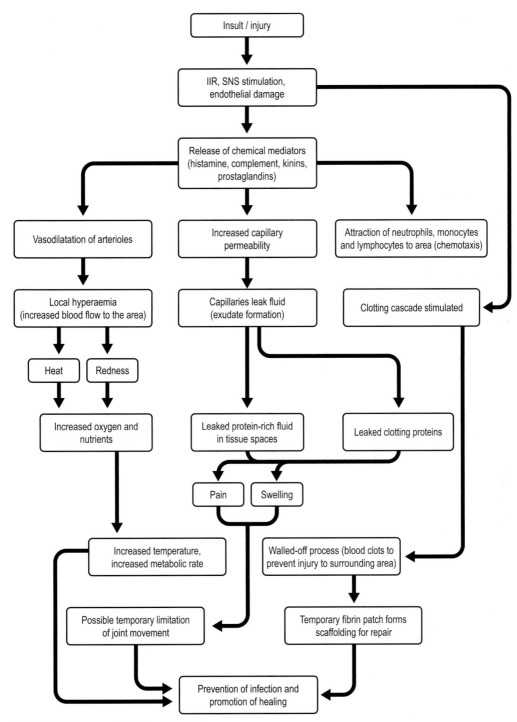

Figure 12.1   The inflammatory immune response.
IIR, inflammatory immune response; SNS, sympathetic nervous system. (Reprinted from Edwards SL. Physiological insult/injury: pathophysiology and consequences. *British Journal of Nursing* 2002; 11: 263–274.)

EFFECT OF STRESS

The results of stress are linked to increased sympathetic nervous system arousal (Marieb, 2004). The body's response to stress is a reaction that involves the whole body and generally consists of a widespread physiological response, which includes a large outflow of adrenal hormones (adrenaline and noradrenaline) in an attempt to defend the body from the insult by:

- increasing heart rate
- increasing blood pressure
- diverting blood from non-essential organs to the vital organs
- converting glycogen to glucose in the liver
- dilating bronchioles
- decreasing digestive system activity
- increasing alertness.

The trauma victim, acutely ill in hospital, is exposed to many stressors simultaneously that tend to act synergistically rather than cumulatively. More long-term responses to stress are controlled by the release of adrenocortical steroid hormones from the cortex of the adrenal gland, resulting in:

- increased blood sugar level
- breakdown of proteins and fat
- retention of sodium and water by kidneys
- increased blood volume and blood pressure.

The general process of hospitalisation is stressful and, for the acutely ill trauma patient, continued exposure to stressors can result in the development of stress ulcers, reduced wound healing, reduced cardiac function and a reduced immune response to infection. More importantly, however, the stress response may mask the development of shock.

EFFECT OF HAEMORRHAGE (HYPOVOLAEMIA)

Hypovolaemia is defined as a diminished circulatory fluid volume (Meyers and Hickey, 1988). Hypovolaemic shock is the state that results from hypovolaemia when there is a decrease in the circulating fluid volume so large that the body's metabolic needs cannot be met. Numerous compensatory mechanisms are activated when the circulating volume is reduced and the venous return is decreased (Meyers and Hickey, 1988).

Losses of 15–30% cause pallor and weakness. A loss of more than 30% of blood volume results in severe shock (see Chapter 13) and may be fatal, as the protective mechanisms eventually cease to function, and circulatory failure and shock ensue (Marieb, 2004).

The principal aetiologies of hypovolaemic states can be classified as haemorrhage, plasma loss, third-space shifts, bleeding disorders, dehydration and high temperatures (Table 12.1).

Haemorrhage causes major disturbances in organ systems and the immune response. In uncompensated hypovolaemia, there is a reduction in circulating volume, which stimulates the release of noradrenaline; this, in turn, decreases the supply of fluid to the muscle beds by vasoconstriction, causing tissue hypoxia. Hypoxia decreases ATP production within the cell, without which the cell membrane sodium pump is disarmed. This shifts extracellular fluid (ECF) and sodium to intracellular fluid (ICF) and sodium, which, in turn, further reduces circulating volume. With the cellular nutrient transport mechanism of the extracellular fluid impaired, biochemical disruption and cell death ensues (see Ch. 13).

EFFECT OF BLOOD TRANSFUSIONS

In the treatment of haemorrhage, whole blood transfusions are often used as a routine, especially when blood loss is substantial.

Blood transfusions have been implicated in immunosuppression and alterations in the IIR (Huddleston, 1992). The changes that occur in stored blood and blood reactions may play a part in the development and potentiation of MSOF.

> Whole blood transfusions should be used where possible in the treatment of severe haemorrhage

Changes that occur in stored blood

Various changes occur in blood as a result of its removal from the body. These changes begin within 24 hours of storage and continue throughout the entire 21 days, after which blood is considered unusable. These changes are many and

Table 12.1 The aetiologies of hypovolaemia

Aetiology	Cause/effect	Outcome/consequences
Haemorrhage	- The loss of whole blood - This is the most common cause of hypovolaemia and hypovolaemic shock - The greater the duration and severity, the more pronounced the overall state of shock. - An acute loss of 10% of total blood volume reduces arterial pressure by 7% and cardiac output by 21% - The loss of 20% of the total blood volume reduces arterial pressure by 15% and cardiac output by 41%	- The loss of red cells decreases the oxygen-carrying capacity of the blood and contributes to hypoxia - Hypoxaemia can develop into an acidosis (reduced pH) and stimulate the vascular chemoreceptors, increasing the rate and depth of breathing
Plasma loss	- This occurs most often in individuals with large partial-thickness burns, full-thickness burns or burns over more than 20–25% of the total body surface area - The rate and volume of plasma deficit are roughly proportional to the extent of the area burned	- There is an increase in capillary permeability leading to a shift of plasma fluid from the vascular space into the interstitial space - This leads to a loss of circulating volume and a reduced cardiac output
Third-space fluid shift	- Owing to stimulation of the IIR, capillaries vasodilate and become more permeable, leading to localised swelling and lymphatic blockage - Trauma or cell damage (e.g. surgical, myocardial infarction, head injury) - It can be external and visible, or internal and invisible - There is movement of fluids, electrolytes and other particles (such as albumin) into the interstitial spaces - This type of hypovolaemia is a relative (rather than a true) hypovolaemic state	- The patient can appear hypovolaemic as fluid has moved into the intravascular spaces, yet may still have the same or excess amount of body water - The vasodilation from the IIR causes a reduction in blood pressure, peripheral vascular resistance and an increase in heart rate - Baroreceptors, volume receptors and osmoreceptors are stimulated in an effort to restore circulating volume and increase blood pressure
Bleeding disorders	- Usually caused by a deficiency in one or more of the clotting factors, an insufficiency of vitamin K, liver disease or disseminated intravascular coagulation - Disorders of platelets include thrombocytopenia and thrombocytosis, and can be caused by drugs, such as anti-inflammatory agents, antimicrobials, antidepressants and adrenergic blocking agents. These disorders can cause or fail to prevent an internal or external haemorrhage	- Coagulation disorders tend to result in more serious bleeding, and are usually caused by a deficiency of one or several clotting factors
Dehydration	- This is more commonly seen in the elderly but, if prolonged, can induce hypovolaemic shock - It may be a consequence of a primary deficit of water, or a primary deficit of salt, or both	- A primary deficit of water leads to cellular dehydration and circulatory failure - A primary deficit of salt leads to reduced extracellular fluid volume, reduced blood volume and increasing difficulty in maintaining an adequate circulating volume
High temperatures	- The vasodilatation observed during a high temperature can make a patient appear hypovolaemic - Fluid space has increased, yet there is still the same amount of circulating volume	- The vasodilation causes a reduction in blood pressure, peripheral vascular resistance and an increase in heart rate and electrolyte imbalance - Dehydration may result owing to fluid loss during sweating and from the lungs owing to increased respiratory rate - Dehydration, together with the profuse vasodilatation of blood vessels, may serve to add to the 'appearance' of a hypovolaemic state

IIR, inflammatory immune response.

varied, and have implications for the trauma patient. These include the following.

Acid–base changes

Stored blood is stored in an air-free container and, as such, aerobic metabolism cannot take place. Anaerobic metabolism and the additional of CPD lead to the accumulation of acids. The longer a unit of blood is stored, the greater the amount of acid it will contain. The citrate phosphate dextrose (CPD) solution used as an anticoagulant adds another acid component to banked blood. The CPD solution added to blood immediately reduces the pH of the blood from a normal body pH of 7.4 to about 7.0. These two processes lead to the accumulation of metabolic acids, and the unit of blood pH continues to decrease to about 6.6 to 6.8 after 14–21 days of storage (Ellerbe, 1981).

Alterations in electrolyte concentration

When blood is stored, the sodium (ECF) and potassium (ICF) concentrations undergo alteration. It can be expected that a unit of stored blood will contain approximately 75–80 mmol/l of sodium and 5–7 mmol/l of potassium (Coltreras, 1992). Patients with normal cardiac and renal function are more likely to be able to handle the increase in sodium and potassium; however, in patients with profound trauma and shock with cardiac and renal dysfunction, the sodium and potassium content of stored blood may have profound effects.

Red cell viability

During blood storage, there is also a progressive loss of red cell viability and the red blood cells tend to take up water (Marieb, 2004). This can cause a leftward shift in the oxyhaemoglobin dissociation curve and cause transfused blood cells to be less capable of releasing oxygen to the tissues than would normal red blood cells.

Microaggregate accumulation

Another significant change that occurs in blood during storage is an increased aggregation of platelets and leucocytes. To prevent these molecules from entering the blood circulation, blood is always filtered through a 170 μm filter. However, electron microscopy studies have now clearly identified the formation of microemboli that are considerably smaller than 170 μm (Edwards, 2001). These are thought to have implications in ARDS. It is now recommended that microfilters with pore sizes ranging from 20–90 μm are utilised.

Trauma is a condition that often requires massive blood transfusions in an emergency and it is recommended that microfilters are always used when large quantities of blood are being administered, especially to those with compromised pulmonary or cardiac status (e.g. those patients in shock (Contreras, 1992).

Depletion of clotting factors

Stored blood is deficient in most of the factors necessary for normal coagulation; it is specifically deficient in factors V, VIII, IX, and platelets (Edwards, 1999). The depletion of platelets and clotting factors will vary in trauma patients. Because of this, it is recommended that clotting screens and bleeding status are closely monitored during transfusion, and platelets and fresh-frozen plasma administered when required.

The temperature of stored blood

Blood is stored at a temperature between 1° and 6°C. The infusion of large quantities of cold blood can cause hypothermia (Edwards, 1999). This compromises the patient's heart rate, blood pressure, cardiac output and coronary blood flow. The heart is the first organ to be exposed to a stream of cold blood. In addition, hypothermia impairs the metabolism of citrate and lactate, and increases the patient's risk of a metabolic acidosis, impaired clotting and a major transfusion reaction.

To safely warm blood, warming coils and controlled-temperature baths have been developed. It is important to note that, when blood is given over the normal 3–4-hour period, it will probably warm sufficiently to prevent complications. However, for trauma patients who are hypothermic, suffering from paralysis, anaesthetised or who are unable to maintain their own body temperature for some other reason, even a single unit of blood should be passed through a warming coil (Contreras, 1992).

Warming devices should always be used when administering blood to victims of trauma

BLOOD TRANSFUSION REACTIONS

When mismatched blood is infused, a transfusion reaction occurs and the donor and recipient's red blood cells are attacked by the recipient's immune system (Higgins, 1994). A severe transfusion reaction can occur with the infusion of as little as 10–15 ml of incompatible blood (Gloe, 1991) and is generally lethal. Minor transfusion reactions include fever, chills, nausea, vomiting and general lethargy (Marieb, 2004).

The administration of blood and blood products is an area of nursing practice in which trauma nurses have to exercise vigilance, both in checking the correct blood group and Rh D antigen factor and in observing for any signs of transfusion reactions. Frequent observations will enable the nurse to detect any reaction at an early stage; these include discomfort, flushing, rash or pain (Glover and Powell, 1996).

Ongoing observation and monitoring are essential to detect the early signs of shock and the early onset of complications

COLLOID AND CRYSTALLOID THERAPIES

It should be note that haemodilution can occur from an over infusion of both crystalloid and colloid solutions not just crystalloid. In an attempt to reduce blood transfusions, other regimes of maintaining circulating volume following trauma have been devised. These include colloid and crystalloid therapies.

The colloid solutions currently available are human albumin solution (Gelofusin®), plasma protein fractions and salt-poor albumin (Haemacell®) and Hespan® (Flanning, 2000). Colloids are used in haemorrhage to achieve the overall primary goal of restoring plasma volume, improving oxygen transport (Ramsey, 1988) and the restoration of cellular function. By administering such 'plasma expanders', there is an improvement in oxygen availability, oxygen consumption, circulating volume, haemodynamic status and tissue perfusion.

There is equivocal evidence to support the argument to give crystalloid solutions in haemorrhage. The crystalloid solutions are Ringer's lactate solution (Hartmann's), sodium chloride 0.9% and dextrose/saline (Flanning, 2000). The main rationale for using crystalloid solutions following haemorrhage is that, during and following hypovolaemic shock, sodium leaks into the surrounding cells and carries with it extracellular water (Edwards, 1998). Therefore, the use of a salt solution is required to restore extracellular fluid volume. However, between two and four times the amount of crystalloid is required, giving rise to possible risks of oedema and haemodilution. This approach thus remains controversial (Edwards, 1998).

EFFECT OF SURGERY AND ANAESTHESIA

Patients undergoing surgical procedures have impaired immunological activity. A surgical procedure is accompanied by anaesthesia, trauma to the body, possible blood transfusion and an overall stress response. These effects may further stimulate the neuroendocrine response, which as previously highlighted may contribute to shock and MSOF.

Surgery is reported to have implications in reducing the cytokine release, which is responsible for the inflammatory response (Tan, 1988). Anaesthesia alone is associated with decreased immune responsiveness, with both decreased phagocytosis and lymphocyte proliferation. It is difficult to isolate which events cause the alterations to the IIR, but the most likely cause is the interactions of all of these events, which operate synergistically to mediate overall host immunosuppression and thus increase susceptibility to infections.

EFFECT OF STARVATION

The recovery from trauma depends upon the consumption and absorption of appropriate amounts of carbohydrates, fats, proteins, minerals and vitamins. Following trauma, a patient may not be allowed to consume any nutrition leading to the start of starvation, although the body can utilise carbohydrates stored as glycogen in the liver and skeletal muscles as a source of energy. To compensate for the lack of a carbohydrate supply, glycogen is converted to glucose (glycogenolysis) and released from the liver. This restores blood glucose levels to normal.

However, despite these mechanisms for supplying blood glucose, they cannot maintain blood glucose levels for very long (12 h). Fat stores provide a large energy deposit, which may be used for energy production. This requires a major physiological adjustment, as all other body tissues must reduce their oxidation of glucose and switch over to fat as the energy source. As the liver metabolises fat, ketone bodies are produced in large quantities. These are oxidised by the body into carbon dioxide, water and ATP. As a result of fat utilisation as a source of energy, hypometabolism occurs so that protein can be spared, and an individual can fast for several weeks, provided water is consumed.

However, if further injury, insult or infection result, hypermetabolism occurs. Starvation in combination with neuroendocrine responses produces hypoalbuminaemia and a malnourished state (Tan, 1998). The body will break down large quantities of muscle protein as a source of energy to maintain cellular functions. Starvation and protein deficiency result in poor immune system function, increasing the risk of infection and reduced wound healing. It is estimated that once protein stores are depleted to about one-half of their normal level, death results.

Clearly starvation contributes to morbidity and mortality in trauma states. It is, therefore, imperative to initiate feeding regimes early (Edwards, 2000). The timing and the route of nutritional support can favourably influence the metabolic response to injury.

OVERSTIMULATION OF THE PHYSIOLOGICAL RESPONSE TO TRAUMA

Patients frequently survive the initial traumatic insult as a result of aggressive treatment. They are, however, at risk of dying days or weeks later of progressive organ failure despite extensive intensive care (Gosling, 1999). This occurs when the physiological protective mechanisms detailed above become overstimulated, causing impaired

gas exchange [adult respiratory distress syndrome (ARDS), systemic inflammatory response syndrome (SIRS) and disseminated intravascular coagulation (DIC)]. These conditions may subsequently cause severe organ dysfunction, which appears unrelated or remote from the original site of injury.

Adult respiratory distress syndrome

Adult respiratory distress syndrome results from injury to the aveolar capillary membrane and pulmonary endothelial damage, which leads to increased pulmonary capillary permeability and leakage of fluid into the interstitial spaces and alveoli. It is caused by an inflammatory response involving neutrophils, macrophages and lymphocytes. Cell adhesion, chemotaxis, chemokinesis, and activation and release of mediators by the cells are important in the pathogenesis of pulmonary tissue damage in ARDS (Takala, 1998). Other important factors in the inflammatory response in relation to ARDS include activation of the complement cascade, alterations in coagulation and fibrinolysis.

The early stages of ARDS are characterised by alveolar oedema resulting from endothelial injury and increased microvascular permeability (Takala, 1998). Destruction of the epithelial cells and leakage of protein into the alveoli reduce the action of surfactant, and gas exchange abnormalities occur. The compliance of the lung decreases substantially, and the resistance of both the airways and the lung tissue increases. Hypoxaemia that does not respond to increasing amounts of inspired oxygen occurs along with decreased pulmonary compliance, respiratory alkalosis, dyspnoea, tachypnoea and the appearance of diffuse fluffy infiltrates on chest x-ray films.

Systemic inflammatory response syndrome

Systemic inflammatory response syndrome is characterised by persistence of the acute inflammatory response due to failure of the down-regulatory mediators to overcome the excessive and persistent IIR. Biochemical mediators released following injury induce a localised IIR that includes mobilisation of neutrophils, monocytes

Table 12.2   Risk factors associated with immune dysfunction

Risk factor	Effect on the immune system
Host-related	
Reduced immune response due to HIV/AIDS	Lives in the CD4 (T-helper) cells and reduces the ability of the body to stimulate the immune system
Leukaemia	Reduces the production of WBC and so the body cannot fight off infection
Treatment-related	
Steroid therapy	Reduces the immune response
Antacids (e.g. Gaviscon) and H_2 receptor drugs (ranitidine)	These can reduce the acid environment within the stomach, which normally kills bacteria and viruses that attempt to enter the body by this route
Insertion of intravenous lines	An intact epidermis is a first line of defence against microorganisms and, as such, prevents entry of bacteria through this route
Prescription of some broad-spectrum antibiotics	These can reduce the normal flora in the vagina, saliva (Candida or thrush) and gut (diarrhoea)
Nil by mouth – undernourishment	Causes changes in phagocytes and in the levels of circulating complement
	May reduce the availability of some organic compounds such as:
	– Vitamin E – assists in stimulating immunoglobulin production, enhancing humoral and cell-mediated immunity
	– Copper – important in maintaining lymphocyte functioning
	– Zinc – implicated in the prevention of wound infections It plays a role in the immune response, as it is required in DNA/RNA synthesis

DNA, deoxyribonucleic acid; RNA, ribonucleic acid; WBC, white blood cells.

and mast cells. However, sometimes the IIR becomes so grossly amplified and distorted owing to prolonged systemic hypoperfusion, it cannot stop. The risk factors associated with immune dysfunction are either host-related or treatment-related (Table 12.2).

Overstimulation leads to immune dysfunction and widespread tissue necrosis. The net effect of the massive assault by these inflammatory mediators is widespread damage to the vascular endothelium resulting in increased vascular permeability, vasodilatation, a pro-coagulant state and progressive destruction of the visceral organs. This response is known as the *systemic inflammatory response syndrome*.

The increased permeability leads to pooling of fluid in the systemic circulation, which, in addition to the release of coagulation factors, influences the formation of microemboli that can cause ischaemic injuries to multiple target organs, particularly the lungs, liver, gastrointestinal tract and kidneys. Thus, SIRS can result in multiple organ failure (MOF), also known as *multiple system organ failure*, which is defined as a failure of at least two distinct organs or organ systems that may be remote from a site of initial injury (Cheevers, 1999).

Disseminated intravascular coagulation

Disseminated intravascular coagulation (DIC) is an acquired coagulopathy, which never occurs as a primary disorder but arises as an intermediary mechanism of disease in numerous underlying conditions (Bell, 1992). DIC can occur due to any illness or injury. Several clinical events, which are known to increase the stimulation of haemostatic mechanisms and predispose the patient to develop DIC are:

- arterial hypotension associated with shock
- hypoxaemia
- acidaemia
- stasis of capillary blood.

Disseminated intravascular coagulation occurs due to overstimulation of normal haemostasis, resulting in disseminated coagulation and excessive fibrinolysis. The overstimulation and dissemination of blood coagulation in DIC produces a unique clinical situation, whereby the patient simultaneously develops microvascular thrombi and haemorrhage.

THE PHYSIOLOGICAL BASIS OF SHOCK

Shock is sometimes defined as the inability of tissues to receive oxygen and nutrients and to rid themselves of waste products (Edwards, 2001). Three components in the body are essential for the transport of oxygen and nutrients to the cells, and for the removal of waste products from the cells – the heart, the vascular system and the blood. Conditions that cause dysfunction of any of these three components may result in shock. When shock occurs, the brain, heart, lungs, kidneys, liver and gastrointestinal tract are affected (see Chapter 13).

> As our understanding of shock increases, it is apparent that it is a very complex syndrome

Following trauma, the development of any form of the five forms of shock, namely, anaphylactic, cardiogenic, septic, neurogenic and hypovolaemic shock (see Chapter 13), must be prevented.

The progress of shock can be divided into three stages: compensated, progressive or uncompensated, and irreversible shock. These stages are not distinct and should be regarded as a continuum.

Compensated shock

The first stage of shock is known as *compensated shock*. The body's compensatory mechanisms are able to maintain cardiovascular dynamic stability and stabilise the circulation in the face of whatever defect is causing the shock. The compensatory mechanisms involved are detailed below.

Sympathetic nervous system

The primary compensatory mechanism is mediated through the sympathetic nervous system and the adrenal glands. This sympathetico-adrenal response is initiated by the decrease in arterial pressure that stimulates baroreceptors located in the aortic arch and carotid sinuses (Marieb, 2004).

Baroreceptors

Baroreceptors respond to any decrease in arterial blood pressure, whether it is due to haemorrhage, peripheral blood pooling or a decrease in myocardial contractility. A decrease in arterial pressure decreases the rate of firing of both the carotid sinus and the aortic arch baroreceptors, which supply sensory information to the cardiovascular centre that regulates blood pressure in the medulla of the brain. This regulating reflex increases sympathetic nervous system discharge, which will increase heart rate; increase myocardial contractility and peripheral resistance by vasoconstriction of blood vessels; increase total peripheral vascular resistance; increase arterial blood pressure, and increase myocardial afterload.

This increase in resistance caused by baroreceptor control is not uniform throughout the body's organ systems. Some systems are given preference, thus varying the distribution of cardiac output with some organs being well perfused and others being hypoperfused. This difference in distribution of cardiac output is due to the distribution of alpha adrenergic receptors, found in the gut, skin and skeletal muscles, and beta adrenergic receptors, found in the heart and brain. These receptors respond to catecholamines liberated from postganglionic sympathetic nerve endings and from the adrenal medulla.

Noradrenaline and adrenaline

Stimulation of the adrenal glands activates the sympathetic nervous system, which causes a release of catecholamines (noradrenaline and adrenaline). Adrenaline is released early in trauma, and shock and circulating concentrations can increase within 3–5 seconds of injury. Adrenaline increases arteriolar resistance, which helps to support perfusion pressure in the face of a relatively low cardiac output. This is done at the expense of certain organs and tissues that will be hypoperfused. The process of selective hypoperfusion causes problems if, and when, shock continues to develop. In addition, adrenaline increases circulating glucose concentrations by inhibiting insulin secretion, stimulating pancreatic glucagon release and gluconeogenesis, and stimulating beta receptors in the heart, increasing myocardial contractility (*inotropic effect*), and heart rate (*chronotropic effect*), which in turn improve cardiac output and increase blood pressure.

Noradrenaline is released more slowly from sympathetic nerve endings and has strong alpha-stimulating effects. Activation of alpha receptors on the cell membranes of vascular smooth-muscle cells causes intense vasoconstriction of the cells in the gut, skin and skeletal muscle, thus tending to preserve perfusion of essential organs, such as the heart and brain. However, the vasoconstriction caused by noradrenaline can soon render circulation and perfusion to these areas inadequate.

The general clinical picture of the patient in the early stages of haemorrhagic shock demonstrating catecholamine release is tachycardia, a narrowing pulse pressure, pale cool skin, decreased urine output owing to selective vasoconstriction of the renal bed, absent bowel sounds, increased blood pressure, increased rate and depth of respiration and alteration in mental state ranging from restlessness to coma.

Venous constriction

Approximately 64% of all blood in the circulatory system is in the systemic veins beyond the capillaries. The systemic veins act as a blood reservoir for the circulation. Even after a loss of 20–25% of the body's total circulating volume, the circulatory system can function almost normally, owing to noradrenaline causing vasoconstriction of the reservoir system of the veins. This increases venous return and increases cardiac pre-load. In this way, sympathetic stimulation helps to maintain cardiac output.

However, the functioning of venous constriction is dependent on vascular compliance. This is the increase in volume a vessel is able to accommodate for a given increase in pressure (Marieb, 2004). The compliance determines the vessel's response to pressure changes. If the patient's veins are stiff from long-term illnesses, such as hypertension, this response may fail to function in a shocked patient.

Renal autoregulation

The kidneys play a complex role in restoring extracellular fluid volume and increasing systemic blood pressure. An elaborate set of interlinked processes involving the renin–angiotensin–

aldosterone system is activated principally when there is a decrease in blood pressure.

A decrease in kidney perfusion activates the *renin–angiotensin–aldosterone mechanism*. Renin is released by the kidneys and converted to angiotensin I. Once in the lungs, angiotensin I is converted to angiotensin II, which has the following two primary actions:

1. It acts as a vasoconstrictor and it stimulates the release of aldosterone.
2. Aldosterone causes increased sodium reabsorption in the renal tubules and, because water follows sodium, there is a subsequent increase in intravascular volume, resulting in increased venous return to the heart, increased cardiac output and increased blood pressure, thus providing a longer term compensation for blood loss.
3. Angiotensin II stimulates the release of noradrenaline (an alpha-receptor stimulator), which causes vasoconstriction of the peripheral vasculature. This vasoconstriction will directly increase the blood pressure by increasing the systemic vascular resistance (SVR) to maintain blood pressure in the face of acute blood loss.

Arterial chemoreceptors

There are further specialised areas within the aortic and carotid arteries that are sensitive to concentrations of oxygen, carbon dioxide and hydrogen ions (pH) in the blood (McCance and Huether, 1997). These receptors are called chemoreceptors and they transmit impulses to the medullary centres of the brain, which regulate blood pressure. There are two types of chemoreceptors: central and peripheral. The central chemoreceptors ar sensitive to changes in carbon dioxide and pH, whereby peripheral chemoreceptors are sensitive to decreases in arterial oxygen. A decrease in arterial oxygen concentration or pH causes vasoconstriction and a reflexive increase in blood pressure (Masasi and Keyes, 1994), whereas an increase in carbon dioxide causes vasodilatation and a decrease in blood pressure. Smooth muscle layers in the vessels carry out these blood pressure changes.

Patients in shock are susceptible to cellular hypoxia owing to a low circulating volume. In addition, trauma patients may be further compromised by chest problems. If hypoxia occurs owing to shock, then patients are at risk of having an increased blood pressure.

Osmoreceptors

To maintain fluid and electrolyte balance, water and electrolytes are in constant motion between intracellular (about 25 litres) and extracellular compartments (divided into interstitial fluid – 12 litres, and plasma volume – 3 litres) (Edwards, 1998). If the concentration of sodium (the major cation in extracellular fluid) is increased, as in the case when there is a loss of extracellular water, osmoreceptors in the hypothalamus are stimulated (Bove, 1994). Osmoreceptors are highly specialised hypothalamic neurons, which continually monitor the solute concentration (and thus water content) of blood. When solutes become too concentrated, as in conditions that cause an increased sodium concentration (e.g. excessive sweating, inadequate fluid intake, burns), the osmoreceptors transmit excitatory impulses to the hypothalamic neurones, which synthesise and release antidiuretic hormone (ADH).

Antidiuretic hormone inhibits urine formation by causing renal tubules to increase water absorption at the renal collecting duct, thus returning it to the circulation. As a result, less urine is produced and blood volume increases, thereby improving venous return to the heart, cardiac output and blood pressure. Urinary output will decrease and a sense of thirst will be aroused (Bove, 1994).

These protective mechanisms, observed in the compensatory stage of shock, will eventually cease to function and circulatory failure will ensue. If the metabolic acidosis, circulatory failure or volume is not corrected or treatment instigated, progressive shock will occur in a short space of time.

Progressive or uncompensated shock

Once shock has developed, the course it takes is complex. Why some shock patients take a progressively downward course despite best efforts at their treatment is not fully understood. Once shock has progressed into this second stage, the outcome is unpredictable but is related to the failure of the compensatory mechanisms to maintain an adequate circulation. The changes associated with this stage of shock are detailed in Chapter 13.

Refractory (irreversible) shock

This is the final stage of shock, and occurs when severe cellular and organ dysfunction develops rapidly leading to death. At this stage, it may be possible to return arterial pressure to normal for a short while, but tissue and organ deterioration continue, and no amount of therapy will reverse the process (Guthrie, 1982). By this stage, so much tissue damage and necrosis has occurred, so many mediators and toxins have been released into the systemic circulation and acidosis is so profound, that even a return of normal cardiac output and arterial pressure will not reverse the downward progression.

At this point there is an almost total depletion of adenosine triphosphate (ATP), essential for the production of energy, and there is usually vasomotor failure owing to central nervous system ischaemia. The vasomotor centres become so depressed that no sympathetic activity occurs. The vascular bed is generally dilated owing to central nervous system (CNS) depression, acidosis and toxins, and so deterioration will continue and death will ensue within a short period of time.

CONCLUSION

Patients surviving the first 24 hours after injury as a result of effective resuscitation continue to be at risk. This may be due to the sequelae of the injury, stress, surgery and anaesthesia, starvation and blood transfusions. Patients remain in danger days or weeks following injury from progressive organ failure from what appears to be an uncontrolled inflammatory process. Thus, when treating trauma victims, it is not only necessary to deliver effective resuscitation, but to also consider other risk factors and the possibility of host response injury.

Shock is a state that can occur following traumatic injury, and it is the responsibility of the nurse to assess and observe for signs of shock. It is important for trauma nurses to understand that early in the shock process, homeostatic compensatory mechanisms maintain blood pressure and cardiac output and, as such, organ and cellular function. Consequently, the nurse may not be easily alerted to the development of shock. Nurses need to observe for more subtle changes in patient colour, perfusion of the skin, heart rate, oxygen saturation, breathing patterns and urine output, as failure to do so may lead to treatment not being provided quickly enough. This could then contribute to the development of progressive or uncompensated shock, irreversible shock and death.

References

Bell TN. Coagulation and disseminated intravascular coagulation. In: Huddleston V (ed.) *Multi-system organ failure: patho-physiology and clinical implications.* St Louis: Mobsy Yearbook, 1992

Bove LA. How fluids and electrolytes shift. *Nursing* 1994; August: 34–39

Cheevers KH. Early enteral feeding of patients with multiple trauma. *Critical Care Nurse* 1999; 19: 40–51

Contreras M. ABC *of transfusion,* 2nd edn. London: BMJ Publishing Group, 1992

Edwards SL. Hypovolaemia: patho-physiology and management options. *Nursing in Critical Care* 1998; 3: 73–82

Edwards SL. Hypothermia. *Professional Nurse* 1999; 14: 253–258.

Edwards SL. Maintaining an adequate circulation. In: Manley K, Bellman L (eds) *Surgical nursing: advancing practice.* Edinburgh: Churchill Livingstone, 2000

Edwards SL. Maintaining optimum nutrition. In: Manley K, Bellman L (eds) *Surgical nursing: advancing practice.* Edinburgh: Churchill Livingstone, 2000

Edwards SL. Shock: types, classifications and exploration of their physiological effects. *Emergency Nurse* 2001; 9(2): 29–38

Edwards SL. Physiological insult/injury: pathophysiology and consequences. *British Journal of Nursing* 2002; 11: 263–274

Edwards SL. Cellular pathophysiology. Part 1: changes following tissue injury. *Professional Nurse* 2003; 18: 562–565

Flanning H. Fluid and electrolyte balance. In: Manley K, Bellman L (eds) *Surgical nursing: advancing practice.* Edinburgh: Churchill Livingstone, 2000

Gloe D. Common reactions to transfusions. *Heart Lung* 1991; 20: 506–514

Glover G, Powell F. Blood transfusion. *Nursing Standard* 1996; 10: 49–54

Gosling P. The metabolic and circulatory response to trauma. In: Alpar EK, Gosling P (eds) *Trauma: a scientific basis for care.* London: Arnold, 1999

Guthrie M. (ed.) *Shock.* New York: Churchill Livingstone, 1982

Higgins C. Blood transfusions: risks and benefits. *British Journal of Nursing* 1994; 3: 986–991

Hoffman WD, Natanson C. Endotoxin in septic shock. *Anaesthesia Analgesia* 1993: 77: 613–624

Huddleston V. *Multisystem organ failure: patho-physiology and clinical implications.* St Louis: Mobsy Yearbook, 1992

Lehmann S. (1993) Nutritional support in the hypermetabolic patient. *Critical Care Nurse Clinics of North America* 5: 97–103

McCance KL, Huether SE. *Patho-physiology: the biologic basis for disease in adults and children,* 3rd edn. St Louis: Mosby, 1997

Marieb EN. *Human anatomy and physiology,* 6th edn. Redwood City: The Benjamin Cummings, 2004

Masasi RS, Keyes JL. The patho-physiology of hypoxia. *Critical Care Nurse* 1994; 14: 55–64

Meyers KA, Hickey MK. Nursing management of hypovolaemic shock. *Critical Care Nursing Quarterly* 1988; 11: 57–67

Ramsey G. Intravenous volume replacement: indications and choices. *British Medical Journal* 1988; 296: 1422–1423

Reilly E, Yucha CB. Multiple organ failure syndrome. *Critical Care Nurse* 1994; 14: 25–31

Skowronski GA. Circulatory shock. In: Oh TE. *Intensive care manual,* 4th edn. Hong Kong: Butterworth Heinemann, 1998

Takala J. Acute respiratory distress syndrome. In: Oh TE. *Intensive care manual,* 4th edn. Hong Kong: Butterworth Heinemann, 1998

Tan IKS. Metabolic response to illness, injury and infection. In: Oh TE. *Intensive care manual,* 4th edn. Hong Kong: Butterworth Heinemann, 1998

Chapter **13**

Pathophysiological mechanisms of shock

Sharon Edwards

INTRODUCTION

This chapter provides a comprehensive review of the classifications and types of shock that can occur following trauma (neurogenic, hypovolaemic, cardiogenic) and during or following treatment (septic, anaphylaxis). It provides an overview of the physiological changes that occur in the cell, at organ level, to oxygen consumption and demand, and coagulation. Nurses are responsible for assessing and observing for signs of shock, therefore, it is essential that they understand the underlying pathophysiological mechanisms.

CLASSIFICATION AND TYPES OF SHOCK

Shock is a condition where the cardiovascular system fails to perfuse the body tissues adequately, thereby bringing about a widespread disruption of cellular metabolism, which results in functional disturbances at organ level (Edwards, 2001). There are many causes of shock; however, they all affect either blood volume, blood pressure or cardiac function.

Blood pressure can be used as a basis for defining different types of shock as follows.

1. Hypotensive shock, which is further subdivided into:
   a. low cardiac-output shock characterised clinically by cold skin
   b. high cardiac-output shock characterised by warm skin.

2. Normotensive or hypertensive shock – blood pressure is compensated.

This classification of shock may be helpful for accident and emergency staff to use, as it is based on parameters that are relatively easy to measure (Guthrie, 1982).

A more traditional way to classify shock is according to the primary cause. With this system of classification, there are five forms of shock: anaphylaxic, septic, neurogenic, cardiogenic and hypovolaemic.

Anaphylactic shock

Anaphylaxis occurs when a sensitised person is exposed to an antigen, to which he or she is allergic. The antigen enters the body and combines with immunoglobulin E (IgE) antibodies on the surface of the mast cells and basophils (Khun, 1990). Mast cells and basophils are primarily found in the lungs, small intestines, skin and connective tissue. An antigen–antibody reaction then occurs, which induces the release of histamine, causing extreme vasodilatation and increased capillary permeability (Howarth, 1998; Jarvis and Burney, 1998). This results in reduced cardiac output and low arterial pressure. Cellular perfusion fails to meet the metabolic demands, resulting in acidosis, coagulopathies and capillary pooling (O'Neill, 1990).

Histamine also has selective vasoconstrictor effects in the pulmonary bed, on the hepatic and other large veins, and causes movement of circulating fluids into the interstitial space, causing a relative hypovolaemia and shock (Hollingsworth and Giansiracusa, 1992). This results in bronchospasm, oedema in the glottis and pharynx, oedema in the lungs and in subcutaneous tissue. It also causes changes in cardiac function, such as reduced contractility and dysrhythmias.

Septic shock

Septic shock is caused by an overwhelming infection following severe injury or in an immuno-compromised patient. The most common causal organisms are Gram-negative enteric bacilli, such as *Escherichia coli*, *Pseudomonas* and Gram-positive staphyloccoccal infections (Bone, 1991). These organisms enter the vascular system and promote the release of endotoxins, which cause interstitial fluid leak, increased vascular permeability and vasodilatation leading to shock (Hoffman and Natanson 1993).

The result of septic shock is tachycardia and a high cardiac output. In this state, the patient may feel warm, have a high temperature, a low circulating volume owing to venous pooling, increased capillary permeability and third-space fluid shift (Bone, 1991). Cardiac output is maintained at a normal or high level by the increasing tachycardia but, if the volume loss is not corrected, hypovolaemia will persist, cardiac output will decrease and the skin will become cool. As in all other types of shock, the primary problem is tissue hypoperfusion, resulting in organ failure.

Neurogenic shock

Neurogenic shock may be the result of a severe brainstem injury at the level of the medulla, an injury to the spinal cord or spinal anaesthesia. Neurogenic shock causes changes to the smooth muscle tension in the walls of blood vessels, and an imbalance between parasympathetic and sympathetic stimulation. There is loss of sympathetic tone causing peripheral vasodilatation, resulting in severe hypotension. There is decreased vascular tone and systemic vascular resistance (SVR), inadequate cardiac output, reduced tissue perfusion and impaired cellular metabolism (Figure 13.1).

> Neurogenic shock may mask signs and symptoms of other types of shock

Cardiogenic shock

Cardiogenic shock occurs when the heart, usually owing to impaired myocardial performance, cannot produce an adequate cardiac output to sustain the metabolic requirements of body tissues. Myocardial infarction is the most common cause of cardiogenic shock as, depending on the size of the infarction, stroke volume and cardiac output may decrease with a concurrent increase in left ventricular end-diastolic pressure (Anderson, 1982).

Compensatory mechanisms are stimulated by the decrease in blood pressure and catechol-

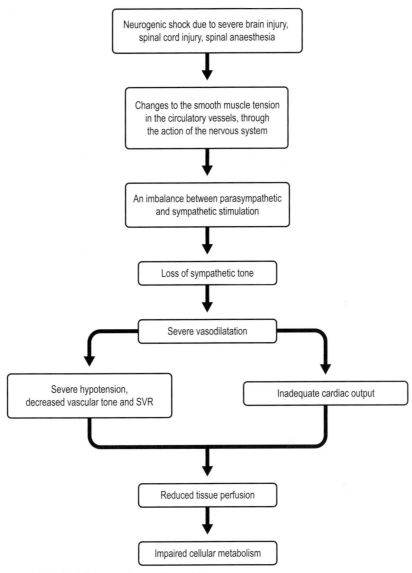

Figure 13.1 Neurogenic shock. SVR, systemic vascular resistance.

amines are released. This causes an increase in heart rate, contractility, blood pressure and SVR to maintain arterial pressure.

Shock occurs if:
– circulating blood volume falls (hypovolaemic)
– the heart does not pump adequately (cardiogenic)
– circulatory capacity exceeds circulating volume (neurogenic, septic, anaphylactic)

The compensatory mechanisms improve blood flow for a time, but more oxygen is required by the already ischaemic cardiac muscle to pump blood into the constricted systemic circulation. The heart ultimately becomes more ischaemic and cardiac failure worsens. The result is that potentially viable tissue is jeopardised and left ventricular function worsens. As cardiac output continues to decline, blood pressure and tissue perfusion decreases, which results in cardiogenic shock and ends with the patient's death (Figure

13.2). Cardiogenic shock is often complicated by arrhythmias or pulmonary oedema.

Hypovolaemic shock

Hypovolaemic shock is the most common type of shock. It is the state that results from severe hypovolaemia; shock is the result of a decrease in the circulating fluid volume so large that the body's metabolic needs cannot be met.

The degree of shock depends on the amount of blood lost, the rate at which it was lost, the age and general physical condition of the patient, and the patient's ability to activate compensatory

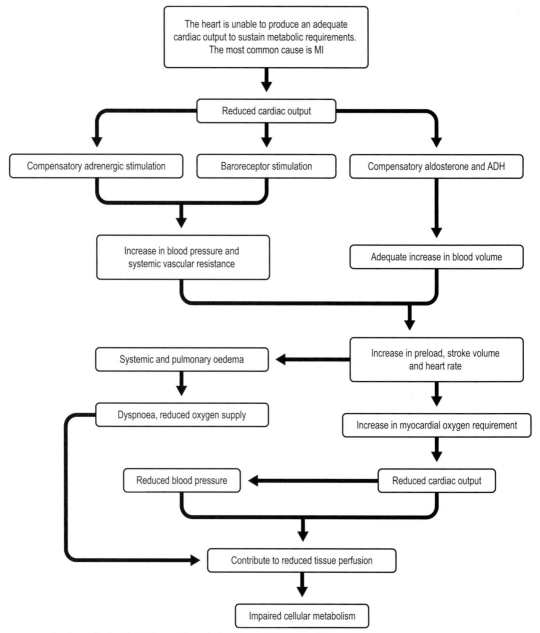

Figure 13.2   Cardiogenic shock. ADH, antidiuretic hormone; MI, myocardial infarction.

mechanisms. Numerous compensatory mechanisms are activated when the circulating volume and venous return is decreased (see Ch. 12) (Meyers and Hickey, 1988). As a result, venous capacity is decreased to match the smaller blood volume, and adequate transport of oxygen and nutrients is maintained.

If the fluid loss exceeds the ability of homeostatic mechanisms to compensate for the loss, the central venous pressure (CVP), diastolic filling pressure, stroke volume and systemic arterial blood pressure will fall. As the severity of shock increases, blood is pooled in the capillary and venous beds, with further impairment of the effective vascular volume available for oxygen transport and tissue perfusion (Figure 13.3).

Patients in shock will not uncommonly have components of more than one of the forms of shock. For example, patients in cardiogenic shock may also be hypovolaemic owing to loss of fluid into the tissues, as a result of high venous pressures or increased capillary permeability. Hypovolaemia is also frequently a complication of septic shock and, in the late stages of hypovolaemic shock, patients usually have some degree of cardiac failure and vasomotor collapse complicating their shock picture.

The signs of compensated and decompensated shock are given in Table 13.1.

PHYSIOLOGICAL PROCESSES COMMON TO ALL FORMS OF SHOCK

As shock progresses, there are deleterious changes that occur in the cells to energy production, to the cell membrane and to coagulation processes.

Table 13.1 Signs of compensated and decompensated shock

	Compensated	Decompensated
Skin	Pale, cool and moist	Chalky white, cold and wet
Pulse	Tachycardia	> 140 beats/minute or bradycardia
Conscious level	Normal	Confused → unresponsive
Blood pressure	Normal	Reduced

Cellular changes

Cellular shock can be caused by any of the types of shock mentioned above. However, before shock occurs at the level of the cell, specific vascular changes begin as described above. All shock states interfere with tissue perfusion, oxygen transport and the synthesis of adenosine triphosphate (ATP), all of which lead to a reduction in the availability of nutrients, energy and oxygen, leading to serious cell damage.

Cellular energy production

Nutrients and oxygen enter the cell across the cell membrane. Shock results in an inadequate flow of nutrients and oxygen to the cell. If tissue perfusion continues to be insufficient, hypoxia occurs and the cells resort to anaerobic metabolic pathways for energy production. This produces several changes in cell function. There is a lack of oxygen for glycolysis, as a result of which lactic acid is produced. This rapidly builds up in the cell and in the blood, lowering the pH. The drop in pH diminishes mitochondrial activity and cellular ATP stores become rapidly used up.

Poor blood flow also impairs the normal removal of carbon dioxide, which is converted to carbonic acid, further lowering blood pH. Consequently, the results of anaerobic metabolism are the production of lactic acid and a reduction in the energy available for cell work.

Lactic acidosis reduces myocardial contractility and arteriolar responsiveness to adrenaline and noradrenaline release, thus potentiating vasomotor collapse, and stimulates the intravascular clotting mechanism. However, acidaemia has the beneficial effect of shifting the oxyhaemoglobin dissociation curve to the right, thereby facilitating the release of oxygen from haemoglobin (Marieb, 2004). Eventually, a large number of cytotoxic, vasodilator, vasoactive and other substances are released from the cell into the circulation, resulting in progressive vasodilatation, myocardial depression, increased capillary permeability and, eventually, intravascular coagulation. These substances include histamine, serotonin, kinins, lysosomal enzymes and endogenous mediators (Huddleston, 1992). If cellular acidaemia becomes extreme, cellular dysfunction becomes

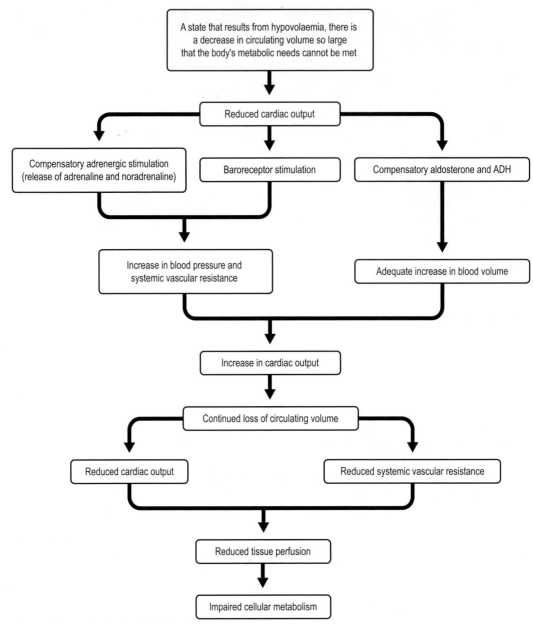

Figure 13.3 Hypovolaemic shock. ADH, antidiuretic hormone.

intemperate and, if permitted to continue, may finally become irreversible.

Cellular membrane disruption

The high intracellular potassium, and low intracellular sodium and calcium concentrations are maintained by active transport systems: the sodium/potassium adenosine triphosphatase (ATPase)-dependent pump, and the ATP-dependent calcium transport pump. Thus, one of the most rapid effects of hypoxia, and of a shortage of ATP, is disruption of the normal ionic gradients across the cell membrane, with a rapid efflux of potassium from the cell, and movement of sodium and chloride into the cell (Gosling,

1999). Increased intracellular sodium results in water entering the cell through osmosis, causing cellular swelling and distortion, which may interfere with organelle function (Buckman et al., 1992). The cytoplasmic membrane of cells becomes increasingly permeable to larger molecular weight proteins, not simply owing to direct cellular injury but also owing to the systemic intracellular energy debt.

The influx of calcium into the cell during shock has a different cause than the initial membrane permeability change involving sodium and potassium. The mechanisms by which the calcium content of cells is regulated are disrupted by a lack of ATP (Gosling and Alpar, 1999). Intracellular calcium is responsible for activation of phospholipases and proteases, and its derangement results in membrane disruption. As a result, calcium accumulates in the mitochondria, causing structural derangements of the organelles, which contributes to irreversible cellular injury and eventually cell death (Buckman et al., 1992).

Cellular fluid shifts

Any type of trauma or cell damage (e.g. surgical, myocardial infarction, head injury), whether it is external and visible, or internal and invisible, will automatically trigger an inflammatory response (Edwards, 2002). The normal body response will be to send nutrients, fluids, white blood cells and clotting factors to the damaged site to repair tissue, prevent infection and, if necessary, to stem blood loss (Huddleston, 1992). Capillaries vasodilate and become more permeable to allow these factors to reach the site of injury, leading to localised swelling and lymphatic blockage.

The increase in permeability causes movement of fluids, allowing water, electrolytes and other particles (such as albumin) into the interstitial spaces, and is known as a *third-space fluid shift* (Edwards, 2002). When third-space fluid shift occurs, patients can appear paradoxically 'dry' or hypovolaemic as fluid has moved into the interstitial spaces, yet they may still have the same amount, or indeed, an excess amount of body water.

Vasodilation is caused by the release of cell mediators (e.g. histamine, kinins, complement) from the damaged endothelium, and causes a reduction in blood pressure, peripheral vascular resistance and an increase in heart rate, further compounding the appearance of a hypovolaemic state (Huddleston, 1992). This relative (rather than true) hypovolaemic state stimulates baroreceptors, volume receptors, and osmoreceptors to reabsorb sodium and water to cause vasoconstriction, in an effort to restore circulating volume and increase blood pressure.

The role of lysosomes

Lysosomes are important intracellular structures and are affected by shock. Lysosomes contain enzymes, which contribute to the breakdown of cell waste (Marieb, 2004). The lysosomal membrane is ordinarily quite stable, but it becomes fragile when the cell is injured or deprived of oxygen. Lysosomal membrane instability is made worse by the lack of ATP and the cell starts to use its own structural phospholipids as a nutrient source. Eventually, the lysosomal membrane becomes more permeable and may rupture, allowing the release of lysosomal enzymes, resulting in self-digestion of the cell. The use of steroids in shock is thought to help stabilise the lysosomal membrane and prevent lysosomal enzyme damage to the cell (Guthrie, 1982).

Coagulation defects

Early in shock, changes in blood coagulation can be seen. A state of hypercoagulability occurs as a result of the IIR and release of thromboplastic substances and as a result of the effects of catecholamines, lysosomal enzymes and acidosis. Platelet aggregation is increased in response to stress. The process of hypercoagulability may at first be compensatory, if the cause of the shock is haemorrhage, but later it can cause significant problems. The combination of hypercoagulation and stagnation of blood in the capillaries may be responsible for microemboli developing during shock (Anderson, 1982). These microemboli further contribute to tissue ischaemia and the progression of shock by decreasing the already poor blood flow through the capillaries.

Late in shock, a state of hypocoagulability may develop, owing to lack of clotting factors through haemorrhage, replacement of lost volume by blood deficient in clotting factors, and/or crystalloid/non-crystalloid solutions causing haemodilution and a decrease in the production of clotting factors owing to poor tissue perfusion.

ORGAN DYSFUNCTION DURING SHOCK

The progressive stage of shock is predominately marked by continuing hypoperfusion and deteriorating organ function. How far the deterioration in organ function goes will vary from person to person, but organ function will largely determine the course and outcome. Some organs bear the brunt of the body's effort to compensate for a decrease in systemic pressure and, as a result, these organs will suffer damage and dysfunction early in the shock syndrome. The point at which organ dysfunction becomes irreversible is not clear.

Kidneys

The kidneys are the most important organs affected early in shock. Renal blood flow is quickly reduced even in moderate haemorrhage. As the total renal blood flow falls, the glomerular filtration rate (GFR) is reduced and renin will be released by the kidney (Marieb, 2004). The GFR is preserved for a time but, nevertheless, oliguria occurs owing to antidiuretic hormone (ADH) and aldosterone secretion.

The renal tubules have a high ATP requirement, which makes them susceptible to ischaemic damage, and when a reduction in oxygen and energy within tubular cells occurs, the reabsorptive function of the tubules is lost (Buckman et al., 1992). With continued ischaemia, the tubules undergo necrosis. Acute tubular necrosis and even cortical necrosis of the kidney commonly occur in shock and, if severe, may lead to acute renal failure. Acute renal failure may contribute to late deaths following resuscitation.

Liver

The liver is a highly complex organ having multiple metabolic, synthetic and immunologic functions. The liver plays a key role in carbohydrate and lipid metabolism, and synthesises many plasma proteins, including albumin, protease inhibitors, transport proteins and coagulation factors (Marieb, 2004). It has a high-energy requirement and is sensitive to ischaemia. Both hepatic arterial and portal venous blood flow are reduced in shock. Early in shock, the liver releases large amounts of glucose as the result of adrenaline-induced glycogenolysis and gluconeogenesis.

In decompensated shock, all liver functions, including bile and cholesterol formation, protein synthesis, gluconeogenesis, lactate metabolism and detoxification are impaired, and the phagocytic activity of the Kupffer cells are depressed (Buckman et al., 1992). With continued shock, the parenchymal cells suffer a reduction of transmembrane potential with cellular swelling, reduced production of high-energy phosphates, loss of lysosomal stability and cellular necrosis. The liver, however, has considerable reserve capacity and removal of up to 90% of liver function is compatible with life, since it has a remarkable ability to regenerate (Gosling, 1999). In general, the liver appears to cope well with shock, and liver failure is frequently of late onset and is more often due to multiple organ failure in association with pulmonary and renal function.

Gastrointestinal tract

The gut suffers an early reduction of oxygen delivery in hypovolaemia and other forms of shock as a result of the effects of vasopressin, angiotensin II and catecholamines (Buckman et al., 1992). This may be because the overall oxygen extraction ratio for the gut is only in the region of 20%. It can thus accommodate major flow reductions before oxygen delivery becomes inadequate. There is, however, a threshold beyond which the reduction in blood flow produces lactate in large amounts. Catabolism of both fat and carbohydrates is inhibited, and there is increased reliance on skeletal muscle amino acids as a fuel source; this further increases lactic acid production owing to mitochondrial dysfunction and hypoxia. The gut is the major source of lactic acidosis in haemorrhagic shock.

The gut contains bacteria and bacterial toxins together with potentially harmful secretions, such as hydrochloric acid and enzymes. The mucosa of the gut forms an essential barrier between the intestine and the bloodstream to which nutrients must be delivered (Elia, 1995). In shock, the gut's mucosal barrier loses its integrity, and becomes permeable to bacteria and endotoxins from the intestinal lumen, probably because of insufficient energy to produce the protective coating of mucin. This results in damage to and necrosis of the intestinal wall by digestive enzymes.

The increased permeability may then allow pathogens to enter the portal and systemic circulation, causing infection and multiple organ failure (Adam, 1994). The translocation of bacteria into the portal and systemic circulation has been proposed as a compounding mechanism of acute shock and as a cause of septic syndromes occurring after resuscitation. In addition, there is mounting evidence that gastrointestinal failure not only closes an avenue for nutrition, but may initiate or perpetuate mechanisms that contribute to remote multiple organ failure and death (Huddleston, 1992).

Lungs

In shock, reduced pulmonary blood flow results in an imbalance between oxygen supply and tissue demands (Gosling, 1999). This is compensated for by hyperventilation, initiated by peripheral chemoreceptor stimulation, which maintains the arterial partial pressure of oxygen.

In advanced shock, where there is a further reduction in the pulmonary circulation, ventilation and/or perfusion and gas exchange does not take place. This results in progressive atelectasis, adult respiratory distress syndrome (ARDS), respiratory muscle fatigue from respiratory muscle hypoperfusion and respiratory failure. Respiratory failure is the primary cause of death following successful initial resuscitation of shock. Factors such as cellular dysfunction, changes in membrane permeability, and shifts in vascular and interstitial fluid volumes, as well as changes in local hormonal responses, all play a role in the development of respiratory failure and shock lung (Buckman et al., 1992). Pre-existing lung disease, chest trauma and cardiac failure may contribute.

Heart

Early deaths from shock are usually associated with unsupportable reductions in cardiac function. The heart muscle relies on the delivery of oxygen and nutrients to its cells via the coronary arteries, and has a very high oxygen requirement (Marieb, 2004). Thus, a major reduction in cardiac blood flow quickly renders the heart muscle ischaemic.

Cardiac blood flow during shock is preserved as a result of homeostatic compensation, even when blood flow to other organs suffers. Consequently, myocardial dysfunction only occurs if there is a reduction in coronary blood flow exceeding the limits of coronary vascular autoregulation. As blood supply to the coronary arteries continues to decrease, myocardial contractility and compliance are reduced. The heart muscle becomes dysfunctional, and the heart ceases to function adequately as a pump, thus causing a decrease in cardiac output (Gosling, 1999). Failure of the circulatory pump intensifies the deficient oxygen delivery throughout the remainder of the body, as well as to the heart itself.

Except in cardiogenic shock, major effects on myocardial function do not occur until the very late stages of shock. The additive effects of acidosis and hypoxia result in a decrease in myocardial contractility, and a further reduction in cardiac output. These effects may also produce dangerous cardiac arrhythmias.

Brain

Of all organs of the body, the brain is both the most intricate and most susceptible to hypoxic injury (McCance and Huether, 1997). The brain is primarily affected because it depends on glucose and oxygen to function. Although it is protected by homeostatic vasoconstriction and by its own autoregulation, the capacity for autoregulation is exceeded if the systolic blood pressure falls below 60 mmHg.

Mental state abnormalities, often associated with poor outcome, occur as respiratory alkalosis, hypoxaemia, and electrolyte disturbances start to appear. If blood flow continues to deteriorate, autoregulation can no longer maintain normal cerebral metabolism and unconsciousness rapidly occurs. With severe degrees of reduction of blood flow, the brain becomes ischaemic and irreversible brain injury occurs. When the cerebral blood flow is reduced below the critical level, all areas of the brain suffer equal deprivation of flow.

OTHER CONSIDERATIONS

There are a number of variables that affect the course of shock. These include age, the general state of health, hypothermia, hyperthermia and pain.

Age

Elderly injured patients require special attention in relation to shock, as they generally have a sluggish circulation, structural and functional changes in the skin, and an overall decrease in heat-producing and heat conservation activities (Moddeman, 1991). In addition, the elderly have a decrease in shivering response (delayed onset and decreased effectiveness), slowed metabolic rate, decreased vasoconstrictor response, diminished or absent sweating, desynchronisation of circadian rhythm, poor nutrition, and decreased perception of heat and cold. They are at more risk of developing late-stage shock following injury quicker than a younger person.

In addition, the elderly patient is more likely to be suffering from dehydration, which, if prolonged, can enhance hypovolaemic shock. Dehydration itself is a critical state and, added to any other form of shock, can precipitate and progress very quickly to multiple organ failure.

General state of health

A patient suffering from a concomitant medical condition is likely to develop shock earlier than a healthy patient. For example, hypertension can affect the circulation by damaging the wall of the systemic blood vessels. Prolonged high pressure within these vessels causes the vessels to thicken and strengthen to withstand the stress (Shephard and Fox, 1996). The thickening gradually becomes sufficient to narrow the blood vessel, thus reducing the patient's ability to compensate during shock states.

Heart failure reduces the supply of nutrients of body tissues, causes circulatory stasis, pulmonary congestion and increased stress on the body (Williams and Bristow, 1995). This is a serious condition, which, in situations that cause shock, can disturb the normal physiological responses and influence the patient's recovery.

Arteriosclerosis and atherosclerosis frequently affect the peripheral arteries. These can influence the survival of the body's extremities, most commonly the lower extremities, during shock. It is imperative, therefore, that those patients who are prone to peripheral vascular disease are identified early following trauma, as they may be more susceptible to low flow states, microemboli and limb loss.

Pain

The goals of trauma teams have expanded to include the control of pain (Cheevers, 1999). Pain can interfere with obtaining accurate and reliable clinical measurements, and may lead to false or inaccurate readings (e.g. increase in blood pressure, heart and respiratory rate) and, as a result, the detection of shock can be delayed. Therefore, pain needs to be identified and treated early (Hollinworth, 1994). Baillie (1993) suggested that because of the subjective nature of pain, only patients can measure their own pain accurately, and so nurses should provide tools to help them assess and communicate their pain. For information on pain and analgesia during trauma and shock, see Chapter 23.

Hypothermia

A large majority of trauma patients will suffer from some form of hypothermia, which is a result of prolonged exposure to cold environments. Hypothermia is characterised by a marked cooling of core temperature below 35°C (Edwards, 1999). A temperature of below 35°C is below the hypothalamic 'set point', and results in attempts to conserve and generate body heat. Vasoconstriction occurs and muscle tone increases, providing an increase in heat production and a decrease in heat loss, thus maintaining body temperature. In extreme cold, these mechanisms cannot produce enough heat to maintain normal temperature and so hypothermia ensues.

Hypothermia affects virtually all metabolic processes in the body (Fritsch, 1995), and produces vasoconstriction, alterations in microcirculation, coagulation and ischaemic tissue damage. These effects can delay the diagnosis of shock.

Hyperthermia

Following traumatic brain injury, hyperthermia may occur. This is caused by hypothalamic injury, when overheating overwhelms the heat loss mechanisms (Holtzclaw, 1993). This condition is critical and may develop quickly, when there is dysfunction of the temperature thermoregulatory mechanism (Walton, 1994).

The increasing body temperature seen in hyperthermia fails to activate compensatory cooling mechanisms and increases cellular metabolism, oxygen consumption and carbon dioxide production. As cerebral metabolism increases, the brain has great difficulty keeping up with the increase in carbon dioxide production (Edwards, 2003). This causes cerebral vasodilation, which can increase intracranial pressure in already neurologically compromised patients. An increased temperature between 41° and 43°C produces nerve damage, coagulopathy, convulsions and death (McCance and Huether, 1997). Unless the temperature is monitored carefully and cooling measures are instituted, irreversible brain damage and death occur (Holtzclaw, 1993).

> In the assessment of the traumatised patient, it is essential to recognise the potential for shock and identify its signs early. Early effective treatment is vital to prevent the progression of shock

STAGES OF SHOCK

The severity of shock is sometimes described as being at a certain 'stage'. The stages range from one to four. They are often associated with a level of loss of circulatory volume and the clinical appearance of the patient as the fluid loss reaches a given amount. The stages and clinical appearance in fit adults are summarised below.

Stage 1

Up to 15% blood volume loss. The patient exhibits:

- pale skin
- normal capillary refill – less than 2 seconds
- no change in blood pressure
- increased pulse rate – up to 100 per minute.

At this stage, peripheral venous constriction and a slight increase in heart rate maintain normal systolic blood pressure.

Stage 2

A total of 15–30% blood volume loss. The patient exhibits:

- pale, cool and clammy skin
- capillary refill – more than 2 seconds
- blood pressure – systolic normal, diastolic elevated, pulse pressure narrowed
- increased pulse rate – more than 100 beats/ minute
- increased respiratory rate.

At this stage the body's compensatory mechanisms are at their limit.

Stage 3

A total of 30–40% blood volume loss. The patient exhibits:

- anxiety and agitation
- lack of cooperation or belligerence
- systolic blood pressure – less than 100 mmHg
- increased pulse rate – more than 120 beats/ minute
- increased respiratory rate.

At this stage the patient is in decompensated shock.

Stage 4

More than 40% blood volume loss. The patient exhibits:

- reduced conscious level
- markedly increased pulse rate – 140+ beats/ minute
- absent radial pulse
- systolic blood pressure 70 mmHg
- respiratory distress.

At this stage the patient is in a critical condition.

The 'stages' described here relate to fit adults. The changes are often delayed in children and pregnant women and may be altered in the elderly.

CONCLUSION

It is clear that, when dealing with shocked patients, knowledge of the signs and symptoms is not enough. Depending on the type of shock, its aetiology and stage, shock can present with any number of haemodynamic changes; its early stages may be difficult to detect owing to compensatory mechanisms or the nature of the shock.

The assessment skills of trauma nurses need to be well developed to enable them to become expert in picking up subtle changes in a patient's condition. Knowledge of the pathophysiology of shock, the course of shock and its probable complications allows trauma nurses to make sense of the changes they observe in patients, and to take appropriate action.

References

Adam SK. Aspects of current research in enteral nutrition in the critically ill. *Care of the Critically Ill* 1994; 10: 246–251

Anderson CS. The pathophysiology of shock: an overview. In: Guthrie M. (ed) *Shock*. New York: Churchill Livingstone, 1982

Baillie L. A review of pain assessment tools. *Nursing Standard* 1993; 7: 25–29

Bone RC. Gram-negative sepsis: background, clinical features, and intervention. *Chest* 1991; 100: 802–808

Buckman RF, Badellino MM, Goldberg A. Pathophysiology of hemorrhagic hypovolaemia and shock. *Trauma Quarterly* 1992; 8: 12–27

Cheevers KH. Early enteral feeding of patient with multiple trauma. *Critical Care Nurse* 1999; 19: 40–51

Edwards SL. Hypovolaemia: pathophysiology and management options. *Nursing in Critical Care* 1998; 3: 73–82

Edwards SL. Hypothermia. *Professional Nurse* 1999; 14: 253–258

Edwards SL. Shock: types, classifications and exploration of their physiological effects. *Emergency Nurse* 2001; 9(2): 29–38

Edwards SL. Physiological insult/injury: pathophysiology and consequences. *British Journal of Nursing* 2002; 11(4): 263–274

Edwards SL. Temperature regulation. In: Brooker C, Nicol M (eds) *Nursing adults: the practice of caring*. Edinburgh: Mosby, 2003: Ch. 5

Elia M. Changing concepts of nutrient requirements in disease: implications for artificial nutritional support. *Lancet* 1995; 345: 1279–1284

Fritsch DE. Hypothermia in the trauma patient. *AACN Clinical Issues* 1995; 6: 196–211

Gosling P. The metabolic and circulatory response to trauma. In: Alpar EK, Gosling P (eds) *Trauma: a scientific basis for care*. London: Arnold, 1999

Gosling P, Alpar EK. Shock. In: Alpar EK, Gosling P (eds) *Trauma: a scientific basis for care*. London: Arnold, 1999

Guthrie M. (ed.) *Shock*. New York: Churchill Livingstone, 1982

Hoffman WD, Natanson C. Endotoxin in septic shock. *Anaesthesia and Analgesia* 1993; 77: 613–624

Hollingsworth HM, Giansiracusa DF. Anaphylaxis. *Emergency Medicine* 1992; 24: 145–146, 148

Hollinworth H. No gain! *Nursing Times* 1994; 90: 24–27

Holtzclaw BJ. Monitoring body temperature. *Clinical Issues in Advanced Practice Acute and Critical Care* 1993; 4: 44–55

Howarth PH. ABC of allergies: pathogenic mechanisms: a rational basis for treatment. *British Medical Journal* 1998; 316: 758–761

Huddleston V. Multisystem organ failure: pathophysiology and clinical implications. St Louis: Mosby Yearbook, 1992

Jarvis D, Burney P. ABC of allergies: the epidemiology of allergic disease. *British Medical Journal* 1998; 316: 607–610

Khun MAM. Anaphylaxis versus anaphylactoid reactions: nursing interventions. *Critical Care Nurse* 1990; 10: 121, 123–126, 128

Marieb EN. *Human anatomy and physiology*, 5th edn. Redwood City: Benjamin Cummings, 2004

McCance KL, Huether SE. *Pathophysiology: the biologic basis for disease in adults and children*, 3rd edn. St Louis: Mosby, 1997

Meyers KA, Hickey MK Nursing management of hypovolaemic shock. *Critical Care Nursing Quarterly* 1988; 11: 57–67

Moddeman G. The elderly surgical patient – a risk of hypothermia. *American Operating Room Nursing Journal* 1991; 53: 1270–1272

O'Neill SP. Anaphylactic shock. *American Journal of Nursing* 1990; 90: 40

Shephard TJ, Fox SW. Assessment and management of hypertension in the acute ischaemic stroke patient. *Journal of Neuroscience Nursing* 1996; 28: 5–12

Walton J. Nurse-aid management of hyperthermia. *British Journal of Nursing* 1994; 3: 239–242

Williams JF, Bristow MR. Guidelines for the evaluation and management of heart failure. *JACC* 1995; 26: 1376

Chapter 14

Applied pharmacology pertaining to the trauma patient

Ann Richards

INTRODUCTION

The administration of drugs is a vital part of the care required by the trauma patient, be it simple analgesia that is needed or, in an extreme situation, emergency resuscitation drugs. Whatever the drug or the situation it is used in, it is essential for the nurse to understand how the drug works.

> Drugs should only be used when really needed, as they often have severe adverse effects

Pharmacology is a branch of medical science that deals with the properties and characteristics of drugs. A drug can be defined as any chemical that alters the function of a living system. Pharmacology includes the study of the actions and the effects of drugs on the body as well as the distribution of drugs inside the body.

After a drug is administered to a patient, a number of events occur before any observable effect is produced. *Pharmacodynamics* refers to the mechanisms by which drugs interact at their site of action and elicit a pharmacological response. Pharmacokinetics refers to the movement of drugs within the body, including absorption, distribution, metabolism and excretion.

This chapter looks at both these vitally important areas and relates their understanding to some of the conditions faced in nursing the trauma patient. The scope of the chapter is, however, limited and the reader should refer to other publications for detailed guidance on the use of specific drugs. Analgesia and anaesthesia are covered in Chapter 21.

THE HISTORICAL USE OF DRUGS IN SOCIETY

Drugs have been used for medicinal and recreational purposes from the beginning of human history, but the first recorded systematic register of drugs dates back to the ancient Greek and Egyptian civilisations. Individuals who made these agents possessed power and influence over their fellows, which could be reflected in the power of the major drug companies of today.

Early drugs were naturally occurring substances and alcohol is an example of such a substance that is still widely used today. Pottery from Mesopotamia made around 4200 BC shows the process of fermentation in illustrations but it is not clear whether the alcohol was given any medicinal properties. Later documented usages of alcohol include its use as a skin antiseptic, an appetite stimulant, an analgesic and an anaesthetic. The social use of alcohol today overshadows any therapeutic application.

Plant derivatives, such as bark, roots, seeds, flowers and leaves, have all been used therapeutically in virtually every culture throughout history. Examples of drugs extracted from these sources include atropine, ergotamine, morphine, cocaine, marijuana, digitalis and caffeine. Curare (tubocurarine), used to paralyse skeletal muscle, especially in surgery, is used by Indians in British Guiana as an arrow poison and is derived from plants belonging to the genus *Strychnos*. This drug cannot be absorbed when given orally, a fact that allowed the Indians to eat the meat that had the poison infiltrated within it.

Antibiotics are derived from certain fungi and bacteria, which produce secretions to protect themselves; in ancient times, it was known that the application of mouldy bread to a wound could help to cure wound infections. There must be very many potential drugs still undiscovered and natural sources of therapeutic substances are still being investigated. Some modern anticancer drugs are derived from plants, such as the periwinkle and the bark of the yew tree. Most modern drugs, however, are made synthetically and are mass-produced relatively cheaply in large laboratories.

DRUG CLASSIFICATION

A drug is generally classified according to either its therapeutic use, mode of action or molecular structure. For example, if a patient is suffering from depression, the type of drug likely to be prescribed is an antidepressant (therapeutic use) and could be a selective serotonin reuptake inhibitor (SSRI) (mode of action) or a tricyclic antidepressant (molecular structure).

The same drug may have more than one therapeutic use, for example, propranolol is a 'beta blocker' and may be used to treat high blood pressure, an overactive thyroid gland, migraine, angina or anxiety.

> Drugs may have more than one therapeutic use

The mode of action describes how the drug actually exerts its effects on the body. A drug usually only has one mode of action; propranolol, for example, exerts its effects by competitively blocking the beta-receptors for norepinephrine in the body, thus it is often called a 'beta blocker'.

Chemists tend to group drugs according to their basic chemical structure, for example, tricyclic antidepressants belong to a group of drugs with a similar three-ringed chemical structure.

DRUG NOMENCLATURE

Drugs have at least three different names by which they may be recognised. These are:

- the chemical name
- the generic name or non proprietary name
- the trade name or proprietary name.

All drugs have a *chemical name*, which is usually very long, and only used by the chemist and pharmacologists involved in their development. An example of a chemical name is 7-chloro-1, 3-dihydro-1-methyl-5-phenyl-2H-1, 4-benzodiazepin-2-1. To overcome this, the original manufacturers of the drug, together with the appropriate drug authorities, derive a simplified chemical name from the full name. This is known as the *generic or non-proprietary name* and is the one that should always be used by those prescribing and administering drugs. The above-mentioned drug became known by the much simpler generic name 'diazepam'.

When a drug manufacturer markets a new product, he gives the drug yet another name, its *trade or proprietary name* used only by that manufacturer. Thus 'diazepam' was known as 'Valium®'. When first developed drugs are sold under patent, usually for 10 years and, after this time, other companies can make the drug but must give it another trade name. As there may be many different trade names, the generic name is the one that should be used in the health service.

> Using the generic name of a drug reduces the potential for confusion

Generic and trade names applied to the drug vary across the world. There is a move to try and make generic names standard throughout the world but this has not yet been accomplished. One example is the drug lidocaine, which was called lignocaine until recently in Britain, and lidocaine in the USA. Furosemide and frusemide is an example where one name was adopted world-wide, with all countries now calling the drug furosemide.

Occasionally, there are drugs with very simple chemical names that can be used (e.g. potassium chloride), thus a shorter generic name is not required.

DRUG FORMULATIONS AND ADMINISTRATION

Pharmaceutics is the branch of pharmacology that deals with the formulation of drugs. Most drugs are administered in very small quantities, often less than a milligram, and inert materials have to be added, for ease of handling, when a tablet is made. Starch may also be added as this swells when in contact with fluids, and thus aids the disintegration of the tablet and its subsequent absorption from the gut.

The aims of administration of a drug are:

- to establish optimal drug concentration at the target site
- to maintain optimal concentration for the required period of time
- to minimise adverse drug reactions owing to general distribution.

To achieve the optimum benefit of the drug according to these aims, different formulations and routes of administration are used.

ROUTES OF ADMINISTRATION

Oral

In a non-emergency situation, most drugs are administered via the mouth in a solid or liquid form. They may be given as tablets or capsules, elixirs or liquids. Drugs may be formulated so that they are released slowly into the gastrointestinal tract by using sustained release preparations or enteric-coated tablets.

Topical

Topical formulations are applied to the body surface to have a direct local effect, as illustrated by the application of ointment to the skin, drops to the eye or ear, and antibiotics to body cavities in surgery.

Transdermal

The skin is tough and relatively impermeable to many drugs: however, some drugs, such as oestrogen creams, have been devised to be absorbed through the skin. Only drugs that are highly lipophilic (fat soluble) may be given via this route. They are often administered as a 'patch'.

Sublingual or buccal

These terms describe a route of administration where drugs are absorbed directly from the sub-lingual or buccal mucous membranes. It avoids the mixing of the drug with gastric contents and allows the drug to reach the bloodstream without it first being partially metabolised in the liver following absorption from the gut. This is very important in some medications (e.g. glyceryl trinitrate; GTN), which are metabolised the first time they pass through the liver and are thus ineffective when given orally. If given sublingually, they are absorbed through the mucous membrane into the capillaries and so reach the vascular system.

Rectal

Drugs formulated for rectal use are usually in the form of suppositories, although some are given in enema or cream form. The rectal mucosa has a good blood supply and lipophilic drugs are absorbed well. This route holds many advantages, as drugs can be easily given to the unconscious patient, the nauseous patient, those with difficulty in swallowing and those where venous access is difficult. It also largely avoids first-pass metabolism in the liver.

Inhalation

This route is used for drugs that exert their effects directly on the respiratory tract (e.g. salbutamol) but may also be used when a systemic action is required, as in general anaesthesia. The lungs provide a large surface area for absorption.

Parenteral

This term describes any method of administration other than oral or via the alimentary tract, but is usually reserved for injections.

Subcutaneous (SC) injection

This describes injections that are given into the subcutaneous layer of the skin. This route is not frequently used because the blood supply to the subcutaneous tissue is poor and absorption of the drug is slow. Examples include insulin and heparin, which are given by this route.

Intramuscular (IM) injections

Intramuscular injections enter directly into the muscle. They are more rapidly absorbed as skeletal muscle normally has a good blood supply and the capillaries contain small pores, allowing drugs of small molecular weight to pass into the bloodstream.

Intravenous (IV)

Intravenous administration involves the direct injection of a drug into a vein. It avoids absorption and thus usually results in a faster drug action. In an emergency, when speed is essential, this is the route of first choice and drug action may sometimes commence seconds after administration. The maintenance of asepsis is important when drugs are administered by this route.

> Intravenous injection is the route of choice in most emergency situations

Intraosseous (IO)

With the IO technique, drugs are injected through a cannula directly into the bone marrow cavity. In pre-adolescent children this is an alternative to intravenous infusion and, in those under the age of seven, is usually the route of first choice. Access can be established very rapidly.

Intrathecal

Drugs are injected directly into the cerebrospinal fluid around the spinal cord, usually at the level of the fifth lumbar vertebra, in order to avoid damaging the spinal cord. This method allows drugs direct access to the central nervous system, avoiding the blood–brain barrier.

Epidural

This method is often used for anaesthesia and analgesia. The drug is deposited above the dura mater and not into the cerebrospinal fluid. It allows the patient to remain fully conscious whilst receiving anaesthesia for surgery or childbirth.

Administration of emergency drugs will in most cases be by the oral, intravenous, intraosseous or inhaled routes. Patients requiring resuscitation have compromised tissue perfusion that makes intramuscular administration not only ineffective but also potentially dangerous, as subsequent resuscitation with restoration of the circulation may lead to rapid absorption of the drug and overdosage.

Oral administration may be the only way of giving some drugs (e.g. soluble aspirin) but the dangers of a subsequent general anaesthetic should never be forgotten and intake of fluid with medication should, therefore, be limited.

PHARMACODYNAMICS

Pharmacodynamics is the mechanism whereby drugs exert their effect on the body, and is concerned with the pharmacological effect of the drug at its site(s) of action. It considers mechanisms of action for both therapeutic and adverse effects of the drug.

> Drugs modify physiological processes with the aim usually being to restore the body's homeostatic balance

All bodily functions occur as a result of the interaction of various chemicals, and drugs interfere with these processes to produce a pharmacological response. To affect the functioning of cellular molecules, the drug must approach the molecules closely and usually combines with a particular chemical to modify its effects on the body. This combination is usually temporary and can be reversible but is occasionally permanent. Chemicals in the body vary from simple inorganic ions to complex biochemicals and proteins, such as enzymes and receptors.

Receptors

Receptors are complex proteins present on cell surfaces, in cells and on DNA. They are responsible for normal physiological functioning within the cell and communication between the cells. Neurotransmitters and hormones bind to receptors to influence the activity of the cells. For most drugs, the site of action is at this specific biological molecule – the receptor.

Drug receptors

The drug has to bind to a receptor to produce an effect. This is analogous to a key opening a lock: the drug molecule has to be the correct shape to activate the receptor. Many endogenous hormones, neurotransmitters and other mediators exert their effects as a result of high-affinity binding to specific protein receptors in plasma membranes or cell cytoplasm. The receptor is connected to elements of the cell that can produce a response, such as enzymes or ion channels.

Agonists and antagonists

If a drug fits into a receptor, the receptor will either respond or be blocked. A drug that activates a receptor is an *agonist* and it mimics the effect of the natural mediator. For example, the adrenergic receptor norepinephrine is an agonist. On binding, norepinephrine produces a change in configuration of the receptor that is linked to enzyme systems within the cell that produce the subsequent biological effects. The maximum response to an agonist is usually achieved without all the receptors on the cell surface being occupied. There are thus excess receptors, known as 'spare receptors'.

Partial agonists bind with a receptor but in a relatively inefficient manner. They do not fit the receptor perfectly and the interaction always produces less than a maximal response, even at 100% receptor occupancy. Partial agonists are capable of blocking the effects of a full agonist acting at the same receptor.

A drug that blocks the effect of the natural mediator is an *antagonist*. An antagonist will bind to the receptor, but will not activate it and thus prevents the natural chemical from producing a response. A well-known example is an antagonist at the beta-adrenergic receptor (beta blocker) propranolol. This drug binds with the beta-adrenergic receptor and prevents the body's natural mediator, norepinephrine, from binding to the receptor. The antagonist, although binding to the receptor, does not change the receptor in such a way as to produce the cellular response of the natural mediator. This means that, by giving a patient a beta blocker, the effects of norepinephrine on the body can be much reduced.

As most drug binding is reversible, there will be competition between the drug and the natural chemical. The more antagonist that is present, the less chance of the natural chemical producing an action. Competitive antagonism is surmountable and the maximum response of the agonist is not reduced if it is present in a high enough concentration.

Morphine exerts its action via the opioid receptors. These receptors are blocked by the competitive antagonist naloxone. This means that in cases of morphine overdosage with respiratory depression, naloxone provides the ideal antidote. It has to be borne in mind, however, that the action of naloxone is shorter than morphine, and so repeat injections or an infusion containing naloxone may be needed.

Occasionally, drugs bind very firmly, or irreversibly, to receptors and antagonism continues until the drug is destroyed. There is no antidote to a drug like this.

Transduction effects – receptor–effector linkage

This describes how the actual chemical changes in the cell occur. Transduction mechanisms are the ways in which receptors are coupled to systems that regulate cell function (i.e. receptor–effector linking).

Receptors are coupled to many types of cellular effect. Some may be very rapid, such as those involved in synaptic transmission – a millisecond time scale. Those produced by thyroid or steroid hormones are very slow, and may occur over hours or days. Intermediate time scales include catecholamines (epinephrine and norepinephrine), which act in seconds.

Receptor regulation

Certain receptors, when exposed to an agonist, can repeatedly *down-regulate* and decrease in number, or become desensitised. This is the case when salbutamol inhalers are overused for the treatment of asthma and become less effective. *Tachyphylaxis* is the term used for loss of efficacy that occurs with repeated doses of a drug. It is believed that the receptors are destroyed by endocytosis of patches of the cell membrane.

Prolonged contact with an antagonist can lead to supersensitivity to the agonist and the formation of new receptors – *up-regulation*. An example of this is when the abrupt discontinuation of a beta blocker leads to the occurrence of angina or dysrhythmias. This result is due to an increase in adrenergic receptors following the persistent blocking of the receptors by the drug. When the drug is discontinued, there are now more receptors available to respond to the body's natural norepinephrine.

Drug potency

Two important properties are associated with an agonist – affinity and efficacy. *Affinity* is the tendency of the drug to bind to its receptor and *efficacy* is the ability of the drug, once bound, to activate the receptor and produce a response. An agonist at a receptor has both affinity and efficacy. An antagonist has affinity but no efficacy. A partial agonist has affinity but low efficacy. These two factors determine the potency of a drug. *Potency* is the concentration of a drug that produces a pharmacological response. The more potent a drug, the less one has to administer to produce the desired effect. The log concentration of the drug is usually plotted, producing a convenient sigmoid-shaped curve. Such plots can be used to compare the potencies of different drugs.

Receptor classification

Major receptor types are classified in terms of the transmitter they recognise. For example, norepinephrine acts at adrenoreceptors, histamine acts at the histamine receptor and acetylcholine acts at the acetylcholine (cholinergic) receptor.

In the 1960s, it was discovered that some of the effects of histamine and catecholamines were strongly antagonised by the competitive antagonists known, but that other actions were not.

This led to the discovery that there was more than one subtype of receptor:

- adrenergic – alpha and beta and even subdivisions of these – α_1 and α_2, β_1 and β_2
- histamine – H_1, H_2 and H_3
- acetylcholine – nicotinic and muscarinic receptors – muscarinic M_1, M_2 and M_3.

> Major receptor types are classified in terms of the transmitter they recognise

Selectivity and specificity

Selectivity occurs when a drug activates one receptor type at a lower concentration than another. Specificity is the ability of a drug to produce an action at a specific site. There are two main subtypes of adrenergic receptor: alpha (α) and beta (β). There are also further subtypes of each of these: α_1, α_2, β_1 and β_2. Salbutamol stimulates the β_2 receptor at lower concentrations than the other receptors and is selective for this receptor type. It is known as a beta$_2$-adrenergic agonist. Selectivity is very useful in the drug industry, but it is still nearly impossible to find drugs that are truly specific and will only work at one receptor subtype, even if high concentrations are present.

In general, the lower the potency of a drug, and the higher the dose needed, the more likely that sites of action other than the primary one will assume significance. This is often associated with the appearance of unwanted side effects, of which no drug is free.

Pharmaceutical companies are trying very hard to manufacture drugs that are more selective and thus less dangerous to other tissues.

> All drug-dosing regimens are aimed at achieving plasma concentrations of a drug that will produce the optimal therapeutic effect with minimal toxicity

Therapeutic index

This is a ratio used to evaluate the safety and usefulness of a drug. Some effects of drugs in the body are desirable and known as the *therapeutic effects*; others are undesirable and known as *adverse effects*. Virtually all drugs produce some adverse effects that we hope will be mild and are usually dose dependent. The *therapeutic index* is a measure of the concentration of a drug required to have the desired action against the concentration that will result in adverse effects. It is calculated by dividing the minimum toxic concentration of the drug by the minimum effective concentration. Ideally, the therapeutic index should be large, which indicates that the drug will have a wide margin of safety. A drug has a low therapeutic index if it can only produce its effects at a nearly toxic concentration. Some anticancer drugs have a very low therapeutic index. Figure 14.1 illustrates the therapeutic safety range of a drug dose when compared to its 'toxic' threshold.

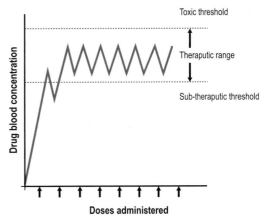

Figure 14.1 Therapeutic safety range of a drug dose.

Ion channels

Ions such as calcium, sodium and potassium are transported into or out of the cell to produce various physiological events. They travel via ion channels that are transmembrane proteins and span the cell membrane. The proteins allow the passage of selective ions, when the channel is open. If the passage of ions is obstructed, this will have an effect on the cellular physiology. An example of drugs that work in this way are the calcium-channel blockers, such as nifedipine, which 'block' calcium channels and prevent calcium entry into the cell. This, in turn, causes relaxation of smooth muscle and, if this is vascular smooth muscle, vasodilation will follow with a resultant drop in blood pressure. Thus nifedipine is used to control high blood pressure. Some drugs may modulate the channel opening, either increasing or decreasing the opening probability. Some antiarrhythmic drugs work in this way.

Enzymes

Enzymes are biological catalysts that enable and speed up chemical reactions within the cell. They themselves are unchanged in the reaction but are essential for the reaction to occur. All chemical reactions in the body are catalysed by enzymes. Each enzyme is a potential target for drugs that may either mimic the effect of the enzyme's substrate or inhibit the enzyme's activity. Angiotensin-converting enzyme inhibitors prevent the enzyme that converts angiotensin I to angiotensin

II from working and thus inhibit the effects of angiotensin II on the body (vasoconstriction and sodium retention). These drugs, therefore, produce vasodilation and have a small diuretic effect. They are used to control hypertension and in cardiac failure to reduce both preload and afterload.

Many other common drugs work by enzyme inhibition, one example being aspirin. Non-steroidal anti-inflammatory drugs such as aspirin prevent the formation of chemicals in the body known as prostaglandins. Prostaglandins have many physiological actions and this explains the multitude of clinical effects that aspirin has – both good and bad.

PHARMACOKINETICS

Pharmacokinetics is the study of the movement of a drug through the body, and includes the time course of drug absorption, distribution, metabolism and excretion. It is the study of what the body does to the drug.

Some understanding of these processes is essential, if one is to consider why some drugs work almost immediately whilst others may take many hours, or why some drugs are only effective when given by continuous infusion, yet others are effective when given only once daily.

We need to know the optimal route of administration, but also need to know how the plasma concentration of the drug relates to its therapeutic and toxic actions, and how the drug is metabolised and eliminated. It is possible that trauma and disease states may affect all stages of this process. It is also possible that the metabolism of a drug may be affected by the administration of another drug.

Absorption

Absorption is the passage of a drug into the bloodstream before it can be distributed around the body. The administration of drugs by the majority of routes has to be followed by absorption before a drug has access to the internal compartments of the body, although there are cases when we actually do not want a drug to reach the systemic circulation. One such example

is the administration of steroid inhalers for asthma: the less steroid that is absorbed, the less the risk of side effects of the drug, such as osteoporosis or reduced growth in children. Other examples would include topical preparations, such as skin creams or eye drops, given for their local action.

Most drugs that are given are designed to be absorbed into the bloodstream, a process that involves the crossing of membranes, usually by simple diffusion. *Diffusion* is the passage of a substance from an area of high concentration to one of lower concentration and it is this crossing of membranes that presents most problems to drug molecules. This problem is avoided when a drug is given by the intravenous route, as it is given directly into the bloodstream and absorption is not necessary. If a drug is given by intramuscular injection, although absorption still has to occur, it is by entry into the capillaries via small pores, and the chemical nature of the drug is not so important.

There are several factors that determine the ease with which a drug is absorbed from the gut into the bloodstream (Box 14.1).

The size of the drug molecules
Smaller molecules diffuse more easily.

The lipid solubility of the drug
Cell membranes are fatty bilayers and drugs that are lipid soluble cross such membranes more quickly.

The extent of ionisation of the drug
Ions are charged particles and do not readily cross cell membranes. An example of ionisation

---

Box 14.1   Factors affecting absorption

- The size of the drug molecules
- Lipid solubility
- Extent of ionisation
- The pH of the drug
- Extent of transportation across membranes
- The area available for absorption
- The rate of stomach emptying
- The rate of gastrointestinal blood flow

preventing the absorption of a drug is the case of curare mentioned earlier. The molecules are so heavily charged that, if contaminated meat is eaten, the curare cannot pass through the membranes from the gut to reach the bloodstream and so is harmless, although, if injected, it would produce paralysis of skeletal muscle.

The pH of the drug
A weakly acidic drug, such as aspirin, will remain unionised in an acidic environment such as the stomach, and so can be absorbed through the gastric mucosa. A weakly basic drug, such as morphine, will ionise in the acidic environment of the stomach and so will not be absorbed, but it will be unionised in an alkaline environment such as the small intestine, where it will be more readily absorbed.

Transportation
Some naturally occurring compounds, such as thyroxine and levodopa, are transported by carriers across membranes.

The area available for absorption
The small intestine has a very large surface area (approximately equivalent to that of a tennis court) and the drug molecules spend more time here than in the stomach. This means that most drug absorption (even of mildly acidic drugs, such as aspirin) occurs in the small intestine and not in the stomach.

The rate of stomach emptying
The rate of stomach emptying and the presence of food in the stomach will affect the rate of absorption. Medication, in most instances, will be more rapidly absorbed when taken without food but with a glass of water. There are some instances, when drugs are gastric irritants, where it is best to take medication with or after food, an example being aspirin.

The rate of blood flow through the gut
This affects the rate of absorption of a drug and, in a shocked patient, there will be minimal blood flow and slow absorption of oral medication.

Bioavailability and first-pass metabolism

Bioavailability is a measure of the percentage of the administered dose of a drug that reaches the systemic circulation. A drug has 100% bioavailability if the entire administered dose reaches the bloodstream, as in the case of intravenous administration. In the case of a drug given orally, bioavailability will depend on the extent of absorption from the gut lumen into the bloodstream but also on the extent of metabolism that occurs when the drug passes through the liver, after absorption from the gut, before it enters the systemic circulation. This is known as *first-pass metabolism*. It is very high in some drugs, such as glyceryl trinitrate, which are completely destroyed on their first pass through the liver and so, if given orally, are ineffective.

Drug distribution

Once a drug is absorbed into the systemic circulation, it will then enter various tissues and organs to a variable extent. This is dependent upon the chemical properties of the drug and the amount of drug that is bound to proteins within the blood thus not being 'free' to leave the bloodstream and have an action on the tissues. Lipid-soluble drugs (e.g. diazepam) tend to distribute widely in the body, as they are more able to cross cell membranes and are also able to enter the central nervous system more readily. Highly 'bound' drugs, such as warfarin, usually have a limited distribution.

Protein binding

Albumin is the main protein in the bloodstream to which drugs bind. The drug molecules attach to binding sites on the albumin molecule and only free drug, not bound, is able to leave the bloodstream and reach the tissues. The stronger the protein binding is, the less free drug is available in the plasma. Protein binding varies and, in some cases, may be over 90%, and even up to 99%. Binding is only temporary as equilibrium exists and there is always some free drug in the plasma. As free drug leaves the bloodstream and enters the tissues, more drug molecules are released from the albumin to maintain the equilibrium.

Some drugs compete for binding sites on the albumin molecules and, very occasionally, this may be important in drug interactions.

Body fluid compartments

Most drug molecules are very small and leave the circulation readily by capillary filtration. Body water is distributed into three main compartments:

- extracellular fluid
- intracellular fluid
- transcellular fluid.

Extracellular fluid is made up of the plasma and interstitial fluid, *intracellular fluid* is the sum of the fluid found inside the cells, and *transcellular fluid* includes cerebrospinal, peritoneal, pleural and synovial fluids.

A few drugs are confined to the plasma because their molecules are too large to cross the capillary wall easily (e.g. heparin). Some polar (ionised) compounds only distribute in the extracellular fluid (e.g. vecuronium and gentamycin). This is because they have very low lipid solubility and cannot readily cross cell membranes. They do not usually cross the placenta or reach the brain. Some relatively lipid-soluble drugs that readily cross membranes may distribute throughout the body water (e.g. ethanol and phenytoin).

The blood–brain barrier

The brain is inaccessible to many systemically acting drugs because of a continuous layer of endothelial cells joined by tight junctions within the capillary system. This barrier is protective of the central nervous system and prevents the entry of some toxic substances from the bloodstream into the brain. Drugs that are highly lipid soluble enter the brain most readily (e.g. thiopentone). Water-soluble drugs often cannot gain access (e.g. aminoglycosides, such as gentamycin, and many anticancer drugs). In inflammation, as in meningitis, the blood–brain barrier may be more easily crossed and this allows systemic penicillin that would not usually cross the barrier to be used in this instance. The barrier is also 'leaky' in certain areas of the brain, such as the chemoreceptor trigger zone or vomiting center, and drugs may reach this area without entering other parts of the brain.

An example of a drug crossing the blood–brain barrier and this leading to unwanted side effects is the antihistamine chlorpheniramine (Piriton®). Drowsiness is an adverse effect caused by entry into the central nervous system. Drug companies have now made compounds that are not lipophilic enough to cross the barrier and thus do not cause drowsiness.

The placental barrier

This is not very efficient and allows the passage of most drugs. It should always be assumed that drugs will cross over the placenta to the fetus and will also enter breast milk, unless there is definite proof that they do not.

Drug elimination

This is the removal of a drug from the body, and may involve both metabolism and excretion. *Metabolism* is the changing of a drug chemically and normally occurs in the liver. *Excretion* is the transfer of the drug (or metabolites) from the inside of the body to the outside, usually via the renal system in the urine. Drug elimination is affected by many factors including:

- age
- sex
- pregnancy
- genetics
- disease processes
- other drugs.

Drug metabolism

The body takes in many unwanted chemicals during daily life, and these are dealt with and made less toxic before they are excreted. Drugs are processed in the same manner as other unwanted chemicals. It is not necessary just to detoxify the drug, but also to make it more water-soluble so that it may be excreted in the urine and not reabsorbed back into the body. The liver is the major organ involved in drug metabolism but a number of other tissues, including the kidney and lung may contribute.

The liver is the major organ involved in drug metabolism

Drug metabolism occurs in two phases as listed below.

- *Phase I metabolism* brings about chemical changes within the molecule that may make it inactive, but sometimes can result in a more active metabolite or a metabolite with biological activity but a different half-life. It my also result in a toxic metabolite as in the case of paracetamol overdosage.
- *Phase II metabolism* is the conjugation of the Phase I metabolite with polar molecules, thus increasing water solubility.

Factors affecting drug metabolism

Enzymes involved in drug metabolism may be stimulated by alcohol and some drugs, for example, rifampicin and phenytoin. This may lead to the more rapid breakdown of certain drugs but the enzymes may be inhibited by other drugs, such as cimetidine. The latter will result in slower metabolism of some drugs in the body and greater likelihood of their toxic accumulation. Other factors affecting metabolism include the following.

- Liver disease, which results in reduced metabolism.
- Age may have an effect, metabolism being reduced in the very young and very old.
- Some inherited conditions are important. One example is pseudocholinesterase deficiency. The neuromuscular blocking action of suxamethonium is terminated by an enzyme in the plasma called pseudocholinesterase. Some individuals produce so little of this enzyme that their metabolism of suxamethonium is greatly reduced and they fail to breathe spontaneously after its use. Assisted ventilation may have to be undertaken for many hours.

Drug excretion

The majority of drugs are excreted either unchanged or as metabolites in the urine or bile. Drugs may also leave the body in the saliva, sweat, breast milk, tears and expired air.

The kidneys are involved to some extent in the elimination of virtually every drug or drug metabolite. Whether or not renal excretion is the major contributor depends on the polarity of a drug. Non-polar, lipid-soluble drugs are efficiently reabsorbed from the renal tubule. Very polar compounds, such as mannitol, are too water soluble to be reabsorbed and are eliminated virtually without any reabsorption. Reabsorption of weak acids and bases depends on the pH of the tubular fluid. For acidic drugs, the more alkaline the urine, the greater the renal clearance as the metabolite is ionised in the alkaline urine and cannot be effectively reabsorbed. This explains why the alkalisation of the urine by the administration of sodium bicarbonate increases the rate of salicylate excretion in cases of aspirin overdosage. Some drugs are actively secreted into the filtrate in the proximal tubule and benzylpenicillin is such an example.

Renal impairment reduces the elimination of drugs, such as digoxin and aminoglycoside antibiotics, that rely on glomerular filtration for their clearance.

The kinetics of drug elimination

Many drugs are eliminated at a rate proportional to their concentration. This is first-order elimination and most drugs are eliminated this way. The half-life (see later) is constant and the rate of elimination depends on how much drug is present, with elimination being higher when there is more drug in the plasma. A constant fraction of the drug is being eliminated in unit time.

Drugs that show non-linear kinetics are the exception rather than the rule. This is often due to the saturation of an enzyme involved in the conversion to an inactive metabolite. Elimination may be first order at low concentrations of the drug but changes to zero order when more drug is present, as is the case with alcohol. The rate of elimination is constant and is independent of the drug concentration.

Plasma half-life

If a drug exhibiting first-order elimination is injected continuously into the arm via a syringe driven by a constant infusion pump, a plot of plasma concentration against time can be constructed. Concentration rises rapidly at first, then more slowly, until a steady state is reached whereby the rate of input of drug into the body is equal to the rate of elimination of the drug from the body. The plasma concentration at this point is the *steady-state concentration*. When the infusion is stopped, the plasma concentration declines towards zero. The time taken for plasma concentration to halve is the *plasma half-life* ($t_{1/2}$).

After a second half-life has passed, the concentration of the drug will have again halved and so on. The increase in concentration when the drug is started is also exponential, and this means that the half-life not only determines the time course of its disappearance when the infusion is stopped but also the time course of its accumulation when the infusion is started. The faster the elimination of a drug, the less time it will remain in the circulation and be available to the body tissues. This type of drug will need to be given more frequently than a drug with a longer elimination time.

Drug dosage

If the concentration of a drug is 600 µg/l at a certain time and this level drops to 300 µg/l in 2 hours, the drug's half-life is 2 hours. This means that in another 2 hours the concentration will have halved again to 150 µg/l, etc. Half-lives are useful when calculating how frequently a drug needs to be given. If a drug is given at approximately half-life intervals, it will reach a steady-state concentration after about five repeat doses have been given. For drugs with long half-lives this could be a long time. As an example, if the half-life is 48 hours, a steady state concentration of the drug would not be achieved for 2 weeks. A way round this is to give a 'loading dose' of the drug. This is usually double the normal dose and its effects are illustrated in Figure 14.2.

Repeated doses of any drug will result in significant drug accumulation, if the drug is ingested at intervals more frequent than twice the plasma half-life. It must be realised that the above is an oversimplification and does not take account of drug distribution into different body compartments and other physiological changes.

The fact that different drugs in a therapeutic group have different half-lives can be therapeutically useful. For example, if a patient has a

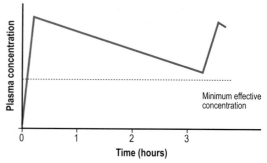

Figure 14.2   The effects of a loading dose of a drug.

problem falling asleep, a hypnotic drug with a short half-life will be more beneficial, whereas if the problem is early wakening, a drug with a longer half-life would be more suitable in helping the patient to sleep through the night.

Chemical transmission

Chemical substances are vitally important in mediating the communication between cells that is essential for coordinated activity within the body. Pharmacological interference with these chemicals is a very common form of drug action and can induce a wide range of effects. This does mean that an understanding of how these natural body mediators work is essential to the understanding of their pharmacological manipulation and therapeutic applications.

Chemical signalling molecules can be divided into three types (Box 14.2).

Neurotransmitters are released from nerve terminals at specialised junctions called synapses. They mediate rapid short-lived actions and, once they have activated the post-synaptic receptor, they are inactivated, often by the action of enzymes.

Hormones are released from endocrine glands directly into the bloodstream and exert an effect on a distant target cell, which has receptors for the

---

Box 14.2   Types of chemical signalling molecules

1. Neurotransmitters
2. Hormones
3. Autocoids (local transmitters)

hormone. Communication via this route is slower and less specific than by neurotransmitters.

Autocoids are chemicals that produce their effects locally. They are very important in the inflammatory process (e.g. prostaglandins) but mediate many other physiological actions.

Some substances may actually belong to more than one category, for example, norepinephrine which is an important hormone as well as a neurotransmitter.

THE AUTONOMIC NERVOUS SYSTEM

The nervous system along with the endocrine system maintains homeostasis, and is the means of control and communication in the body. It is divided into the central nervous system (CNS) and the peripheral nervous system (PNS).

The *central nervous system* is the brain and spinal cord. The *peripheral nervous system* is that part of the nervous system outside the brain and spinal cord, and has motor and sensory branches. One part of the peripheral nervous system is the *autonomic nervous system* and we have little control over its functioning. The autonomic nervous system controls our internal environment and our physiological functions. It represents the motor innervation of smooth muscle, cardiac muscle and glandular cells. It is responsible for regulating the contraction and relaxation of smooth muscle, all exocrine and some endocrine secretions, the heartbeat and some steps in metabolism.

The autonomic nervous system has two main branches, *the sympathetic system* and *the parasympathetic system*, both of which are working continuously within the body to maintain homeostasis and to control our bodily functions finely. In very general terms, the two branches are antagonistic and the sympathetic nervous system is associated with the 'flight and fight' response, whereas the parasympathetic nervous system is associated with 'resting and digesting'. The effects of the parasympathetic and sympathetic divisions on various organs are shown in Table 14.1.

Acetylcholine and norepinephrine are the two important neurotransmitters in the autonomic nervous system. A nerve that releases acetylcholine is said to be *cholinergic* and one that releases norepinephrine is said to be *adrenergic*.

Adrenergic pharmacology

Norepinephrine is released by most sympathetic nerve endings as well as by the adrenal gland. Epinephrine is released by the adrenal gland in stress. Adrenoreceptors are widely distributed throughout the body and mediate almost all actions of the sympathetic nervous system. Norepinephrine and epinephrine are both natural agonists at these receptors. Drugs that mimic the actions of epinephrine or norepinephrine are known as *sympathomimetic* drugs.

It was Ahlquist in 1948 that rationalised a large body of observations and conjectured that catecholamines act via two principal receptors that he called alpha and beta receptors. The physiological properties of the various subtypes of adrenoreceptors are shown in Table 14.2.

Epinephrine stimulates all subtypes of the receptor and so produces all the effects shown in this table. Norepinephrine is a stronger stimulant at the alpha receptor than epinephrine and so will result in a greater increase in blood pressure. Soon after the demonstration of separate alpha and beta receptors, it was found that there are at least two subtypes of beta receptors, designated β_1 and β_2. These receptors are operationally defined by their affinities for epinephrine and norepinephrine. β_1 receptors have approximately equal affinity for epinephrine and norepinephrine, whereas β_2 receptors have higher affinity for epinephrine. A third subtype, the β_3 receptor, has now been cloned. Following the demonstration of the beta subtypes, it was found that there were also subtypes of the alpha receptor.

α_1 receptors

These receptors are located on blood vessels, and influence both blood pressure and tissue perfusion. The diameter of these blood vessels determines resistance to blood flow. Stimulation of the alpha receptors produces vasoconstriction and a rise in peripheral resistance and, therefore, blood pressure. In many vessels, this stimulation provides resting vasomotor tone.

Clinical application

- Control of hypotension especially as an emergency measure. The danger is that blood

Table 14.1 The effects of the autonomic nervous system

Target organ/system	Parasympathetic effects	Sympathetic effects
Eye (iris)	Constricts pupil	Dilates pupil
Lens of eye	Accommodation	None
Glands (nasal, lacrimal, salivary, gastric, pancreatic)	Stimulates secretory activity	Inhibits secretory activity
Sweat glands	No effect	Stimulates sweating
Adrenal medulla	No effect	Stimulates secretion of epinephrine and norepinephrine
Erector pili muscles attached to hair follicles	No effect	Stimulates contraction – hairs stand on end and goose pimples occur
Heart muscle	Decreases rate	Increases rate and force
Coronary blood vessels	Constricts	Dilates
Bladder	Causes contraction of smooth muscle in the bladder wall, relaxes the urethral sphincter and promotes voiding	Causes relaxation of smooth muscle of bladder wall; constricts urethral sphincter and inhibits voiding
Lungs	Constricts the bronchioles	Dilates bronchioles and mildly constricts blood vessels
Digestive tract	Increases peristalsis and secretion by digestive organs. Relaxes sphincters and allows movement of food along tract	Decreases activity of glands and muscles of digestive tract and constricts sphincters
Liver	No effect	Stimulates the release of glucose into the bloodstream
Gall bladder	Causes contraction and release of bile	Relaxation and no release of bile
Kidney	No effect	Causes vasoconstriction; decreases urine output; promotes renin formation
Blood vessels	Little or no effect	Constricts most blood vessels and increases blood pressure
		Constricts vessels in skin and abdominal viscera to divert blood to the muscles, brain and heart
		Dilates vessels of skeletal muscle during exercise
Blood coagulation	No effect	Increases coagulation
Cellular metabolism	No effect	Increases metabolic rate
Adipose tissue	No effect	Stimulates fat breakdown
Mental activity	No effect	Increases alertness
Penis	Causes erection	Causes ejaculation

pressure may be raised at the expense of perfusion to vital organs such as the kidneys.

- Use as a vasoconstrictor in combination with another drug. Local anaesthetics may be combined with epinephrine or norepinephrine for this purpose.

β_1 receptors

These receptors are present on the myocardium, and stimulation results in increased rate and force of cardiac contraction. This leads to an increase in cardiac output that can result in a rise in blood pressure. Any drug that results in an increase in heart rate is said to have a *positive chronotropic effect*. A drug that results in an increase in the force of cardiac contraction is said to have a *positive inotropic effect*. Stimulation of β_1 receptors has both a positive inotropic and a positive chronotropic effect.

Clinical application
- Cardiac arrest – epinephrine is used because of its stimulatory effects on the cardiac muscle.
- Dobutamine is a β_1 agonist and produces direct myocardial stimulation, increasing

Table 14.2 A summary of some responses following stimulation of each subtype of adrenoreceptors

α_1 receptors	β_1 receptors	β_2 receptors
Vasoconstriction (increases blood pressure and relieves congestion)	Increase heart rate, stroke volume and cardiac output	Bronchodilation
Pupil dilation	Lipolysis (fat breakdown)	Fine skeletal muscle tremor
Decreased gut motility and secretions	Decreased gut motility and secretions	Vasodilation of blood vessels to skeletal muscle
Glycogen breakdown (increases blood glucose levels)	Renin release from the kidney (increases blood pressure)	Glycogen breakdown (increases blood glucose levels)
Urinary retention		Relaxation of the pregnant uterus
Facilitates sperm emission and ejaculation		Mast cell stabilisation

cardiac output, stroke volume and heart rate with minor effects on peripheral resistance. It may be used for short-term treatment of cardiac decompensation occurring after cardiac surgery or following an acute myocardial infarction. All β_1 agonists are arhythmogenic and may increase the size of a myocardial infarction. One serious problem encountered is that any prolonged and vigorous beta stimulation leads to receptor down-regulation and so reduced inotropic response with time.

- A β_1 agonist such as norepinephrine that has additional alpha effects will also increase peripheral resistance and afterload. Increased blood pressure is thus gained at the expense of increased cardiac work so that cardiac output is likely to decline.

β_2 receptors

These receptors are distributed on the smooth muscle of the bronchioles, skeletal muscle, blood vessels supplying the heart, lungs, kidneys and skeletal muscle and on the uterus. Stimulation results in bronchodilation but will also result in increased skeletal muscle excitability resulting in a fine muscle tremor. This is seen as a side effect of drugs that stimulate the β_2 receptors. Stimulation of the β_2 receptor may also lead to hypokalaemia carrying with it an arrhythmogenic potential.

Clinical application
- Treatment of bronchoconstriction. Salbutamol is a β_2 agonist widely employed in the treatment of asthma and chronic obstructive

pulmonary disease, and is usually administered by inhalation.
- Salbutamol may also be used to reduce raised serum potassium and to relax the uterus in premature labour.

Adrenoreceptor antagonists

These drugs reduce the effectiveness of sympathetic nerve activity and prevent the naturally occurring agonists from interacting with their receptors.

Alpha–adrenoreceptor antagonists

Administration results in a fall in blood pressure but some alpha antagonists may cause quite severe postural hypotension. There are drugs now developed that are selective α_1 antagonists and do not have these side effects to any degree. Examples are prazosin and doxazosin, which are used in the treatment of hypertension.

Beta–adrenoreceptor antagonists

The most important actions of these drugs are on the cardiovascular system. They decrease heart rate, myocardial contractility, cardiac output and conduction velocity within the heart. They also result in a reduction in blood pressure, when administered over a period of time, by complex actions not totally understood, but including a reduction in the release of renin from the kidney and alterations in baroreceptor activity. Propranolol is an example of an adrenergic antagonist.

Owing to the wide distribution of beta receptors, these drugs have many uses that include cardiac disease, hypertension, migraine prophylaxis, anxiety and hyperthyroidism. They should not be given to patients with asthma, as they will be antagonistic at both the β_1 and the β_2 receptor and may provoke severe bronchoconstriction. Some drugs, such as atenolol, are β_1 selective and are less likely to provoke an asthma attack. They are used for their action on the cardiovascular system in angina and hypertension.

EPINEPHRINE

Epinephrine is an agonist at both the alpha and beta adrenergic receptors, but has a stronger beta effect. Epinephrine is also referred to as 'adrenaline', a term more often used in the UK in the past; however, the move towards internationally agreed nomenclature has resulted in a change to 'epinephrine'. 'Norepinephrine' was known as 'noradrenaline'.

Uses

Cardiac arrest
Epinephrine 1 in 10 000 (1 mg/10 ml) is recommended in a dose of 10 ml by intravenous injection through a central line. The procedure for cardiac arrest is given in Chapter 16 and this section explains why epinephrine is the drug of choice in this instance. Direct effects on the heart are largely determined by the β_1 receptor. Activation of this receptor results in increased calcium influx in cardiac cells, which has both electrical and mechanical consequences. Pacemaker activity, both normal (sinoatrial node) and abnormal (e.g. Purkinje fibres), is increased (positive chronotropic effect). Conduction velocity is increased in the atrioventricular node and the refractive period is decreased. Intrinsic contractility is increased (positive inotropic effect) and relaxation is accelerated.

Anaphylactic shock
This is a severe systemic allergic reaction that involves either respiratory difficulty (owing to laryngeal oedema or bronchoconstriction) or hypotension. Other features, such as urticaria, are usually present. Common causes of anaphylaxis include the administration of a drug (e.g. peni-

cillin), an insect sting or the ingestion of certain foods (e.g. nuts). The reaction is a result of mast-cell deregulation and the release of inflammatory mediators, including histamine. Administration of epinephrine is often life saving. It should be given intramuscularly and the adult dose is 0.5 ml of a 1 in 1000 (1 mg/ml) solution. A second dose may be given in 5–10 minutes if there is no improvement. The intramuscular route is used as absorption of the drug, if given subcutaneously, is not as predictable and, if there is peripheral shutdown in a shocked patient, the epinephrine will not work quickly. Inhaled epinephrine may be used in pre-hospital environments and emergency personnel may also use nebulised epinephrine if intramuscular epinephrine has not been given. It is effective for mild to moderate laryngeal oedema but is not a substitute for intramuscular epinephrine. Intravenous administration is not used in anaphylaxis except under exceptional circumstances, such as profound life-threatening shock.

> Epinephrine should only be administered intravenously by those experienced in its use

A dilute solution (1:10 000) is always used with a maximum initial dose of 100 µg and cardiac monitoring is essential.

Epinephrine is very safe when given intramuscularly but there are risks associated with its use intravenously. Intravenous injection increases the risk of inducing myocardial infarction, ischaemia or a fatal cardiac arrhythmia. Increased myocardial oxygen consumption may induce angina, ischaemia, myocardial infarction and arrhythmias, including ventricular fibrillation. It may also cause greatly increased systolic and diastolic blood pressure, and there is an increased risk of intracerebral bleeding.

In anaphylaxis, the alpha-receptor action of epinephrine reverses vasodilation and capillary leak, reducing mucosal and cutaneous oedema as well as shock. There is a decrease in angio-oedema and urticaria. β_1 adrenergic stimulation has positive inotropic and chronotropic effects on cardiac activity: blood pressure improves and coronary artery perfusion is increased. β_2 receptor action dilates the airway smooth muscle and, therefore, promotes bronchodilation. Epinephrine also inhibits further mediator release from the mast cells.

The administration of epinephrine in anaphylaxis is followed by the administration of chlorphenamine (chlorpheniramine) (Piriton®) and hydrocortisone. Chlorphenamine is an antihistamine and an antagonist at the histamine receptor. Hydrocortisone suppresses the immune response and is most useful in preventing a late relapse.

Other uses of epinephrine include use as an adjunct with local anaesthetics. It reduces circulation to the site, which results in a slowing of vascular absorption. This promotes the local effect of the anaesthetic and prolongs its duration of action.

ACETYLCHOLINE

All parasympathetic effectors, some sympathetic effectors, all autonomic ganglia and voluntary muscles bear cholinergic receptors. Cholinergic drugs may, therefore, affect the functions of both divisions of the autonomic nervous system as well as the somatic nervous system. Acetylcholine is the transmitter that interacts with the cholinergic receptor and is inactivated by an enzyme within the synapse, called acetylcholinesterase.

Two main subtypes of cholinergic receptor have been identified:

- nicotinic receptor
- muscarinic receptor.

Nicotinic receptors respond to stimulation by nicotine and *muscarinic receptors* respond to stimulation by muscarine. Both types of receptor can be activated by acetylcholine but, because of subtle structural differences, pharmacologists have been able to develop cholinergic agents specific to one subtype of receptor.

Nicotinic receptors are located centrally, in autonomic ganglia and at the neuromuscular junction of skeletal muscles. Muscarinic receptors are located centrally and on the surfaces of effectors of the parasympathetic nervous system.

Drugs acting at the nicotinic receptor

The main drugs of interest are the neuromuscular blocking agents, used to relax skeletal muscle.

Most anaesthetics involve the use of muscle relaxants to facilitate intubation, to relax muscles sufficiently to make surgery possible or to enable easier artificial ventilation of the lungs. The drugs act at the neuromuscular endplate and block transmission of impulses from nerve to muscle. Acetylcholine is released when a nerve impulse reaches the synapse with a muscle. The acetylcholine then causes depolarisation to occur; this results in muscular contraction. The acetylcholine is then rapidly broken down by the enzyme cholinesterase, repolarisation occurs and the muscle is ready to be stimulated again. Should depolarisation persist, the muscle would remain unresponsive to further stimuli.

Muscle relaxants may work in two ways at the nicotinic receptor. Suxamethonium is a depolarising nicotinic agonist. It is similar to acetylcholine and acts as an agonist at the nicotinic receptor, but is not destroyed by acetylcholinesterase. This means that, when it stimulates the cholinergic receptor, its action is sustained, preventing repolarisation of the muscle endplate and resulting in paralysis. The agonist action of suxamethonium can be seen as soon as it is injected and all the muscles from toe to scalp go into spasm. The spasm lasts only for a second or so, and then the patient goes flaccid. This is because the cholinergic receptor is occupied by the suxamethonium and the muscle cannot be stimulated again because repolarisation has not occurred. The enzyme pseudocholinesterase terminates the action of suxamethonium after about 4 or 5 minutes.

A common side effect following administration of suxamethonium is muscle pain and tenderness, particularly in the chest and abdomen. Suxamethonium may also cause hyperkalaemia. One in 2800 of the population will have a prolonged paralysis of up to 2–3 hours following administration. This is due to a genetic abnormality when insufficient of the enzyme pseudocholinesterase is produced to break down the drug. A rare side effect is malignant hyperthermia, resulting in severe muscular rigidity and temperatures of over 41°C. This is a life-threatening condition and requires prompt treatment to reduce body temperature and to reverse muscle spasm by using intravenous dantrolene.

Another type of action is shown by the non-depolarising neuromuscular blocking agents. These are competitive muscle relaxants and antagonists of acetylcholine at the nicotinic receptor. The receptor is blocked, resulting in non-depolarisation of the muscle endplate and complete paralysis. The release of acetylcholine is ineffective as the nicotinic receptors are blocked. Examples of these drugs include tubocurarine, alcuronium, pancuronium, vecuronium and atracurium. Some of these agents can cause histamine release that can result in a fall in blood pressure as well as bronchospasm. One advantage of these agents is that their action can be reversed. They compete with acetylcholine for the receptors and, by increasing the amount of acetylcholine available at the neuromuscular junction, their action will be reversed. This is possible by blocking the action of cholinesterase, the enzyme that destroys acetylcholine. Neostigmine is an example of one such acetylcholinesterase inhibitor.

Drugs acting at the muscarinic receptor

The action of acetylcholine in the parasympathetic nervous system takes place at the muscarinic receptor. Stimulation of these receptors also induces the sympathetic response of sweating. The actions of the parasympathetic nervous system are shown in Table 14.1. Drugs used in emergencies do not include agonists at the muscarinic receptor but do include the antagonist, atropine.

ATROPINE

Epinephrine is an example of a drug that stimulates the adrenergic receptors, and so is an agonist and enhances the actions of the sympathetic nervous system. Atropine produces its effects not as an agonist but as an antagonist of the parasympathetic nervous system. Atropine blocks one type of acetylcholine receptor, the muscarinic receptor. It is sometimes referred to as anticholinergic in action or, more correctly, as an antimuscarinic agent because of its antagonist action at the muscarinic receptor. Competitive antagonism of the muscarinic receptor with atropine prevents the normal effector responses occurring.

There are two naturally occurring muscarinic antagonists, atropine and hyoscine; both are alkaloids found in plants of the nightshade species (solanaceous). Deadly nightshade (*Atropa belladonna*) contains mainly atropine and the thorn apple contains mainly hyoscine.

The main effects of atropine are summarised in Box 14.3.

Clinical application of antimuscarinic drugs

Bradycardia

Bolus injections of 0.3 mg up to a maximum of 2.0 mg of intravenous atropine are useful in bradyarrhythmias with atrioventricular block, particularly common after an inferior myocardial infarction.

Atropine may also be used in sinus or nodal bradycardia with hypotension, or when there are multiple ventricular ectopic beats related to severe bradycardia. Following administration of low doses of atropine, paroxysmal bradycardia may occur owing to central action and stimulation of the cardioinhibitory centre.

Prophylactic atropine for uncomplicated bradycardia has been largely abandoned because reduced parasympathetic activity may unmask latent sympathetic overactivity and contribute to tachyarrhythmias, including ventricular tachycardia and fibrillation.

Treatment of poisoning by anticholinesterase agents

Antimuscarinic drugs are used in the treatment of poisoning by anticholinesterase agents (organophosphorus compounds) and some mushrooms.

Anaesthesia

Antimuscarinic drugs are used as an adjunct for anaesthesia, producing reduced secretions and bronchodilation.

Antispasmodic and smooth muscle relaxant

Antimuscarinic drugs are used as an antispasmodic and smooth muscle relaxant in the gut. They are not used frequently for this purpose because of the potential side effects.

Pupil dilation

Antimuscarinic drugs are used to dilate the pupil, most often used for ocular examination.

Box 14.3   The effects of atropine

- The inhibition of secretions. Salivary, bronchial and sweat glands are inhibited by very low doses, producing an uncomfortably dry mouth
- Modest tachycardia (up to 80–90 beats/minute). This is due to inhibition of parasympathetic tone. Greater tachycardia is not produced, as there is no stimulation of the sympathetic nervous system, only blockage of the cardiac muscarinic receptors
- Arterial blood pressure is unaffected following oral or intramuscular atropine, as most resistance vessels have no cholinergic innervation. Intravenous administration may increase total peripheral resistance
- Dilation of the pupil (mydriasis) and loss of pupil response to light. The ciliary muscles relax and this leads to paralysis of accommodation and impairment of near vision
- Gastrointestinal motility is reduced but not totally, as its action is inhibited by the effects of other excitatory transmitters
- Relaxation of bronchial, biliary and urinary smooth muscle. Reflex bronchoconstriction in anaesthesia is prevented by atropine, but bronchoconstriction due to local mediators such as histamine and leukotrienes in asthma is unaffected.
- Excitation of the central nervous system producing mild restlessness at low doses and agitation and disorientation with higher doses. Atropine also affects the extrapyramidal system, reducing the involuntary movement and rigidity of some patients with Parkinson's disease and counteracting the extrapyramidal side effects of antipsychotic drugs.

Bronchodilation

Antimuscarinic drugs are used for bronchodilation in airways disease (e.g. ipratropium bromide – Atrovent®).

Motion sickness

Antimuscarinic drugs are used as treatment for motion sickness (e.g. hyoscine).

Parkinsonism

Antimuscarinic drugs are used in the treatment of parkinsonism, especially to counteract movement disorders caused by antipsychotic drugs (e.g. benzhexol, benztropine).

Urinary incontinence

Antimuscarinic drugs are used in the treatment of urinary incontinence (e.g. oxybutinin).

Side effects of atropine

Side effects include constipation, transient bradycardia followed by tachycardia, palpitations and arrhythmias, reduced bronchial secretions, urinary retention, dry mouth, flushing and dryness of the skin, and dilatation of the pupil. Occasionally, confusion may occur, especially in the elderly.

> Atropine poisoning is sometimes seen in children eating deadly nightshade

Marked excitement and irritability result in hyperactivity and an increase in body temperature; this is accentuated by the loss of sweating.

The action of atropine is opposed by physostigmine, which inhibits the cholinesterase enzyme responsible for destroying acetylcholine, thus preventing its destruction and allowing it to compete effectively with atropine at the muscarinic receptor.

ANTICONVULSANTS

Post-traumatic epilepsy may follow both open and closed head injuries. It occurs in approximately 5% of patients with closed injuries and in approximately 15% with severe head injuries. Seizures in the first week following trauma carry a low risk of future epilepsy, but may cause severe hypoxic brain damage. Some neurosurgeons may use prophylactic anticonvulsants for the first week in severe head injury.

The neurochemical basis of epilepsy is not totally understood but seizures are most likely to be due to an imbalance of neurotransmitters in the brain. Neurotransmitters in the brain fall into two broad categories, excitatory and inhibitory. They are released from the endings of neurones (nerve cells); an excitatory transmitter stimulates neurons connected to it, whereas an inhibitory one does not.

As long ago as 1972 it was found that the amino-acid content of the cortex removed from patients with epilepsy was deficient in gamma aminobutyric acid (GABA) and aspartate, two inhibitory neurotransmitters. The epileptic focus contained a greatly raised concentration of glycine, an excitatory neurotransmitter. Drugs that have an inhibitory effect on the action of GABA cause convulsions to occur. Some anticonvulsants work by increasing the inhibitory aspects of GABA but the mechanism of action of all anticonvulsants is not clearly understood.

Therapy is aimed at controlling seizures both immediately and in the longer term. Only the drugs seen in an emergency situation are discussed below.

Phenytoin

Phenytoin is an anticonvulsant; it was first used in 1935 and is structurally related to barbiturates. Although it has been studied in detail, its mode of action is not totally understood. The drug acts on the cell membrane, rather than the synapse, stabilising it and thus preventing excessive neurotransmission and decreasing excitability of the neurones. It appears to block the sodium channels and also has some local anaesthetic and antiarrhythmic properties.

Phenytoin is suitable for partial and generalised convulsions, but not absence seizures. It is well tolerated orally but may also be given intravenously as a loading dose to prevent further seizures in the post-trauma patient. A 10–15 mg/kg bolus may be given over 20 minutes but both electrocardiogram (ECG) and blood pressure monitoring are needed. This may be followed by an intravenous infusion of 250–500 mg over 4 hours. Thereafter, 100 mg may be given every 8 hours, IV or orally.

Phenytoin causes an increased rate of metabolism of some other drugs (e.g. anticoagulants); the metabolism of phenytoin can itself be affected by the administration of other drugs in an unpredictable manner. It is a drug that is slowly metabolised and takes about a week for a regular oral dose to give stable blood levels, if no loading dose is given.

Phenytoin is metabolised at different rates by different individuals. Plasma concentrations vary widely between patients receiving the same dosage, necessitating monitoring of the serum levels

The effective plasma concentration is 10–20 mg/l and the oral dose is adjusted accordingly. If the plasma concentration is higher than this, side effects will occur. Once patients achieve levels within the target range, the majority require once a day dosage.

Mild side effects include vertigo, ataxia, headache and nystagmus, but not sedation. If larger doses are given, marked confusion and mental deterioration occur, but these are quickly reversible. Hypersensitivity reactions, especially skin rashes, are common. Over a longer period, hyperplasia of the gums and hirsutism may occur, and are probably due to increased androgen secretion. Phenytoin has been implicated in the increase in fetal abnormalities in the babies of women with epilepsy.

Benzodiazepines

These drugs bind to the GABA ion channel and increase the action of the inhibitory neurotransmitter. Diazepam and lorazepam may be used to control seizures in an emergency but cause too much drowsiness to be used as regular anticonvulsants. Clonazepam is relatively selective as an anticonvulsant, and is used in absence and tonic clonic seizures.

Following trauma, intravenous diazepam, lorazepam or clonazepam may be used to control seizures acutely but may cause respiratory depression necessitating mechanical ventilation. Clonazepam 0.25 mg IV may sometimes be given incrementally after each seizure.

DIURETICS

A diuretic is any substance which increases urine output. A diuretic usually increases the output of sodium as well as water, necessary because they are often used to remove fluid in oedema, which is composed of water and solutes, sodium being the most important. Diuretics may also be used as antihypertensive agents.

Mannitol

This is a polyhydric alcohol with a small molecular weight. It is an osmotic diuretic and, as such, is small enough to be filtered by the glomerulus but cannot be reabsorbed by the renal tubule, thus increasing the osmolarity of the tubular fluid. The principal site of action in the kidney is the proximal convoluted tubule and the loop of Henle. Mannitol prevents the reabsorption of water from these parts of the kidney and urine volume will increase in proportion to the load of diuretic given.

Mannitol also encourages the movement of water from inside the cells to the extracellular fluid. This means it can be used for the rapid reduction of intracranial or intraocular pressure, and to maintain urine flow to prevent tubular necrosis. It is contraindicated in heart failure, where it may acutely increase the blood volume.

A typical dose of mannitol in cerebral oedema is 1 g/kg as a 20% solution given by rapid intravenous infusion. It should not be given in large doses to a hypotensive patent, as it can aggravate hypovolaemia.

Furosemide (frusemide)

This is a loop diuretic with high efficacy. It can cause 5–25% of filtered sodium to be excreted and impairs the powerful urine concentrating mechanism of the loop of Henle. It is a 'high-ceiling' diuretic meaning that an increase in dose results in a larger diuresis.

> Overtreatment with furosemide can rapidly dehydrate the patient

Furosemide remains effective at glomerular filtration rates below 10 ml/minute (normal 120 ml/minute). It also causes urinary potassium loss and hypokalaemia may occur, especially in prolonged use. Magnesium and calcium loss are also increased. Furosemide is highly successful for the treatment of oedema and, given intravenously, action is within 30 minutes. It also has a vasodilator action; this occurs prior to diuresis and aids its action in acute pulmonary oedema.

ANTIEMETICS

Antiemetics are drugs given to relieve nausea and vomiting. The vomiting centre in the medulla of the brain is involved in coordinating the act of emesis, whatever its cause. Near this centre is an area known as the *chemoreceptor trigger zone* (CTZ), which is extremely sensitive to the action of drugs and other chemicals, and stimulates the vomiting centre. There are many muscarinic and histamine receptors in the vomiting centre and dopamine receptors in the CTZ. Serotonin (5-HT) is also involved. Drugs that are antiemetics block one or more of these receptor types.

Antiemetics that are dopamine antagonists include metoclopramide (Maxalon®), which also increases the tone of the oesophageal sphincter, relaxes the pylorus, and increases peristalsis and gastric emptying, and prochlorperazine (Stemetil®). They do have extrapyramidal side effects and can cause severe oculogyric crises in some patients, especially those under the age of 20.

Domperidone (Motilium®) is also a dopamine antagonist that increases the rate of gastric emptying, but does not cross the blood–brain barrier and so is less likely to cause an oculogyric crisis.

Serotonin (5-HT$_3$) receptors are in the gastrointestinal tract, CTZ and vomiting centre, and serotonin antagonists are very effective antiemetics. They include ondansetron, a drug that is very effective in anticancer therapy.

RESPIRATORY DRUGS

Drugs are used to maintain the patency of the respiratory tract, and ensure effective gas exchange between the blood and the tissues.

> Obstruction in the respiratory tract can be due to bronchoconstriction, increased mucus production and oedema

Stimulation of the parasympathetic nervous system and the release of acetylcholine increases bronchial secretions and contracts bronchial smooth muscle, causing bronchoconstriction. Stimulation of the sympathetic nervous system, release of norepinephrine and its action on the beta-adrenergic receptors in the respiratory tract relaxes bronchial smooth muscle and encourages the clearance of mucus by the movement of cilia. This would be indicated in asthma and other conditions associated with reversible airways obstruction.

β_2 agonists

The most widely prescribed bronchodilator is salbutamol (Ventolin®). This is a β_2 adrenoreceptor agonist that antagonises bronchial muscular contraction even when there are several different spasminogens involved, as in asthma.

The development of a relatively specific β_2 agonist was an exciting step forward in the treatment of respiratory disease, as β_1 receptor stimulation is associated with cardioacceleration, an effect that is both not required and undesirable.

Salbutamol is usually given by inhalation, which enhances selectivity by increasing concentration of the drug in the airways and reduces the chances of systemic side effects. The drug is usually taken by aerosol inhalation from a metered dose inhaler – 100–200 µg (1–2 puffs) as needed and up to 3–4 times daily. The maximum effect is within 30 minutes and the duration is up to 4–6 hours. In a severe asthma attack or in other forms of bronchoconstriction, the client will need higher doses of β_2 stimulant. This is given in the form of a nebuliser, where up to 5 mg of salbutamol may be used, made up with 4 ml of normal saline. The drug may also be given orally or by slow intravenous injection or infusion, but systemic side effects will be greater. There is increasing evidence that beta agonist tolerance can develop in asthma. Steroids can help this because they inhibit beta receptor down-regulation

Side effects of β_2 agonists do occur. Salbutamol may cause tachycardia, as it is not totally β_2 specific. In high doses it also causes fine muscular tremors, and may lead to muscle cramps and hypokalaemia. The latter may be potentiated by concomitant treatment with diuretics, steroids or theophylline. Other adverse effects may include palpitations and peripheral vasodilation, resulting in hypotension, headache and dizziness

Muscarinic receptor antagonists

Ipratropium bromide (Atrovent®) is an antagonist at the muscarinic receptor and is a synthetic drug that is structurally related to atropine. The drug reverses bronchial constriction caused by increased smooth muscle tone due to parasympathetic stimulation. It inhibits mucus secretion, may increase mucociliary clearance of bronchial secretions and is particularly useful in chronic obstructive pulmonary disease.

Ipratropium is given as an inhaled dose via an aerosol or nebuliser, and drug action can be expected within 45 minutes, lasting about 3–4 hours. Common adverse reactions are antimuscarinic in nature and include a dry mouth, constipation and occasionally urinary retention. Ipratropium can be given with β_2 adrenoreceptor agonists and the two agents together produce a greater degree of bronchodilation. They may be administered in the same nebuliser.

Xanthines

This group of drugs are powerful relaxants of smooth muscle. They cause bronchodilation but are rather less effective than the β_2 agonists. They have been used in the treatment of asthma, since it was observed that a cup of strong coffee helped to relieve the symptoms of asthma at the turn of the century. Coffee contains naturally occurring xanthines.

The main xanthine used clinically is theophylline, sometimes administered in the form of aminophylline. They are believed to inhibit the enzyme phosphodiesterase and so prevent the breakdown of cyclic adenosine monophosphate (AMP), resulting in smooth muscle relaxation. Xanthines have some central action and are weak respiratory stimulants. They are not usually used for this purpose, although caffeine is occasionally used in neonates. They do have a stimulant action on the central nervous system, causing increased alertness, but may cause nervousness and interfere with sleep. They have a small diuretic action.

Aminophylline is given orally but sometimes as a slow infusion, with constant cardiac monitoring, in acute asthma. The main problem with the use of xanthines is their relatively low therapeutic index, and there is little difference between the therapeutic dose and the toxic dose. The concentration required for effective bronchodilation is 10 µg/l, but 20 µg/l is associated with adverse reactions, such as nausea, arrhythmias and convulsions.

Aminophylline should never be given to patients already receiving theophyllines, as the risk of fatal cardiac dysrhythmias is high

ANTIARRHYTHMIC AGENTS

Most antiarrhythmic drugs work by impeding the movement of ions across the membrane of myocardial cells. They act to stabilise and suppress the excitable myocardial tissue, and may achieve this by suppressing automaticity, by depressing the rate of depolarisation, by slowing impulse conduction through tissue, by prolonging the action potential or by increasing the refractory period (Galbraith et al., 1999). They are not suitable for the treatment of all forms of arrhythmia and may be contraindicated in certain circumstances such as heart block.

Drugs are grouped into four groups. This is not a perfect system and some drugs fall into more than one class (e.g. amiodarone). Clinicians may prefer to group drugs into the arrhythmias they are used to control.

Class I
Class I drugs inhibit the movement of sodium into the cell associated with depolarisation. They are relatively selective to arrhythmogenic cells rather than normal cardiac cells. They are also local anaesthetics.

Lignocaine (lidocaine) is a Class I drug with little atrial activity. Its use is limited to arrhythmias of ventricular origin, usually those associated with myocardial infarction and cardiac arrest. It is effective in suppressing ventricular tachycardia and fibrillation after cardioversion, cardiac surgery and anaesthesia. It is largely ineffective in the treatment of supraventricular arrhythmias except when associated with Wolff–Parkinson–White syndrome or digoxin toxicity. The drug should not be given in bradycardia.

At therapeutic doses, lignocaine is the least cardiotoxic of the currently available Class I drugs. The most commonly reported adverse reactions are at high doses and affect the central nervous system. They include paraesthesia, tremor, nausea, slurred speech, hearing disturbances and convulsions.

Flecainide is also a Class I drug used to treat ventricular arrhythmias. It also blocks some potassium channels and this may account for its efficacy in the treatment of atrial arrhythmias. It is more proarrhythmic than lignocaine (lidocaine).

Class II
Class II drugs have beta-adrenoreceptor antagonist action and include the beta blockers *sotalol* and *propranolol*. They are useful in arrhythmias associated with exercise or emotion, and may be used to treat sinus tachycardia, paroxysmal atrial tachycardia, exercise-induced ventricular arrhythmias and those occurring in the hereditary prolonged QT syndrome.

Class III
Class III agents lengthen the cardiac action potential duration and hence the effective refractory period. They also block potassium channels in cardiac muscle.

Amiodarone is the most important drug in this category. It also has sodium channel-blocking activity with very little negative inotropic action. Amiodarone is a complex antiarrhythmic drug that shares some of the properties of all four classes of antiarrhythmic drug. It is a unique wide-spectrum antiarrhythmic agent with chiefly Class III effects, *but also powerful Class I activity and ancillary Class II and Class IV activity*. It lengthens the effective refractory period by prolonging the action potential duration in all cardiac tissues and blocks sodium channels, mainly when they are in the inactivated state. It non-competitively blocks beta-adrenergic receptors and has a calcium antagonist effect, which might explain the bradycardia, the atrioventricular nodal inhibition and the relatively low incidence of *torsades de pointes* it produces.

It is a powerful inhibitor of abnormal automaticity, and also has coronary and peripheral vasodilator properties. It is one of the drugs of first choice in preventing life-threatening ventricular arrhythmias and recurrent cardiac arrest. It is also effective in the treatment of atrial fibrillation, atrial flutter and paroxysmal supraventricular tachycardia.

Amiodarone has an exceptionally long half-life of 25–110 days. A steady state may not be established for several months unless large loading doses are given. Even given intravenously, its full electrophysiological effect is delayed.

Amiodarone is lipid soluble and extensively distributed in the body, being highly concentrated in many tissues, especially the liver and lungs. This leads to the persistence of adverse effects long after the drug is discontinued. These include the following:

- Abnormalities in thyroid function may occur. Amiodarone contains high concentrations of iodine and is structurally related to thyroxine.
- It may also cause nausea and vomiting.
- Neurological side effects include peripheral neuropathy, insomnia, headache and ataxia.
- After prolonged high-dose therapy, a photosensitive slate-grey or bluish discoloration of the skin may occur. This slowly improves on withdrawal of the drug.
- The most serious complication, probably dose-related, is pulmonary fibrosis.

Class IV

Class IV drugs are calcium channel antagonists, such as *verapamil* and *diltiazem*, which inhibit slow calcium-channel-dependent conduction through the atrioventricular node and are effective in supraventricular arrhythmias. They are not effective in the treatment of ventricular tachycardia and can be lethal in wide complex ventricular tachycardia.

Class V

Class V has been added recently to include drugs that do not fit into the four classes above and include digoxin, adenosine, magnesium and potassium.

Adenosine is a naturally occurring nucleotide with a complex mechanism of action. It is given as an intravenous bolus and inhibits atrioventricular nodal conduction, also increasing the atrioventricular nodal refractory period. It has a short duration of action following intravenous administration. The peak action occurs in 10 seconds and the effect lasts about 10 seconds. It is given as a rapid intravenous bolus for the treatment of paroxysmal atrial and nodal tachycardias, including those associated with Wolff–Parkinson–White syndrome. It can be given safely to patients with broad complex tachycardia, and poor left ventricular function or hypotension owing to its short duration of action. It is useful in differentiating between broad complex tachycardias of ventricular or supraventricular origin. Ventricular tachycardias do not respond usually, unless they are related to exercise. It is not useful in the treatment of atrial fibrillation or flutter, and may exacerbate the arrhythmia.

CONCLUSION

Pharmacology is a complex and intricate subject. This chapter has outlined some of the basic concepts of pharmacodynamics and pharmacokinetics, and the use of some of the drugs used in emergency situations.

It will be appreciated, however, from reading this chapter that the pharmacology of drugs used in the care of trauma victims is a huge subject and that no single chapter can do justice to such a subject. The reader is, therefore, strongly encouraged to refer to specific texts on therapeutics for advice when treating patients.

References and further reading

Galbraith A, Bullock S, Manias E, Hunt B, Richards A. *Fundamentals of pharmacology*. Harlow: Addison Wesley, 1999

Gilman A, Rall T, Nies A, Taylor P. *The pharmaceutical basis of therapeutics*. Oxford: Pergamon, 2001

Neal MJ. *Medical pharmacology at a glance*, 4th edn. London: Blackwell Scientific, 2002.

Page C. *Integrated pharmacology*, 2nd edn. London: Mosby, 2002

Rang H, Dale M, Ritter J. *Pharmacology*, 5th edn. Edinburgh: Churchill Livingstone, 2004

Readers should also be familiar with the following journals and books that are issued on a frequent basis: *The British National Formulary*, *Prescriber's Journal* and *Prescriber*.

Chapter **15**

The pathogenesis of disease and infection control

Lynn J. Parker

INTRODUCTION

Microbes are thought to have been the first living organisms on the planet. Largely invisible, they inhabit areas of the world where other organisms cannot survive. They are found in soil, water, dust, air, food, in our clothes, and in and on our bodies. The majority of microbes are beneficial to humans and are used in biotechnology, and perform useful functions in the ecological chain in breaking down dead matter of plants and animals. They are also used in food production.

When considering the pathogenesis of disease, resistance, immunity, age and nutritional status of the individual exposed, plus the virulence of the organism and the level of exposure, all play a role in deciding whether an individual will develop a disease or not. This chapter discusses the pathogenesis of infectious disease and outlines the simple measures that can be taken to prevent the occurrence of such diseases.

PATHOGENESIS OF INFECTIOUS DISEASE

Pathogenic organisms that cause disease include viruses, bacteria, chlamydia, rickettsiae, mycoplasma, fungi and protozoa. There is a classification system that has evolved for identification of individual organisms, grouping them together according to their similarities in structure. With advances in scientific knowledge, microbes can sometimes be reclassified and moved into other groupings and be renamed.

Viruses are different from other organisms in that they can only replicate inside living cells, usually destroying the host cell in the process. Bacteria replicate mainly by binary fission dividing into two, although there are other methods by which they transfer genetic information, known as conjugation, transduction or transformation. Fungi are more complex than bacteria and are plants lacking the green pigmentation of chlorophyll. Both chlamydiae and rickettsiae are obligate intracellular parasites with deoxyribonucleic acid (DNA) and ribonucleic acid (RNA) multiplying by binary fission.

Skin is normally colonised by a stable population of microbes, which assist the natural defence mechanisms of the body against infection. Some areas in the body are sterile and microbes should not be present there. Details of the normal flora and common pathogens associated with particular body sites are given in Table 15.1.

Pathogenicity is dependent upon the virulence of an organism and host defence factors, which include the person's age, genetic factors and general and local host defences (see Box 15.1). Conversely colonisation by microbes occurs when they are found to be growing and multiplying on or in the body, but without invading the surrounding tissues and causing damage. Such coexistences can be found to a different degree

with them being further defined as resident or transient flora. Resident flora can be found in certain areas of the body on a regular basis; they can be reduced but rarely eliminated on a permanent basis as they always re-establish themselves. Transient organisms can inhabit the body for hours, days or weeks, surviving or multiplying until they are removed by normal bodily hygiene or functions, and do not normally cause disease.

Other terms used to describe colonisation by microbes are intermittent and chronic carriage. Intermittent carriage occurs when microbes stay longer than transient organisms, disappear and then recur at a later date. Chronic carriage of microbes occurs when a pathogenic organism persists without incurring illness in the host, such as *Salmonella* in the gut.

All microbes that cause disease in humans can be considered as opportunistic in nature, as disease is not the normal state of being. Opportunistic organisms can be considered as those organisms that rarely cause disease in healthy individuals, or they are part of the normal body flora but cause disease when introduced to another part of the body. An example is *Escherichia coli*, which is normally found in the gut but which causes urinary tract infection when introduced into the urinary tract.

Table 15.1 Body sites, their normal flora and common pathogens. (Reproduced from Lawrence J, May D, 2002)

Site	Normal flora	Specimen	Common pathogens
Central nervous system	Normally sterile	Cerebrospinal fluid	S. pneumoniae, N. meningitidis, H. influenzae, other Gram-negative rods
Bladder and urinary tract	Normally sterile	Urine	E. coli, Strep. faecalis, M. tuberculosis
Lower respiratory tract	Normally sterile	Sputum	S. pneumoniae, H. influenzae, M. tuberculosis, viruses
Upper respiratory tract	S. epidermidis, S. aureus, H. influenzae, bacteroides	Throat swab	S. pyogenes, viruses
Skin and hair	S. epidermidis, S. aureus, diphtheroids	Swab from wound lesion	S. aureus, S. pyogenes
Perianal skin	Ent. faecalis, Bacteroides fragalis, yeasts	Swab from wound lesions	Gram-negative rods, anaerobic gram negative rods, dermatophytes
Small bowel and colon	Coliforms, yeasts, bacteroids sp., Ent. faecalis, Clostridium perfringens	Faeces	Salmonella sp., Shigella sp., Campylobacter sp., Yersinia sp. ova, cysts and parasites, viruses
Vagina (adult)	Lactobacillus sp., S. epidermidis, Group B Streptococcus, yeasts, Gram-negative rods	High vaginal swab	N. gonorrhoeae, Trichomonas vaginalis, Candida albicans, Gardnerella sp.

Box 15.1   Risk factors for acquiring infection

General factors
- Age: the very young and the very old
- Nutrition: the emaciated, thin, obesity, dehydration
- Mobility: limited, immobile, temporary, permanent
- Mental state: confused, depressed, senile
- Incontinence: urine and/or faeces, temporary, permanent
- General health: weak, debilitated
- General hygiene: dependence, mouth/teeth, skin

Local factors
- Oedema: pulmonary, ascites, effusion
- Ischaemia: thrombus, embolus, necrosis
- Skin lesions: trauma, burns, ulceration
- Foreign body: accidental, planned

Invasive procedures
- Cannulation: peripheral, central, parenteral
- Catheterisation: intermittent, closed drainage, irrigation
- Surgery: anaesthesia, wound, wound drainage, wound/colostomy, implant
- Intubation: endobronchial suction, humidification, ventilation

Drugs
- Cytotoxics, antibiotics, steroids

Disease
- Carcinoma, leukaemia, aplastic anaemia, diabetes mellitus, liver disease, renal disease, AIDS

It is impossible to determine from a clinical specimen if an individual has an infectious disease or is colonised by a microbe, especially if that microbe would be considered as part of the normal body flora

The clinical condition of the patient must determine whether the individual has an infection or not. Consideration must be given to visible signs of infection present in the patient, other investigations that might support the diagnosis of infection, and whether there are appropriate symptoms.

Infections are the result of organisms being transmitted from one host to another, where they replicate and cause disease

---

The degree of dependence by the parasite on the host can be considered as a continuum from those organisms considered as saprophytes, which are fairly independent and only incidentally cause disease in the host, to those pathogens that are dependent on the host cells for their reproduction. Such organisms can range from those producing toxins that cause the disease in the host (such as botulism), to bacteria that cause infection in the body's tissues (such as staphylococci and streptococci), to rickettsiae and viruses, which cannot grow in the absence of body tissue. These examples of the variety and degree of parasitism show that the changes in the relationships between the host and parasite can be a continuous evolutionary process.

Microbes often show an adaptability or preference to a specific host species. It is unlikely that microbes that infect plants are likely to infect animals or vice versa. However, natural infection of a secondary host may occur leading to severe or fatal disease. Rabies is an example of a disease highly fatal in humans but is found as an asymptomatic infection in bats.

Most infectious diseases are preventable, usually by preventing contact and transmission of the infection between the host and the source of infection, and by making the host unsusceptible to the disease by use of natural or artificial immunity. The efficacy of the preventive measures varies from one disease to another. This can all be summarised as the 'infectious process', defined by Osterholm et al. (1995), which suggests that, apart from serious pathogenic microbes, people and microbes coexist in harmony for most of the time. Only when the equilibrium is disrupted do the microbes enter the body past the defence mechanisms and cause an infection; thus the development of a disease depends upon both the host and the agent.

It is stated that, for an infection to occur, six components have to take place at the same time (Horton and Parker, 2002). These are:

- a microbe likely to cause infection
- a reservoir where the microbe can survive and/or multiply
- a portal of exit or means by which the microbe can leave the reservoir

- a mechanism to transfer the microbe from the reservoir into the susceptible person
- a portal of entry or means by which the microbe can enter the host
- a susceptible person.

Thus the formula for an infection to occur can be described as:

$$\text{Risk of infection} = \frac{\text{Dose + time + virulence of microbe}}{\text{Host susceptibility}}$$

As stated earlier, it is the vulnerability of the human host that determines whether the combination of the above factors produce an infection.

A list of organisms causing infection in humans, detailing the disease, morphology and reservoir, mode of transmission and prevention for each organism, is provided in the Appendix at the end of the book.

A great hope of the 20th century was the possibility of eradicating infectious diseases throughout the world by the year 2000, following on from the success of the eradication of smallpox in the 1970s. Currently, infectious diseases are responsible for the majority of deaths worldwide, with an increase in the numbers of tuberculosis and human immunodeficiency virus (HIV). Success in the eradication of polio and measles in Europe is thought to be possible, but political changes in Eastern Europe have seen an upsurge in infectious disease, particularly diphtheria, during the 1990s. What this demonstrates is that, whilst the impression has been that such diseases have been defeated and controlled, owing to the advances of scientific knowledge, the reality is different. We are now looking at the possibility of re-emergence of past infections with the added problem of antimicrobial resistance.

Infectious diseases can have a serious effect on people's health if they spread unchecked, as epidemics may develop. There are a number of infectious diseases that are notifiable by law to the public health authorities in the UK (Box 15.2; Horton and Parker, 2002). Many diseases can be controlled by setting up environmental control measures, as they are food- and water-borne infections. Other infections may be controlled by vaccination and effective treatment of cases.

Box 15.2   Notifiable diseases

Under the Public Health (Control of Disease) Act (1984)
- Cholera
- Plague
- Relapsing fever
- Smallpox
- Typhus

Under the Public Health (Infectious Diseases) Regulations (1988)
- Acute encephalitis
- Acute poliomyelitis
- Anthrax
- Diphtheria
- Dysentery (amoebic or bacillary)
- Leprosy
- Leptospirosis
- Malaria
- Measles
- Meningitis
- Meningococcal septicaemia (without meningitis)
- Mumps
- Ophthalmia neonatorum
- Paratyphoid fever
- Rabies
- Rubella
- Scarlet fever
- Tetanus
- Tuberculosis
- Typhoid fever
- Viral haemorrhagic fever
- Viral hepatitis
- Whooping cough
- Yellow fever

This system of recording infectious diseases cases was introduced at the beginning of the last century as a method of controlling outbreaks. There is a statutory responsibility for local authorities to control infectious diseases within their own boundaries. The diseases that are listed above have to be reported to a person called the 'proper officer', who is often the consultant for communicable disease control based at the local health authority. The responsibility usually falls on the doctor who makes the original diagnosis. Reporting such infections allows for contact tracing of family and friends, who may also have been exposed to the same infection, as in meningococcal meningitis or pulmonary tuberculosis, so that prophylactic treatment may be offered or monitoring for signs of infection can be carried out.

Finally, local and national analysis of the data is made to consider the effects of vaccination programmes (such as MMR), detecting epidemics and the planning of preventative programmes.

STANDARD PRECAUTIONS AGAINST INFECTIOUS DISEASE

Three factors are required for cross-infection to occur in an institution: these are a source where the microorganism can be found, a susceptible host and a means of transmission.

Source of infection

The source is the place where microbes can be found, either in humans or inanimate objects in the environment that are contaminated. Human sources can be other patients, staff or visitors, who can be colonised with organisms, have an acute infection or be incubating an infection. Other sources may be the individual patient's own body organisms that colonise the gut, skin and respiratory tract. Animals may provide a reservoir for some microbes, such as *Salmonella* and *Campylobacter*, and the environment of soil, dust and water may be reservoirs for other microbes, such as *Clostridium* and *Legionnella*.

Individuals vary in their susceptibility to infections. Some people, once exposed to an infection, become immune; others may become carriers of the disease, or may actually succumb and show clinical symptoms.

Standard precautions must be taken by all health care workers when in contact with patients to reduce the risk of transmission of infection between patients, from patient to staff, and from staff to patients regardless of their presumed infection status or diagnosis. The precautions are aimed at reducing the risk of transmission of microbes from both recognised and unrecognised sources of infection.

> Standard precautions apply to all situations when the health care worker may come into contact with blood, other body fluids, secretions and excretions except sweat

Transmission of infection

Most organisms use a single route of transmission to a new host; some organisms can use more than one route. The essentials of standard precautions are to prevent transmission of microbes by the common transmission routes of direct and indirect contact, airborne and droplet spray, fomites and ingestion, and vector-borne transmission.

Certain basic measures can be taken to decrease the risk of transmission. These are the essentials of standard precautions and include handwashing, wearing gloves, use of protective clothing (aprons and gowns) and face protection. Additionally, the decontamination of equipment after use, and the safe disposal of linen and clinical waste are important factors in the prevention of infectious disease.

The most common route of transmission for infections, and the most important are direct or indirect contact. Direct contact is the physical transfer of infective material from body surface to body surface between an infected or colonised person and a susceptible host. This can occur between patients or by staff to patients, when performing patient care activities. Indirect contact involves the susceptible host having contact with an intermediate object – either contaminated instruments, needles, and dressings, or hands that have not been washed or gloves that are not changed between patients.

Droplet spread is sometimes confused with the airborne route for the transmission of infections. Droplets are produced by an infected person by coughing, sneezing, talking or singing. Droplet spread can also occur when certain procedures, such as bronchoscopy or tracheal suctioning, are performed. Microbes cannot be transmitted through the air by themselves but need something to carry them. Droplets are composed mainly of saliva and can contain small numbers of microbes and, depending upon their size, they quickly fall to the ground. Most respiratory infections like colds and flu are spread through contact with respiratory secretions on tissues, handkerchiefs and hands (Ansari et al., 1991).

Airborne transmission carries microbes by droplet nuclei (small particle residue) or by dust particles composed of dead skin scales, fibres from clothing and other fabrics carrying microbes. Air currents carry the particles dispersing them widely in the environment, where they may be breathed in by a susceptible host or settle on horizontal surfaces. Most microbes are unable to survive in the environment and die quickly without access to nutrients and water (Rhame, 1992), but some bacteria form spores that enable them to lie dormant and survive this stage for many months in such circumstances. Tetanus is such an example and another more familiar to hospitals is *Clostridium difficile*, which is released from the faeces of infected patients (Hoffman, 1993).

Infection by the route of ingestion is another method by which microbes gain access to the body by using food or water as a transport medium. The organisms are excreted in the faeces and passed on as result of poor hygiene. This is often referred to as the faecal–oral route of transmission. Food becomes contaminated by hands that have been in contact with faeces through lack of, or poor, hand washing and the infective agent is then transferred on to food that someone else will eat. If the food is cooked after handling, it is less likely to transmit infection because the infective agents will be killed by the cooking process. However, food that is cooked and then eaten cold may become contaminated by poor hand hygiene or cross-contamination.

Contamination of water from the faeces of animals or humans has been responsible for a number of outbreaks of hepatitis A, Norwalk virus, cholera, cryptosporidiosis and *Giardia*.

The inanimate environment, often referred to in the literature as fomites, includes beds, curtains, toys, bedpans, tables and washbowls. Infections are usually spread by the indirect contact route with the hands of the staff acting as vectors (Ansari et al., 1991). Hands have been shown to become readily contaminated when performing what is perceived as a clean task, such as bed making (Parker, 1999a). Wet environments are a greater hazard, with microbes able to survive and multiply more easily to become a larger source of infection. Equipment filled with water, such as humidifiers or washbowls, quickly become contaminated.

It is important to differentiate between sources and reservoirs of infection, as many bacteria may be found in washbasins but are unlikely to be transferred to a patient, whereas bacteria that contaminate, say, a nebuliser, which acts as a reservoir, could easily be inhaled into the respiratory tract of a patient.

Safe practice

Hand washing and gloves

Hand washing is considered to be the primary method of controlling the spread of infection, although it is acknowledged as only one factor in preventing cross infection (Parker, 1999a). Hands should be washed after being in contact with blood, body fluids, secretions and excretions, and contaminated articles, regardless of whether gloves have been worn. Washing hands at the start of a shift and between patients protects the patients *and* the nurse, and hand washing before breaks and at the end of shifts is good protection for the nurse.

Gloves are frequently worn by all health care workers, both in hospital and in community settings, as they provide a protective barrier and prevent gross contamination of the hands of staff from blood or body fluids. They are also worn so that microbes on the hands of staff are not transferred to patients during invasive procedures, or other procedures that require touching of broken skin or mucous membranes. For clinical procedures, non-powdered latex gloves are recommended, although alternatives, such as nitrile gloves, can be used if either the patient or the member of staff is allergic to latex.

Finally, they are worn to reduce the risk of cross-infection by staff from patient to patient or from contaminated equipment. Gloves must be changed between contacts with patients and hands should be washed after they have been removed.

> The wearing of gloves does not replace hand washing

Gloves tear during use, they are not impermeable to all microbes and can contaminate hands when they are being removed. Failure to change gloves between patients is a serious infection control hazard.

Personal protective clothing

The choice of protective clothing depends upon the task being undertaken. The amount of microbes transferred to clothing when caring for patients is usually small and most will not survive for long periods of time. For the majority of situations, a plastic apron gives better protection than cotton gowns and, even though they do not cover the arms and shoulders of staff, they do cover effectively the middle part of the body, which gets maximum contamination (Babb et al., 1983). There are now various types of masks, goggles and face protection available, and the wearing of these is recommended by a number of regulatory bodies to protect a member of staff from contamination by splashes of blood and body fluid as well as disinfectants.

> The benefit of wearing masks, even in operating theatres, is considered to be of little benefit in reducing the spread of infection (Orr, 1981; Department of Health, 1997)

Isolation of infected patients

In preventing the spread of infections, it is not normally necessary that every patient be isolated in a room on their own. However, if they are, precautions are much more likely to be complied with by all staff members (Wilson, 2001). Those patients who are non-compliant with precautions or who have poor personal hygiene, those who are likely to contaminate the environment because of diarrhoea, severe vomiting or bleeding, or are suspected of having an infection transmissible by airborne spread, such as tuberculosis or chicken-pox, are best placed in a single room.

'Cohort nursing', when patients with the same infection are nursed together in a double sideroom or a bay area on a ward, can be used provided the patients have only one transmissible infection.

Patients requiring investigations and treatments in other hospital departments, or who are transferred to another hospital should not be denied such treatment because of an actual or suspected infection. What is important is that the correct precautions are taken to reduce the risk of cross-infection by understanding how the infection normally spreads. Those involved with trans-porting patients, such as porters and ambulance personnel, should be informed of the necessary precautions to be taken and the importance of good hand-washing techniques. The receiving department or hospital must also be informed of the precautions to be taken and the investigation performed immediately without the patient waiting in reception rooms or in corridors so that the risk of transmission to other patients is minimised.

Isolation precautions are usually considered to be a nursing responsibility (Jackson and Lynch, 1985). It is now taught alongside the other universal precautions in nursing curricula, but the principles of asepsis and isolation techniques are often excluded from medical school curricula (Worsley et al., 1990). Isolation systems have grown out of the concept of fever nursing, as described by Florence Nightingale, when she separated patients with infectious diseases from others and stressed the importance of avoiding contact with body substances (Parker, 1999b). Up to date infection control and isolation guidelines are regularly produced by the Centre for Disease Control (CDC) in Atlanta, Georgia, and the Hospital Infection Control Programme Advisory Committee (HICPAC), and are based on the latest epidemiological information on transmission of infection in hospitals. UK Standard precautions (DoH, 2001) are published by the National Institute for Clinical Excellence (NICE).

> Clinicians should consult the NICE guidelines if there is any concern about the care of an infected patient in their care

Wound healing

Human skin in healthy individuals is inhospitable to pathogenic organisms. The normal flora of the skin plays a vital role in maintaining the microbial balance, which, if disrupted, can lead to invasion of the body by opportunistic or pathogenic organisms. Skin provides both a mechanical and chemical barrier to organisms, as they cannot penetrate the horny keratin layer, if it is unbroken. Resident flora of the skin produce antimicrobial substances that are bactericidal and the secretions of the skin are acidic in nature; thus they provide additional protection.

> A wound occurring from any accidental or deliberate trauma that breaks the surface of the skin creates the risk of infection

All soft tissue injuries heal using the same basic biochemical and cellular processes whether they are chronic ulcerative leg ulcers and pressure sores, lacerations, abrasions, burns or surgical wounds. Wound healing can be classified into the three stages of primary, secondary and tertiary intention.

Wounds caused by breaks in the skin due to trauma or surgical procedures normally heal by *primary intention*. Here the edges of the skin are brought together and healing is often quick with minimal scarring. Chronic and long-standing wounds heal by *secondary intention* and may become infected. These include leg ulcers, pressure sores, burns and delayed primary suturing (DPS) for blast injuries or gunshot wounds. Healing by *tertiary intention* occurs in wounds that have broken down, usually following surgery, and often require further surgical intervention to remove the cause of infection (Russell, 2000). The large amounts of degrading tissue found in such chronic wounds and the exudate containing bacterial toxins often delay wound healing (Wysocki, 1996).

THE PRINCIPLES OF ASEPSIS

To prevent the transmission of microbes entering a wound and infection occurring when wound care is being delivered, it is normal practice to apply the principles of the aseptic technique. This involves using sterile equipment, cleansing agents, dressings and sterile gloves and, where possible, a 'no-touch' technique, and is recognised as standard best practice (Lund and Caruso, 1993; Horton and Parker, 2002).

A variation to this approach is now being advocated suggesting that, for certain wounds and in certain situations, using a clean rather than an aseptic technique may be acceptable. This involves wearing non-sterile gloves when dealing with certain wounds and irrigating some chronic wounds using solutions such as tap-water (Riyat and Quinton, 1997; Hollinworth and Kingston, 1998).

As hand washing is the cornerstone of good infection control practice, a variety of bactericidal skin-cleansing agents are available for use, but most transient flora are quickly removed by thorough washing with soap and water and hand drying. It must be remembered that excessive hand washing may damage the skin and increase the risk of hand colonisation with pathogens (Ayliffe et al., 1992; Gould, 1993). It has been suggested that, when removing dressings from surgical wounds more than 24 hours old, gloves do not need to be worn, if adequate hand washing has taken place (Chintz et al., 1989).

It should be remembered that it is necessary to wash hands after wearing gloves, to remove any bacterial growth on the hands under the gloves, and on removing dirty gloves, as there is a risk of contaminating the hands (Ayliffe et al., 1992).

The debate as to whether to use non-sterile or sterile gloves for wound care is currently very active, and it has been suggested by a number of studies that, for routine wound care and change of dressings, clean non-sterile gloves may be used safely (Rossoff et al., 1993; Hollinworth and Kingston, 1998).

Wound cleansing

The routine cleansing of wounds must be questioned, as it goes against the principles of moist wound healing (Pudner, 1997). The traditional method of wound cleansing using a variety of sterile or antiseptic solutions to remove exudate from the surface of the wound may delay its healing.

Alternatives, such as bathing and showering, have been shown as a suitable method for cleansing sacral and perianal wounds, and also for leg ulceration (Bucknole, 1996). Hydrotherapy and whirlpool baths are an aggressive form of bathing, using turbulent water to dislodge debris from the wound (Williams, 1999). The risk of cross-infection must be considered, and baths must be cleaned before and after use. A polythene liner should be placed in buckets or bowls if they are used to wash a patient.

Tap-water has been recommended for cleansing wounds in A&E departments in patients with open traumatic wounds (Riyat and Quinton,

1997). It is essential that there is access to a clean water supply and that its safety is regularly monitored, and individual patients should be assessed for their risk of acquiring an infection; it may be considered a safe practice to follow (Hollinworth and Kingston, 1998).

Sterile dressings

Most sterile dressing packs and occlusive dressings are commercially prepared and, as long as the packaging remains intact, the contents should remain sterile. Before being used, they should be checked for evidence of damage or moisture and, if found, they should not be used (Ayliffe et al., 1993).

A vital component in creating the most effective environment for wounds to heal is to maintain the surface temperature of the wound. Reducing the temperature of the wound may hinder the healing activity of certain cells, such as leucocytes, if the wound temperature drops from the optimum of 37°C to 28°C. Such a drop in temperature can easily be achieved by removing dressings to look at wounds when they could be exposed for periods of time; therefore, dressings should not be removed unnecessarily.

Dressings should prevent microbes entering the wound and allow the normal body defence mechanisms to act, whilst still keeping the tissue moist (Winter, 1962). Infection in a wound results in an increased production of exudates, and the dressing may need to be chosen or changed to ensure optimum absorbency or antimicrobial properties (Thomas, 1997). The function of the ideal dressing is to remove excess fluid from the immediate vicinity of the wound. The state of hydration of a wound would normally decrease as it progresses towards healing; continuous and regular evaluation of wounds and the dressings used to match the patient and the wound is necessary (Krasner and Sibbald, 1999).

Types of dressings

Dressings are divided into conventional dressings, which include gauze, non-adherent gauze and gauze impregnated with topical agents, and advanced dressings, such as alginates, collagen, films, foams, hydrocolloids and hydrogels. There is a wide range of products available in each of these categories, which ensure an ideal moist environment that also absorbs exudate (Krasner and Sibbald, 1999).

DECONTAMINATION OF EQUIPMENT

Equipment should be decontaminated between patients as an essential part of routine infection control procedures and, in most cases, normal decontamination procedures are sufficient.

Equipment that has been in contact with blood and body fluids may transmit infection to those who have to service or repair it. It must, therefore, be decontaminated thoroughly before it is inspected or repaired, and certificates stating what method of decontamination and the precautions need to be taken when handling it must accompany the item to the repair facility [NHS Management Executive (NHSME), 1993].

Items such as commodes and patients' trolleys that become contaminated with body fluids should be cleaned with hot water and detergent after each use. It is not usually necessary to throw away unused disposable items that have not been opened or contaminated with the patient's body fluids.

Within an A&E department, the principal priority is to manage the cubicle or patients' bed area with a rapid throughput of patients. The infectious status of these patients will often be unknown and so the risk of cross-infection is high. Therefore, there is a need to ensure that single-use items are used where possible and those items that can be reused are decontaminated appropriately after every use. Consideration must be given to cleaning trolleys between use, and to changing linen and pillows.

All waste contaminated with blood or body fluids is considered to be clinical waste and, within the UK, a national colour-coding system dictates that it is placed in yellow bags for incineration (NHS Estates, 1995). There is no need for 'double bagging' of waste, as the outer surface of the bag should not become significantly contaminated (Maki et al., 1986).

Sharps from all patients must be segregated from other waste

Sharps are a major cause of transmission of blood-borne viruses (Heptonstall et al., 1993) and containers for disposal must conform to British Standard 7320 or its equivalent.

Used linen must be disposed of according to health service guidelines (NHSME, 1995); these recommend a national colour-coding standard allowing for easy segregation of used linen from infected linen. Infected linen is placed in a water-soluble bag before being placed in a red bag with white or off-white bags being used for other linen.

If relatives take personal items home for washing, they should be informed that they should be transported in a plastic carrier bag and that they should normally be washed at a temperature greater than 65°C.

After patients have been discharged or removed from a cubicle/bed area following isolation, the area should be cleaned thoroughly before being used by other patients. Curtains should be changed and washed, if contaminated; walls are no longer routinely washed when the patient has been discharged from the room. Attention should be paid to cleaning the trolley/bed, bedrails, locker, tables, chairs, door handles, sinks, taps and all horizontal surfaces. Suction and oxygen equipment on the wall behind the bed area should also be cleaned.

There is no evidence to support the use of disposable plates, cutlery and cups, as microbes are unable to survive on the surfaces of normal cutlery or crockery (Maki et al., 1979). The combination of hot water and detergent is sufficient to decontaminate all eating and drinking implements, especially when cleaned in a dishwasher.

Decontamination processes

During the 1940s, the concept of using a central sterile services system was first developed. The purpose of such systems is to standardise the aseptic procedure and to prepare, sterilise and distribute pre-packaged materials and instruments to wards and departments in a hospital so that they are ready for immediate use.

Guidance from the Department of Health reminds chief executives of the importance of implementing existing guidance on the cleaning and sterilisation processes of medical devices (Health Service Circular, 1999a). The guidance collates all relevant guidance and legislation on which safe practice is based.

It is the role of the Medicines and Healthcare Products Regulatory Agency (MHRA) on behalf of the government to be the competent authority to carry out the requirements of European Union (EU) Directives. These require tighter statutory controls on almost every aspect of sterilisation with past practices no longer being acceptable or lawful today. The legislation for this area is contained in the Health Technical Memorandum (HTM) 2010 (NHS Executive, 1994).

The essential requirements that are set out in the Directives are that medical devices must not compromise the health or safety of the patient, user or any other person, and any risks associated with the device are compatible with patient health and protection. The current definition of a medical device can be all encompassing, and includes not only the device but any accessories that may be used with it (Box 15.3).

These devices carry the 'CE' marking that can be seen on the packaging of current sterile devices. The CE marking shows that the product is fit for its intended purpose and that the manufacturers have provided full details on how

---

Box 15.3 Definitions of medical devices – Council Directive 93/42/EEC quoted in HTM 2010 (NHS Executive, 1994).

The Directive defines a medical device as any instrument, apparatus, appliance, material or other article, whether used alone or in combination, including the software necessary for its proper application intended by the manufacturer to be used on human beings for the purpose of:

a. diagnosis, prevention, monitoring, treatment or alleviation of disease
b. diagnosis, monitoring, treatment, alleviation or compensation of an injury or handicap
c. investigation, replacement or modification of the anatomy or of a physiological process
d. control of conception

and which does not achieve its principal intended action in or on the human body by pharmacological, immunological or metabolic means, but which may be assisted in its function by such means.

to decontaminate the product that they supply. Since 1993, all medical devices that need to be inspected, serviced, repaired or transported all need a declaration of contamination status (Health Service Guidance, 1993). If this certificate of decontamination does not accompany equipment, staff may refuse to handle such items until they have been decontaminated and a declaration provided.

Emerging diseases such as new variant Creutzfeldt–Jakob disease (nvCJD) have raised concerns in the general population and have resulted in guidance being issued on how to minimise the risk of transmitting the infection from one patient to another (Health Service Circular, 1999b). Now reclassified as variant CJD (vCJD), concerns surround the risk of cross-infection in health care settings, since the abnormal prion proteins of vCJD have been found in the lymphatic tissue (including tonsils) of those patients who are confirmed as having the disease. Advice on the safe handling of instruments used on known or suspected cases of vCJD patients is given by the Advisory Committee on Dangerous Pathogens (ACDP) Spongiform Encephalopathy Advisory Committee (1998). This includes the use of single-use disposable kits for all lumbar punctures and the use of single-use instruments wherever practicable for surgical procedures. Current practice in sterile services departments is to monitor surgical instruments through the decontamination processes, which are then documented and recorded in the records of the department and the patient on whom the instruments are used. The ideal is that the patient, instrument and decontamination process is matched allowing for traceability, should the need arise.

Different equipment requires different processes for decontamination. Each item of equipment should be assessed according to its risk and then the appropriate process of cleaning, disinfection or sterilisation undertaken (Box 15.4). Items of equipment are grouped together under high, medium, low and minimal risk and then matched to the most appropriate process before they are used on patients (Box 15.5).

When considering safe practice and the decontamination of equipment, the following points should be remembered:

Box 15.4 Definitions of cleaning, disinfection and sterilization (Medical Devices Agency, 1996)

Cleaning
A process which physically removes contamination but does not necessarily destroy microorganisms. The reduction of microbial contamination is not routinely quantified and will depend upon many factors, including the efficiency of the cleaning process and the initial bioburden. Cleaning removes microorganisms and the organic material on which they thrive. It is a necessary pre-requisite of effective disinfection or sterilisation.

Disinfection
A process used to reduce the number of viable microorganisms but which may not necessarily inactivate some microbial agents, such as certain viruses and bacterial spores. Disinfection may not achieve the same reduction in microbial contamination level as sterilisation.

Sterilisation
A process used to render an object free from viable microorganisms, including viruses and spores.

---

1. Look for the CE mark on new pieces of equipment and, if in doubt of the compatibility of disinfectants and processes, contact the manufacturers.
2. Speak to the hospital's sterile services department to ensure that they are familiar with the equipment you wish them to process for you and that you provide them with the appropriate sterilisation containers to prevent shock damage to sensitive items.
3. Involve the hospital's infection control team in your purchases of equipment and the decontamination processes proposed.
4. Check with hospital's health and safety officers as to the precautions required under the COSHH regulations for the safe handling of disinfectant solutions.
5. Ultrasonic cleaning is recommended for removing debris from small intricate components in devices.
6. Autoclaving must be the process of choice for all equipment providing that it is compatible. If autoclavable instrument trays are available, they should be used to hold equipment safely during processing.

Box 15.5   Decontamination of items according to level of risk (Horton and Parker, 1997)

High-risk items
Items in contact with breaks in the skin or mucous membranes, or introduced into a sterile body area. These items should be cleaned and then sterilised. Items include surgical instruments, laparoscopes, arthroscopes, cardiac catheters, implants, infusions, injections, needles, syringes and surgical dressings.

Medium-risk items
Items in contact with intact mucous membranes, damaged skin, infected lesions, blood and other body fluids, or that have been contaminated with virulent or readily transmissible organisms. These items should be cleaned and then disinfected. Items include respiratory and anaesthetic equipment, gastroscopes, endoscopes, bronchoscopes, vaginal speculae, body fluid spillages, dirty instruments before reprocessing, and bedpans.

Low-risk items
Items in contact with normal and intact skin. Cleaning is usually sufficient; disinfection should be used if there is an infection risk. Items include trolley tops, operating tables, washbowls, baths, toilets, bedding, patient items (e.g. Patslides), slide sheets, hoists.

Minimal-risk items
Items are not in direct contact with patients and cleaning alone is sufficient to remove any risk they may hold for patients. Items include floors, walls, furniture and drains.

7. Regular maintenance is essential to ensure maximum life and efficiency from equipment with basic procedures, such as lubrication undertaken on a frequent basis to prevent sticking of moving parts, particularly after ultrasonic cleaning.

Since 1995, the reuse of medical equipment has been regulated by the Medical Devices Agency (MDA), which states that such devices have to be designated as single or multiple use. Castille (1999) highlighted the dubious practice of retaining items, such as opened packs of wound-care products, and saving unused swabs and dressings from packs. She also commented on the risks of cross-contamination associated with sharing topical creams and lotions between patients, reusing nebulizers, oxygen masks, breathing circuits and masks, and failing to change sheets, pillowcases, blankets and duvet cases between patients.

If a product has been designated by the manufacturer for single-patient use, then it should *never* be reused

In 1988, a major piece of legislation 'The Control of Substances Hazardous to Health', known as the COSHH regulations, came into force; this has been regularly amended since then (HSC, 2004). It requires employers to undertake risk assessment systematically for all hazardous substances, either chemical or biological, that may be met as a result of work activity.

When considering the chemical products used in hospitals and other institutions, it is important to remember that they should all have been assessed according to this legislation and manufacturers are required to provide data sheets to accompany their products. Staff need to have some understanding of chemical compatibility of the products that they use, and that chemicals used for cleaning and the management of spillages in accordance with hospital policies should be treated with respect. No cleaning product should be brought into the hospital from the home environment. Current policies recommend the use of sodium hypochlorite and/or clear soluble phenolics to cover the widest range of pathogenic microbes.

All biological specimens and body fluids should be regarded as potentially infectious, with the aim being to contain, neutralise and dispose of the material safely. Staff who manage spillages should always check their own local policies or contact their infection control teams for specific advice.

MANAGEMENT OF SHARPS RISKS

Potential hazards will always exist, where devices that penetrate the human body are present. All hospitals have policies that give guidance to all members of staff who have to handle such devices during their working day.

'Sharps injuries' are common sources of inoculation with blood borne infections, such as hepatitis B virus, hepatitis C virus and human immunodeficiency virus to staff in health care centres

Special care should be taken when handling sharps, when cleaning used instruments, and disposing of used needles and other sharps. Containers specifically made for such implements to be disposed in must conform to the British Standards Institution (BSI) specification 7320 (BSI, 1990).

This regulation requires devices to:

- be puncture resistant and leak proof
- be capable of being handled and moved while in use with minimal danger of the contents spilling or falling out
- have a handle that is not part of the closure device
- have an opening, which, in normal use, will inhibit removal of the contents
- have a closure device attached for sealing when the container is three-quarters full
- be marked with the words 'Warning – do not fill above the line'
- be made of material that can be incinerated
- be yellow in colour
- be clearly marked with the words 'Danger', 'Contaminated sharps only', 'Destroy by incineration' or 'To be incinerated' (Health Service Advisory Committee, 1992).

STAFF HEALTH

Whilst both patients and staff are at risk of contracting infections from each other, staff members have more control over the circumstances in which such incidents occur than do patients. Hazards to staff are associated with clinical practices as well as simple exposure to microbes and it is almost impossible to legislate for all eventualities when an exposure to infection may occur. Mandatory reporting of occupational exposures following needlestick injuries remind staff that many disease producing microbes may be present in the blood, body fluids, secretions and excretions of an otherwise healthy and undiagnosed person (Horton and Parker, 2002).

Occupational health and infection control personnel work closely together to ensure that staff are neither at risk of contracting infectious diseases from patients or patient care practices, or transmit their infections to vulnerable patients in their care. It is important that staff report illnesses, such as diarrhoea and vomiting, as they may need to be excluded from work for 48–72 hours following their symptoms subsiding, depending upon local policy. Contact with other infectious conditions, such as chickenpox and shingles, should also be reported to ensure that they pose no risk to immunocompromised patients. The good practice of covering cuts and abrasions with waterproof plasters, and reporting skin conditions and allergies should also be encouraged.

The employer has the responsibility to ensure that staff have access to an occupational health department. They also have the responsibility to report injuries, diseases and dangerous occurrences to appropriate authorities (Health and Safety Executive, 1995; NHSME, 1994).

A staff member's immune status to infectious diseases, such as hepatitis B, tuberculosis, rubella and polio, must be assured.

Hepatitis B

It is a requirement that staff involved in exposure-prone procedures must be immunised against hepatitis B virus (HBV) unless natural immunity to HBV, as a result of infection, has been documented. It must be remembered that there are approximately 7–10% of people who do not respond to vaccination despite repeated doses. Such people are usually checked for core antigen to obtain an indication of infectivity, as they may have already been infected prior to immunisation. They may also be carriers of the virus and, as such, pose a risk to patients. Non-responders without previous infection or exposure to HBV may be at risk of infection and will require counselling on prevention (Horton and Parker, 2002).

Government guidance on this matter requires that any inoculation incidents are reported, treated and followed up according to standard guidelines. There is also an issue that staff who are already positive for HBV surface antigen must not undertake 'exposure-prone procedures' until their e-antigen status has been established (Department of Health, 1996).

Hepatitis C

There is estimated to be an exposure risk to hepatitis C virus, following needlestick injury, of between 3% and 10%. There is no effective routine postexposure treatment or vaccine available (British Medical Association, 1996).

Human immunodeficiency virus

The risk for HIV infection following percutaneous exposure is estimated to be approximately 0.3% (Tokars et al., 1993). The risk is thought to increase if the exposure involves a larger quantity of blood identified by the device being visibly contaminated by the patient's blood, the procedure involved a needle placed directly into a vein or artery, or a deep injury was sustained (CDC, 1995).

The giving of zidovudine for postexposure prophylaxis for HIV relies on the fact that, when in the body, zidovudine's active metabolite inhibits viral replication by competitive inhibition of HIV reverse transcriptase. Current guidance in the UK suggests that it may be protective for staff, if given as postexposure prophylaxis, and that, to be effective, it must be available during the initial viral replication cycle (Department of Health, 1992). Treatment should commence within 2 hours of exposure, particularly when percutaneous inoculation with a concentrated preparation of the virus or HIV culture material, transfusion or injection of blood infected with HIV and from HIV-positive patients has occurred (Jefferies, 1991). It must be remembered that side effects from the drug include nausea, vomiting, lethargy, insomnia and headaches, and the safety of zido-vudine in pregnancy and during breastfeeding has not been established (Jefferies, 1991).

Rapid reporting of injuries should be followed by a general assessment of the circumstances surrounding the exposure. Blood specimens should be taken from the patient and the member of staff following counselling and consent. Refusal by the patient must be respected, in which case the assessment of possible treatment of the member of staff should be based on the clinical likelihood of HIV in the patient.

Tuberculosis

The incidence of tuberculosis has declined during the past century owing to the improvement in living conditions, nutrition and chemotherapy. It is a chronic progressive infection that most commonly affects the lungs, but also affects the kidneys, intestine, skin and bone. Patients can often be asymptomatic but may have general malaise, weight loss, fever and cough.

Miliary tuberculosis occurs when tubercle bacilli are carried in the blood causing small foci of infection described as the size of millet seeds around the body. Transmission occurs by inhaling the tubercle bacilli in droplets spray spread by the air when an infected person coughs or speaks.

'Open tuberculosis' occurs when there are large numbers of the organism found in the sputum of an infected patient under direct microscopy. If the organism cannot be seen in three separate sputum specimens, the patient may still have tuberculosis but, as they are not likely to be exhaling enough of the organism, they are considered not to be infectious to others.

Non-pulmonary tuberculosis is not considered to be infectious and so patients do not require to be isolated from others; however, all patients diagnosed with tuberculosis require treatment and monitoring of the compliance of that treat-ment to ensure that multidrug resistance does not occur.

Those patients who are considered to be infectious, if nursed in hospital, should be isolated from other patients in a single room for the first 2 weeks of their therapy. The main risk of infection is to those patients who are susceptible to infec-tion owing to their impaired immune system. Standard universal precautions should be under-taken by staff with added respiratory precautions as described by The Interdepartmental Working Group on Tuberculosis (DoH, 1997). Gowns and masks are not necessary as there needs to be prolonged close contact for the disease to be spread to healthy people.

The risk to hospital staff of contracting tuber-culosis from patients is extremely small especially as the policy, employed by most occupational health departments, of prevention by vaccination and monitoring staff who come into contact with such patients limits the potential for infection. If a case of open pulmonary tuberculosis is found within a hospital community, the immunity of the staff will be checked. Staff with a previously positive Heaf test or evidence of successful BCG immunisation require no further tests, but all contacts should be told to report if they develop a chronic cough over the next 6 months. Contact tracing of family and other close contacts of the patient is coordinated by the consultant in communicable disease control (CCDC).

Methicillin–resistant *Staphylococcus aureus* (MRSA)

Acquired resistance to antibiotics has occurred since they were first used. Most pathogenic organisms are not sensitive to all antibiotics and one of the roles of the laboratory is to identify which are the most appropriate antibiotics to use. Concern arises when the bacteria is found to be resistant to the antibiotic of choice.

Staphylococci have an ability to develop resistance to the antibiotics in their environment. Initially, in the 1960s, methicillin was the antibiotic of choice to treat staphylococcal infections. Because it had to be given parenterally it was soon replaced by flucloxacillin, which could be given orally and became the established antibiotic of choice, since resistance to other penicillins was widespread. Methicillin is now only used in the laboratory to test for sensitivities. Methicillin use increased until the 1970s, when there was a decrease in the number of reported outbreaks. By the 1980s, it had re-emerged after the introduction of the third-generation cephalosporin antibiotics, and new penicillin derivatives were introduced (Wilson, 2001).

The variety of infections caused by MRSA are the same as those caused by *S. aureus*. These range from mild infections, boils and abscesses to severe systemic infections, septicaemia, bacteraemia and wound infections. As well as causing infections, *S. aureus* normally colonises the nose, axillae, groin and perineum. It will also colonise parts of the skin that are damaged; these include pressure sores, leg ulcers and infusion sites. Infection may not occur but these areas may become sources for spread to other patients. The most important route of spread is on the hands of staff, who acquire it by direct and indirect contact from the infected or colonised skin of patients. Removal of such transient organisms is achieved by an effective hand-washing technique.

Most hospitals have a policy covering the treatment of patients colonised with MRSA that requires the patient to be isolated in a single room and a course of topical treatment given to remove the MRSA from the colonised sites of the skin. Once this has been achieved and screening swabs confirm that the MRSA can no longer be identified in the laboratory, the patient's isolation is stopped. Patients' notes should be annotated so that, if a readmission occurs, further screening swabs can be taken to verify that the MRSA is no longer colonising the patient.

The incidence of staff acquiring MRSA is low and is usually of a transient nature, with the organism generally disappearing after a few hours (Cookson et al., 1989). Screening of staff is now undertaken when there is an outbreak, usually coordinated by an infection control team, or as part of employment screening for new employees. Treatment is usually arranged through the occupational health department.

Viral haemorrhagic fevers

There are a number of viral infections that do not occur in the UK but may be seen on rare occasions in patients who have recently travelled abroad.

> Viral haemorrhagic fevers pose a high level of risk to staff

These illnesses are Lassa fever, Marburg and Ebola viruses, and Argentinian and Bolivian fevers, which are named after the places where they were first identified. Rodents are known to be the source of the virus for transmission to humans in the cases of Lassa, Argentinian and Bolivian fevers, but the natural habitat for the Marburg and Ebola viruses is unknown. Such viruses have been known to infect health care workers by transmission, presumably through the handling of blood and body fluids of patients infected with the virus. There is a high fatality rate associated with viral haemorrhagic fevers (VHFs) and, in cases where this diagnosis is suspected, strict isolation precautions must be taken, usually involving the transportation of the patient to specialist isolation units.

Initially, a patient may be admitted to the A&E department of a general hospital; however, if VHF is suspected, the patient is considered to be highly infectious to others, and should be immediately isolated and then transferred to one of the previously mentioned isolation units in the UK. The person in charge must contact the infection control doctor, who will give specific instructions for the management of the patient and arrange for the transfer of the patient. Specimens should not be routinely taken from these patients and, following the transfer of the patient, the room must be decontaminated and potentially contaminated materials disposed of appropriately.

If a case of VHF is suspected, a 'major outbreak committee' meeting must be held and the CCDC informed so that all contacts of the patient can be traced. The admission to a general hospital of a patient suspected with VHF must be avoided if at all possible. Any patient with a history of pyrexia of unknown origin and symptoms of VHF 3 weeks after travelling abroad, particularly to West Africa, should be visited at the patient's home by the infectious diseases consultant and the CCDC, and quarantine arrangements made.

Meningitis

Meningitis can be caused by a number of organisms both bacterial and viral. Much of the public and staff concern around meningitis relates to the publicity surrounding meningococcal meningitis owing to its sudden onset and sometimes fatal outcome.

The organism responsible for meningococcal disease is *Neisseria meningitides*. It is spread by droplets from the upper respiratory tract from person to person. The carriage rate is about 10% of the general population who will normally carry one of a number of strains in the nasopharynx. The risk of transmission to staff is thought to be very low, but prophylaxis or vaccination may be considered in exposed staff, if there is exceptionally close contamination, such as occurs in mouth to mouth resuscitation (Communicable

Disease Report, 1995). The prophylaxis of choice is rifampicin and people who are given this must be informed of the following side effects:

● reduction of effectiveness of hormonal contraceptives
● body fluids of urine, tears and sputum will colour red
● soft contact lenses could be permanently stained
● occasional rash
● gastrointestinal disturbances.

Vaccination in the UK provides protection against the meningococcal serogroups A and C. Vaccination for serotype B is not yet available. A new vaccine specifically for type C is now available for all children up to university age. A vaccination programme for group C meningococcal infection was introduced in 1999 to reduce the incidence of group C meningococcal disease, which causes 40% of cases of the disease in the UK and is one of the major causes of death in young people.

BIOTERRORISM

The deliberate release of biological agents in light of recent worldwide events has become a possibility. Bioterrorism is not exclusively about the epidemiology of emerging diseases, but about fear and disruption. Owing to the high infectivity of many of the diseases associated with the agents used, multiagency contingency plans need to be developed.

Consideration has always been given to how we manage cases of viral haemorrhagic fevers should they present to a hospital. The biological agents thought to be associated with bioterrorist attacks are category A agents of anthrax, smallpox, botulism, plague and tularaemia. They are easily transmitted between people, and cause high morbidity and mortality. Contingency plans include the role of hospitals and staff for the safe management of patients and their contacts, which are already included in many major accident plans.

In the short term, there is a need to consider the following:

● organising on-call rotas so that appropriately trained staff are available should an emergency occur

Table 15.2 Treatment for specific diseases associated with bioterrorism. (*Biological threats: a health response for Ireland 2002*, www.ndsc.ie)

Disease	Treatment	Prophylaxis	Immunisation
Anthrax	Antibiotics	Yes	Not indicated
Smallpox	Antibiotics for skin infections	No	Yes
Botulism	Antitoxin	No	Antitoxin
Tularaemia	Antibiotics	Yes	Not indicated
Viral haemorrhagic fevers	Antivirals	Antivirals	Not indicated

Table 15.3 Infection control precautions required for patients with bioterrorism-related illnesses. (*Biological threats: a health response for Ireland 2002*, www.ndsc.ie)

Organism	Single room	Precautions	Immunisation of staff
Anthrax	No	Standard	No
Smallpox	Negative-pressure isolation room	Airborne	Yes
Botulism	No	Standard	No
Plague	For 72 hours	Droplet	No
Tularaemia	No	Standard	No

- stockpiling appropriate antibiotics, antivirals, antitoxins and vaccines, and arranging for appropriate storage
- arranging for adequate supplies of personal protective clothing and equipment to be available to staff
- considering vaccination of staff for front-line services
- preparing and having available information material on the various biological agents for staff.

Table 15.2 summarises the method of treatment for specific diseases associated with bioterrorism. All patients including symptomatic patients with suspected or confirmed bioterrorism-related illnesses should be managed using standard precautions. Further precautions may also be required, should the suspected illness be transmitted by the droplet or airborne route. Table 15.3 summarises the appropriate infection control precautions required.

CONCLUSION

The much hoped for eradication of infectious diseases in the 20th century has not been achieved. In reality, there is a re-emergence of past infections, such as tuberculosis, and new infections of HIV and *E. coli* 0157. Most diseases are preventable by either stopping contact and transmission from people and the source of the infectious organism, or by providing the host with a natural or artificial immunity to the organisms. The use of standard precautions, whilst important, supports this essential infection control practice. Current infection control practices are based upon informed best practice by experts in the field and, as such, 'informed best practice' should be complied with until proved otherwise. Compliance to standard precautions and relevant legislation, and to infection control policies will help to control infection.

References and further reading

Advisory Committee on Dangerous Pathogens. *Management and control of viral haemorrhagic fevers*. London: The Stationery Office, 1996

Advisory Committee on Dangerous Pathogens Spongiform Encephalopathy Advisory Committee. *Transmissible spongiform encephalopathy agents: safe working and the prevention of infection*. London: The Stationery Office, 1998

Ansari SA, Springthorpe S, Sattar SA, et al. Potential role of hands in the spread of respiratory infections: studies with human parainfluenza virus 3 and rhinovirus 14. *Journal of Clinical Microbiology* 1991; 29, 2115–2119

Ayliffe GAJ, Lowbury EJL, Geddes AM, Williams JD. *Control of hospital infection: a practical handbook*, 3rd edn. London: Chapman & Hall, 1992

Ayliffe GAJ, Collins BJ, Taylor LJ. *Hospital – acquired infection. Principles and prevention*. 2nd edn. Oxford: Butterworth-Heinmann, 1993

Babb JR, Davies JG, Ayliffe GAJ. Contamination of protective clothing and nurses uniforms in an isolation ward. *Journal of Hospital Infection* 1983; 4: 49–57

British Medical Association. *A guide to hepatitis C*. London: BMA, 1996

British Standards Institution. *Specification for sharps containers*. BS 7320 HCC/34. London: British Standards Institution, 1990

Bucknole W. (1996) Treating venous ulcers in the community. *Journal of Wound Care* 1996; 5: 258–260

Castille K. (1999) To reuse or not to reuse – that is the question. *Nursing Standard* 1999; 13(34): 48–52

Centers for Disease Control. Case–control study of HIV seroconversion in health care workers after percutaneous exposure to HIV-infected blood: France, United Kingdom and United States: January 1988–August 1994. *Morbidity and Mortality Weekly Report* 1995; 44(50): 929–933

Chintz H, Vibits H, Cordtz TO, et al. Need for surgical wound dressing. *British Journal of Surgery* 1989; 76: 204–205

Communicable Disease Report. *Control of meningococcal disease: guidance for consultants in communicable disease control*. CDR Review, Vol. 5, no. 13. London: PHLS, 1995

Cookson BD, Peters B, Webster M, et al. Staff carriage of epidemic methicillin resistant *Staphylococcus aureus*. *Journal of Clinical Microbiology* 1989; 27: 1471–1476

Department of Health. *Occupational exposure to HIV and use of zidovudine: a statement from the expert advisory group on AIDS*. PL/CO (92) 1. London: HMSO, 1992

Department of Health. Addendum to HSG (93) 40: *Protecting health care workers and patients from hepatitis*. B EL (96) 77. Wetherby: Department of Health, 1996

Department of Health. The Interdepartmental Working Group on Tuberculosis: *UK recommendations for the prevention and control of HIV, tuberculosis and drug resistant tuberculosis*. London: The Stationery Office, 1997

Department of Health. The EPIC Project: developing national evidence based guidelines for preventing healthcare associated infections. *Journal of Hospital Infection* 47(suppl): S1–S82

Garner J. Guideline for isolation precautions in hospital. *American Journal of Infection Control* 1996; 24: 24–52

Gould D. Assessing nurses hand decontamination performance. *Nursing Times* 1993; 89(25): 47–50

Health and Safety Commission. *Control of Substances Hazardous to Health (amendments) Regulations (2004)*. London: The Stationery Office, 2004

Health and Safety Executive. (1995) *Reporting of Injuries, Diseases & Dangerous Occurrences Regulations (RIDDOR)*. London: HMSO, London. 1995

Health Service Advisory Committee. *Safe disposal of clinical waste*. London: HMSO, London, 1992

Health Service Circular. *Controls assurance in infection control: decontamination of medical devices*. HSC 1999/179, NHS Executive. London: Department of Health, 1999a

Health Service Circular. *Variant Creutzfeldt–Jakob disease (vCJD): minimising the risk of transmission*. HSG (95) 18, HSC 1999/178, NHS Executive. London: Department of Health, 1999b

Health Service Guidance. *Decontamination of equipment prior to inspection, service or repair*. HSG (93) 26, NHS Management Executive. London: Department of Health, 1993

Heptonstall J, Porter K, Gill N. *Occupational transmission of HIV. Summary of published reports*. PHLS AIDS Centre. London: CDSC, 1993

Hoffman PN. *Clostridium difficile* and the hospital environment. *PHLS Microbiology Digest* 1993; 10: 91–92

Hollinworth H, Kingston JE. Using a non-sterile technique in wound care. *Professional Nurse* 1998; 13, 4: 226–229

Horton R, Parker L. *Informed infection control practice*, 2nd edn. New York: Churchill Livingstone, 2002

Jackson MM, Lynch P. Isolation practices: a historical perspective. *American Journal of Infection Control* 1985; 13: 21–31

Jefferies DJ. Zidovudine after occupational exposure to HIV. *British Medical Journal* 1991; 302, 1349–1350

Krasner DL, Sibbald RG. Nursing management of chronic wounds. *Nursing Clinics of North America* 1999; 34: 933–955

Lund C, Caruso R. Nursing perspectives: aseptic techniques in wound care. *Dermatology Nursing* 1993; 5: 215–216

Maki DG, Alvarado CJ, Hassemer CA, Zilz MA. Relation of the inanimate environment to endemic nosocomial infection. *New England Journal of Medicine* 1979; 307: 1562–1566

Maki DG, Alvarado C, Hassemer C. Double bagging of items from isolation rooms is unnecessary as an infection control measure: a comparative study of surface contamination with single and double bagging. *Infection Control* 1986; 7: 535–537

Medical Devices Agency. *Sterilization, disinfection & cleaning of medical devices & equipment. Guidance from Microbiology Advisory Committee to Department of Health, Medical Devices Agency, Part 2 protocols*. London: HMSO, 1996

NHS Estates. Health Service Guidance Note. *Safe disposal of clinical waste whole hospital policy guidance*. HMSO, London, 1995

NHS Executive. *Sterilization*. Health Technical Memorandum (HTM) 2010, NHS Estates. HMSO, London, 1994

NHS Management Executive. *Decontamination of equipment prior to inspection, service or repair*. HSG (93) 26, HMSO, London, 1993

NHS Management Executive. *Occupational health services for NHS staff*. HSG (94) 51. London: Department of Health, 1994

NHS Management Executive. *Hospital laundry arrangements for used & infected linen.* HSG (95) 18. London: Department of Health, 1995

Orr NW. Is a mask necessary in the operating theatre? *Annals of Royal College of Surgeons in England* 1981; 63: 390–392

Osterholm MT, Hedberg CW, McDonald KL. Epidemiology of infectious diseases. In: Mandell GL, Bennett JE, Dolin R (eds) *Principles and practice of infectious diseases,* 4th edn. New York: Churchill Livingstone, 1995

Parker LJ. Importance of handwashing in the prevention of cross infection. *British Journal of Nursing* 1999a; 8: 1162–1166

Parker LJ. Current recommendations for isolation practices in nursing. *British Journal of Nursing* 1999b; 8: 881–887

Pudner R. Wound cleansing. *Nursing Standard* 1997; 11(20): 47, 49–51

Rhame FS. The inanimate environment. In: Bennett JV, Brachman PS (eds) *Hospital infections,* 3rd edn. Boston: Little, Brown & Co, 1992

Riyat MS, Quinton DN. Tap water as a wound cleansing agent in Accident and Emergency. *Journal of Accident Emergency Medicine* 1997; 14: 165–166

Rossoff LJ, Lam S, Hilton E, et al. Is the use of boxed gloves in an intensive care unit safe? *American Journal of Medicine* 1993; 94: 602–607

Russell L. Understanding physiology of wound healing and how dressings help. *British Journal of Nursing* 2000; 9: 10–21

Thomas S. Assessment and management of wound exudate. *Journal of Wound Care* 1997; 6: 327–330

Tokars JI, Marcus R, Culver DH. Surveillance of HIV infection and zidovudine use among health care workers after occupational exposure to HIV-infected blood. *Annals of Internal Medicine* 1993; 118: 13–19

Williams C. Wound irrigation techniques: new steripod normal saline. *British Journal of Nursing* 1999; 8: 1460–1462

Wilson J. *Infection control in clinical practice,* 2nd edn. London: Baillière Tindall, 2001

Winter G. Formation of the scab and the rate of epithelialisation of superficial wounds in the skin of the young domestic pig. *Nature* 1962; 193: 293–294

Worsley MA, Ward KA, Parker L, Ayliffe GAJ, Sedgwick J. *Infection control guidelines for nursing care.* Infection Control Nurses Association, 1990

Wysocki AB. Wound fluids and the pathogenesis of chronic wounds. *Journal of Wound Ostomy Continence Nurse* 1996; 23: 283–290

SECTION 3

Resuscitation and stabilisation of the critically ill

SECTION CONTENTS

Chapter 16

Aetiology of cardiac arrest in trauma

John Horton

INTRODUCTION

The two types of cardiac arrest are those due to ventricular fibrillation (VF) or pulseless ventricular tachycardia (VT), and those due to non-VF/VT causes, namely asystole and electromechanical dissociation, which is also known as pulseless electrical activity. The general management of these conditions is discussed in Chapter 18.

Few traumatic cardiac arrests are likely to respond to defibrillation owing to massive underlying blood loss, although the outcome may be different if the initial cause of arrest was a primary cardiac event, i.e. the driver of a car having had a cardiac arrest, which caused the car crash.

The survivors are those whose condition is recognised early and, rather than being transported to definitive care, *definitive care is transported to them*. A recent study by the helicopter emergency medical service (HEMS) from the Royal London Hospital demonstrated only one survivor in a pre-hospital study of 466 traumatic cardiac arrest patients. The patient in question survived following a thoracotomy and insertion of a finger into a single hole in the ventricle, thus tamponading the blood loss.

CARDIAC ARREST IN TRAUMA

The recognition of cardiac arrest in trauma differs from conventional primary cardiac events in two important respects:

1. Generally there is a history or evidence of massive haemorrhage caused by blunt or

penetrating injury, or there is an associated deceleration injury.
2. The prognosis of survival is poor owing to widespread tissue destruction.

Fatalities from trauma are often found in the first of the three peaks of the 'trimodal distribution of death', as described by Donald Trunkey in 1983. This occurs within seconds to minutes of injury. Instantaneous death can be the direct result of massive blood loss from large vessels or organs such as the liver, spleen, heart and great vessels, such as the aorta. Destruction of the spinal cord or brain matter will also result in the same outcome. Public education is possibly the only significant way of reducing this peak of trauma-related deaths, as survival from trauma is only possible in areas within a few minutes of transportation time to a trauma centre.

The second peak occurs within minutes to several hours, and accounts for those individuals with untreated airway obstruction, severe un-treated blood loss and head injuries. Training courses, such as 'Advanced Trauma Life Support™', 'Pre-Hospital Trauma Life Support', 'Battle Trau-matic Life Support', and 'Pre-Hospital Emergency Care' have reduced preventable deaths by providing a logical process that rapidly identifies and treats life-threatening conditions, allowing patients to reach definitive treatment, such as surgical intervention, as quickly as possible.

The third peak accounts for late deaths, occurring days to weeks after the initial event. These are often the result of sepsis and/or multiple organ failure. Deaths at this time may be the long-term consequence of inadequate initial management of the airway leading to cerebral hypoxia or may be due to circulatory crisis.

It can, therefore, be seen that the majority of deaths in trauma can be attributed to hypoxia and circulatory failure.

> The majority of trauma deaths can be attributed to hypoxia and circulatory failure

HYPOXIA

Hypoxia denotes a state of reduced oxygen in the tissues and can be attributable to hypovolaemia.

Other causes of hypoxia include hypoventilation, airway obstruction, sudden apnoea and alveolar anoxia.

Hypoventilation

Hypoventilation leads to a reduction in alveolar ventilation. This produces an increase in arterial PCO_2 (hypercarbia) and a decrease in arterial PO_2 (hypoxaemia). Hypoventilation may be a symp-tom of partial airway obstruction or a short-lived event in total airway obstruction, and will, if not resolved, result in apnoea (i.e. temporary cessa-tion of breathing) and asphyxia. Asphyxia results from a combination of hypoxaemia and hypercarbia.

Airway obstruction

Airway obstruction may be due to compromise of the upper or lower airway, each of which have a range of causes (Box 16.1). Obstruction of the upper airway is most often caused by soft tissue obstruction as a consequence of malpositioning of the head, altered anatomy as a consequence of head or facial trauma (e.g. Le Fort type I and II fractures), or laryngeal trauma. Alternatively, obstruction or compromise of the lower airway and its passages is most often caused by tracheal trauma, bronchospasm (such as that which occurs in an asthmatic crisis), chronic obstructive pulmonary disease and adult respiratory distress syndrome.

Box 16.1   Causes of airway obstruction

Upper airway
- Soft tissue obstruction of the airway caused by malpositioning of the head.
- Altered anatomy as a result of head or facial trauma, e.g. Le Fort type I and II fractures
- Laryngeal trauma

Lower airway
- Tracheal trauma
- Bronchospasm (asthmatic crisis)
- Chronic obstructive pulmonary disease
- Adult respiratory distress syndrome

> **Box 16.2   Mechanical causes of airway obstruction**
>
> **Upper airway**
> - Obstruction caused by foreign body, e.g. vomitus, food bolus, blood, broken teeth
> - Cellulitis of the floor of the mouth, epiglottis and croup
>
> **Lower airway**
> - Inflammatory swelling from aspiration of stomach contents, inhalation of superheated air (fires)

The tongue is the most common cause of airway obstruction

Airway obstruction may also be due to a variety of mechanical causes, some of which affect the upper airway and others which affect the lower airway (Box 16.2). Those affecting the upper airway include foreign bodies, such as blood, vomitus, foodstuffs, blood, teeth or cellulitis of the floor of the mouth, such as that which occurs in epiglottitis or croup. Those affecting the lower airway include inflammatory swelling owing to aspiration of gastric contents, or the inhalation of gases and hot air.

Hypoxia-induced apnoea associated with foreign matter may cause laryngospasm and subsequent airway obstruction, although relaxation of the larynx in such cases may occur just prior to cardiac arrest.

Partial airway obstruction, such as that which occurs in bronchospasm, initially causes a rise in respiratory rate and effort. As the patient tires or the obstruction becomes more severe, asphyxia develops. Hypoxaemia and hypercarbia rapidly follow, leading to secondary apnoea and cardiac arrest.

Complete airway obstruction initially causes a rapid rise in respiratory rate and effort. Intercostal and suprasternal recession is then seen, caused by fluctuations in intrathoracic pressure. Arterial hypertension and tachycardia ensue as a result of sympathetic stimulation. Within two minutes, the patient becomes unconscious, as the PaO_2 drops to approximately 30 mmHg ($SaO_2 < 50\%$). Apnoea follows in 2–6 minutes. As the PaO_2 reaches 10 mmHg, pulselessness occurs and asystole develops within 5–10 minutes. Circulatory failure occurs as a consequence of hypoxia, acidosis from the rapid rise of CO_2 and the build-up of lactic and carbonic acid in the blood and tissues. The pH of arterial blood at this stage has fallen to 6.5–6.8.

If cardiopulmonary resuscitation is started within 2–5 minutes of cardiac arrest, the prognosis of recovery with an intact central nervous system is reasonably good. Beyond 20 minutes, the outlook is poor owing to the severe acidosis.

In cases of slow asphyxiation, such as crush injury to the chest, as little as 1–2 minutes of arrest, either respiratory or cardiac, have been shown to cause permanent neurological deficit. The prognosis is also generally poor when associated with pre-existing conditions or other injuries, which may have caused a prolonged decrease in PaO_2 and cardiac output *prior* to airway obstruction. The assumption is that an acute rise in cerebral acidosis during asphyxiation leads to comparatively greater brain damage than the same period of primary VF-induced cardiac arrest.

Sudden apnoea may occur as the result of high-voltage electric shock or an intravenous injection of opiates. Anaesthetic agents, hypnotics and paralysing doses of depolarising/non-depolarising muscle relaxants (as used during anaesthesia) will have the same effect. Head injuries that lead to marked increases in intracranial pressure can result in cerebral herniation and acute respiratory depression.

Alveolar anoxia is rare and is only found in patients who have been subjected to oxygen-free gas, such as in mining or cave incidents, industrial accidents and rapid decompression emergencies, such as those experienced by divers and pilots.

Hyperventilation is spontaneous in the oxygen-free environment. The sudden change from breathing oxygen to breathing oxygen-free gas causes rapid cerebral failure, respiratory arrest, hypotension within one minute, bradycardia, pupillary dilation and, ultimately, cardiac arrest (asystole) within 3–7 minutes. Metabolic processes, such as carbon dioxide removal from anoxic tissues, will continue until the oxygen debt stops the heart. The associated respiratory and metabolic acidosis may be lower than those levels found in conventional asphyxia.

Survival in high-altitude or mixed-gas (low oxygen concentration) environments is limited and death is imminent, if the period of exposure is prolonged.

The mechanism of death by alveolar hypoxia is the same as that of hypoxaemia from pulmonary disease. When the PaO_2 reaches 30 mmHg, cerebral vessels have reached their maximum dilation. Any further reduction in PaO_2 will result in cerebral anaerobiosis. Cardiac arrest is likely to occur when the PaO_2 is approximately 15–25 mmHg. In the presence of such pronounced hypoxaemia, cardiac and cerebral function will cease. Survival is dependent on early removal from the hostile environment or by the provision of a resuscitation system that can provide significantly raised FiO_2 levels.

CIRCULATORY FAILURE

> Shock is a momentary pause in the act of death
> John Collins Wadden 1895

Shock is defined as an inadequate supply of oxygen or nutrients to the tissue following trauma and can be caused by any or all of the following conditions:

- reduced venous return
- hypovolaemia
- cardiac contusion
- neurogenic dysfunction
- sepsis.

Reduced venous return

The amount of blood returning to the heart is dependent on the pressure gradient created between the high hydrostatic pressure in the peripheral veins and the low hydrostatic pressure in the right atrium. If the relationship is altered, say by higher pressure in the right atrium, such as that caused by tension pneumothorax or cardiac tamponade, there will be a reduction in the venous return to the heart and subsequent circulatory failure leading to death.

Hypovolaemia

If there is loss of blood from the arterial or venous circulation (haemorrhage), the circulating blood volume will escape into a cavity (e.g. thorax, abdomen, pelvis, retroperitoneum or muscles), or externally (e.g. open fractures or lacerations), once again compromising venous return. Haemorrhage is the most common cause of shock in trauma patients.

Cardiac contusions

Cardiac contusions caused by blunt trauma to the thorax have a negative inotropic effect on the heart, thus reducing cardiac output. Concomitant use of antiarrhythmic agents with a negative inotropic affect may compromise such situations further. At least 40% of the left ventricular myocardium must be damaged before true cardiogenic shock occurs.

Neurogenic dysfunction

The reflex tachycardia that is vectored by the sympathetic nervous system in response to hypovolaemia is dependent on the effective functioning of the spinal cord above T6. An injury to the spinal cord above this level will result in widespread vasodilatation, bradycardia, dysfunctional temperature control and the state of neurogenic shock. Neurogenic shock will also cause a decrease in blood supply to the spinal column, thus increasing damage to the nervous tissue. Spinal blood flow will be further reduced by any other associated haemorrhage.

Sepsis

Gram-negative bacteria, often associated with dirt-laden injuries, are responsible for most cases of septic shock. Circulating endotoxins, originating from bacteraemia or sepsis, cause vasodilatation and adversely affect the use of energy. The endotoxins make the capillary walls leaky, allowing sodium and water to move freely from the interstitial space into the intracellular space, further compounding any pre-existing hypovolaemic state. In the late stages of sepsis, it may be almost impossible to differentiate between the various potential causes of shock, as several may be attributable.

SUMMARY

Cardiac arrest following trauma has a bleak prognosis.

Shock following trauma need not be a permanent state: patients die if it is not treated, but many will survive if shock is aggressively treated by early controlled fluid resuscitation and early surgical intervention. If management is not instigated early, an ever-increasing compromise in tissue oxygenation will develop. Cells will revert to anaerobic respiration and the build-up of lactic acid that develops will lead to intracellular and systemic acidosis. The toxins that are released as the condition continues to deteriorate will ultimately lead to multiple organ failure and cardiac arrest. Often it is predictable where there has been inadequate fluid resuscitation in the early stages of shock. This decline is a common cause of late death amongst trauma patients. Patients who survive the second peak of the trimodal distribution of death often go on to die in the third peak of death as a direct result of poor initial shock management.

Aggressive resuscitation must be instigated immediately to provide a clear airway and adequate ventilation with high-flow concentrated oxygen, and circulatory support must be given. The only true hope of survival depends on rapid transportation of the patient to definitive care, where expert help may be of benefit.

Further reading

Safer P. *Cardio Pulmonary Resuscitation*, 1976
Driscoll, PA, et al *Trauma resuscitation – the team approach.*
  Macmillan Press Ltd, 1993

Chapter **17**

Basic life support in adults

Brenda Cottam

INTRODUCTION

The term 'basic life support' (BLS) refers to the essential and simple techniques for assessing and determining life-threatening problems with airway patency, breathing and circulation, then treating these with no additional equipment. If equipment such as a faceshield, pocket mask or active compression–decompression device (ACD) is used, then the term becomes 'basic life support with airway adjunct/ACD...' etc.

BLS guidelines ensure optimal rescuer ability to maintain life, giving oxygen via expired air ventilation and circulating this to vital organs, particularly the heart and brain. This chapter presents the European Resuscitation Council (ERC) guidelines for adult BLS as published by Handley et al. (2001) and is included to reflect the overall important of BLS in the management of the trauma patient. Some modifications to the techniques outlined in the guidelines have been noted, where appropriate. Of key importance is the need to remember that the object of BLS is to sustain the essentials of life until more advanced assistance is available to definitively treat the cause of the problem.

These basic techniques also form the backbone of more advanced resuscitation techniques outlined in Chapter 18 and do not cease to be important when more advanced help arrives.

Andréasson et al. (1998) highlight studies discussing outcomes of sudden cardiopulmonary arrest. Survival rates vary with a mean of 15% for in-hospital arrests having been identified. This figure is less for out of hospital arrests, mainly due to delayed essential cardiopulmonary resuscitation (CPR). De Vos et al. (1998) indicate difficulty in predicting outcome from cardiopulmonary arrest whilst Varon et al. (1998) remind us that some reversible conditions have better outcomes. In the absence of a complete medical history, documentation of 'do not attempt resuscitation' (DNAR) orders or a definitive immediate reason not to start CPR (McIntyre, 1980), it is advisable to attempt resuscitation even though it may not be successful.

Although BLS tends to be considered a 'holding' management option, maintaining oxygen delivery primarily to the heart and brain, simple techniques may be the definitive treatment required and recovery may occur without further intervention.

> Complete neurological recovery is doubtful unless cerebral ischaemia is reversed within minutes

Emphasis is on assessing and treating as quickly as possible after onset of cardiac arrest. Following a simple A (airway), B (breathing), C (circulation) sequence of assessment and 'treat what you find' management, the possibility of recovery is increased.

EUROPEAN RESUSCITATION COUNCIL (ERC) GUIDELINES 2000 FOR ADULT BASIC LIFE SUPPORT

In relaying the European Resuscitation Council guidelines, any reference to the victim is written in the masculine form for ease of reading, but applies equally to both males and females.

Safe approach

As trauma is the leading cause of death under approximately 40 years of age (Driscoll et al., 1993), any rescuer attempting to approach any victim must ensure *their own safety first*. A traumatic event causing injury to the victim could also cause injury or worse to the rescuer. If possible, the environment should be made safe. If not, the relevant emergency services should be summoned immediately for expert help. Although unfortu-

nate, the victim could lose their life, but many media reports have also documented the loss of rescuers' lives in attempts to save others. Once the situation is perceived safe, the rescuer can assess the victim.

> Personal safety is paramount

Response

Check for any response from the victim. Speaking to him on approach to assess conscious level may be all that is required. If he responds, leave him in the position found and determine the nature of the problem. If any first-aid measures are required, for example, pressure on a bleeding wound, perform this and summon immediate medical assistance. With no first-aid equipment to hand, it is better to leave the victim as found to ensure *no further harm*. Reassurance will help, particularly the knowledge that emergency medical assistance is en route.

If the victim does not respond to verbal stimuli, his upper arms should be grasped carefully and squeezed tightly, simultaneously speaking to him again. In traumatic situations, it is important to avoid shaking or movement, thus preventing unnecessary cervical spine movement. If this generates a response assess breathing then send for immediate assistance. Perform any first-aid measures required and monitor him closely. Repeated checks of airway patency, respiratory effort and circulation are required, noting any improvement or deterioration.

If the victim is completely *unresponsive* to verbal or tactile stimuli, the rescuer should shout for help but remain with the victim and start the ABC assessment.

Airway

Assess airway patency. If trauma is suspected, it is important to leave the victim in the position initially found, and then check for breathing for no longer than 10 seconds. If breathing is present and unlaboured, this indicates that he is maintaining his own airway. In this situation, help should be summoned and the patient monitored.

If there is *any difficulty in breathing* or breathing is absent, the airway must be cleared to allow adequate respiration. The mouth should be opened slightly and a check made for any obvious visible obstructions. Particulate matter should be removed using a finger sweep. The removal of liquids may be facilitated by briefly turning the head to one side to drain them. This may mean having to log roll the victim if there are sufficient rescuers to assist.

Leave *well-fitting* dentures in place

To open the airway and raise the tongue from the posterior wall of the pharynx, the advised technique is the head tilt–chin lift manoeuvre. One hand should be placed across the forehead, preventing rotational movement of the head, and the head tilted back, simultaneously lifting the chin with two fingers of the other hand (Figure 17.1). In unconscious individuals, this manoeuvre alone may be all that is required to allow adequate respiration.

If trauma is suspected, particularly to the cervical spine, then this technique should be modified. Using one hand to stabilise the forehead, the chin lift alone can be used to lift the tongue from the back of the airway. Preferably, the safer jaw-thrust manoeuvre allows adequate airway opening whilst providing in-line stabilisation of the cervical spine (Figure 17.2).

Breathing

Once the airway is open, this should be maintained and regular checks for breathing carried out. This may be performed by looking along the victim's chest and abdomen for movement, listening at his nose and mouth for breath sounds, and feeling for air movement. This should be performed for 10 seconds, observing for respiration beyond the occasional agonal gasp.

If the victim is breathing airway maintenance takes priority

The recovery position is used to allow the victim to lie in a position that ensures the tongue falls to the side of the mouth and allows drainage of secretions, which could collect in the pharynx if the victim remains supine (Figure 17.3). Much debate surrounds the preferred recovery position to use (Higginson and Beale, 1998; Turner et al., 1998). The ERC recommendations are shown in Box 17.1.

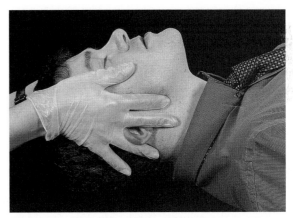

Figure 17.2   Jaw-thrust manoeuvre.

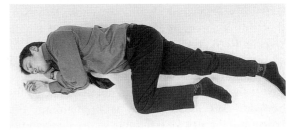

Figure 17.3   Recovery position.

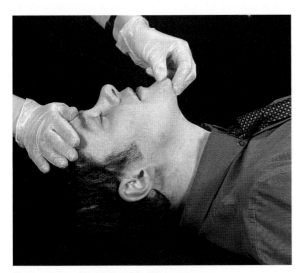

Figure 17.1   Head tilt–chin lift manoeuvre.

Box 17.1   Recovery position

Step 1
Straighten the victim's legs. Remove any spectacles and objects in the pockets nearest to you. (Keep these items with him!).

Step 2
Lay the near arm out at right angles to his body – shoulder high, palm facing upwards. Bend the elbow up at a right angle or to the nearest comfortable position.

Step 3
Bring the far arm across his chest. Lay the palm of your hand against the palm of his hand and hold the back of his hand against his near cheek. Keep this hand in position, otherwise it will fall back on to his chest.

Step 4
With your other hand holding just above the knee, bend the far leg up until his foot rests flat on the floor. Pull *towards* you, moving back slightly to allow his body to roll over under its own momentum. *The hand holding his palm allows you to control the way his head turns.* Move his upper leg forwards off his lower leg, and rest this with hip and knee bent at right angles.

Step 5
Tilt the head back, ensuring the hand under the cheek assists in maintaining the airway.
In this position, it is possible to check breathing and circulation as necessary.

In trauma-related situations where cervical spine injury is suspected, the recommended modification is to avoid moving the victim to prevent potential further harm. However, the airway is the priority; if possible, this should be maintained using the jaw-thrust manoeuvre and manual in-line cervical spinal immobilisation until help arrives. It should be noted, however, that this manoeuvre can be tiring for a single rescuer. Roth et al. (1998) describe a technique of maintaining the airway by stabilising the head (one hand on the forehead) and lifting the lower jaw at the chin. Again, this is not always easy to perform. The *absolute need* is to maintain the patency of the airway. If the above two manoeuvres are not possible, or the rescuer is tiring or losing

the airway, the recovery position should be employed.

Expired air ventilation

If the victim is *not* breathing or an occasional gasp only is detected when assessing breathing, then immediate emergency medical assistance should be summoned. If no one has responded to the initial shout for help, the victim must be left alone at this stage if there is a telephone/help nearby. On returning to the victim, there is no need to reassess him. Apnoea has already been established, so should be managed using expired air ventilation techniques. To perform expired air ventilation, the victim should be on his back and the airway reopened.

Using one hand, the mouth should be kept slightly open, remembering not to allow the lower jaw to drop. The forehead should be supported and the fleshy part of his nose pinched with the other hand to occlude the nostrils. Taking a breath in, the rescuer should place his/her mouth over the victim's, completely covering it and sealing his mouth. Breaths should be given steadily over 2 seconds, observing his chest for movement. The aim is to deliver two breaths that cause the chest to rise and fall visibly, as would be noticed with unlaboured, normal, spontaneous respiration.

Five attempts are initially allowed to achieve two adequate breaths. Sometimes one or two attempts are required to open the airway adequately or to achieve a good seal. Excessive chest movement should be avoided but adequate chest movement should be visualised. In an adult, this indicates that the desired volume of 700–1000 ml of air has been delivered (Handley et al., 2001). After each inflation, the rescuer should take his/her mouth away from the victim's. The chest should be allowed to fall and expired air felt on the cheek. This may take 1 or 2 seconds, and possibly longer. The chest should be allowed to fall fully before delivering the next breath. Rescue breaths can be difficult to perform; however, some problems can be easily corrected (Table 17.1). After two effective breaths have been delivered, the victim should be assessed for signs of circulation. If, after five attempts to deliver rescue breaths, no chest movement is detected, the rescuer should move

Table 17.1   Some problems encountered during mouth-to-mouth expired air ventilation attempts

Problem	Solution(s)
High level of resistance felt when attempting to breathe into victim	Recheck mouth for obstructions. Readjust the airway – it may not be fully open. Perform rescue breaths more gently and slowly
Air leaking from nose/mouth	Pinch fleshy part of nostrils. Ensure mouth covers victim's mouth fully. Do not 'blow' into victim too quickly
'Vibration' or 'gurgling' in victim's throat	Check breathing again. Victim may be attempting spontaneous respiration. Readjust airway. Check for secretions in back of mouth; clear if necessary
No chest rise in victim	Check mouth for obstruction. Readjust airway. *Slightly* increase force of breath into victim

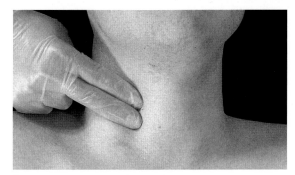

Figure 17.4   Carotid pulse check.

on to chest compressions (see choking guidance later).

Circulation

The optimal site to assess the 'circulatory motorway' to the brain is the main carotid artery located in the hollow between the Adam's apple and the sternocleidomastoid muscle in the neck (Figure 17.4). The pads, not the tips, of two or three fingers should be placed into this hollow, checking for the presence of a pulse for 10 seconds. Owing to documented discrepancies in assessing carotid pulse (Eberle, 1996; Mather and O'Kelly, 1996), it is also recommended that other signs of perfusion to the brain are checked. Whilst checking for a pulse, the victim should be observed for signs of movement, breathing, cough reflex, swallowing, etc., all of which are suggestive of cerebral perfusion.

> If there are *definite* signs of life/circulation, then continue rescue breathing as necessary

As an average expired air ventilation cycle takes several seconds, ten rescue breaths should be given (approximately 1 minute of mouth-to-mouth resuscitation) followed by a 10-second reassessment to detect any signs of circulation, repeated as necessary.

Trauma-related events can lead to difficulty in performing expired air ventilation. The mouth may be damaged and mouth to nose ventilation may provide an alternative [American Heart Association and International Liaison Committee on Resuscitation (ILCOR), 2000]. The whole face may be damaged, making basic expired air ventilation measures impossible, in which case compression-only CPR is better than no CPR at all (Kern et al., 1998).

An airway can be maintained by a rescuer if cervical spine injury is suspected, as described earlier, but it is unlikely that a single rescuer could perform adequate mouth-to-mouth ventilation using a jaw-thrust. A pocket facemask adjunct would allow jaw-thrust manoeuvres and expired air ventilation to be performed. If no such adjunct is available, the priority is to ensure that expired air ventilation is carried out.

If the casualty is not breathing, use the safest technique possible. Some may find that the only way to provide this is to perform a *minimal* head tilt, chin lift manoeuvre but this *must* result in *adequate* ventilation.

Chest compression

If, on assessment of an unconscious apnoeic adult, there is doubt about signs of circulation or circulation is absent, chest compressions should be commenced to perfuse the heart and brain. External cardiac compression allows blood to be expelled from the heart and thorax via patent arteries, thereby providing around 25–30% of normal cardiac output, sufficient to supply the heart and brain (American Heart Association and ILCOR, 2000).

Kneeling beside the victim, the rescuer should use the hand nearest the victim's legs to locate the lower margin of the ribcage. Using the middle and index fingers to trace up the costal margin until the junction between this and the base of the sternum is located, the middle finger should be placed on this junction and the index finger next to it on the lower end of the sternum itself.

The *heel* of the hand nearest to the victim's head should be slid down the sternum until it meets the index finger at the lower end of the sternum. The index and middle finger should *not* be covered. This should ensure that the heel of the hand is in the middle of the lower half of the sternum, thus avoiding the weaker xiphisternum and positioning the hand over the heart to max-imise efficiency of external cardiac compression.

The heel of the other hand should be placed on top of this, and the palm and fingers raised from the chest wall, leaving only the heel of the hand in contact with the sternum. Elbows should be straight. The rescuer, kneeling close to the victim, should have his or her shoulders, arms and wrists in a vertical line down on to the sternum. Kneeling up and looking vertically down on the victim's far arm may help achieve the correct position.

The victim's chest should be compressed rhythmically to a depth of 4–5 cm at a rate of around 100 per minute. Compression:relaxation of the chest should be equal in both time and depth. The hands should not be lifted off the chest during compressions. Fifteen compressions should be performed before returning to perform two venti-lations. A rate of fifteen compressions in 10–12 seconds achieves the approximate rate required (Handley et al., 2001).

Common problems in chest compression technique and the possible resulting consequences are listed in Table 17.2.

> The ratio of compressions to ventilations CPR is 15:2, however many rescuers are available

Once full CPR has been commenced, there is no need to pause and check the victim. The likeli-hood of chest compression restarting the heart is remote. If, however, any of the following occur, resuscitation should be stopped and the situation re-assessed:

- the victim shows some sign(s) of life (e.g. cough, gasp, movement, gag reflex, swallowing)
- CPR trained help arrives to assist
- the rescuer becomes too tired to continue and would, therefore, be ineffective
- the environment becomes unsafe and the rescuer needs to leave the victim.

It is interesting to note the effects of rescuer fatigue. Depth and rate of compression can

Table 17.2 Some problems noted with external cardiac compression techniques and possible consequence to the victim

Technique fault	Consequence
'Bouncing' on chest	Incorrect hand placement, if not remeasured, resulting in possible sternal or rib fractures/dislocations. Incorrect hand placement reduces efficiency of output achieved
Incomplete relaxation of chest	Heart unable to refill fully, therefore, reduced 'stroke volume' per compression
Rate too fast	Heart unable to refill fully
No landmark check for hand placement	Potential damage to sternum, ribs and underlying organs Reduces quality of output, if located incorrectly
Arms bending at elbows	Early rescuer fatigue, less effective compression
'Rocking' over chest	Potential/reduced output as directional force through chest will vary

deteriorate within less than 5 minutes of commencing resuscitation. Therefore, there should be no embarrassment or guilt if a rescuer tires quickly and either requires someone else to take over or, if alone, has to stop (Ochoa et al., 1998).

Adjuncts in the form of active compression–decompression devices for performing external chest compression–decompression are available. Mauer et al. (1999) studied the advantages and disadvantages, and note that training is required to use these effectively; an approach highly recommended by Baubin et al. (1999) to prevent potential thoracic injury.

In the context of trauma, chest injuries may cause problems for the rescuer. The rescuer should follow guidance to do the best s/he can without creating further harm, remembering that to do something is better than to do nothing. Suominen et al. (1998) describe a paediatric study suggesting that survival from trauma-related cardiopulmonary arrest is very poor. However, some attempt should be made and delivery of the best care within the constraints of BLS attempted.

Summoning help

The importance of summoning more advanced medical assistance and access to definitive care cannot be emphasised enough. Once the need for medical assistance has been established, help must be mobilised. In the conscious victim, a brief overview only of the problem should be carried out and help summoned. In the unconscious victim, the airway should be opened to check for breathing. If the victim is apnoeic, medical help must be summoned immediately. In adult cardio-respiratory arrest situations, the primary cause tends to be cardiac in nature. If due to a dysrhythmia, such as ventricular fibrillation or pulseless ventricular tachycardia, the only definitive treatment is defibrillation.

> Sending for assistance to mobilise a defibrillator is vital, owing to the significance of time lapse reducing the chance of successfully terminating dysrhythmias

When more than one rescuer is present, one should commence relevant resuscitation, whilst the other goes for help. The difficulty arises when there is only a single rescuer. In this situation, the rescuer must leave the victim unattended, if there is a telephone nearby. If the environment is isolated with no resource for obtaining help, the rescuer should treat as able for as long as able, while realising that the efforts may be futile, but *may* also be enough to sustain life until definitive help becomes available.

A number of occasions have been identified where a single rescuer should commence resuscitation first, *then* go for help after approximately one minute. These are:

- trauma-related incidents
- drowning incidents
- choking incidents
- intoxication by alcohol or drugs
- paediatric patients.

The rationale for this is that the cause of arrest is *unlikely* to be cardiac in origin and, therefore, possibly secondary to a respiratory problem. If this is the case, one minute of resuscitation may help to mediate the effects of hypoxia (American Heart Association and ILCOR, 2000).

Choking

This chapter on basic life support would not be complete without guidance for choking. This can be immediately life saving and, should an unconscious victim be found with an airway obstruction, offers the rescuer a chance to relieve this effectively.

If the victim is *conscious* and choking, he should be encouraged to cough, as this is often effective in removing partial obstructions. If he becomes weaker or if the obstruction is complete (no air passing in or out of the nose/mouth), a sequence of five back blows followed by five abdominal thrusts should be given. To deliver effective back blows, the heel of the hand should be used between the scapulae. For abdominal thrusts the side of the fist of one hand should be placed in the space between his navel and the costal margins, sharply pulling inwards and upwards by placing the other hand over the fist to do so. This forces the diaphragm upwards. Both back blows and abdominal thrusts are performed by approaching the victim from behind; therefore, it is important to explain what is being done, reassuring him and ensuring that he leans forward to help move any dislodged foreign body towards the mouth. These cycles should be continued as necessary.

Nowitz et al. (1998) identify associated risks with abdominal thrusts; these should, therefore, only be performed where necessary, ceasing treatment once the obstruction is relieved. The patency of the airway and breathing should be reassessed and constantly monitored.

Should the victim become unconscious, he must be laid on his back, the airway opened and breathing checked. Any *obvious* obstruction should be removed from the mouth by a finger sweep. Rescue breaths should be attempted as described earlier, aiming to deliver two effective rescue breaths. In an unconscious victim, the airway may relax a little, so it may be possible to administer some expired air into his lungs.

If attempts at rescue breaths are unsuccessful, 15 chest compressions should be commenced as described earlier *without* checking for signs of circulation. The compressions in this situation aim to relieve the obstruction. After this, the mouth should be rechecked and two rescue breaths attempted before returning to chest compressions and continuing as required. Medical assistance should be summoned after approximately 1 minute (approximately four cycles of breaths:compressions). This sequence should be continued until help arrives or the obstruction is relieved and the victim starts breathing *effectively*; signs of circulation should then be sought and the patient placed in the recovery position, monitoring breathing and circulation.

SUMMARY

Assess the airway, breathing and circulatory (ABC) needs of the victim, and treat whatever is found at the time of assessment (Figure 17.5). Trauma-related situations can present difficult management options but, with modification *not*

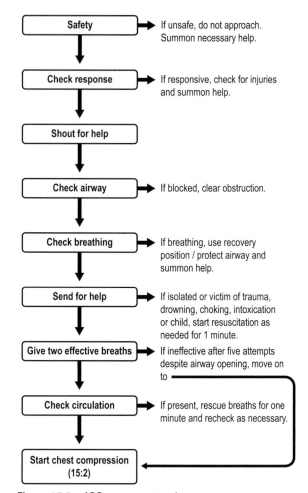

Figure 17.5   ABC assessment and treatment.

compromise of technique, basic life support may still be effective. The need for medical help is vital as soon as any individual is found to be unconscious in order to diagnose and treat the cause. Help must, therefore, be sought as soon as possible within these guidelines.

Resuscitation guidelines are refined and updated regularly as science and evidence guide optimal patient management. It is important to keep up to date with current guidelines. Updates are widely publicised in national nursing and medical press.

References

American Heart Association in collaboration with the International Liaison Committee on Resuscitation (ILCOR). Guidelines 2000 for cardiopulmonary resuscitation and emergency cardiac care – an international consensus on science. *Resuscitation* 2000; 46: 29–71

Andréasson AC, Herlitz J, Bång A et al. Characteristics and outcome among patients with a suspected in-hospital cardiac arrest. *Resuscitation* 1998; 39: 23–31

Baubin M, Sumann G, Rabl W, Eibl G, Wenzel V, Mair P. Increased frequency of thorax injuries with ACD-CPR. *Resuscitation* 1999; 41: 33–38

de Vos R, Koster RW, de Haan RJ. Impact of survival probability, life expectancy, quality of life and patient preferences on do-not-attempt-resuscitation orders in a hospital. *Resuscitation* 1998; 39: 15–21

Driscoll PA, Gwinnutt CL, Le Duc Jimmerson C, Goodall O. *Trauma resuscitation. The team approach.* London: Macmillan, 1993: 1.

Eberle B, Dick WF, Schneider T et al. Checking the carotid pulse check: diagnostic accuracy of first responders in patients with and without a pulse. *Resuscitation* 1996; 33: 107–116

Handley AJ, Koenraad GM, Bossaert LL. European Resuscitation Council guidelines 2000 for adult basic life support. *Resuscitation* 2001; 48: 199–205

Higginson I, Beale P, Covey L, Kerwin-Nye A. Haines recovery position. *Pre-hospital Immediate Care* 1998; 2(2): 115 (letters).

Kern K, Hilwig RW, Berg RA, Ewy GA. Efficacy of chest compression – only BLS CPR in the presence of an occluded airway. *Resuscitation* 1998; 39: 179–188

Mather C, O'Kelly S. The palpation of pulses. *Anaesthesia* 1996; 51: 189–191

Mauer DK, Nolan J, Plaisance P, et al. Effect of active compression–decompression resuscitation (ACD–CPR) on survival: a combined analysis using individual patient data. *Resuscitation* 1999; 41: 249–256

McIntyre KM. Medicolegal aspects of CPR and emergency cardiac care. *Journal of the American Medical Association* 1980; 244: 511–512

Nowitz A, Lewer BMF, Galletly DC. An interesting complication of the Heimlich manoevre. *Resuscitation* 1998; 39: 129–131

Ochoa FJ, Ramalle-Gómara E, Lisa V, Saralegui I. The effect of rescuer fatigue on the quality of chest compressions. *Resuscitation* 1998; 37: 149–152

Roth B, Magnusson J, Johansson I, Holmberg S, Westrin P. Jaw lift – a simple and effective method to open the airway in children. *Resuscitation* 1998; 39: 171–174

Suominen P, Räsänen J, Kivioja A. Efficacy of cardiopulmonary resuscitation in pulseless paediatric trauma patients. *Resuscitation* 1998; 36: 9–13

Turner S, Turner I, Chapman D, et al. A comparative study of the 1992 and 1997 recovery positions for use in the UK. *Resuscitation* 1998; 39: 153–160

Varon J, Marik PE, Fromm RE. Cardiopulmonary resuscitation: a review for clinicians. *Resuscitation* 1998; 36: 133–145

Chapter **18**

Advanced life support in adults

Brenda Cottam

INTRODUCTION

The guidance for basic life support (BLS) discussed in Chapter 17 leaves little room for interpretation and manipulation. However, guidelines for advanced life support (ALS) have been simplified greatly over the past 5–10 years to enable multidisciplinary groups to provide essential life-saving measures within individual abilities.

The guidelines presented here are those of the European Resuscitation Council (ERC), as agreed by the International Liaison Committee on Resuscitation (ILCOR) in 2000 and finalised by de Latorre et al. in 2001. Depending on the level of staff training, resources available and capacity for more advanced continued care, these guidelines can be more widely interpreted.

Various aspects of advanced resuscitation will be considered in this chapter. Varon et al. (1998) remind us that some causes of cardiac arrest are associated with better outcomes. The more reversible causes will be discussed along with specific guidance for emergency treatment.

> The value of defibrillation is unquestioned, particularly in witnessed cardiac arrest with shockable rhythms

Difficulty is often experienced in interpreting cardiac rhythms. A synopsis of the recommended system of interpretation proposed in the *Advanced life support manual* (Resuscitation Council, 2000) will be considered, in addition to the treatment of non-fatal but potentially life-threatening periarrest dysrhythmias.

Decisions regarding when to cease a resuscitation attempt are often difficult. The process of making this decision and how it can be achieved will be highlighted.

ADULT ADVANCED LIFE SUPPORT GUIDELINES 2000 (ERC)

Historically, many countries and continents published their own guidelines for resuscitation. In response to this, an international group of experts recognised the need for a consensus in the treatment of cardiac arrest. This culminated in an International Liaison Committee on Resuscitation (ILCOR) being convened in 1992 to achieve this consensus. The ERC guidelines 2000 are based on this consensus and appear as a simple algorithm (Figure 18.1). This algorithm enables Advanced Life Support (ALS) to begin whether delivered by a first-responder with only BLS capabilities plus defibrillation or by a fully equipped trauma resuscitation team with back-up medical and surgical facilities.

Establishing cardiac arrest and initiation of cardiopulmonary resuscitation

Irrespective of whether cardiopulmonary resuscitation (CPR) is ongoing as the patient is received into hospital, or whether his or her status changes whilst in care, assessment to establish cardiac arrest is the same. The guidance outlined in relation to BLS should be followed based on assessing conscious level, airway patency, breathing and circulation. BLS measures should be commenced as appropriate.

The main modification with regard to ALS is airway maintenance incorporating cervical spine control, described in more detail later. Maintaining BLS is vital as a 'holding' measure until the underlying cardiac rhythm and possible cause of arrest is established. The one occasion when this assessment and initial treatment differs slightly relates to the situation where a patient has suffered a witnessed cardiac arrest, usually characterised by sudden loss of consciousness and no central pulse, or if electrocardiogram (ECG) monitoring shows a sudden rhythm change to ventricular fibrillation (VF) or pulseless ventricular tachycardia (VT). In this event, a precordial thump may terminate the event quickly, reversing the dysrhythmia and

hopefully restoring *return of spontaneous circulation* (ROSC). Robertson (1992) provides evidence to support the potential benefit of the precordial thump. Caldwell et al. (1985) also cite witnessed successful termination of pulseless VT in 17 patients and VF in five patients from a significant number of cardiac arrest events. The precordial thump is delivered to the area where chest compression is performed, once only, and can generate around 10–20 joules (J) of energy through the chest.

Establish cardiac rhythm monitoring

Several methods of monitoring the patient exist. As the rapid treatment of VF or pulseless VT is one of the most significant factors influencing survival from cardiac arrest, monitoring and defibrillation (if indicated) should be carried out as soon as possible (Bossaert et al., 1997). One person can maintain BLS, whilst another establishes cardiac monitoring. This monitoring can be established via standard three-lead or five-lead ECG monitoring, defibrillator paddles or adhesive pads.

The operator *must* be familiar with the equipment and ensure it is functioning correctly

Once monitoring is established, the decision regarding which 'arm' of the algorithm to follow can be made.

Pulse checks

Pulse checks to confirm cardiac arrest are carried out in association with establishing cardiac monitoring or as prompted by automated external defibrillators (AEDs). Pulse checks are performed for 10 seconds. As each side of the algorithm loops, or if rhythm changes are noted, a pulse check should be performed. It is, however, reasonable to omit pulse checks if, in the VF/VT protocol, defibrillation plus CPR has made *no difference* to the rhythm. If the rhythm was pulseless before defibrillation, it is unlikely to have a pulse afterwards, if the rhythm is unchanged.

VENTRICULAR FIBRILLATION/VENTRICULAR TACHYCARDIA

Bossaert et al. (1997) state that the only definitive treatment for VF or pulseless VT is electrical

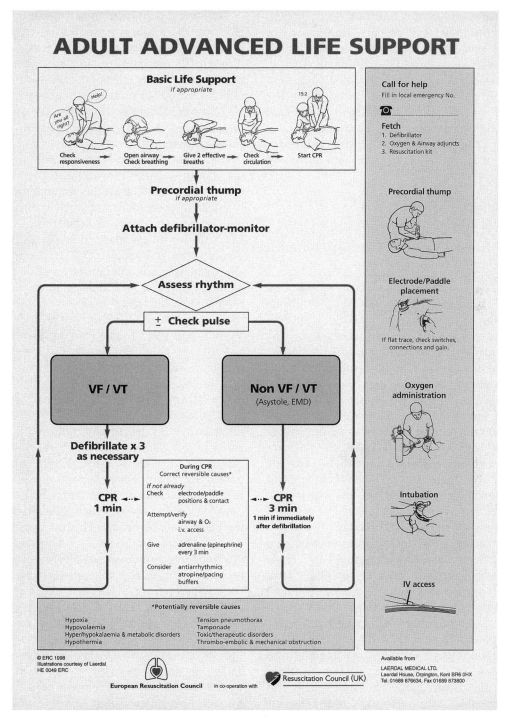

Figure 18.1   Adult advanced life support treatment algorithm. (Reproduced with permission from Laerdal Medical.)

defibrillation and maintenance of oxygenation. The identification of these two rhythms relies either on staff at the scene interpreting a monitored rhythm, or on an AED analysing the rhythm. Once established, it must be confirmed the patient is not only pulseless but is also unconscious. The diagnosis of cardiopulmonary arrest is a *clinical* one based on this assessment. Parish et al. (2003) state that VF usually occurs as a result of coronary artery disease, so may be a rarer complication of trauma-related events.

> Initial defibrillation should be performed as soon as possible to influence survival (Varon et al., 1998)

Defibrillation

If VF/VT occur as a monitored event, defibrillation should be carried out without delay for BLS, if equipment is at hand. The only acceptable delay to defibrillation is performing a precordial thump, which takes seconds. If equipment is not ready or immediately available, then BLS should be commenced until defibrillation is possible.

Many emergency departments use manual defibrillators requiring the user to place conductive pads on the patient's chest (to improve the chance of successful defibrillation), place the paddles over these and manually charge and discharge the defibrillator. All of this requires the user to be competent at recognising VF and VT, and in using the manual defibrillator.

Automated external defibrillators are becoming more widely available (Bossaert et al., 1997). These allow a wider range of users to potentially treat cardiac arrest definitively once relevant training has been provided. One advantage is the reduced need for the user to interpret cardiac rhythms; the AED is prompted to analyse the rhythm and in-built software recognises the 'shockable' rhythms (Cobbe et al., 1991). The 'human' element involved in using these machines is the assessment and confirmation of an unconscious and pulseless patient, and the correct positioning of pads. The patient should also be kept still during analysis to prevent artefact. General safety factors associated with manual defibrillation must also be observed with AEDs.

The aim of defibrillation is to send an external electrical shock (direct current) through the chest. If correctly performed, the current will pass through the myocardium and cause a simultaneous contraction of most of the myocardium. This will hopefully stop the fatal dysrhythmia and allow a natural pacemaker within the conduction system to regain control of the cardiac rhythm and restore output.

If the initial shock sequence fails to convert the rhythm to one compatible with a perfusing output, then CPR must be recommenced. This re-establishes cerebral and cardiac oxygenation, which is also vital in influencing survival. Defibrillation is less likely to be successful, if the myocardium is hypoxic. CPR is performed for approximately one minute followed by reassessment of rhythm and further defibrillation, if indicated, continuing cycles as required. As recommended by Kloeck et al. (1997): 'defibrillate VF/VT until VF/VT is no longer present'.

Varon et al. (1998) succinctly reviewed the management of cardiopulmonary arrest, describing the rationale behind the energies used in defibrillation. The ERC recommend an initial monophasic shock energy of 200 J, repeated immediately if unsuccessful, followed by a third shock of 360 J (Robertson et al., 1998). Shocks then continue in groups of three at 360 J as required using the recommended paddle positions of below the right clavicle at the sternal edge and over the cardiac apex in the mid-axillary line on the chest wall (American Heart Association and ILCOR, 2000) (Figure 18.2). Alternative paddle positions (e.g. anterior/posterior) can be used, if repeated defibrillation attempts are unsuccessful (Resuscitation Council UK, 2000).

The American Heart Association (AHA) and ILCOR (2000) describe the advent of biphasic defibrillators, and present impressive evidence of their effectiveness. This technology allows smaller energy levels to be used owing to the shock waveform delivering the current more efficiently through the heart. Torok (2003) highlights an evidence-based review suggesting that biphasic defibrillation is the preferable option.

Guidelines describe the 'biphasic equivalent' of 200 J but, to date, there appears to be no definitive evidence for recommending a particular energy

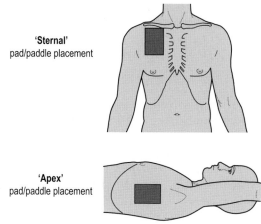

'Sternal'
pad/paddle placement

'Apex'
pad/paddle placement

Figure 18.2   Placement of conductive pads on chest for defibrillation.

level. Relevant manufacturer recommendations for their particular defibrillator should be followed, as waveforms vary with different types.

It is important to remember safety factors

Attention to safety factors is vital. Others must not be in contact with the patient or bed at the time of defibrillation. Oxygen flowing into the immediate environment can support combustion, if a spark occurs. Implanted pacemakers may be adversely affected. Fluids on the chest may result in arcing of the current. This list is by no means exhaustive, and relevant training in manual and automated defibrillation is highly recommended.

Cardiopulmonary resuscitation

Without adequate spontaneous circulation, the patient's heart and brain will not be perfused. The only way to support this in the emergency treatment phase is to ventilate the patient actively and perform external chest compression. Depending on the airway adjuncts available, the patient may be ventilated in a variety of ways, which will be discussed under airway management later in this chapter. Chest compression should be performed as described in Chapter 17.

Active compression–decompression devices may be available. Mauer et al. (1999) provide details of a large study indicating rationale for using these. It is important to remember rescuer

fatigue during CPR; the team and team leader should be vigilant and rescuers should not be afraid to ask for another to take over chest compression (Ashton et al., 2002). Cardiac output generated by external chest compression is limited; a tiring rescuer will reduce this output significantly after only a few minutes.

Other options for cardiac compression include the 'thumper' (a pneumatically driven external chest compressor), 'vest' CPR (again mechanical) or open chest cardiac massage. These require expert technique and equipment, but are employed as necessary in centres equipped to use these methods.

Cardiopulmonary resuscitation must be *effective*, that is, each ventilation should cause the chest to rise and fall adequately, and compressions should generate a palpable output, often monitored at the femoral pulse. If there are airway and ventilation problems, these *must* be managed to ensure adequate ventilation of the patient. CPR should continue with a ratio of 15 compressions to two ventilations. Once the airway is protected definitively (ideally with an endotracheal tube), chest compressions should be performed *continuously* at a rate of 100 per minute and ventilations delivered at a rate of 10–12 breaths per minute. The rationale for this is that coronary and cerebral perfusion pressures remain constant, as opposed to the drop in pressure whilst ventilations take place during the 15:2 ratio of CPR (Resuscitation Council UK, 2000). Continuous compressions are only indicated after the airway is secured because of the risk of regurgitation.

Non–ventricular fibrillation/ventricular tachycardia

Asystole and pulseless rhythms ('pulseless electrical activity'; PEA) *other* than VF/VT are managed in this 'arm' of the algorithm. Parish et al. (2003) identify PEA as being more common than VF/VT in hospital-based cardiac arrests. It occurs as a result of tissue hypoxia or anoxia for a variety of reasons, trauma-related issues being one. The focus of care in a non-shockable cardiac arrest, therefore, is optimal oxygenation of the heart and brain, then searching for, and treating, the cause of arrest. In this non-VF/VT section, with the exception of asystole and agonal rhythms, the conduction system of the heart in PEA is attempting to cause cardiac contraction. However, no output is detected; therefore, the cause of this disturbance should be found and treated, if possible, to enable the return of a spontaneous output.

The guidelines, therefore, show one absolute ongoing requirement – CPR. This maintains the coronary and cerebral blood flow whilst measures are taken to treat reversible causes and administer any drugs required. If the initial rhythm shown is non-VF/VT, 3 minutes of CPR is recommended. As previously mentioned, this must be *effective* CPR.

An exception to the 3 minutes of CPR in the non-VF/VT 'arm' occurs if defibrillation was the *last* intervention before non-VF/VT occurred. Having determined pulselessness, *1 minute* of CPR should be performed prior to a 10-second reassessment of the pulse. If there is still no output, CPR should be continued for the remaining 2 minutes of that cycle and drugs administered. If there *is* a pulse, this precludes the need for further chest compression or adrenaline. Sometimes a 'straight line' appears on the ECG monitor after defibrillation – this could indicate asystole or possible temporary myocardial stunning (Robertson et al., 1998). It is recommended that 1 minute of CPR *without* additional drugs is performed and reassessment carried out. Oxygenating and supporting the myocardium may generate an output. Should a rhythm *compatible* with an output appear after defibrillation but have no associated palpable pulse, the treatment is as above. Following a period of CPR, myocardial contractility may increase and generate a palpable pulse.

During CPR – a window of opportunity for other interventions

The two 'arms' of the advanced life support algorithm show the ongoing continuous treatments required to treat cardiopulmonary arrest based on the rhythm. Whilst CPR is in progress, several interventions can improve the chance of survival.

ELECTRODE/PADDLE POSITIONS AND CONTACT

During the window of opportunity whilst CPR is ongoing, several common management options

are available, whatever the cause of arrest. ECG lead placement to display continuous rhythm is important. In the *initial* stages of assessment, defibrillator paddles/adhesive pads may be used to identify the rhythm. Potential problems using *manual* defibrillator paddles to monitor patients during cardiac arrest have been highlighted (Chamberlain, 1999) but, if this allows VF to be identified and treated quickly, it is a reasonable action to take. Robertson et al. (1998) note that the most common problems associated with defibrillation are incorrect paddle placement and poor chest wall contact. Nurmi et al. (2004) verify this, showing evidence of incorrect paddle/adhesive pad placement despite guidelines placing this high in the priority of interventions to assist successful outcome.

AIRWAY AND OXYGENATION AND/OR INTRAVENOUS ACCESS

'Valid scientific evidence supports only three interventions as unequivocally effective in adult cardiac resuscitation' (Kloeck et al., 1997):

- basic CPR
- defibrillation – if the rhythm is VF or pulseless VT
- tracheal intubation.

Baskett et al. (1996) produced detailed guidance for airway management from basic airway opening techniques and expired air ventilation to more advanced techniques, including surgical airway. These have been only minimally modified in the latest ERC guidelines (de Latorre et al., 2001). Mechanical airway opening devices, such as oral or nasal airways (Figure 18.3), laryngeal mask airways (LMA), Combitube and endotracheal tubes (Figure 18.4) are all described. Guidance emphasises the need to use the best available approach depending on the individual situation. Ventilation thereafter follows the same guidance – the best system available should be used.

Deakin (1997) identifies airway problems as a significant cause of *preventable* pre-hospital death in trauma. He further highlights airway obstruction as being a major cause of death that *could* have been prevented by simple foreign body

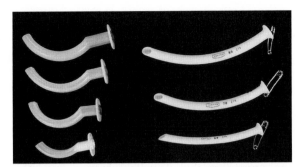

Figure 18.3 Oropharyngeal (left) and nasopharyngeal airways (right).

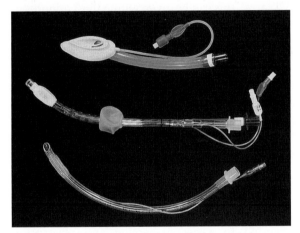

Figure 18.4 Laryngeal mask airway (top), combitube (middle) and endotracheal tube (bottom).

removal or simple airway opening techniques, and reviews the relative benefits of LMA, combitubes and endotracheal intubation.

The LMA is widely used in anaesthesia as an alternative to endotracheal intubation in certain cases, but most importantly in *fasted* patients. A disadvantage to using this adjunct is the possibility of regurgitation and aspiration of stomach contents, as the LMA does not definitively protect the trachea. Its advantages are, however, that it is relatively easy to use and can be used in patients with suspected cervical spine injury, where endotracheal intubation may be difficult. It also offers better protection of the airways than a self-inflating bag–valve–mask technique (Stone et al., 1998).

The combitube is used more frequently in Europe than in the UK, but has the similar advantage of requiring less training for use and is a potentially valuable alternative to intubation.

Disadvantages include its expense and possible regurgitation (Resuscitation Council UK, 2001).

Tracheal intubation is viewed as the optimal desirable goal of airway management to provide the best possible oxygenation. It is, however, a skill requiring training, practice and expertise, particularly when faced with difficult airway problems associated with some trauma cases and cervical spine immobilisation. Some techniques to facilitate intubation in cervical spine injury can be employed (e.g. fibreoptic intubation).

Cervical spine immobilisation in trauma is considered vital in cases where neck injury is suspected. This can be achieved *initially* by manual in-line stabilisation, securing the neck and preventing movement whilst also providing a jaw-thrust to open the airway. Adjuncts, such as the application of a rigid cervical collar with sandbags placed at either side of the head, and tape used to secure the head to the spinal board/stretcher, can be used once the airway is cleared. It is interesting to note that, despite the common belief that rigid cervical collars restrict cervical spine movement, this may not be as useful as first thought. Houghten and Driscoll (1999) provide evidence suggesting that a collar *must* be used in association with head blocks and strapping to provide effective cervical spine immobilisation. However, Deakin (1997) reaffirms that cervical spine management must not compromise airway management.

Oxygenation and ventilation are vital to survival. Robertson et al. (1998) recommend an inspired oxygen concentration of 100% oxygen. A bag–valve–mask system can provide greater than 90% inspired oxygen, if used correctly, while endotracheal intubation and mechanical ventilation provide the best possible oxygenation. As before, the best technique available should be used. Studies suggest that the bag–valve–mask technique may cause regurgitation when compared to use of the LMA (Stone et al., 1998). However, in the absence of the LMA option, correct bag–valve–mask technique using a two-person approach can provide adequate oxygenation (Figure 18.5). Advice for tidal volumes should be considered to help prevent regurgitation of stomach contents in unprotected airway management (AHA and ILCOR, 2000).

All airway and ventilation techniques have their own advantages and problems. The aim is to obtain the best airway and oxygenation possible.

Intravenous (IV) access should not create the same dilemmas as airway management. Access is recommended to enable IV blood sampling and the delivery of drugs and fluids as required. Any existing cannulae should be checked for patency with a saline flush to prevent drugs (e.g sodium bicarbonate) causing potential tissue necrosis. If there are no existing cannulae, access should be attempted as centrally as possible without causing disturbance to CPR. Most often the antecubital vein is recommended (Varon et al., 1998). Central venous cannulation has advantages in that the drug reaches the central circulation quicker but associated complications (e.g. misplacement) mean a higher level of expertise is required to perform this (Resuscitation Council UK, 2000). Peripheral cannulation requires either a continuous infusion fluid or a saline flush to ensure the drug reaches the central circulation. When establishing IV access, blood should be drawn for analysis of electrolytes, particularly potassium levels, and blood grouping, if hypovolaemia is suspected.

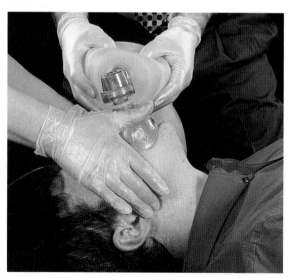

Figure 18.5 Two-person technique for performing bag–valve–mask ventilation.

ADRENALINE/EPINEPHRINE EVERY 3 MINUTES

The use of adrenaline/epinephrine is advocated to help increase coronary and cerebral blood flow owing to its alpha-agonist vasoconstrictive effect. Cairns and Niemann (1998) suggest that the first bolus is the most important, subsequent boluses having less effect. This assists CPR; however, there is no scientific evidence to support or refute the suggestion that its administration improves survival outcome. The recommended regime for administration is every 3 minutes. In the non-VF/VT 'arm', this can be given within the 3 minutes of CPR. In the VF/VT 'arm', it is important to give shock sequences without interruption. Administration is, therefore, recommended during the 1 minute of CPR as absolute timings are unlikely to occur.

Intravenous administration is preferred, however adrenaline/epinephrine can be given endo-bronchially, delivered as a fine spray via a catheter through an endotracheal tube, if IV administration is not possible. The dose administered via the endotracheal tube should be twice to three times the IV dose, diluted to a volume of around 10 ml. Hyperventilation with five breaths is recommended to assist dispersion and absorption (Robertson et al., 1998). A study by Paret et al. (1998) suggests that the endotracheal dose may be too low, while Robertson et al. (1998) emphasise that this route is to be considered a second-line intervention when IV access is not possible, noting problems with questionable absorption. In cases of thoracic trauma, ILCOR (1997) do not recommend using endotracheal drugs owing to the possibility of blood within the lungs.

AMIODARONE, ATROPINE/PACING, BUFFERS

Antidysrhythmic agents are considered owing to their possible role in helping to prevent ventricular ectopy/dysrhythmia. The ERC indicates that there is too little evidence to propose any one agent being superior to another. In the absence of any clear data, recommendations suggest that *amiodarone* may be of use in cases of VF or pulseless VT unresponsive to defibrillation attempts. A bolus of 300 mg IV is recommended but this exceeds current datasheet advice so should be used in pulseless patients only (de Latorre et al., 2001). It should also be noted that antidysrhythmic agents may also *generate* dysrhythmias (ILCOR, 1997).

Atropine may be considered for asystole or, in the presence of a pulseless bradycardia, a bradycardic rate of less than 60 beats per minute. The dose recommended to block vagal effect on the sinoatrial and atrioventricular nodes completely is 3 mg. This single dose has been reported to reverse asystole but there are no studies to prove its benefit. It is, however, unlikely to cause harm. *Cardiac pacing* may help in some cases. In the first instance, external pacing can be commenced followed by transvenous pacing, when equipment and skilled help are available. Similarly, percussion pacing, involving gentle fist blows just to the left of the precordium, can assist cardiac output until electrical pacing is available (Resuscitation Council UK, 2000).

The use of *buffers* also remains controversial during the management of cardiac arrest. The ERC recommends use in cases where blood gas analysis demonstrates an arterial blood pH of less than 7.1 (de Latorre et al., 2001). Special situations, such as hyperkalaemia or an overdose of a tricyclic antidepressant agent, can create a metabolic acidosis, which may benefit from the use of sodium bicarbonate. It is also suggested as an option for use if the patient has been in cardiac arrest for over 20 minutes. Sodium bicarbonate liberates carbon dioxide; therefore, optimal ventilation must be achieved to allow venting of carbon dioxide to prevent worsening of the acidosis. Most cardiac arrest patients show a degree of respiratory acidosis, thus efforts should concentrate on optimising ventilation.

All agents/techniques described above tend to be considered when treatments within the algorithm fail. There is a level of expertise required in determining the potential benefits of these interventions. In the absence of obvious need for the above, a policy of keeping treatment as simple as possible may be prudent.

The ERC guidelines for ALS are now simple and concentrate on scientifically proven interventions. The algorithm is a dynamic process of flow and may move from one side to the other. Return of spontaneous circulation may not be sustained, or even occur, however these guidelines provide a simple framework of action based on the best clinical evidence available to date.

REVERSIBLE CAUSES

The more commonly reported reversible causes of cardiac arrest are identified in an easy to remember 4Hs and 4Ts format (Box 18.1). Others identify different methods for recall, including Hughes and McQuillan (1998), all of which recommend ruling out the more treatable problems first.

> Rapid detection and treatment of problems can save lives

In 2000, AHA and ILCOR published detailed advisory statements for treating some possible causes of cardiopulmonary arrest. These identify specific treatments that can assist in these 'special resuscitation situations'. It is valuable to gain a detailed history if possible. Clues may lie in the preceding events, for example, a patient involved in a motor vehicle accident with multiple injuries may have initially experienced chest pain and signs of a myocardial infarction, possibly causing the accident.

Hypoxia

Hypoxia can occur as a result of many factors. All apnoeic patients should be considered hypoxic until proven otherwise, using blood gas analysis or pulse oximetry. All should be treated with the best available airway and ventilation systems,

> **Box 18.1   Reversible causes of arrest ('4Hs and 4Ts')**
>
> - Hypoxia
> - Hypovolaemia
> - Hyperkalaemia/hypokalaemia and metabolic disorders
> - Hypothermia
> - Tension pneumothorax
> - Tamponade
> - Toxic/therapeutic disorders
> - Thromboembolic and mechanical obstruction

whether as simple as pocket masks or as definitive as endotracheal intubation. The highest concentration of oxygen available should be administered and adequate chest movement observed to ensure effectiveness of ventilation. Breath sounds should be checked to verify equal lung expansion. Recommended tidal volumes with, and without, added oxygen are included in the guidance from AHA and ILCOR (2000). A more recent study by Dorph et al. (2004) makes further recommendations to ensure adequate *ventilation* of carbon dioxide, another key factor in the management of hypoxia. If the history indicates primary hypoxia as the cause of arrest (e.g. toxic inhalation, asthma, near drowning, foreign body obstruction), the cause must be treated as quickly as possible. Driscoll et al. (1993) describe five life-threatening respiratory problems, which are associated with thoracic trauma, each of which should be ruled out:

- airway obstruction
- tension pneumothorax
- open pneumothorax
- massive haemothorax
- flail chest.

Hypovolaemia

If haemorrhage is obvious, the first treatment is to *stop* the source of blood loss and replace lost volume – preferably with blood. Some blood loss can be hidden (e.g. closed fractures or within chest or abdominal cavities). Surgical assistance will be required urgently to stop this loss definitively. For other causes, e.g. burns, dehydration or problems of fluid distribution (sepsis, neurogenic shock), fluid replacement should first be started followed by attempts to definitively treat the cause.

Much debate surrounds the fluid to use, how much to use and how quickly to administer this (Deakin, 1997). A recent consensus view for *prehospital* trauma patient fluid management was published in 2002 by Revell et al., which provides useful evidence-based guidance. Two sites of intravenous access with large-bore cannulae should be gained as centrally as possible. The recommendation is that saline is used in the first instance (Revell et al 2002). For blood loss, red cell replacement should be commenced as soon as available considering cross-matching require-

ments, blood availability and balancing risks of transfusion against the catastrophe of the loss (Driscoll et al., 1993). Fluid replacement should be monitored and the effects of treatment regularly evaluated. In cardiac arrest, it is difficult to estimate the exact loss and the volume required to replace this. Regular re-evaluation of blood count can help but observation of clinical signs can provide more immediate feedback (American College of Surgeons, 1997).

Hyperkalaemia/hypokalaemia

Unless there is any obvious history indicating hyperkalaemia/hypokalaemia as the main cause (e.g. diabetic ketoacidosis, renal history), the search for this cause tends to be carried out as a 'rule-out' option. Potassium imbalance is the most rapidly fatal electrolyte disturbance (AHA and ILCOR, 2000). Definitive diagnosis is dependent on laboratory results, although ECG changes and history can influence the index of suspicion, and treatment started before results are available. IV access should be gained as soon as possible, obtaining blood samples before administering fluids or drugs. A potassium level can be analysed relatively quickly. Other electrolyte analysis takes longer (e.g. calcium, magnesium). Potassium imbalance can be treated quickly; various regimes (e.g. calcium chloride, insulin and glucose or dialysis) can quickly reduce a hyperkalaemia, with potassium replacement improving a hypokalaemia. Similarly, blood glucose levels can be quickly estimated and treated, being a common concurrent complication of other causes of arrest. It may be useful to consider the effect of cardiopulmonary arrest in that it can result in hypokalaemia owing to several factors, including adrenaline administration and potassium shift during VF. Roffey et al. (2003) highlight the importance of checking potassium levels *during* cardiac arrest management, even if it is not suspected as a primary cause.

Hypothermia

From extensive reviews of accidental hypothermia, Lloyd (1996) suggests that actual body temperature offers no guidance for survival potential. Silfvast and Pettila (2003) also note that there is currently no method available to help predict survival from hypothermia. Hypothermia should be strongly suspected in any patient who feels centrally cold to the touch. Many patients in cardiac arrest are *peripherally* shut down and feel cold. Lloyd recommends feeling the axilla as an *immediate* indicator, with a core-temperature evaluation performed as soon as possible (rectal, oesophageal), acknowledging that this may take a few minutes to achieve. If the history is obvious, cold wet clothing should be removed and the patient taken to a warm environment. Excessive movement of the patient can trigger arrhythmias (e.g. VF), so care must, therefore, be taken and movement restricted to the minimum required. Resuscitation is modified slightly in the following ways.

Airway and breathing

Airway management should include cervical spine management, if injury is suspected. Ventilation should be carried out as able, with warmed humidified gases delivered as soon as possible, preferably via endotracheal tube. Hypothermia also causes stiffening of the chest, resulting in the need for increased tidal volumes to achieve chest movement.

Circulation

Pulse checks should be performed, allowing extended time for assessment (i.e. 30–45 seconds) (AHA and ILCOR, 2000). This will allow extreme bradycardias or very low blood pressures to be detected, therefore, obviating the need for unnecessary chest compression. Chest compressions are performed as normal, if indicated, again bearing in mind that chest stiffness may make these more difficult.

Defibrillation

> The heart may not respond to defibrillation attempts

The AHA and ILCOR (2000) recommend three initial shocks and, if core temperature is less than 30°C, to continue CPR and carry out rewarming measures to increase body temperature. The heart may not respond to defibrillation, even above 30°C, thus rewarming should continue.

Drugs

The algorithm recommends administration of adrenaline/epinephrine every 3 minutes. The AHA and ILCOR (2000) identify that this could cause problems in hypothermia. Blood levels of drugs could become dangerous, so extended times between administrations should be observed or even withheld in temperatures less than 30°C. The focus should be on rewarming efforts.

Rewarming methods

Lloyd (1996) provides detailed guidance for rewarming measures. Depending on facilities available, the best methods possible should be used. The main principles involve prevention of further heat loss (removal of wet, cold surroundings/clothing) and actively rewarming by providing heat externally, centrally or both. Surface heating is normally the most readily available, using warmed blankets, heated air mattresses, etc. Lloyd reasserts that rewarming the body *surface* leads to increased oxygen demand of the *peripheral* tissues. Surface rewarming will not assist core rewarming, thus these measures may only be effective in patients with a spontaneous circulation. Central rewarming also warms the core. This can be achieved using warmed humidified oxygen or air for ventilation, warmed IV fluids, warmed fluids to flush the stomach via nasogastric tube (intubation to protect the airway is vital first) and warm bladder irrigation via an irrigation catheter. Surgical techniques involving the insertion of peritoneal catheters and chest drain(s) can facilitate warmed peritoneal and pleural cavity lavage.

Cardiopulmonary bypass allows the quickest method of core rewarming, but is the most difficult to perform and establish. If available, however, this should be considered. The combination of core and surface rewarming is best, using the facilities and techniques available within the department. A review of data by Silfvast and Pettila (2003) on the management of hypothermic patients over 10 years in Finland found that cardiopulmonary bypass performed after prolonged periods of conventional CPR still had positive outcomes. This suggests that patients can still be optimally managed, being transferred to a suitable facility with CPR ongoing in transit.

> In hypothermia, resuscitation attempts will be prolonged and there is no 'normal' time limitation

A case study published in 2002 describes the management of a 37-year-old male who had a core temperature of 17°C. He survived to discharge from hospital. The authors do note that this will not always be the case but highlight the need to allow prolonged resuscitation efforts to continue (Ko et al., 2002).

Tension pneumothorax

Tension pneumothorax can be due to spontaneous rupture of fragile bullae in the lung or to a thoracic injury. It may also be iatrogenic (e.g central venous cannulation attempt). This is a life-threatening problem that can be relieved in an emergency situation, creating immediate restoration of spontaneous circulation. With a tension pneumothorax, air is entrained into the pleural cavity but cannot escape, therefore causing collapse of the lung with mediastinal shift. This compresses the heart, thereby significantly decreasing venous return and diminishing cardiac output to the degree where it becomes undetectable.

Diagnosis is made by clinical examination. Looking at equality of chest movement and listening to breath sounds may reveal diminished movement and sounds on the affected side. A later sign is tracheal displacement *away* from the affected side. The neck veins may be distended owing to the obstructive increase in pressure in the thorax. To establish the difference between tension pneumothorax and possible haemothorax, percussing the chest will reveal hyper-resonance over the affected side indicating an air filled space. Dullness is indicative of the presence of fluid. A recent case study contends that *looking at equality of chest movement and expansion cannot be emphasised enough*, especially when other signs are not conclusive (Leigh-Smith and Davies, 2003).

Immediate treatment is indicated and easily achievable with needle decompression. A large-bore cannula should be inserted into the second intercostal space in the mid-clavicular line, resulting in the sound of escaping air. The needle should be removed, leaving the plastic cannula in place, taking care to avoid it kinking. This will allow the immediate release of trapped air and decompression of the pneumothorax. The cardiac monitor should be observed for any rhythm change and pulse checks performed. Return of circulation can be immediate (American College of Surgeons, 1997). Definitive treatment is conventional chest drain insertion, which can be performed later. Continuous reassessment is advisable until this is achieved. Chest x-ray should only be performed *after* decompression to evaluate the effect of treatment. It is inappropriate to perform chest x-ray as a diagnostic aid in such a life-threatening condition (American College of Surgeons, 1997).

> The diagnosis of tension pneumothorax is based on *clinical* evidence

Tamponade

Pericardial tamponade can be due to trauma-related incidents, penetrating or blunt injury to the thorax, or from ruptured coronary vessels or ventricles. If the heart is compressed within its fibrous pericardial sac by a collection of fluid, its own ability to fill and create a palpable output is impaired. Pericardial effusion can have the same effect.

Diagnosis can be difficult. A history of injury and a high index of suspicion, associated with signs of full neck veins, may lead to considering cardiac tamponade as the primary cause of cardiac arrest. Muffled heart sounds can be indicative of tamponade but, in the case of total loss of output, these may be inaudible. Echocardiography may assist in diagnosing tamponade.

Driscoll et al. (1993) describe the technique for pericardiocentesis (i.e. draining fluid from the pericardial sac). This requires a degree of expertise and involves the insertion of a long needle into the chest 1 to 2 cm below and to the left of the xiphisternum, moving towards the ipsilateral scapular tip. Fluid, blood or effusion aspirate can then be removed to alleviate the pressure on the heart. The cannula should be kept in place, with repeated aspiration performed as necessary to regain return of spontaneous circulation. Cannula removal could recreate tamponade. Early surgical intervention is recommended. ECG monitoring is essential during the procedure, as some changes may be noted which could indicate myocardial irritation. If so, the needle should be withdrawn until the ECG resumes its previous pattern. Complications can include rupture of coronary vessels or the ventricular walls.

Thromboembolic/mechanical obstruction

The two most notable conditions in this category are myocardial infarction (MI) and pulmonary embolism (PE). The main problem is that the cause of arrest cannot be definitively removed or reversed, but the resulting damage *can* be limited and resuscitation efforts can resume circulation. Diagnosis will tend to be guided by the history prior to cardiac arrest.

> In some cases, the first manifestation of heart disease can be cardiac arrest

A history of chest pain, known ischaemic heart disease, angina or deep vein thrombosis can focus attention on possible MI or PE. ECG changes can also provide clinical indicators, namely ST segment changes. Dysrhythmias should be treated in accordance with appropriate guidelines. If the dysrhythmia is VF, defibrillation should be performed as quickly as possible. Thrombolysis may be considered where indicated. CPR is no longer an absolute contradiction to thrombolysis as long as there is no associated traumatic injury. Interventions, such as arterial blood gas analysis and large, non-compressible venous puncture, should be avoided, if possible, to minimise complications of thrombolysis.

Survival from these causes is variable and unpredictable. Resuscitation efforts are, therefore, worthwhile, although survival possibility from massive PE tends to be poor. Treatment options include thrombolysis, however this cause may require cardiothoracic surgery to remove the clot, which is not available in many centres (Resuscitation Council UK, 2000). Debate reigns regarding the use of thrombolysis, owing to complications of haemorrage, however Janata et al. (2003) contend that the benefits of treatment may outweigh the risk of bleeding.

Toxic/therapeutic disturbance

The AHA and ILCOR (2000) list the more common drugs causing cardiac arrest, ranging from antidepressants to opiates, and from agents such as cyanide to organophosphates. Some agents are more readily treatable than others. Diagnosis of these as primary causes may be difficult in the absence of a clear history. Treatment involves removing the cause while ensuring personal safety precautions. Most toxins require specific antidotes for successful treatment and most accident and emergency departments have rapid access to advisory guidance. Contacting regional poison centres is recommended for specific treatment.

An overdose of opiates and benzodiazepines can be quickly treated 'blindly' by giving naloxone or flumazenil. If it transpires that these were *not* indicated therapies, they are unlikely to cause further harm but, in the absence of clear evidence of what toxin was taken, they may prove beneficial. Caution should be taken where a combination overdose involving these agents is concerned.

The main priority for these patients is to protect the airway by endotracheal intubation, as soon as possible, to prevent problems associated with aspiration. Patients may already have aspirate in their lungs; in these circumstances, endobronchial suctioning will be made more accessible via the endotracheal tube.

Some readily reversible causes of arrest may be obvious, particularly in trauma situations. However, in searching for these eight causes, it is possible that one or several may be found on further examination.

ECG RHYTHM INTERPRETATION

Cardiac arrest dysrhythmias are divided into two areas: VF/pulseless VT, and any other rhythm.

> It is important to recognise the absence of pulse and to follow the relevant side of the cardiac arrest algorithm, aiming to restore circulation as soon as possible

The rhythm itself requires no special intervention beyond what has been described; however, if the patient has a pulse, periarrest guidelines should be used, outlined in algorithmic form later. It is important to establish what ECG rhythm is displayed. This section briefly outlines a system described within the *Advanced life support manual* (Resuscitation Council UK, 2000) to assist in determining some of the more common dysrhythmias appearing on an ECG rhythm strip or cardiac monitor. Specialised electrocardiography texts are recommended for more detailed information on lead settings, monitoring systems, rate calculation, complex identification and the conduction system.

Several important components should be considered when interpreting cardiac rhythms, as listed below:

- *QRS rate*: simplify to > 100 tachycardia, 60–100 normal, < 60 bradycardia.
- *QRS rhythm*: regular or irregular – map this out between R waves.

- *QRS complex width*: narrow/normal = < 0.10 seconds or 2.5 small squares on ECG graph paper; widened / prolonged = > 0.10 seconds/ 2.5 small squares. Narrow QRS complexes are conducted from above the division of the bundle of His in the conduction system and are, therefore, atrial or supraventricular in origin. Widened QRS complexes either arise from within the ventricles or reflect some type of conduction delay down one or more of the bundle branches.
- *Atrial activity*: P waves – upright, inverted or biphasic, 'saw-tooth' flutter waves, irregular fibrillation waveform.
- *Relationship of atrial activity to ventricular activity*.

Some samples using this system follow. Each strip is monitored in lead II, the optimal lead for showing atrial and ventricular depolarisation.

Fast rhythms – tachycardias

ECG trace 1

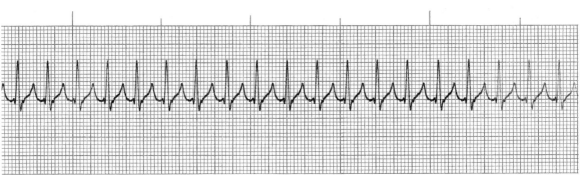

- QRS rate: fast.
- QRS rhythm: regular.
- QRS width: < 0.10 seconds (normal).
- Atrial activity: too fast to identify clearly. Smaller deflections could be P waves or T waves. P waves could be hidden in QRS or T complexes.

- Relationship: unable to distinguish clear atrial activity.

Rhythm is a narrow complex tachycardia or supraventricular tachycardia based on the first three points.

ECG trace 2

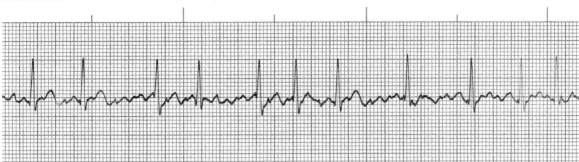

- QRS rate: normal to fast.
- QRS rhythm: irregular.
- QRS width: < 0.10 seconds (normal).
- Atrial activity: wavy baseline between QRS complexes, therefore, fibrillating.
- Relationship: differing 'lengths' of 'fibrillating'

baseline between QRS complexes. QRS complexes normal, therefore, conducted from the atria.

Rhythm is atrial fibrillation (normal to rapid ventricular response).

ECG trace 3

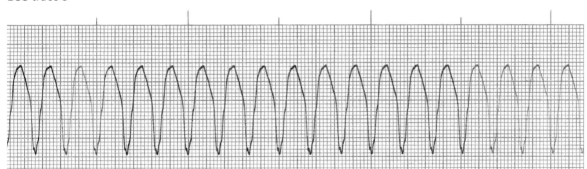

- QRS rate: fast.
- QRS rhythm: regular.
- QRS width: > 0.10 seconds (widened).
- Atrial activity: none identifiable, possibly hidden.
- Relationship: not possible to elicit owing to non-identifiable atrial activity.

Rhythm is a broad complex tachycardia – probably ventricular tachycardia. (This could be an atrial rhythm with bundle branch block but the important factor here is patient status – stable or not – therefore, consider ventricular tachycardia *first* as this can be life threatening.)

ECG trace 4

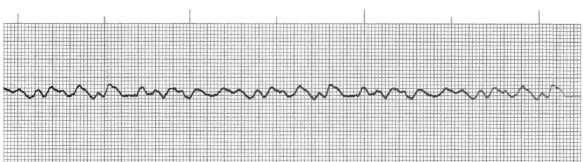

- QRS rate: fast.
- QRS rhythm: irregular, random, no identifiable QRS complexes.
- QRS width: no identifiable normal QRS complexes.

- Atrial activity: none identifiable.
- Relationship: not able to assess

Rhythm is ventricular fibrillation. (No organised pattern recognizable.)

Slow rhythms – bradycardias, heartblocks

ECG trace 5

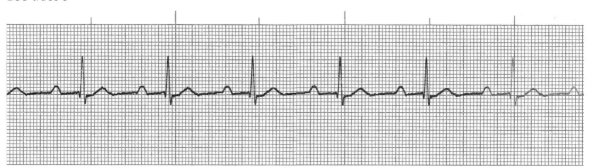

- QRS rate: slow.
- QRS rhythm: regular.
- QRS width: <0.10 seconds.
- Atrial activity: P waves (upright).
- Relationship: every QRS complex has an upright P wave preceding it. Sinus node firing producing upright P wave. Slightly prolonged interval between P wave and normal QRS complex suggests some delay in conduction through the atrioventricular node.

Rhythm is first-degree atrioventricular block.

ECG trace 6

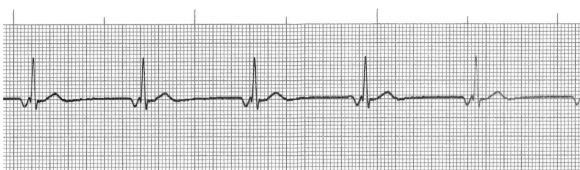

- QRS rate: slow.
- QRS rhythm: regular.
- QRS width: < 0.10 seconds.
- Atrial activity: inverted P waves. No flutter or fibrillation waveforms.
- Relationship: an inverted P immediately precedes each QRS. The QRS rhythm complex is narrow, therefore, conducted from the atria.

The inverted atrial complexes suggest retrograde conduction through the atria. Normal sinus activity is not apparent; therefore, the rhythm is arising from the atrioventricular node or junction between the atria and ventricles.

Rhythm is junctional or nodal bradycardia.

ECG trace 7

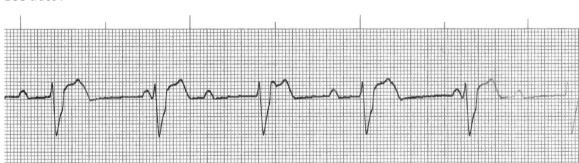

- QRS rate: slow.
- QRS rhythm: regular.
- QRS width: > 0.10 seconds.
- Atrial activity: P waves, upright.
- Relationship: no identifiable relationship between P waves and QRS complexes. No pattern. P waves march along regularly from P wave to P wave, with some hidden within QRS complexes. QRS complexes do the same. This suggests atria are contracting at intrinsic rate, but QRS also regular at a much slower rate. Widened QRS suggests they are not being

conducted from the atria and the rate suggests intrinsic ventricular automaticity.

Rhythm is complete (third-degree) atrioventricular block.

Whilst it is not possible to demonstrate all rhythms within this section, these rhythm strips give a brief introduction to very simple rhythm interpretation. Reading one of the simpler electrocardiography texts available is highly recommended.

PERIARREST DYSRHYTHMIA MANAGEMENT

Periarrest dysrhythmias can lead to, or follow, successful management of cardiac arrest. They are split into tachyarrhythmias and bradyarrhythmias. Several principles should be followed when evaluating the significance of these dysrhythmias. The algorithms shown provide guidance on management in the immediate stages until expert help is available. The Resuscitation Council UK (2000) remind us that drugs used for *treating* dysrhythmias can also generate dysrhythmias.

It is relatively useless to use drugs recommended for periarrest dysrhythmias, if there is *no cardiac output*; therefore, treat the cause of arrest first, then the rhythm once circulation is restored

PRINCIPLES OF MANAGEMENT FOR ALL ARRHYTHMIAS

Always check the patient first. Time must not be spent interpreting rhythms, if the patient is unconscious and pulseless. If *pulseless*, treatment follows the advanced life support algorithm. If the patient *has* a pulse, the haemodynamic status should be assessed to determine its stability and the presence of adverse clinical signs (e.g. hypotension, chest pain, pallor, deteriorating conscious level).

In all cases, there is no harm in giving oxygen first. Hypoxia itself may worsen the dysrhythmias. Intravenous access should be established as soon as possible. It is easier to achieve this before the patient is haemodynamically compromised to ensure it is available for immediate use if needed.

Tachyarrhythmias

Tachyarrhythmias can lead to the heart being unable to refill adequately owing to an excessive heart rate. This in turn reduces blood flow to the coronary and cerebral circulation, which culminates in the patient showing symptoms of underperfusion (listed under adverse signs within the algorithms). The key is to differentiate between broad and narrow complex tachycardias.

Broad complex tachycardias are mostly ventricular in origin. Treatment is, therefore, aimed at managing the ventricular arrhythmia. If *pulseless*,

treatment is immediate defibrillation. If there is a pulse and the patient is haemodynamically stable, IV antidysrhythmic agents can be used. If these have no effect, synchronised cardioversion is indicated. If the patient is *unstable*, cardioversion should be performed after giving sedation (Figure 18.6).

Expert assistance is advised before performing cardioversion

Narrow complex tachycardias occur for various reasons, the most important of which is to rule out a supraventricular tachycardia. Vagal manoeuvres may help initially, noting the associated cautions, followed by an adenosine regime which may terminate the problem. The patient *must* be monitored and warned that they may feel hot and dizzy, and may experience chest pain briefly when adenosine is administered.

If these efforts fail to terminate the dysrhythmia, expert help is recommended and other antidysrhythmic agents considered if the patient is haemodynamically stable. If the patient shows evidence of adverse clinical signs, sedation and synchronised cardioversion are advised (Figure 18.7).

Atrial fibrillation has been included as a periarrest dysrhythmia and, in 2000, was classified into low, intermediate and high-risk patients. In the context of advanced life support, only the high-risk section is included here. High-risk patients require early cardioversion under sedation, as they show signs of hypoperfusion and need definitive treatment of the dysrhythmia. They should receive heparin first to minimise the risk of thromboembolic complications that can occur with atrial fibrillation (AHA and ILCOR, 2000). If cardioversion is unsuccessful, antidysrhythmic agents may be indicated (Figure 18.8).

Bradyarrhythmias

After administering oxygen, it is vital to assess the patient for the risk of asystole. If the patient is not considered to be at risk of asystole and is haemodynamically stable, no intervention beyond observation is required. If the patient is unstable and there is any risk of asystole, the patient should

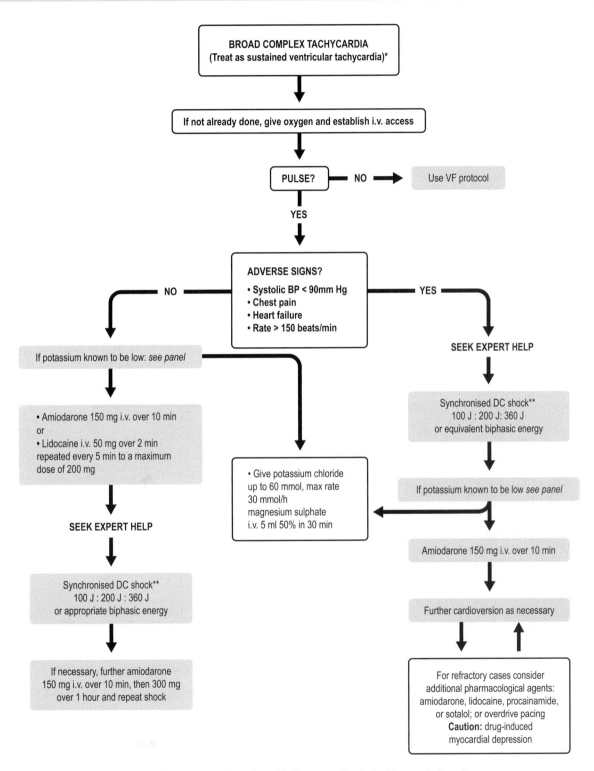

Figure 18.6   Algorithm for management of broad complex tachycardia. Doses throughout are based on an adult of average body weight. (Reproduced with permission from the Resuscitation Council UK.)

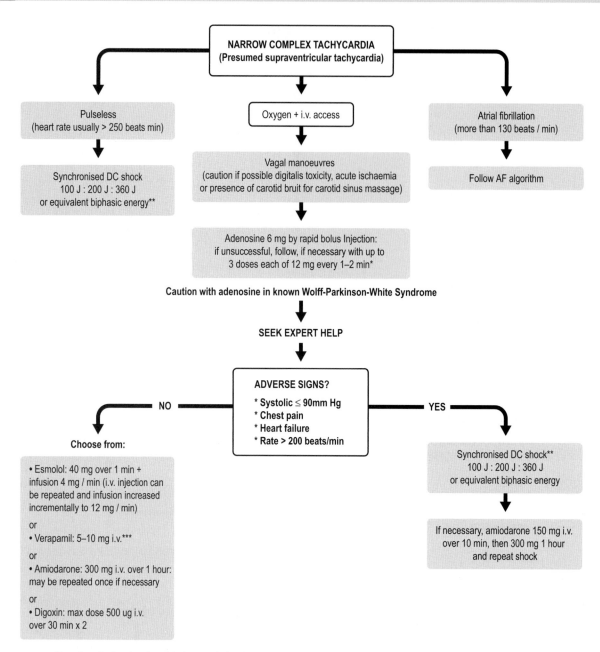

Figure 18.7 Algorithm for management of narrow complex tachycardia. Doses throughout are based on an adult of average body weight. A starting dose of 6 mg adenosine is currently outside of the UK licence for this agent. (Reproduced with permission from the Resuscitation Council UK.)

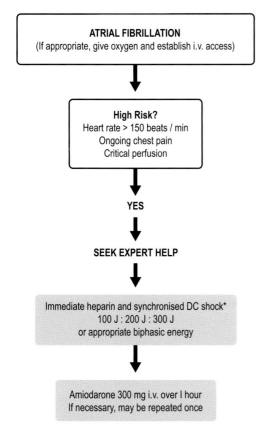

Figure 18.8 Algorithm for management of high-risk patients with atrial fibrillation. Doses throughout are based on an adult of average body weight. (Reproduced with permission from the Resuscitation Council UK.)

be treated with atropine and expert assistance summoned in case any form of pacing is required (Figure 18.9).

The important factors to note for any periarrest dysrhythmia are to maintain optimal oxygenation, gain early IV access and seek expert help as soon as possible. This may help to avoid multiple drugs being used, which could cause further problems.

The information for periarrest arrhythmia management is taken from the guidelines found in the *Advanced life support course provider manual* (Resuscitation Council UK, 2000) and advice from the ERC (de Latorre et al., 2001).

ETHICS AND DECISIONS TO CEASE RESUSCITATION ATTEMPTS

In trauma-related cardiac arrest, it is generally advised to start resuscitation unless there are signs that the patient is irretrievable (e.g. decapitated, rigor mortis, decayed) (ILCOR, 1997). In 2000, the AHA and ILCOR highlighted the need for rapid transfer to a trauma centre and definitive treatment to increase the patient's chance of survival. One other contradiction to starting resuscitation would be some form of documentation from the patient with specific guidance *not* to resuscitate (e.g. living will or advance directive). However, this documentation is often only found after resuscitative efforts have been started and may help a team to make the decision to cease the resuscitation attempt. Specific advice regarding decisions relating to cardiopulmonary resuscitation has been published, jointly written by the British Medical Association, Resuscitation Council (UK) and the Royal College of Nursing. This is comprehensively covered in the appendix to the *Advanced life support course provider manual* (4th edition) 2000.

In terms of survival, various studies reveal the outcomes of cardiac arrest based in accident and emergency departments. Arrests occurring within the department have better outcomes than pre-hospital events requiring resuscitation before arrival in the department (Tunstall-Pedoe et al., 1992; White and Guly, 1999). Pre-hospital event survival outcomes depend largely on the care given in the pre-hospital field. Some factors may be considered to predict outcome (e.g. age, time from collapse to initiation of treatment, and comorbidity factors), but these are not absolute indicators. Mohr et al. (1997) explore the ideal of providing resuscitation only for those patients *expected* to survive, but also warn against not initiating resuscitation, or ceasing attempts prematurely and losing potential survivors.

Efforts, if considered appropriate in the first place, should continue until the team agree that all interventions possible have been performed to no avail

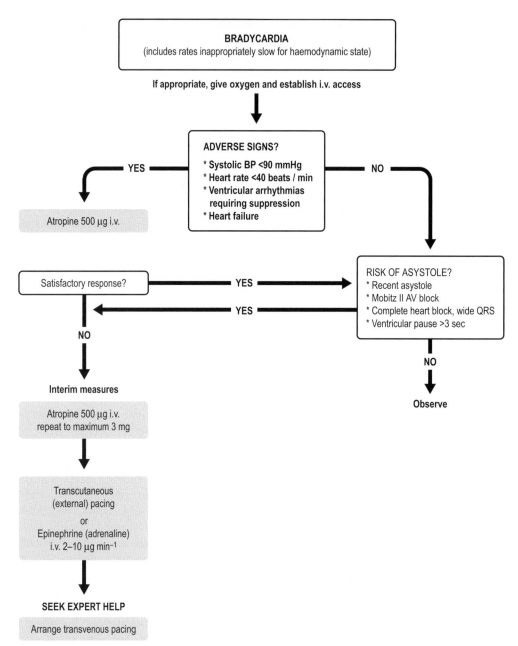

Figure 18.9   Algorithm for management of bradycardias. (Reproduced with permission from the Resuscitation Council UK.)

CONCLUSION

This chapter provides guidance and the rationales for adult ALS as recommended by the ERC, the AHA and ILCOR. It includes a simple method of interpreting ECG rhythms and directs the reader to review this subject in more detail. Sometimes, the prevention of cardiac arrest may lie in the prompt treatment of periarrest dysrhythmias following relevant guidelines. The complex decision on who to resuscitate is touched upon in addition to guidance on when to stop resuscitative efforts. Resuscitation is a team event and all members have a significant role. A greater understanding of the issues involved will help multi-disciplinary teams to work together to achieve a common goal and optimise the patient's chances of survival.

References and further reading

American College of Surgeons. *Advanced trauma life support for doctors, student course manual*, 6th edn. Chicago: American College of Surgeons, 1997: Chapters 1–4

American Heart Association and International Liaison Committee on Resuscitation. Guidelines 2000 for cardiopulmonary resuscitation and emergency cardiovascular care – an international consensus on science. *Resuscitation* 2000; 46: 109–113, 135–163, 253–297

Ashton A, McCluskey A, Gwinnutt CL, Keenan AM. Effect of rescuer fatigue on performance of continuous external chest compressions over 3 min. *Resuscitation* 2002; 55: 151–155

Baskett PJF, Bossaert L, Carli P, et al. Guidelines for the basic management of the airway and ventilation during resuscitation. *Resuscitation* 1996; 31: 187–200

Baskett PJF, Bossaert L, Carli P, et al. Guidelines for the advanced management of the airway and ventilation during resuscitation. *Resuscitation* 1996; 31: 201–230

Bossaert L, Callanan V, Cummins R. Early defibrillation. *Resuscitation* 1997; 34: 113–114

Cairns CB, Niemann JT. Haemodynamic effects of repeated doses of epinephrine after prolonged cardiac arrest and CPR: preliminary observations in an animal model. *Resuscitation* 1998; 36: 181–185

Caldwell G, Millar G, Quinn E, Vincent R, Chamberlain DA. Simple mechanical methods for cardioversion: defence of the precordial thump and cough version. *British Medical Journal* 1985; 291: 627–630

Chamberlain D. Spurious asystole with the use of manual defibrillators. *British Medical Journal* 1999; 319: 1574

Cobbe SM, Redmond MJ, Watson JM, Hollingworth J, Carrington DJ. 'Heartstart Scotland' – initial experience of a national scheme for out of hospital defibrillation. *British Medical Journal* 1991; 302: 1517–1520

De Latorre F, Nolan J, Robertson C, et al. European Resuscitation Council guidelines 2000 for adult advanced life support. *Resuscitation* 2001; 48: 211–221

Deakin CD. Preventable pre-hospital death from trauma. *Pre-Hospital Immediate Care* 1997; 1: 198–203

Dorph E, Wik L, Steen PA. Arterial blood gases with 700 ml tidal volumes during out-of-hospital CPR. *Resuscitation* 2004; 61: 23–27

Driscoll PA, Gwinnutt CL, Le Duc Jimmerson C, Goodall O. *Trauma resuscitation. The team approach*. London: Macmillan, 1993: Chapters 1 and 2

Houghten L, Driscoll P. Cervical immobilisation – are we achieving it? *Pre-hospital Immediate Care* 1999; 3: 17–21

Hughes S, McQuillan PJ. Sequential recall of causes of electro-mechanical dissociation (EMD). *Resuscitation* 1998; 37: 51

International Liaison Committee on Resuscitation. Special resuscitation situations. *Resuscitation* 1997; 34: 129–149

Janata K, Holzer M, Kurkciyan I, et al. Major bleeding complications in cardiopulmonary resuscitation: the place of thrombolytic therapy in cardiac arrest due to massive pulmonary embolism. *Resuscitation* 2003; 57: 49–55

Kloeck W, Cummins R, Chamberlain D, et al. The universal ALS algorithm. *Resuscitation* 1997; 34: 109–111

Ko CS, Alex J, Jeffries S, Parmar JM. Dead? Or just cold: profoundly hypothermic patient with no signs of life. *Emergency Medical Journal* 2002; 19: 478–479

Lloyd E. Accidental hypothermia. *Resuscitation* 1996; 32: 11–124

Leigh-Smith S, Davies G. Tension pneumothorax: eyes may be more diagnostic than ears. *Emergency Medical Journal* 2003; 20: 405–496

Mauer DK, Nolan J, Plaisance P, et al. Effect of active compression-decompression resuscitation (ACD–CPR) on survival: a combined analysis using individual patient data. *Resuscitation* 1999; 41: 249–256

Mohr M, Bahr J, Schmid J, Panser W, Kettler D. The decision to terminate resuscitative efforts: results of a questionnaire. *Resuscitation* 1997; 34: 51–55

Nurmi J, Rosenberg P, Castren M. Adherence to guidelines when positioning the defibrillation electrodes. *Resuscitation* 2004; 61: 143–147

Paret G, Vaknin Z, Ezra D, et al. Endotracheal adrenaline: should the recommended dose be reconsidered? *Pre-hospital Immediate Care* 1998; 2: 66–70

Parish DC, Chandra KMD, Dane FC. Success changes the problem: why ventricular fibrillation is declining, why pulseless electrical activity is emerging, and what to do about it. *Resuscitation* 2003; 58: 31–35

Resuscitation Council UK. *Advanced life support course provider manual*, 4th edn. London: Resuscitation Council UK, 2000: Chapters 5, 7, 8, 10, 12, 13

Revell M, Porter K, Greaves I. Fluid resuscitation in pre-hospital trauma care: a consensus view. *Emergency Medical Journal* 2002; 19: 494–498

Robertson C. The precordial thump and cough techniques in advanced life support. *Resuscitation* 1992; 24: 133–135

Robertson C, Steen P, Adgey J, et al. The 1998 European Resuscitation Council guidelines for adult advanced life support. *Resuscitation* 37: 81–90

Roffey P, Thangathurai D, Mikhail M, Shoemaker W. Implication of epinephrine-induced hypokalaemia during cardiac arrest. *Resuscitation* 2003; 58: 231

Silfvast T, Pettila V. Outcome from severe accidental hypothermia in Southern Finland – a 10 year review. *Resuscitation* 2003; 59: 285–290

Stone BJ, Chantler PJ, Baskett PJF. The incidence of regurgitation during cardiopulmonary resuscitation: a comparison between the bag valve mask and laryngeal mask airway. *Resuscitation* 1998; 38: 3–6

Torok R. Biphasic or monophasic defibrillation for adult ventricular fibrillation. *Emergency Medical Journal* 2003; 20: 464–465

Tunstall-Pedoe H, Bailey L, Chamberlain DA, Marsden AK, Ward ME, Zideman DA. Survey of 3765 cardiopulmonary resuscitations in British hospitals (the BRESUS study): methods and overall results. *British Medical Journal* 1992; 304: 1347–1351

Varon J, Marik PE, Fromm RE. Cardiopulmonary resuscitation: a review for clinicians. *Resuscitation* 1998; 36: 133–145

White SP, Guly HR. Survival from cardiac arrest in an accident and emergency department: use as a performance indicator? *Resuscitation* 1999; 40: 97–102

Chapter **19**

Recognition and management of shock

Matthew Wyse

INTRODUCTION

Shock has several aetiologies; these have been described in previous chapters. Whatever the aetiology, the final outcome at cellular level is a loss of cellular energy production, leading to cellular death and subsequent death of the organism. This chapter looks at the recognition of when an individual is in shock, the universal treatment of shock, specific therapies for specific causes and how one can recognise when the treatment is working or failing.

HAEMORRHAGIC SHOCK

In traumatised patients at initial presentation hypovolaemia is the most common aetiology of shock; however, the principles of initial management of hypovolaemic shock are pertinent to the management of all types of shock.

> Hypovolaemia results from the loss of circulating blood volume, either from external or internal haemorrhage

Initial assessment

The initial assessment of trauma patients follows a well-defined pattern: the A,B,C of resuscitation. Whilst maintaining spinal immobilisation, the patient's airway and ventilation should be controlled and high-flow oxygen administered.

The assessment of circulation and, therefore, consideration of shock comes after the airway and breathing have been attended to

However, shock will lead to death if not detected and treated; thus, the recognition and treatment of shock will always form a high priority in trauma patient management.

Traditionally, it has been stated that patients exhibit sequential changes in haemodynamic parameters such as: pulse, blood pressure, mental state, urine output and skin colour, depending on the percentage blood volume lost (American College of Surgeons Committee on Trauma, 1997) (Table 19.1).

The figures in Table 19.1 were derived from animal and human volunteer models of hypovolaemia; however, there is now a growing understanding that patients who have suffered painful traumatic injuries may not slot into one of these predefined models (Demetriades et al., 1998). Pulse and blood pressure should still be measured and recorded from the earliest contact with the patient, as they may give immediate warning that the patient is grossly hypovolaemic, but normal readings do not rule out the presence of shock. Inevitably, this makes the recognition of shock difficult. Using indicators of a deficit in tissue oxygen delivery and perfusion may assist in the diagnosis of shock (Table 19.2), but many of the tests shown are not immediately available in the resuscitation room and may take an unacceptably long time to provide a result. Perhaps most important of all is to take notice of the mechanism of trauma and keep a high index of suspicion for occult bleeding.

During initial assessment intravenous access is secured. Additionally, blood must be sampled from the patient for cross-matching; all major trauma patients should have the cross-match process started immediately after admission. It is safer for the patient for blood to be requested that subsequently is not required than to wait until the need for blood becomes obvious. Once intravenous (IV) access is secure, fluids may be administered.

Table 19.1   Classes of haemorrhage and associated clinical signs

	Class 1	Class 2	Class 3	Class 4
% blood volume lost	Up to 15%	15–30%	30–40%	> 40%
Respiratory rate	Normal (< 20)	20–30	30–40	> 35
Pulse rate	< 100	> 100	> 120	> 140
Blood pressure	Normal	Normal	Decreased	Decreased
Urine output (ml/hour)	> 30	20–30	5–15	Nil
Mental state	Normal or anxious	Anxious	Confused	Obtunded

Table 19.2   Tests of tissue perfusion

Measure of tissue perfusion	Advantage	Disadvantage
Blood lactate	Quick, available	Debate over significance
Arterial base excess	Quick, available	
Gut pHi[a]	Accurate indicator of gut hypoperfusion	Time consuming; need for nasogastric tube
Arteriovenous O_2 difference or mixed venous PO_2	Indicator of global tissue hypoperfusion	Requires pulmonary artery catheter; time consuming
Tissue CO_2	Potentially quick	Experimental

[a]pHi refers to acid–base status of the mucosa of the stomach, or sigmoid colon, derived from a sample of saline within a balloon in contact with the stomach wall, a process called gastrointestinal tonometry.

Further monitoring

Once the initial assessment is complete, attention can be turned to monitoring the circulation accurately. The ideal situation would be to have precise real-time monitoring of pulse, blood pressure, urine output, cardiac output and tissue oxygenation. This ideal is probably still unobtainable within the resuscitation room. An arterial line should be sited in a convenient artery; the radial, brachial and femoral are commonly used. The larger, more central arteries tend to be used in cases of more profound shock, when the more peripheral arteries can be difficult to palpate. The arterial waveform as displayed on a multifunction monitor will provide an accurate pulse rate and a numerical blood pressure averaged out over each 6–8 heartbeats. The shape of the waveform can give the experienced observer a good clue to the cardiac function and the intravascular volume of the patient. Central venous pressure (CVP) monitoring is often instituted at this stage.

It is important to recall that central intravenous catheters are generally too narrow for fluid resuscitation. The advantages in having a good CVP line *in situ* are multiple, observing changes in the CVP over time will assist in assessing the presence of ongoing intravascular loss (a falling CVP) and the response to infused fluid (a rise in CVP closely following IV fluid administration).

Urinary catheterisation is instituted as soon as contraindications to passing a catheter have been excluded. Once the residual bladder volume has drained, the subsequent urinary output should be accurately recorded via a urometer. The presence of urinary flow in excess of 0.5 ml/kg per hour is taken to show that renal perfusion is adequate, and thus other vital organ perfusion is also adequate.

If there is access to one of the other monitoring modalities detailed in Table 19.2, it may be appropriate to institute them now, providing that there is no delay to definitive treatment of the patient.

Treatment

Once the diagnosis of hypotension consistent with actual or impending shock has been established, there are two questions to be asked: 'What is the cause?' and 'How to treat the shock?' In most cases of hypovolaemic shock the definitive treatment is to stop the blood loss, that is, to 'plug the hole' in the circulation.

Blood loss may be stopped or minimised in a number of ways (Table 19.3).

In 1994, Bickell et al. demonstrated in a study of 598 patients that in penetrating trauma of the torso very early surgery combined with no fluid resuscitation prior to surgery may be the treatment of choice. It is difficult to extrapolate Bickell's results to all trauma patients for two reasons. Primarily, most trauma systems are unable to get trauma patients to the operating theatre as quickly as in Bickell's unit. Secondarily, in blunt trauma, a patient may have more than one bleeding site, in more than one body part; hence, it is not practical to wait until all bleeding has been definitively stopped before commencing fluid resuscitation. Bleeding from a fractured pelvis or from a ruptured kidney may not be amenable to immediate

Table 19.3   Methods for controlling blood loss in traumatic haemorraghic shock

Site of blood loss	To control blood loss
External	Direct pressure, elevation of affected part
Long bone fracture (femur)	Splint in anatomical position, with traction
Pelvic fracture	External fixator ± compression clamp
	Embolisation of bleeding vessels
	(MAST suit, temporary only)[a]
Retroperitoneal trauma (kidneys, pancreas)	Radiographic localisation and embolisation
	Surgery
Intraperitoneal trauma	Laparotomy
Massive intrathoracic bleeding	Emergency thoracotomy

[a]MAST suit (military antishock trousers): pneumatic leggings and lower abdominal suit that, when inflated to 60 mmHg, will increase cardiac output and reduce bleeding from abdominal, pelvic and lower limb sources. Very uncommon in current clinical use.

surgery. So, although the principle of stopping the bleeding is sound, for example, by using an external fixator on a fractured pelvis to reduce the volume of the pelvis and restore anatomical alignment, in practice, the patient's circulation has to be supported in the mean time.

The mainstay of circulatory support in hypovolaemic shock remains intravenous fluid therapy supplemented with blood and blood products. Thus, fluid resuscitation should be considered in two phases: that occurring before definitive haemorrhage control and that occurring after bleeding has stopped.

Whichever fluid is used, certain principles apply. The fluid should be warmed to 37°C, the response to the fluids should be accurately monitored and documented and the volume infused recorded. It is particularly important to warm any blood products as the infusion of blood at 4°C will cause cooling of the patient, leading to hypothermia with all the adverse effects that will have on cardiac function and clotting.

In considering the correct amount of fluid to give, advanced trauma life support (ATLS) guidelines recommend an initial fluid bolus of 2000 ml of Ringer's lactate (20 ml/kg in children) to be repeated once. If after a second bolus further fluid is required, blood should be given. This recipe is based on the assumptions that for each millilitre of blood lost, we need to replace 3 ml of crystalloid solution, the aim being to restore blood volume immediately. Rather than follow a recipe for fluid resuscitation, it is now recognised that prior to definitive haemorrhage control, the aim of fluid resuscitation should be to maintain perfusion of vital organs. This is the concept of *hypotensive or controlled resuscitation* (Burris et al., 1999). The principle is that by not increasing blood pressure too much, the driving force for further bleeding is minimised and the body's own homeostatic and clotting processes are given a chance to work. However, by maintaining vital organ perfusion, the risk of multiorgan failure is reduced.

Pre-haemorrhage control resuscitation

The exact level of blood pressure that is acceptable is unclear; maintaining a radial pulse that is just palpable or a systolic blood pressure of 80 mmHg have both been suggested. These crude levels of blood pressure may be useful in pre-hospital care, but a more targeted approach for in-hospital use is to aim for a urine output > 20 ml/hour, no worsening of arterial base excess and blood lactate (McCunn and Dutton, 2000).

Post-haemorrhage control resuscitation

Once further bleeding has been stopped or contained as far as possible by surgery or any of the other methods mentioned in Table 19.3, the priority is management of shock changes. The aim is now to restore blood volume to normal levels, to maintain a normal blood pressure and to correct any biochemical or coagulation abnormalities that have arisen from the resuscitation to date. The patient should be cared for in an intensive care or high dependency area. If arterial and CVP monitoring have not already been instituted, this should be done. A full biochemical, haematological and coagulation screen should be obtained.

Blood tests required

The blood tests required are the following:

- full blood count
- urea and electrolytes
- prothrombin time (PT), partial thromboplastin time (PTT) and fibrinogen level
- blood glucose.

If any coagulation deficit exists, this should be treated aggressively. After any substantial fluid administration in trauma, the patient's blood clotting is likely to be impaired. This is multifactorial: as a result of consumption of clotting factors, dilution by fluids, adverse effect of administered fluids on clotting processes and hypothermia. It is important to recognise that this may be an ongoing problem and take regular blood samples for platelet counts and clotting studies. In almost all cases of trauma with hypovolaemia it will be necessary to infuse blood-clotting products, such as cryoprecipitate, fresh-frozen plasma and platelet suspensions (Stehling et al., 1998).

The optimum haemoglobin concentration for the patient is a cause of debate. Traditionally a haemoglobin level of 10 g/dl was considered to offer the best compromise between oxygen delivery and good haemodynamics. It is now clear that, in patients with otherwise normal hearts and respiratory systems a much lower haemoglobin concentration (> 7 g/dl) is acceptable (Herbert et al., 1999). Blood transfusion poses a small but definite risk to the patient; therefore, any decision to transfuse must be based on laboratory evidence of anaemia and an assessment of the potential benefit to the patient.

If, despite adequate volume resuscitation, the patient remains hypotensive the circulation may require inotropic support. The possible aetiologies for hypotension are vasodilatation, as in the systemic inflammatory response syndrome (SIRS), and neurogenic shock or diminished myocardial contractility, as in cardiogenic shock. Determining exactly the cause may be difficult and may require expert help; echocardiography may be useful, as may a monitor of cardiac output, such as a pulmonary artery catheter. Once the cause is established, inotropic agents should be used.

The period of stabilisation after the initial life-saving resuscitation may take several days. During this time, the patient should remain in a high dependency or intensive care unit.

Choices of resuscitation fluid

There are many types of intravenous fluid that have been used in resuscitation, the merits of which have been debated at length over the years; the so-called 'crystalloid versus colloid debate' (Table 19.4). In recent years there has been interest not only in the relative volume-expanding merits of the fluids but also in the concept that fluids may have beneficial or harmful effects on the patient unrelated to the effects they have on blood pressure.

Isotonic crystalloid

Isotonic crystalloid solutions, such as 0.9% saline or Ringer's lactate, are widely available and safe in clinical practice. It is assumed that, following IV administration, the crystalloid will be rapidly distributed throughout the extravascular and intravascular spaces, thus only one-third of the solution will remain in the circulation. As a result, crystalloids are often given in large volumes, typically three times the estimated blood loss. Recent work in volunteers suggests that, in the presence of hypovolaemia, isotonic crystalloid is retained in the intravascular space with a slower redistribution to the extravascular space (Hahn, 1999). Rapid large volume infusions will predispose to hypothermia, acute anaemia and rapid expansion of the circulation, causing loss of clot stability and further bleeding.

> A sensible approach to crystalloid resuscitation is to infuse lower volumes than would have been used previously and to monitor the response accurately in line with the principles of controlled resuscitation

Gelatin solutions

Gelatin solutions have a short half-life (3–4 hours) and are excreted by the renal system. This makes them attractive as a fluid for resuscitation; however, meta-analyses in critically ill patients show a potentially worse outcome following colloid use rather than crystalloid use (Alderson, 2000). Gelatins have also been associated with allergic reactions, and interfere with platelet aggregation (Evans et al., 1998) and clot stability (Mardel et al., 1998) in vitro. As a result of the above factors,

Table 19.4 Comparison of commonly available resuscitation fluids

Fluid	Volume effect	Average molecular weight	Half-life
Isotonic crystalloid	25–33%	N/A	Minutes
Gelatins	80%	35 000	3 hours
HES	100–140%	200 000–450 000	8–72 hours
Hypertonic saline	500–700%	N/A	Variable

HES, hydroxyethyl starches.

there is little evidence to support the continued use of gelatin solutions in trauma resuscitation.

Hydroxyethyl starches

A particular class of fluid that may be of benefit in trauma patients is the hydroxyethyl starches (HES). These are synthetic compounds made from amylopectin, a polysaccharide. They are a diverse group of solutions; the older HES compounds had a wide range of molecular weights and as a result of some very large molecules within the solution, the average molecular weight was 450 000 Daltons. These compounds had several side effects, including interference with the clotting cascade, pruritus and concerns regarding the reticulo-endothelial system in the liver where the larger molecules were phagocytosed. The newer HES compounds have an average molecular weight of 200 000 Daltons and a much more homogenous molecular size. When administered early in trauma resuscitation, they have been shown to have a beneficial effect on certain biochemical markers of multiorgan failure (Allison et al., 1999) and may well be associated with less post resuscitation organ failure. The studies published so far are small; it is unclear whether the phenomenon is dose related and whether it only affects certain subgroups of trauma patients. There have been concerns about the effects of HES on coagulation, and current clinical studies are contradictory; it may be that modern HES compounds have less effect on coagulation than older compounds.

Hypertonic saline (HTS)

Hypertonic fluids are solutions of concentrated saline, 7% versus normal saline at 0.9%, usually in a carrier such as dextran. When infused, they cause an osmotic effect within the circulation to cause an influx of extravascular water into the intravascular space, thus expanding the circulating volume. In theory, small volumes infused will lead to a circulatory expansion several times greater than the infused volume. A typical resuscitation dose is in the order of 4 ml/kg, 20% of the ATLS recommended crystalloid dose. They have theoretical attractions in pre-hospital care and military practice where small volume resuscitation is very attractive. Aside from the volume effect, there may be other beneficial effects from

hypertonic saline. Zallen and Moore (2000) have demonstrated in an animal model of shock that resuscitation with HTS reduces neutrophil priming. This may lead to decreased acute lung injury and multiorgan failure after shock. Coimbra et al. (1997) also demonstrated less sepsis after haemorrhagic shock in an animal model. There have been conflicting reports on the effect of HTS on cardiac output after haemorrhagic shock. It is possible that HTS increases cardiac output and myocardial contractility over and above that caused by expanding intravascular volume (Diebel et al., 1998). It is too early to say if this is going to be a significant effect in clinical practice.

Hypertonic saline solutions have attracted interest in specific types of trauma; burns and head injury in particular. It has been postulated that using a small volume of hypertonic fluid will reduce the total resuscitation volume needed and reduce oedema at the injury site (Anderson et al., 1997); so far it appears that any benefit is short term only. Currently the role of hypertonic saline solutions in the resuscitation of haemorrhagic shock needs further delineation.

Intravenous access

In resuscitation it is necessary to use cannulae that permit high flow rates of fluid; the flow rate is usually specified on the cannula packaging. Flow through a tube (cannula) is proportional to the radius to the fourth power and inversely proportional to the length. Thus, doubling the radius of a cannula will increase the flow rate eight times (Table 19.5).

Cannulae should be of wide bore and as short as possible

Table 19.5 Flow rate versus gauge of typical intravenous cannulae

Gauge of cannula	Diameter (mm)	Flow rate (ml/minute)
20	1.0	54
18	1.2	80
17	1.4	125
16	1.6	180
14	2.0	270

In the traumatised patient, it is customary to cannulate large veins in the upper limb. The antecubital fossa is often used because of the relatively consistent nature of the anatomy of the veins in that area. If a peripheral vein cannot be cannulated, conventionally it may be necessary to perform a surgical cut down on to a vein; in this procedure a vein is surgically exposed and incised and a catheter passed in under direct vision. The commonest site for surgical cut downs are the saphenous vein at the ankle, the femoral vein in the groin and the antecubital fossa.

Central venous catheterisation

In all forms of shock, a central venous catheter may be useful, but the procedure of establishing central venous access requires skill and has risks (Table 19.6). The commonly used veins are the internal jugular vein in the neck, the subclavian veins and the femoral veins. The insertion should be performed with full aseptic precautions and using local anaesthetic in the conscious patient. A tilting trolley is useful to enable the patient to be placed head down during cannulation of the upper body veins. In view of the high incidence of complications of central venous catheterisation, the conscious patient should have a full explanation of the procedure. Central venous catheterisation in the major trauma patient may be very difficult; the presence of a cervical collar and a potentially unstable spine limit access to the great veins of the neck. In hypovolaemic patients, the veins may be collapsed and difficult to cannulate. As a result even experienced operators report a higher incidence of complications from central vein cannulation in trauma patients compared with more stable patients.

Table 19.6 Advantages and disadvantages of central vein catheters

Advantages	Disadvantages
Secure intravenous assess	Time for insertion
Can infuse inotropes	Requires skilled operator
Blood sampling	Poor for fluid resuscitation
Monitoring of central venous pressure	Complications of:
	– Pneumothorax/haemothorax
	– Infection
	– Cardiac tamponade

Most central venous catheters are designed for monitoring CVP or infusing low-volume infusions. The exception is a very wide bore cannula used specifically for fluid resuscitation or through which to pass pulmonary artery catheters. These will allow flow rates of several hundred millilitres per minute and should only be used by experienced operators as there is potential for damaging the vein or surrounding structures.

NON–HAEMORRHAGIC SHOCK

There are three types of non-hypovolaemic shock to be considered in the trauma patient:

- neurogenic shock
- cardiogenic shock
- septic shock.

The pathophysiology of these conditions has been covered in previous chapters. In a patient who has sustained trauma, it is vital to exclude haemorrhagic shock before assuming that shock is due to one of the above causes. The history of the trauma and the mechanism of injury will give clues as to the possibility of non-haemorrhagic shock being present.

Initial management

The initial assessment and management of patients with non-haemorrhagic shock will follow the pattern outlined earlier until significant haemorrhage has been excluded. The next priority is to diagnose the cause (Table 19.7) and quantify the extent of the shock. All the markers of tissue perfusion previously mentioned are valid in determining the extent of the shock.

Neurogenic shock

Once diagnosed, the priority is to improve tissue perfusion, in particular, as a partial spinal cord lesion may deteriorate in the presence of hypotension and tissue hypoxia. There may be only a slight or moderate response to the initial fluid bolus and it is important not to over-transfuse a spinal injury patient, as their capacity for dealing with any additional respiratory problems such as pulmonary oedema will be limited.

Table 19.7   Diagnosis of non-haemorrhagic shock

Neurogenic	Cardiogenic	Septic shock (SIRS)
Mechanism of injury	Mechanism of injury	History and mechanism
Spinal fractures on x-ray or CT scan	Past medical history	Other causes excluded
Presence of sensory and/or motor level	Presence of arrhythmias	Tachycardia
Bradycardia and hypotension	ECG abnormalities	Respiratory rate > 20/minute
Peripherally vasodilated	Valvular or wall motion abnormalities	Temperature < 36°C or > 38°C
Low to normal CVP	on echocardiogram	WBC > 12 000 or < 4000/mm^3;
	Poor response to IV fluids	often poor peripheral perfusion
	High CVP	Moderate response to fluids
	Poor peripheral perfusion	Need for inotropic support
		CVP low or high

CT, computed tomography; CVP, central venous pressure; ECG, electrocardiogram; IV, intravenous; SIRS, systemic immune response syndrome; WBC, white blood count.

Table 19.8   Causes and mechanism of injury in cardiogenic shock

Cause of traumatic cardiogenic shock	Mechanism
Myocardial contusion	Fractured sternum, blow to chest
Valvular rupture	Rapid rise in intrathoracic pressure (deceleration)
Penetrating wound causing tamponade	Penetrating wound or aortic dissection
Acute traumatic coronary artery occlusion (myocardial infarction)	Penetrating or severe blunt trauma

If fluids are ineffective, it may be necessary to use drugs to improve the heart rate and blood pressure. Atropine may correct any acute bradycardia. If this is not adequate, the use of inotropes with an alpha receptor agonist action, such as dopamine or noradrenaline via a central line will be required to both increase the heart rate and cause peripheral vasoconstriction.

The patient will need referral to a spinal injury centre but it is important that shock is corrected in the referring centre before transporting the patient. Prior to and following transfer, the patient should be monitored on an intensive care or high dependency unit using arterial and CVP monitoring.

Cardiogenic shock

If cardiogenic shock is suspected, the cause must be elucidated. The patient may well have previous cardiac disease, especially the elderly, in which case the trauma may have caused an acute deterioration such as an acute myocardial infarct (AMI). The cardiogenic shock may be due directly to cardiac trauma.

Diagnosis will be based on mechanism of injury (Table 19.8), clinical examination and markers of cellular hypoperfusion. In addition, a chest x-ray (CXR) and electrocardiogram (ECG) should be obtained. An echocardiogram (ECHO) is very likely to be needed; this can be transthoracic or oesophageal. The ECHO will help to diagnose or exclude structural damage to the heart; it will also provide information on the presence of any blood in the pericardium and any wall motion abnormalities, a marker of acute ischaemia. Treatment of cardiogenic shock may well require surgical intervention to repair structural damage or to revascularise an ischaemic myocardium. The patient should be referred to a cardiac centre as soon as possible and may require urgent transfer.

Septic shock

Septic shock refers to a condition of hypotension, hypoperfusion and sepsis (i.e. infection). Many patients with so-called septic shock have no demonstrable infection, hence the term septic syndrome has been used; one form of the septic syndrome is the systemic inflammatory response syndrome (Consensus Conference, 1992; Brun-Buisson, 2000). Within the first few hours after trauma infection is unlikely to be a problem; however, many trauma patients exhibit signs of SIRS (Table 19.7) within a few hours of presentation. The causes are multifactorial, but are largely thought to be due to the effects of cellular and humoral mediators and cytokines, such as interleukin 1, interleukin 6 and tumour necrosis factor. The process appears to be caused by trauma to tissues, particularly endothelium, but also from the gut wall if it becomes ischaemic (Rowlands et al., 1999).

Treatment follows the principles of shock treatment. Fluids will have a variable effect; SIRS may cause a profound capillary leak, rendering patients hypovolaemic. Inotropes are likely to be required: alpha agonists for correcting vasodilatation and beta adrenergic agonists will be required, as global cardiac dysfunction is common in SIRS, leading to loss of myocardial contractility.

> Patients with SIRS provide a challenge for clinicians and should be looked after in intensive care

CONCLUSION

Shock following trauma has several different aetiologies. It is clear that relying on simple haemodynamic variables will not consistently detect early shock or delineate the severity of shock. The treatment of shock should be concentrated on correcting the cause where possible, and maintaining vital organ perfusion; initially through controlled resuscitation. In cases of severe shock, more than one aetiology may exist, and the management may continue for several days following the initial insult, involving surgeons, intensive care specialists and specialised units, such as cardiothoracic and spinal injury centres.

References and further reading

Alderson P, Schierhout G, et al. Colloids versus crystalloids for fluid resuscitation in critically ill patients. *Cochrane Database of Systemic Reviews* [computer file.](2):CD000567, 2000

Allison KP, Gosling P, et al. Randomized trial of hydroxyethyl starch versus gelatine for trauma resuscitation. *Journal of Trauma-Injury Infection and Critical Care* 1999; 47: 1114–1121.

American College of Surgeons Committee on Trauma. Shock. In: *Advanced trauma life support for doctors*, 6th edn. Chicago: American College of Surgeons, 1997: 108.

Anderson JT, Wisner DH, et al. Initial small volume hypertonic resuscitation of shock and brain injury: short and long term effects. *Journal of Trauma-Injury Infection and Critical Care* 1997; 42: 592–600

Bickell WH, Matthew J, et al. Immediate versus delayed fluid resuscitation for hypotensive patients with penetrating torso injuries. *New England Journal of Medicine* 1994; 331:1105–1109

Brun-Buisson C. The epidemiology of the systemic inflammatory syndrome. *Intensive Care Medicine* 2000; 26(Suppl 1): S64–S74

Burris D, Rhee P, et al. Controlled resuscitation for uncontrolled hemorrhagic shock. *Journal of Trauma-Injury Infection and Critical Care* 1999; 46: 216–222

Coimbra R, Hoyt DB, et al. Hypertonic saline resuscitation decreases susceptibility to sepsis after hemorrhagic shock. *Journal of Trauma-Injury Infection and Critical Care* 1997; 42: 602–606

Consensus Conference. American College of Chest Physicians/Society of Critical Care Medicine: definitions for sepsis and organ failure and guidelines for the innovative use of therapies in sepsis. *Critical Care Medicine* 1992; 20: 864–874

Demetriades D, Chan LS, et al. Relative bradycardia in patients with traumatic hypotension. *Journal of Trauma-Injury Infection and Critical Care* 1998; 45: 534–539

Diebel LN, Tyburski JG, et al. Effects of hypertonic saline solution and dextran on ventricular blood flow and heart–lung interaction after haemorrhagic shock. *Surgery* 1998; 24: 642–649

Evans PA, Glenn JR, et al. Effects of gelatin based resuscitation fluids on platelet aggregation. *British Journal of Anaesthesia* 1998; 81: 198–202

Hahn R. Volume kinetics in hypovolaemia. *Anaesthesiology* 1999; 90: 81–91

Hamilton Davies C, Mythen MG. Comparison of commonly used clinical indicators of hypovolaemia with gastrointestinal tonometry. *Intensive Care Medicine* 1997; 23: 276–281

Herbert PC, Wells G, et al. A multicentre randomised controlled trial of transfusion requirements in critical care. *New England Journal of Medicine* 1999; 340: 409–417

Mardel SN, Saunders FM, et al. Reduced quality of clot formation with gelatin based plasma substitutes. *British Journal of Anaesthesia* 1998; 80:204–207

McCunn M, Dutton R. End points of resuscitation: How much is enough? *Current Opinions in Anaesthesiology* 2000; 13: 147–153

Rowlands BJ, Soong CV, Gardiner KR. The gastrointestinal tract as a barrier in sepsis. *British Medical Bulletin* 1999; 55: 196–211

Stehling LC, et al. for The American Society of Anesthesiologists Task Force on Blood Component Therapy. Practice guidelines for blood component therapy. *Anaesthesiology* 1998; 84: 732–747

Zallen G, Moore EE. Hypertonic saline resuscitation abrogates neutrophil priming by mesenteric lymph nodes. *Journal of Trauma-Injury Infection and Critical Care* 2000; 48: 45–48.

Chapter **20**

Monitoring the trauma patient

Mark Dawes

INTRODUCTION

Management of the seriously injured patient requires a systematic and consistent approach in order to identify and treat life-threatening conditions rapidly, and monitor the response to interventions carried out. The importance of structure during patient assessment cannot be overemphasised, with a disordered approach potentially resulting in failure to diagnose and treat fatal conditions.

Rapid assessment of the patient by the use of monitoring devices indicates baseline observation of physiological status, aids diagnosis of clinical conditions, helps ascertain deterioration in the patient's condition, and indicates and evaluates efficiency of intervention.

This chapter aims to discuss the monitoring devices and diagnostic techniques available in the management of the trauma patient. It will also highlight the indications for and limitations of the various techniques commonly employed.

In order for data obtained to be correctly interpreted and acted upon, trauma nurses must be familiar with the equipment used in their own clinical settings. Nurses require an understanding of the relevant physiological processes affecting interpretation of data obtained and should be aware of the indications for seeking medical assistance in response to relevant changes in observations.

MONITORING OF PHYSIOLOGICAL PARAMETERS

Obtaining vital signs on arrival in hospital forms an important part of the initial assessment of a patient's response to pre-hospital interventions and ongoing priorities for the resuscitation effort.

Non-invasive measures must firstly be relied upon, until more accurate invasive measures can be obtained. The recording of vital signs is a priority for nursing staff within the trauma team. It is essential that they can adequately assess and to some extent evaluate ongoing readings so that a patient's response to treatment is recorded and reported to the relevant medical staff.

The vital signs that can be non-invasively monitored at the bedside include pulse, blood pressure, respiratory rate and temperature.

Pulse

There are a number of different parameters that must be evaluated when taking a pulse. The site usually utilised is the radial pulse and, when it is palpated, it should be assessed for rate, rhythm and volume. The pulse rate is normally within the range 60–100 beats per minute (bpm). An elevated rate may indicate *hypovolaemia* with a reactive sympathetic rise occurring in an attempt to maintain perfusion of the body's vital organs. Tachycardia in the trauma patient should always be assumed to be indicative of shock and fluid replacement initiated accordingly, unless other signs and symptoms suggest otherwise. Tachycardia may also occur as consequence of pain or anxiety; there should be no rise in rate as monitoring continues. An elevated pulse rate can also be caused by *hypoxaemia* owing to a primary airway or ventilatory problem, or inadequate cardiac function of medical origin or secondary to trauma to the heart.

Bradycardia in a fit individual can be normal but, in a trauma patient with known or suspected head injury, may be highly significant. It suggests raised intracranial pressure (ICP), especially if accompanied by a rising or elevated blood pressure. Bradycardia could also be the result of beta-blocker treatment for hypertension but should not be assumed unless there is reliable information to support this.

The rhythm of the pulse is an important factor to assess. A dysrhythmia may precipitate the trauma, or be secondary to cardiac or brain injury. Initially, any irregularity can be detected by palpation and further information later obtained by electrocardiogram (ECG) monitoring later. Pulse volume is also an important parameter that aids diagnosis. A good volume pulse at the radial artery indicates good peripheral perfusion, whereas a low volume pulse, especially when associated with tachycardia, demonstrates that the patient is becoming shocked.

The site of palpable pulses can give a predictive indication of likely blood pressure. Blood pressure can be rapidly *estimated* by the presence of pulses at three main pulse sites – radial, femoral and carotid:

- radial pulse – indicates a systolic blood pressure of 80 mmHg and above
- femoral pulse – indicates a systolic blood pressure of 70 mmHg and above
- carotid pulse – indicates a systolic blood pressure of 60 mmHg and above.

Although these do not give exact figures, the presence of pulses at these sites may provide a useful and rapid indicator of arterial blood pressure.

Palpation of pulses distal to the site of limb trauma is extremely important. The presence of a pulse implies that no major arteries have been disrupted, whilst absence may indicate shock, if combined with contralateral absence, but should alert the team to the need for rapid reduction of a fracture or dislocation, if pulses are asymmetrical. It may also indicate the need for surgery, if a pulse cannot be restored by conservative techniques.

Blood pressure

Frequent assessment and monitoring of the patient's blood pressure is an essential component of patient assessment. Changes in arterial blood pressure in conjunction with other physiological signs may provide early indicators to the emergency nurse of a patient's response to initial treatment or the signs of a patient's deterioration. Blood pressure readings should be recorded accurately and at regular pre-determined intervals, ensuring that any variations in pressure or evolving trends are reported back to the trauma team leader and acted upon appropriately.

Peak systolic blood pressure is directly related to left ventricular systolic pressure, with diastolic blood pressure being maintained by vascular tone (i.e. peripheral vascular resistance). The systolic blood pressure varies by up to 10 mmHg between the left and right brachial arteries. Standing up usually results in a slight decrease in the systolic pressure (up to 20 mmHg) with an associated increase in the diastolic blood pressure (up to 10 mmHg). Blood pressure measurements can be obtained by palpation, auscultation, Doppler or oscillometric methods.

Respiratory rate

A number of clinical abnormalities can be deduced by observing respirations. A raised respiratory rate (tachypnoea) may be caused by failure to ventilate the lungs adequately owing to a blocked airway or failure to transfer oxygen into the blood as a result of chest trauma (i.e. pneumothorax or haemothorax). Pulmonary contusion may also result in inadequate transfer of oxygen.

The respiratory rate will also increase if hypoxaemia is cardiac or circulatory in origin, for example, in cardiac tamponade, pulmonary embolism, cardiac contusion, myocardial rupture and disruption of major arteries. It will also be exacerbated by pre-existing heart failure or lung disease. A decreased respiratory rate may occur as a result of drug ingestion such as opiates.

Depth of respiration may indicate a number of factors. Shallow respirations are often due to pain in the chest wall or abdomen, and may be alleviated by analgesia. Deeper respiratory excursion is an involuntary response to hypoxaemia.

Symmetry of chest wall movement is an important observation; paradoxical movement of a flat segment of chest may suggest a *flail segment*. A unilateral failure of chest wall movement may be indicative of conditions such as pneumothorax (tension or simple), haemothorax or massive pulmonary contusion.

Irregularity of respirations is likely to suggest brain injury involving the respiratory centre and is a poor prognostic sign.

Pulse oximetry or invasive oxygen monitoring, which are discussed later, together with observations of respiratory effort can be used to assess the need for intubation and artificial ventilatory support.

Temperature

Temperature can be measured orally, rectally, in the axilla or electronically with a tympanic thermometer. Rectal temperature is the nearest to a true core temperature that can be obtained but is usually impractical in the trauma patient, especially if the patient is immobilised on a rescue (spinal/long) board.

MONITORING THE PATIENT

There are now many electric devices that can be used in addition to traditional methods for monitoring the trauma patient. It must be emphasised that electrical devices are not a substitute but an adjunct to clinical assessment of a patient.

> 'Treat the patient, not the monitor'

Monitoring devices may be non-invasive or invasive. They may be multifunctional and many different models are available on the market. Familiarity with the use of each is essential. Ideally, equipment should be 'user friendly', light and compact for ease of transfer, and must not rely on mains electricity. It must contain battery back-up in order to function in the event of an electricity failure.

BLOOD PRESSURE

Blood pressure (manual)

The equipment required for blood pressure measurement comprises a stethoscope and a sphygmomanometer with cuff and inflatable bladder.

Blood pressure is ideally taken from the right arm with the patient sitting at a 45° angle. This may be difficult in practice, as the patient may be lying supine on a spinal board, may have intravenous lines and monitoring devices *in situ*, or underlying humeral fractures, which may render measurement impractical.

The sphygmomanometer cuff is placed around the patient's upper arm. It is essential for the cuff to be the appropriate size for the patient. The width of the cuff should ideally be 40% of the upper arm circumference and the length of the cuff should be at least 80% of the upper arm circumference (Kirkendall et al, 1985). A cuff that is too narrow may give a falsely high reading and, if too wide, a lower reading may be obtained. The cuff is inflated until the pressure exceeds the arterial pressure and the radial pulse is no longer palpable.

The diaphragm of the stethoscope is positioned over the brachial artery just below the cuff. The cuff pressure is slowly reduced until sounds (Korotkoff sounds) are heard. This is recorded as the *systolic blood pressure*, and indicates the point at which systolic blood pressure exceeds the pressure in the cuff and blood flow is just returning in the arteries. It is heard because the obstructed flow is turbulent. The cuff pressure is allowed to fall further until the Korotkoff sounds disappear. This is recorded as the *diastolic blood pressure* and indicates that normal non-turbulent blood flow has returned.

The main points to be considered when taking blood pressure are listed in Box 20.1.

Electronic monitoring of blood pressure

This is a reliable method for the non-invasive blood pressure assessment. Many of the automated electronic machines available incorporate addi-

> **Box 20.1   Important considerations when taking blood pressure**
>
> - Ensure all clothing has been removed from the patient's arms
> - Ensure the arm is supported at the level of the heart
> - Use correctly sized cuff
> - Check systolic blood pressure by palpation
> - Release cuff pressure slowly in order to auscultate Korotkoff sounds
> - Record diastolic pressure at the disappearance of Korotkoff sounds
> - Ensure that the sphygmomanometer is serviced and calibrated on a regular basis to ensure accurate measurement

tional monitoring functions, such as pulse rate, pulse oximetry, temperature and invasive monitoring (i.e. arterial, central venous pressure and capnography).

Automated blood pressure monitors comprise a cuff, which can be automatically inflated and deflated as required, or at pre-determined intervals in time. The blood pressure cuff contains a sensor (which may be either a microphone or oscillometer) that is placed over the brachial artery and monitors pulsation through the artery. There are various markings impregnated on to the cuff – such as an arrow, which should be directly over the brachial artery, or pointers to the zone of the cuff in which the artery must lie.

The cuff is inflated automatically by the machine and slowly deflated. Oscillometric monitors detect motion in the blood pressure cuff from the underlying artery. Systolic blood pressure is recorded from a sudden increase in the amplitude of arterial oscillations, diastolic blood pressure being recorded when there is an abrupt decrease in oscillations. Monitors that use a microphone receiver identify Korotkoff sounds and return of blood flow to identify systolic and diastolic pressures.

Some authors have questioned the accuracy of oscillometric methods (Johnson and Kerr, 1985), when it was noted that oscillometric monitors may underestimate systolic pressures when a patient's blood pressure is high and overestimate systolic blood pressure when the blood pressure is low.

Automated machines may be unreliable when there is excessive artefact present, particularly in a combative patient when muscle movement of the arm is marked. Reliability can also be questioned when a patient is profoundly hypotensive and if their peripheral vascular resistance is high, as in extreme hypothermia.

It is imperative that the manufacturers' own cuffs are used with each device and that instructions are followed.

> Devices must be regularly serviced and recalibrated in order to maintain accuracy of readings

PULSE OXIMETRY

This is a simple non-invasive and reliable way of measuring capillary blood oxygenation valuation.

The technique was pioneered in Germany in 1932 by Nicolai, Kramer and Matthes.

Accurate clinical assessment of oxygenation is often difficult, particularly in poor lighting and in patients who are shocked, or hypothermic and in those who have chronic skin discoloration (e.g. polycythaemia)

The pulse oximeter can be both mains- and battery-operated. These devices rely on a probe, which can be applied to the patient's digits, ear or nasal bridge (Figure 20.1). From the probe, pulses of light of two specific wavelengths in the red (660 nm) and infrared (940 nm) ranges of the electromagnetic spectrum are produced by two adjacent light-emitting devices. The light waves are absorbed in differing amounts depending on the total haemoglobin and oxyhaemoglobin present. Waves that are not absorbed are detected by a photodetector in the probe, and converted to an electronic signal and transferred to a processing unit, which is displayed as an arterial waveform and a numerical display indicating oxygen saturation (SpO_2). The majority of machines also demonstrate the pulse rate.

There are a number of advantages and disadvantages in using pulse oximetry devices. The advantages are that these devices are:

- non invasive
- continuous
- do not require calibration
- accurate (within 1–4% if saturation greater than 70%).

The disadvantages are listed below:

- accuracy can be affected by movement artefact, excessive light, hypoperfusion, deep skin pigmentation and nail polish.

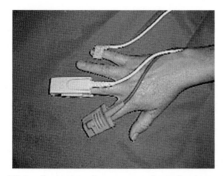

Figure 20.1   Examples of common pulse oximeter probes.

- SpO_2 may be overestimated in the presence of methaemoglobin or carboxyhaemoglobin (i.e. poisoning).
- it provides no indication of carbon dioxide saturations, therefore, is not a good way of assessing adequate ventilation.
- accuracy at saturations < 70% is decreased, leading to a falsely high reading.

Pulse oximetry is useful for diagnosis of trauma related respiratory compromise, although normal oxygen saturation does not exclude pathology, if the patient is compensating by increasing their respiratory rate. Normal values for pulse oximetry are given in Box 20.2.

Pulse oximetry is a widely used and relatively inexpensive monitoring technique, which provides a non-invasive and generally reliable assessment of tissue oxygenation.

CAPNOGRAPHY

Capnography is the measurement of the CO_2 concentration in expired air. It can be utilised in patients who have required intubation either in the pre-hospital field or within the A&E department. The reading obtained is defined as the end tidal CO_2 ($ETCO_2$). The use of capnography was first developed in the mid-1970s by Smalhout and Kalenda.

Capnography is a useful method for:

- assessing correct endotracheal tube placement;
- monitoring and detecting a possible blockage or obstruction within the breathing circuit;
- observing CO_2 levels in a head-injured patient who may require ventilation.

It is a non-invasive technique that has been shown to correlate well with the $PaCO_2$ of the blood. However, it is less accurate when monitoring patients with chronic obstructive

Box 20.2	Normal values for pulse oximetry
97–100%	Adult normal at sea level
90–96%	Mild hypoxia
85–90%	Moderate hypoxia
< 85%	Severe hypoxia

pulmonary disease (COPD) and severe asthma, where gas exchange may be impaired between the alveoli and capillaries.

It must be emphasised that correct placement of an endotracheal (ET) tube should usually be obvious from clinical observation, such as direct visualisation of the tube passing between the vocal cords, palpation of the tube passing through the larynx, absence of leakage around the inflated cuff, bilateral chest expansion, auscultation of breath sounds in the axillae and finally absence of breath sounds in the epigastric area.

> Capnography should be used as a final check rather than relying on it as the sole method of ensuring correct endotracheal tube placement

Detection of higher levels of CO_2 in expired air usually confirms tracheal as opposed to oesophageal intubation.

Capnography equipment and monitors

There are two main types of carbon dioxide detectors available: infrared and colorimetric.

Infrared

Mainstream analyser   This is a transducer placed in line with the ventilation unit (Figure 20.2). It is attached between the ET tube and the catheter mount of the ventilator. It contains an infrared, light-emitting diode (LED) source and a photodetector. It is kept at a constant 40°C to reduce the rate of condensation of the expired air, which may alter the reading. The LED emits a pulsed beam

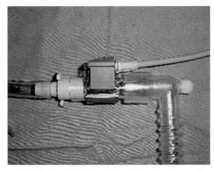

Figure 20.2   Example of a mainstream analyser. Note the analyser is in line with the endotracheal tube and catheter mount.

of infrared waves through a filter, which prevents interference from other gases, such as oxygen and nitrous oxide. The beam is received by the photodetector and turned into an electrical signal, which is shown as a waveform on the monitor and a digital numerical value.

Side-stream analyser   This is also referred to as a 'diverting capnometer'. This device withdraws air from the tip of the ET tube and channels it through a side port and into a sampling tube. The sample is then manually transferred to a separate analyser. This is a slower method and does not allow continuous end-tidal CO_2 monitoring.

Colorimetric detectors   These are disposable devices, which measure pH levels by colorimetry. They are attached in series with the ventilation circuit and simply produce a visible change in colour on a membrane within the device. CO_2 levels of < 0.5% (as in the inspiratory phase of respiration) produce a mauve coloration. Levels between 2 and 5% (as in expiration) produce a yellow colour. These devices are designed to function for approximately two hours.

Capnography devices have a number of limitations (Box 20.3); however, the use of capnography in conjunction with oxygen saturation monitoring is a useful indication of the effectiveness of artificial ventilation and diagnosis of changes in clinical conditions. End-tidal CO_2 monitoring is predominantly used with a conventional ET tube, but new research is being evaluated to determine its usefulness with laryngeal mask airways and bag–valve–mask ventilation (Nakatani et al., 1999) and sampling from intranasal cannula (Fukuda et al., 1997).

ELECTROCARDIOGRAPHY

It is essential that the trauma patient routinely undergoes continuous ECG monitoring. Continuous ECG monitoring should alert the trauma team to changes in heart rate or rhythm, which may occur as a result of:

- pain
- hypovolaemia
- hypoxaemia
- hypercapnia.

Box 20.3   Limitations of capnography

- Recent ingestion of a carbonated drink may lead to artificially high levels of CO_2 in the stomach gas. This may suggest correct placement of the endotracheal tube initially even though the tube is within the oesophagus. Therefore, the patient requires close observation and early readings may need to be ignored
- High levels of CO_2 may occur following aggressive mouth-to-mouth ventilation leading to high CO_2 levels in the stomach. It is suggested that readings during the first six ventilation cycles are disregarded
- During cardiac arrest, CO_2 is not produced and will not be detected, even in a correctly placed tube
- Copious secretions in the airway may impair gaseous exchange and result in a low CO_2 level, which may make the clinician assume oesophageal placement
- Disposable devices may be contaminated by gastric acid, causing a permanent orange colour in colorimetric devices
- Lignocaine (lidocaine) and epinephrine given via the endotracheal tube cause a permanent orange colour in colorimetric devices
- Infrared devices are expensive and delicate

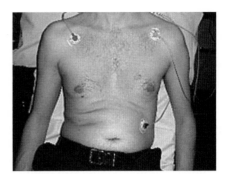

Figure 20.3   Electrocardiograph leads *in situ*.

It can also be used to evaluate the success of treatment strategies, such as intravenous (IV) fluids, drugs and defibrillation

ECG electrode placement

Pre-gelled adhesive electrodes should be positioned in the standard three-lead positions (Figure 20.3) and connected to the ECG leads as follows:

- red: below right clavicle
- yellow: below left clavicle
- green: over cardiac apex/left upper abdomen.

It may be necessary to dry and clean the skin of any water or blood, and remove any chest hair in order to obtain a good contact, thus reducing artefact and a 'wandering baseline' on the ECG trace.

The standard lead used for monitoring is lead II. This records the ECG trace between the electrodes placed over the cardiac apex and the right clavicle. ECG recognition and interpretation is discussed in Chapter 18.

Tachycardia may indicate hypovolaemia or sympathetic activity resulting from pain or anxiety. Bradycardia may indicate hypoxia or extreme hypothermia. Atrial fibrillation, premature ventricular contractions and ST segment changes may indicate blunt cardiac damage (i.e. cardiac contusion). Electromechanical dissociation/pulseless electrical activity (EMD/PEA) may indicate tension pneumothorax, cardiac tamponade or severe hypovolaemia.

INVASIVE MONITORING

Intra-arterial transducers

This invasive method of monitoring oxygen saturation and arterial pressure is commonly used in the management of the seriously injured patient in the hospital environment and during interhospital transfer.

Arterial pressure is dependent on the cardiac output and peripheral vascular resistance. It must be remembered that there are many physiological mechanisms that work to maintain arterial pressure, and oxygenation in the presence of changes in blood volume, cardiac output or respiratory-impaired compensation for these conditions may initially give normal readings and do not exclude pathology.

Arterial lines through which the transducers are passed allow frequent sampling of arterial blood for acid–base balance evaluation, and haematological and biochemical analyses. They avoid the need for recurrent arterial puncture, decreasing the risk of complications and stress to the patient. The line may also be used to introduce radio-opaque dye for radiological investigation of vascular disruption. The choice of puncture site is mainly determined by the ease of fixing it in any given patient and the presence of limb trauma. Commonly used sites are the radial, femoral or dorsalis pedis arteries.

Radial artery

The radial artery is used most often because it is relatively superficial and the line can be secured to the wrist without significant reduction of movement of the arm. It can be easily observed by nursing staff for signs of occlusion, dislodgement or infection.

Prior to insertion of a radial arterial line, it is essential to assess the adequacy of perfusion of the hand by the ulnar artery, which forms an arcade connecting with the radial artery in the palm, giving off branches to the fingers and hand. The Allen's test is performed by simultaneous occlusion of the radial and ulnar arteries by manual pressure against underlying bones. The patient then makes a fist to force blood out of the hand. Pressure on the ulnar artery is released and blood flow should be restored to the ulnar aspect of the palm in 1–2 seconds, if it is adequate (Bedford, 1977). If the hand remains pale for greater than 2 seconds, an alternative site should be considered. The technique for radial artery cannulation is shown in Box 20.4.

The radial artery is also commonly used to obtain arterial blood samples for the measurement of arterial blood gases (Figure 20.4).

Brachial artery

The brachial artery in the antecubital fossa may be used but complications are more common. Damage to the artery may result in decreased perfusion of the limb and ischaemia. This risk will be worsened if a haematoma forms at the site. The proximity of the median nerve to the brachial artery in the antecubital fossa also makes this site less favourable. Splintage of the elbow may be difficult, making dislodgement more likely.

Femoral artery

The femoral artery is a large-calibre and relatively superficial structure, thus facilitating placement of

---

Box 20.4   Technique for radial artery cannulation

1. Perform Allen's test and, if satisfactory, continue with placement
2. Sterile equipment and aseptic technique must be used.
3. The arm is supported with the wrist extended
4. The artery is palpated where it arches over the radial head
5. Local anaesthetic, essential in the conscious patient, is infiltrated at the chosen site
6. An arterial cannula of 20G (adult) or 22G (child) is selected
7. The cannula is introduced at an angle of 30° to the skin and advanced a few millimetres in line with the vessel
8. The cannula is threaded up the artery in a proximal direction and the needle withdrawn
9. Tubing, containing heparinised saline, is connected to the cannula at one end and an oscilloscope at the other. The tubing contains a transducer and flushing device

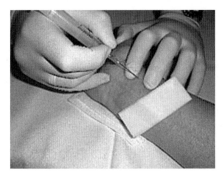

Figure 20.4   Obtaining an arterial blood sample from the radial artery.

---

an arterial cannula. Contraindications to its use are a history giving symptoms of impaired arterial supply to the limb or signs of hypoperfusion of the leg on clinical examination.

Dorsalis pedis

The dorsalis pedis artery is occasionally used for arterial cannulation. It is again relatively superficial and, therefore, accessible to the practitioner. Adequacy of the collateral arterial supply to the foot by the posterior tibialis artery is assessed in a similar way to the Allen's test. Both arteries are compressed and the toes flexed to produce blanching of the foot. Pressure of the posterior tibialis is released and restoration of blood supply noted. The drawback of this site is that owing to its increased distance from the central circulation and relatively narrow calibre, readings of 15–20 mmHg lower than central arterial pressure are often obtained. Distal ischaemia is also a more common complication than at other sites.

Whichever site is chosen, regular inspection for signs of distal ischaemia must be carried out. This may be indicated by impalpable pulses, pallor and decreased skin temperature distal to the site. Any swelling suggestive of an evolving haematoma must be observed closely.

Complications of arterial lines include:

- thrombosis of the vessel and subsequent embolism
- ischaemia and later necrosis distal to the site owing to impaired arterial supply
- accidental use for administration of drugs that could cause vascular occlusion
- disconnection leading to haemorrhage and possible hypovolaemia
- reduction of sepsis and contamination requires a complete change of transducer sets every 48 hours
- accidental damage to surrounding structures such as nerves
- haematoma at site, further impairing blood supply distally and compressing adjacent structures.

Arterial pressure monitoring

The systolic and diastolic pressures can be recorded and mean arterial pressure calculated by placing a transducer in the arterial line. The transducer is a fluid-filled device that detects fluctuations in pressure and converts this into an electrical signal that is transmitted and displayed on the monitor as a waveform and numerical value. Prior to its use, the transducer must be calibrated so that it reads zero in atmospheric pressure; it should be remembered that the elasticity of the tubing might affect the pressure recorded by the transducer.

Although the arterial line is a convenient source for obtaining blood for analysis, user error can significantly affect the results. If there is a significant delay in analysing the sample after it has been obtained (i.e. greater than 15 minutes), the continuing metabolism within the blood sample may lead to the measurement of lower levels of oxygen and increased levels of CO_2 than were present in the arterial blood at the time of sampling. This effect can be reduced by capping the sample and storing it over ice before rapid transfer to the analyser.

The sampling device must be heparinised (0.1 ml per 2 ml blood) to prevent clots forming within the analyser but care must be taken, as too much heparin may cause spurious abnormalities in the acid level results. Air bubbles in the sample may also alter oxygen and CO_2 measurements owing to equilibration of gases between the blood and the air bubbles. This can be minimised by holding the sample vertically and tapping the bubbles to the top of the syringe and then expelling the air.

The arterial line is an invaluable means of monitoring arterial pressures continuously and provides a means of obtaining arterial blood for gas analysis without recurrent, and painful, arterial puncture.

CENTRAL VENOUS CATHETERISATION AND MONITORING

Central venous access has become an increasingly utilised invasive procedure. The prime indications for central venous catheterisation in the resuscitation room are as follows:

1. The assessment of the patient's circulation and intravascular volume during resuscitation and following fluid replacement through measurement of the central venous pressure (CVP).
2. Emergency access to the central circulation when peripheral access may be difficult to establish (i.e. major burns, fractures, severely traumatised extremities and in obese patients). It is not, however, considered a useful means of rapid fluid infusion as a long thin catheter is used, which only allows low

velocity of fluid infusion when compared with a short, larger-diameter cannula; flow rate is directly proportional to the fourth power of the radius and is inversely proportional to the length. Therefore, a short, wide catheter or cannula has a greater flow rate than a long thin catheter.

3. Administration of drugs that are sclerosant, if extravasation should occur (e.g. dopamine).

In order to obtain a CVP reading, the tip of the CVP catheter must be positioned in the thoracic cavity, the catheter having been passed through one of the larger veins (i.e. superior vena cava), entering the heart and lying in the right atrium.

The CVP is defined as the pressure exerted by the blood against the walls of the intrathoracic vena cava. It, therefore, reflects the pressure at which blood is returned to the right atrium and equates with right ventricular end diastolic pressure (filling pressure). It essentially indicates the pressure of blood returning from peripheral veins to the heart.

However, the CVP does not always reflect left heart pressure or the status of the intravascular volume. The CVP may be within normal limits, even when the patient is hypovolaemic, especially in patients who have pre-existing lung disease (i.e. COPD), when blood pressure in the lungs is already raised causing back pressure and thus artificially raising CVP. It is also inaccurate when the patient is peripherally vasoconstricted. It, therefore, has some limitations in the initial stages of monitoring of the critically ill patient.

Central venous cannulation procedures

Central venous cannulation carries a number of risks, thus the practitioner carrying out the technique should possess a detailed knowledge of both the superficial and deep anatomy, and should be aware of the potential complications.

> The site used for CVP cannulations should be dependent on the operator's skill and experience, and on the clinical situation

Sites of insertion
The three main access sites are:

- subclavian vein
- internal jugular vein
- femoral vein.

Subclavian vein   In order to cannulate the subclavian vein, the patient should be supine and in the Trendelenburg position (10–15° head down). The Trendelenburg position is used to reduce the risk of air embolism by increasing positive pressure inside the vein when the needle enters it. It has also been thought that the head-down position increases the dilation of the subclavian vein but this remains controversial.

The right subclavian vein is the most favourable side of insertion, as the pleural dome does not rise as high above the clavicle on this side compared to the left, and there is the added risk of thoracic duct damage with left-sided cannulation. The head should be turned to the contralateral side with a small towel or pillow placed between the scapulae to further open up the sternoclavicular angle, thus improving access from the infraclavicular approach. Strict asepsis must be maintained throughout and the area anaesthetised, if the patient is conscious.

In practice, this positioning cannot always be carried out, if there is any suspicion of cervical spine injury, where manipulation of the head could lead to subluxation of cervical vertebrae and possible spinal cord damage.

There are several approaches to the supraclavicular vein. One common approach is described in Box 20.5.

Internal jugular vein   The internal jugular vein can also be used to gain access. The patient is again placed in the Trendelenburg position to distend the internal jugular vein. If cervical spine injury can be excluded, the head is turned to the

---

Box 20.5   Cannulation of subclavian vein

- Identify the midpoint of the clavicle and the suprasternal notch
- Aim a 20G needle at the suprasternal notch, hooking under the clavicle
- The needle is advanced until it enters the vein and blood is aspirated, flowing freely into an attached syringe

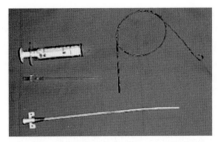

Figure 20.5   Example of a single lumen catheter.

contralateral side. The right side is the preferred side, as it provides a more direct route to the superior vena cava. The technique is summarised in Box 20.6.

Femoral vein   This is occasionally the preferred route of choice for patients who have sustained substantial trauma to the neck or chest, thus making subclavian or internal jugular approaches difficult. This route is also ideal in patients who have coagulopathy problems or who are at risk of arrhythmias.

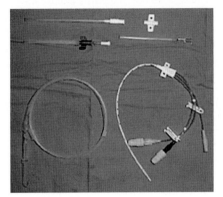

Figure 20.6   Example of a multilumen catheter.

The femoral vein is sited medial to the femoral artery

The needle is inserted 1–3 cm below the inguinal ligament. It should be advanced cephalically parallel to the femoral artery.

Choice of catheter
Catheters available may be single-, double- or triple-lumen (Figure 20.5). Multilumen catheters have luminal exit ports down the length of the cannula (Figure 20.6). These are the catheters of choice in the resuscitation room, as they allow for different drugs to be administered simultaneously, as well as monitoring the CVP.

Catheters are inserted using two different techniques:

- *through cannula*, where the vein is cannulated with an IV cannula, the needle removed and a catheter is then fed through the cannula and sutured into place.
- *'catheter over guide wire'*. This is known as the Seldinger technique (Box 20.7), which was

pioneered by Seldinger in 1953 for the purpose of percutaneous arteriography.

Measuring the CVP

The CVP measurement may be recorded using two methods:

- manual manometer
- CVP transducer.

Manual method
Central venous pressure measurement is performed with the use of a fluid-filled manometer tube. The fluid level is referenced against a fixed external landmark – either the mid-axillary line or the manubriosternal angle. The latter gives a reading 5–7 cm lower than the former but this is not important as long as consistency is maintained.

The patient is placed flat, and the manometer and measuring scale fixed to an intravenous drip stand so that the 10 cm mark is in line with the chosen anatomical point. A three-way tap is used to control normal saline flow into the manometer

---

Box 20.7   Seldinger technique

- A large-bore needle is inserted through the skin into the chosen vein. Venous blood should flow freely back through the introducer.
- A guide wire is inserted through the needle and advanced into the vein.
- The needle is withdrawn leaving the guide wire *in situ*. (The guide wire causes minimal trauma to the vein owing to its flexibility, thus reducing the chances of vein-wall perforation.)
- A dilator is fed over the needle to open up a channel into the vessel
- A CVP catheter is then passed over the wire to the desired distance and the wire removed.
- Catheter position must be verified by the easy aspiration of blood.
- The catheter is then flushed with saline or heparinised saline to ensure patency is maintained.
- The catheter is then sutured to the skin and covered with a transparent semipermeable dressing.
- A chest x-ray *must* be performed to verify the position of the catheter
- Following verification of the position, drugs may be administered and CVP measurements carried out.

---

tubing. The tube is filled to the 30 cm level – well above the predicted CVP reading. The three-way tap is then positioned to allow free flow of fluid into the patient. The fluid level will descend and swing up and down with respiration until it settles.

The CVP is measured in centimetres of water in the tube when referenced against the previously agreed landmark. Normal values are:

- 0–5 cmH$_2$O sternal angle
- 5–10 cmH$_2$O mid axilla point.

This manual method only allows for intermittent measuring of CVP, as the manometer tubing must be refilled each time.

CVP transducer
The transducer method, identical to that described in arterial pressure monitoring, allows direct CVP measurements by the use of a pressure monitor. This allows continuous observation of CVP trends in the compromised patient. When connected to

the CVP line, the transducer converts the pressure from the vessel into an electrical waveform and digital reading, which can be observed on any compatible electronic monitoring device.

It is essential that the CVP line and transducer set are zeroed, calibrated and free from air bubbles prior to taking a reading

CVP readings are not without their problems, and it is possible that certain physiological states or clinical problems may cause incorrect readings.

Causes of high CVP readings

- Cardiac tamponade – venous return to the heart is impaired.
- Tension pneumothorax – increased intrathoracic pressure impedes blood return.
- Fluid overload.
- Abnormal right ventricular function as in chronic cardiac failure, acute right ventricular failure or large pulmonary embolism.
- Malposition of the CVP tip – the tip may be resting against a physical obstruction.
- Raised venous tone (e.g. when catecholamines are released in response to trauma).

Causes of low CVP readings

- Hypovolaemia.
- Peripheral vasodilation (i.e. sepsis; drug therapy/overdose).

Complications of central venous cannulation

There are a number of potential complications that can arise when a CVP line is *in situ*. These are summarised in Box 20.8.

Care of the CVP line

It is essential that CVP lines are properly cared for and maintained. Simple checks, as listed below, will ensure that the line functions with the minimum of problems.

- Maintain asepsis at all times.
- Check patency of the line – observing for kinks or extravasation at regular intervals.
- Ensure the line is secure.

Box 20.8   Complications of central venous catheters

1. Pneumothorax, especially when using subclavicular access
2. Haemorrhage/haematoma – increased risk with internal jugular vein, which lies close to the carotid artery
3. Infection – local/systemic
4. Air embolisms
5. Haemothorax
6. Central vein thrombosis/embolism
7. Dysrhythmias
8. Catheter malposition/knotting
9. Myocardial perforation, which may lead to cardiac tamponade

---

- Observe vital signs and temperature, as they may affect readings.
- If using a transducer, ensure it is zeroed and calibrated before each recording.
- Observe for cardiac dysrhythmias by continuous ECG monitoring.

DIAGNOSTIC INVESTIGATIONS

As part of the investigation of any trauma patient, it is essential that blood be drawn in order to carry out specific laboratory studies.

Blood grouping and cross-matching

This is essential when anticipating blood replacement in the case of severe hypovolaemic shock. Such investigations can take some time before blood becomes available; a guide is given in Table 20.1.

Full blood count

A full blood count is taken to give a baseline blood count. Although the haemoglobin concentration indicates to some extent how much blood has been lost, initial readings in acute haemorrhage may not reflect the true picture because, although the blood volume has decreased, the concentrations of constituents remains the same in the acute stage. If the remaining blood has been 'diluted' by crystalloid or colloid infusions, the haemoglobin

Table 20.1   Times required for grouping and cross-matching blood

Type of blood	Time for preparation
Full cross-match	30–40 minutes
ABO compatible (type specific)	10 minutes
Uncross-matched O Rh negative	Immediate

concentration and haematocrit will give a more accurate indication of blood loss. A full blood count will also allow identification of sickle cell disease in susceptible groups.

Urea and electrolytes

Urea and electrolytes are also checked to give a baseline count. Abnormal results may indicate pre-existing renal disease but may also indicate hypovolaemia that has not been adequately treated, as poor perfusion of the kidneys leads to a rise in urea and potassium, followed by a rise in creatinine. Amylase levels may also be important, if there is a strong suspicion of abdominal trauma and the potential for pancreatic injury.

Toxicology and blood alcohol levels

If there is a strong suspicion of drug or alcohol ingestion, bloods must be drawn and analysed. Results from these tests may explain some abnormal physiological findings, such as peripheral vasodilation, pupillary constriction or dilation, or unexpectedly low Glasgow Coma Scale (e.g. opiate abuse).

Blood glucose

Blood glucose may identify compounding factors, such as diabetic ketoacidosis or hypoglycaemia, both of which may affect the patient's level of consciousness.

Children are particularly likely to develop hypoglycaemia, requiring urgent treatment, as a result of trauma

Clotting profile

A clotting profile may identify impending disseminated intravascular coagulation following blood replacement with fluids containing no clotting factors. Clotting studies may also identify if the patient is taking anticoagulation therapy (e.g. warfarin), which could be reversed, if necessary.

Beta human chorionic gonadatrophin (BHCG) (pregnancy test)

A pregnancy test should be considered for all females of childbearing age. This can be easily performed by carrying out a simple urine test. It must be emphasised that BHCG levels fall after 16 weeks gestation and may be undetectable after 20 weeks gestation. In this situation, a careful history and clinical examination should exclude pregnancy.

RADIOGRAPHY

Radiographic investigations are essential in the correct management of the severely injured patient; however, the timings of such investigations must never compromise care by delaying resuscitation measures. The three essential x-rays that must be obtained are:

- anteroposterior (AP) chest
- lateral cervical spine
- anteroposterior pelvis.

These can be initially performed in the resuscitation room with a portable x-ray machine. They can rapidly provide the trauma team with information to aid early diagnosis and management, but are usually of poor quality compared to those obtained in the radiology department.

After life-threatening injuries have been identified and resuscitation established to the point where the patient is in a stable condition, further x-rays may be carried out in the radiology department. It is essential that constant monitoring of vital signs be continued throughout this process.

Further x-rays that may be indicated include skull, thoracic and lumbar spine, limbs, and possibly abdominal films. If there are life-threatening but treatable conditions that have already been identified by clinical or initial radiographic investigations, intervention must not be delayed. Portable x-rays may be obtained perioperatively in theatre.

Chest x-ray

A number of deaths following major trauma are due to thoracic damage. Therefore, a chest x-ray is considered to be the most essential of the three initial x-rays. Ideally, the best view is the position anterior erect view but, in the resuscitation room, a supine AP view is usually the only practical option. It is limited by apparent enlargement of the mediastinum by distended great vessels (gravity effect) and poor inspiration in this position.

> There is often poor correlation between external evidence of chest wall injury and the actual severity of intrathoracic injury

Any observations noted on chest x-ray may often underestimate intrathoracic injury (Staik, 1993).

Trauma-related conditions that may be demonstrated on chest x-ray are:

- haemothorax
- pneumothorax
- airway (bronchial or tracheal) disruption
- diaphragmatic rupture
- rib fractures
- surgical emphysema.

A systematic approach to the interpretation of the chest x-ray is advisable. This approach can be remembered by the saying 'always be cautious and sensible':

A adequacy and alignment
B bones
C cartilage and joints
S soft tissues

Adequacy and alignment
Adequacy of inspiration is confirmed by visualisation of ten posterior ribs above the hemidiaphragm. Penetration of the film is of importance and is usually confirmed by visualisation of two intervertebral spaces behind the mediastinal shadow. Proper alignment of the x-ray can be checked by looking for equidistant spaces between the medial ends of the clavicle and the manubrium sterni.

Bones
Clavicles, scapulae, ribs and usually the humerus can be examined for fractures. The establishment

of the site of rib fractures can be of use in predicting likely coexisting trauma. The fifth to ninth ribs are most commonly injured. When lower ribs are fractured, there is a risk of coexisting splenic, hepatic and renal damage. Fractures of the first two ribs imply a considerable force has been sustained, and there is likely to be associated intrathoracic injury with airway or great vessel disruption.

Fractures of ribs 4–9 are often associated with pneumothorax, haemothorax and pulmonary contusion. If fractures of two or more adjacent ribs in two or more separate places are seen, a 'flail chest' can be diagnosed, even if it is not evident on clinical examination. Sternal fractures are likely to predict underlying pulmonary or cardiac contusion.

Cartilage and joints

All visible joints including shoulders, acromioclavicular, costochondral and sternoclavicular joints can be examined for dislocation and congruity of their articular surfaces.

Soft tissues

This encompasses the lung fields, mediastinum, skin overlying the chest wall and diaphragm. Parenchymal damage or contusion may be seen as consolidation on the x-ray, and may be patchy, homogenous or diffuse in nature. It could also be confused with coexisting lung disease such as pneumonia or COPD. If shadowing is confirmed in the upper lobes, particularly on the right side, aspiration must be considered. Acute or chronic congestion of the hilar regions shown as a 'bat wing' appearance indicates pulmonary oedema.

Pleural space collections may indicate a haemothorax, or splenic or hepatic lacerations, if noted basally. A large haemothorax may shift the mediastinum to the contralateral side. Air seen at the lateral margins of the thoracic cavity indicates a pneumothorax. Collapse of a lobe or whole lung field with consequent shift of the mediastinum towards the affected side may be seen in a tension pneumothorax. Mediastinal air is indicated by a line parallel to the mediastinal border or surrounding the heart. This may be the result of penetrating, blunt or deceleration injuries, and indicates disruption of the major airways or oesophagus.

Major vascular or cardiac injuries may be represented by a widened mediastinal shadow. Loss of definition of the aortic knuckle and right tracheal dilation are indicative of aortic rupture. If subsequent x-rays show the enlargement of the heart shadow, a haemopericardium or a pneumopericardium is suggested.

Diaphragmatic rupture is indicated by a raised hemidiaphragm, air in the stomach or intestine above the hemidiaphragm, and often a shift of the mediastinum toward the affected side. An ill-defined hemidiaphragm indicates overlying fluid or soft tissue masses. This may be caused by the bowel, liver, kidney, spleen or pancreas. The skin outlining the thoracic cavity may show air within it, indicating airway or lung disruption and subsequent surgical emphysema

The chest x-ray may also be of use in post-intervention evaluation. Adequacy of treatment of a tension pneumothorax can be evaluated. The siting of a CVP line may be observed for its position and absence of a complicating pneumothorax. Nasogastric and ET tube placement may also be assessed.

Cervical spine x-ray

In the patient with multiple injuries, 'it must always be assumed that a cervical spine injury could have been sustained' (American College of Surgeons Committee on Trauma, 1997).

> Adequate cervical spine immobilisation must be established as rapidly as possible in the pre-hospital field and maintained in the A&E department until bony trauma has been satisfactorily excluded by clinical examination and radiographic investigation

A lateral cross-table view is usually obtained in the resuscitation room. The x-ray must reliably include the base of the skull, all seven cervical vertebrae and the cervicothoracic junction (C7/T1). Caudal traction on the patient's arms (i.e. a pull in line with the axis of the body towards the feet), may improve success, as the clavicles and scapulae may obscure the view. An alternative is the 'swimmer's view', where one arm is raised above the head with traction applied to the contralateral limb, whilst x-rays are directed through the axilla. This may compromise cervical spine control and will be difficult with upper limb injury.

It is important to know that only 70–90% of cervical injuries are demonstrated by the lateral view (Perry et al., 1996). It is, therefore, essential to perform supplemental anterior, odontoid peg and oblique views. These are better carried out in the radiology department.

When examining x-rays of a cervical spine, always inspect the lateral view first and apply the ABCS mnemonic.

Adequacy
This is as detailed earlier but it is most important to remember that the top of T1 must be seen.

Alignment
Trace three important lines:

1. anterior vertebral margins;
2. posterior vertebral margins
3. spinolamina line.

Bones
Check that the vertebral bodies are of the same height at the anterior and posterior margins (crush injury). Any bone fragment may signify a fracture. The spinous processes should be intact.

Cartilage and joints
The disc spaces should be roughly equal in height, and of same distance anteriorly and posteriorly. Inspect facet joints for dislocation:

Soft tissue
Observe for any abnormal widening of the pre-vertebral spine. Swelling occurs in approximately 50% of cases with a bone damage (Miles and Finlay, 1988).

Other cervical spine views

A similar approach is used in looking at AP views, particularly looking for spinous process alignment.

On the open-mouth odontoid 'peg' view, look for a fractured odontoid peg. Artefacts, such as overlying teeth, the occiput and soft tissue may mimic a fracture. Also check the symmetry of the spaces between the peg and body of C1.

> Failure to immobilise an injury to the cervical spine may lead to preventable irreversible spinal cord damage

Pelvis

A pelvic x-ray should be the final x-ray to be obtained in the resuscitation room. The film is obtained via the anteroposterior approach and provides the team with evidence of any pelvic fracture or disruption.

The ABCS approach should again be utilised.

Adequacy
Ensure that the whole pelvis can be observed. The film should include the iliac crests and the femurs distal to the lesser trochanters.

Alignment
The pubic symphysis should be in line with the midline of the sacrum.

Bones
Fractures may appear as low- or high-density areas, or merely as a disruption in the trabecular pattern. Examine each of the three bones that make up the pelvis: the sacrum and the two inominate bones joined by the pubic symphysis and sacroiliac joints.

The next observation is the three elliptical curves of the pelvis: the pelvic brim in the centre, and the two obturator foramina inferolaterally. Check the pelvic brim for a continuous line all the way round. It cannot be breached in one place alone, as it is a rigid structure. The obturator foramina are rarely broken in one place alone.

> If one pelvic fracture is found, look for more disruption elsewhere

Cartilage and joints
As well as the joints mentioned above, it is also important to check the acetabular rims within which the three parts of each inominate bone come together. Examine them especially for fragments lying behind the femoral heads.

Soft tissues

Haematomas may appear as dense areas within the soft tissue shadows inside and outside the bony structures. Where the psoas muscles bridge the pelvis to join the femur, a black line is seen representing a small plane of fat between intra-peritoneal and extraperitoneal structures. Loss of this line indicates extraperitoneal haemorrhage or soft tissue oedema. Deviation of the line suggests intraperitoneal haemorrhage.

COMPUTED TOMOGRAPHY

Computed tomography (CT) was developed in the early 1970s and is widely available in many radiology departments. It involves the use of a radiation-emitting source directed across the body and picked up by a detector opposite. The source and the detector are rotated around the body, and the recorded wave attenuations processed by computer to produce an accurate two-dimen-sional image of both bony structures and the soft tissues.

Computed tomography scanning has an impor-tant role in trauma care. It is non-invasive and reliable in its diagnostic capabilities concerning all body areas and different tissue types. Examples of its uses in trauma are highlighted in Box 20.9.

There are a number of advantages of CT scanning, which include the following:

- They are non-invasive.
- They are very accurate (in abdominal trauma, the diagnostic rate is approximately 95%).
- They demonstrate soft tissue as well as bony injuries.
- Two-dimensional 'slices' are obtained, which overcome the problem of overlying structures obscuring views, as is the case with plain x-rays.

Equally there are some disadvantages. In most cases, CT scans necessitate transport out of the trauma department away from monitoring devices and resuscitation tools, exposure to high levels of ionising radiation – an abdominal CT scan is equivalent in radiation exposure to approximately 400 plain x-rays – and they are time consuming and may delay intervention. Scanning the chest, head, abdomen and pelvis may take in excess of 30 minutes, not including

> **Box 20.9 Summary of uses of computed tomography (CT) in trauma**
>
> **Head**
> Identification of fractures, cerebral haematomas, oedema and contusion injuries. It can also be useful in the diagnosis of maxillofacial bone injuries.
>
> **Neck**
> It is more reliable than the plain x-ray in diagnosis of cervical spine injuries. Soft tissues, pharynx and tracheal disruption are also more readily demonstrated.
>
> **Chest**
> The plain chest x-ray may well fail to give accurate information about the size of pneumothoraces or haemothoraces. With mediastinal injuries that may have been crudely diagnosed on plain films, the actual structures can be defined to allow therapeutic interventions to be better planned. Lung contusions may show as non-specific high-density patches on x-ray and can be seen in better detail on a CT scan.
>
> **Abdomen**
> Plain x-rays are a non-specific guide to visceral trauma. A bleeding solid organ, such as the spleen, may be missed easily on an x-ray but is easily seen with a CT scan. The retroperitoneal structures are also better demonstrated with CT.
>
> **Limbs**
> Most fractures should be diagnosed on plain x-rays, but associated vascular injury and hidden bleeding may be missed. A useful adjunct to diagnosis is the injection of contrast media into the circulation to identify sites of disrupted blood supply. The vascular systems of any area in the body can be seen in this way.

transport and set-up times. CT scans require a cooperative or anaesthetised patient, as move-ment artefact is a considerable problem. The scan must not compromise patient monitoring and, therefore, a doctor or nurse should be present throughout the procedure, a fact that may expose the carers themselves to radiation risks. Rarely, contrast media, if used, can cause an anaphylactic response. CT scanners have thereby been referred to as the 'doughnut of death'.

Another disadvantage is that CT scans are expensive investigations. Additionally, CT scan-ning is relatively contraindicated in pregnancy and so the threshold for this examination is higher. Finally, metal objects, such as pacemakers or joint prostheses, may obscure views.

MAGNETIC RESONANCE IMAGING

Magnetic resonance imaging (MRI) has become more widely available in recent years and is increasingly used in the diagnosis of trauma as well as in many other clinical settings.

It differs from CT scanning in that it does not use ionising radiation and is thus much safer. It uses changing magnetic fields applied across the body to set up movement of electrically charged atoms within cell nuclei. The positively charged proton is most often used and, when stimulated to move within the attenuating field, emits waves that can be detected by a transducer. The presence and abundance of charged protons can be detected by altering the frequency of the alternating magnetic field. Changes in the chemical environment of tissues due to trauma are easily demonstrated. It is more sensitive than CT scanning, which relies on tissue density alone.

The advantages of MRI scanning are that there is no ionising radiation damage, structures surrounded by bone are well demonstrated (e.g. pituitary fossa), and the scanner can be moved in any plane to provide three-dimensional images (CT is confined to one plane only).

There are, however, some disadvantages. These include its expense and the fact that the patient must be moved to the radiology department. MRI scans cannot be used in patients with metallic objects within the body (e.g. pacemakers, joint replacements, aneurysm clips and cochlear implants). Metallic monitoring devices or pumps cannot be in the same room and this may compromise care. The MRI scanner is also a very claustrophobic environment for patient and allows only limited access by the carers. It is less accurate than CT for acute intracranial haemorrhage and the long-term sequelae are not known, particularly in pregnancy, although in comparison with CT it is relatively safe (Royal College of Radiologists, 1998).

ULTRASOUND

Ultrasound involves directing very high frequency (1–10 MHz) sound waves across the body

and detection of the reflected waves by the same device. It can penetrate tissues but does not cause ionisation within the cells. The sound waves cause particles within tissues to move backwards and forwards. Waves are reflected back in different amounts, depending on the density of the structure and so demonstrate boundaries between adjacent structures.

Ultrasound imaging has had a major impact on the non-invasive diagnosis of trauma, particularly within the abdominal cavity. It is the only imaging method, which provides a real-time continuous picture. It can show free fluid within a body cavity, blood or oedema in the solid organs, and collections within confined structures. It has a diagnostic rate comparable to that of CT scanning and diagnostic peritoneal lavage, when looking at abdominal trauma.

It is useful because the portability of devices allows it to be taken to the bedside, thus not compromising the monitoring of vital signs. It is without significant effect on the tissues, is not contraindicated in pregnancy, and is inexpensive in comparison with other imaging modalities.

Images, however, may be impaired by a large fat layer between the skin surface and underlying structures and ultrasound will not demonstrate structures lying behind the bowel, as gas within it does not transmit waves effectively. Additionally, bones reflect large amounts of waves and structures behind them cannot be demonstrated. Pelvic cavity views may be significantly impaired by the pelvic bones and a full bladder is required to give the best chance of good pelvic views. Encapsulated organs may be surrounded by collections of blood obscuring views of the parenchyma of the organ.

> The interpretation of ultrasound images requires specialist training and so the diagnostic rates vary with operator experience

Doppler

This method of scanning employs the effect of ultrasound waves hitting a moving object. Waves are emitted from Doppler devices by the use of a piezoelectric device. Any object moving towards the source reflects waves at a higher frequency than an object moving at right angles to the wave, which in turn reflects at a higher frequency than waves reflected from an object moving away from it. Movement of blood within vessels can be demonstrated effectively and is often converted into an audible signal or displayed on a screen, which may be enhanced by the use of colour to distinguish between movement towards or away from the device.

In the resuscitation room, it is useful for evaluating blood flow to certain structures, particularly limbs, where vascular disruption is suspected. It is more sensitive than conventional devices to measure blood pressure, particularly in hypovolaemic patients. Blood flow at a pressure as low as 30 mmHg may be demonstrated. It is also used to identify the viability of a fetus from 6 weeks gestation onwards in a pregnant woman.

Images are enhanced by the use of 'acoustic gel' to aid transmission between the device and the skin surface. Any water-soluble gel is adequate for this purpose. Where peripheral pulses are being assessed, a superficial site of a vessel is identified. Some pressure must be applied to aid transmission of waves but it must not impede the flow of blood. It is used in conjunction with a sphygmomanometer cuff to assess systolic and diastolic pressures.

PAIN ASSESSMENT

Pain is an unpleasant sensory and emotional experience. Its assessment and treatment is of a high priority following preservation of life and treatment of major injuries. Pain alone can cause significant deterioration in clinical conditions. An example would be a chest injury leading to pain on movement causing the patient to take shallow breaths. This decreases tidal volume, which in turn can lead to hypoxia.

Pain also causes the release of catecholamines, such as epinephrine, which may increase the work of the myocardium, increase oxygen demand and increase blood pressure, with the higher blood pressure leading to increased haemorrhage.

Trauma is almost invariably associated with pain but is unfortunately often neglected on initial assessment. Because the perception of pain differs so widely between individuals, objective measure-

---

Box 20.10 Factors influencing pain

1. *Biological factors* – multifocal and complex types of pain are often present in the elderly
2. *Fatigue* – decreases pain tolerance level
3. *Psychological factors* – stress and anxiety alone exacerbate pain perceived; and vulnerability and lack of control over the situation are important common contributory factors
4. *Personality type* – often affects the way in which pain is felt and expressed. Anxious patients may have low pain thresholds but may also be reluctant to express this
5. *Cultural factors* – religion or culture are important factors affecting the individual's perception and expression of pain

---

ment of severity is difficult. Factors that may affect the perception of pain are detailed in Box 20.10. It is important that previous experience of particular patient groups does not prejudice staff and have an adverse effect on accuracy of pain assessment.

Pain is as severe as the patient says it is

There are a number of different ways in which an evaluation of severity of pain can be made.

1. subjective measures
2. physiological measures
3. behavioural observation.

Subjective measures

This is the most valuable way of assessing pain but is obviously dependent on the patient's condition. It is based on a rating of severity expressed by the patient. A number of different scales are available that can be tailored to the patient as necessary.

An example is an ascending series of numbers from 0 to 10, where 0 represents 'no pain' and 10 represents 'the worst pain every experienced'. This can also be expressed on paper as a horizontal line, where pain level is marked along the line and can be given a numerical value by measurement from the start of the line to the point marked by the patient (McCaffrey and Beebe, 1994).

Another widely approved model is the Burford Pain Thermometer, which combines a verbal and visual concept to express the patient's level of pain (Burford Nursing Development Unit, 1984).

Categorical verbal rating scales are another method used, which differ from the above analogue scales in that they assign a numerical value to a limited set of responses (e.g. severe 3, moderate 2, sharp 1 and none 0). The main criticism of these is that the limited responses force a less than accurate description of the parameter measured.

Each of the above scales may be combined with a body outline on which the individual sites and intensities of pain can be separately assessed.

Physiological measures

These are useful for young children, and head-injured and confused patients, who are unable to understand an analogue or categorised scale.

Known responses to pain are:

- increase in blood pressure
- increase in pulse rate
- increase in respiratory rate
- diaphoresis (sweating).

Their interpretation is very difficult owing to compounding factors such as anxiety, pre-existing medical conditions or trauma-related responses.

Behavioural observation

This is sometimes used in the assessment of children, where a quiet smiling child can be assumed to be in little pain, whereas the screaming restless child is more likely to be experiencing pain. Again this method has limitations, as, for example, with the extremely unwell child, who will be still and quiet, or the patient who has been sedated.

> Assessment of pain provides an invaluable framework for setting standards of care

For accurate results, methods of pain assessment must be tailored to the individual patient. As the severity of trauma increases, options for assessment techniques become progressively more limited. There are, however, very few patients in whom no rating is possible. Use of multiple methods of assessment improves accuracy of interpretation. It must be remembered that the same person should perform the assessment on each occasion, although, in practice, owing to shift patterns of staff and environmental changes, this is often impossible.

Every health professional should be competent in reliable and ongoing assessment of pain in order to minimise suffering.

TRAUMA SCORING

The concept of a trauma scoring system was devised to predict the likelihood of survival of a patient following trauma. The uses of trauma scoring are listed in Box 20.11.

In developed countries, trauma is the leading cause of death in children and young adults. In the UK, approximately 10 000–10 600 people suffer major injuries per annum (Burdett-Smith et al., 1995). Approximately 9000 die per annum as a result of their injuries (Department of Transport, 1996). The cost of trauma to the National Health Service is approximately £1.2 billion per annum (Department of Health, 1998).

There are three main categories of scoring systems; those that:

1. consider the extent and anatomical site of injury
2. indicate the degree of physiological disturbance

Box 20.11   Uses of trauma scoring

1. Evaluation and improvement of pre-hospital triage
2. Monitoring hospital care and response to treatment
3. Ranking of injuries according to mortality rates to focus priorities for treatment
4. Grouping cases for clinical research
5. Epidemiology, i.e. identification of preventable deaths
6. Evaluation of cost effectiveness of hospital treatment and appropriate allocation of resources

3. combine both anatomical and physiological parameters.

Some systems are more appropriate in the pre-hospital environment using observations alone, whilst some can only be used in hospital where more invasive parameters are used. The various systems are listed below.

1. *Anatomical:*
   abbreviated injury scale (AIS)
   maximum abbreviated injury score (MAIS)
   probability of death score (PODS)
   injury severity score (ISS).
2. *Physiological:*
   Glasgow Coma Scale (GCS)
   trauma index
   pre-hospital index
   triage index
   revised trauma score (RTS)
   trauma score and injury severity score (TRISS).
3. *Combined:*
   major trauma outcome study (MTOS).

Abbreviated injury scale (AIS)

This, first published in 1971 by The American Association for the Advancement of Automotive Medicine, provided the first universally acceptable method for rating tissue damage caused from vehicle accidents. A more recent update of the AIS was introduced in 1990. It comprises a six-digit score, the first five of which identify the specific injury, the basis of which can be obtained from a database publication. The sixth figure represents the severity of the injury ranked from 1 (minor) to 6 (fatal) (Table 20.2). There is obviously no linear correlation between score and mortality rate as, for example, a score of 4 does not indicate a mortality rate double that of a score of 2.

Table 20.2	The abbreviated injury scale (AIS)
AIS code	Description
1	Minor
2	Moderate
3	Serious
4	Severe
5	Critical
6	Unsurvivable

Maximum abbreviated injury scale (MAIS)

This is used in the multiply injured patient where only the most severe injury is ranked by the AIS system.

Probability of death score (PODS)

This takes into account the two most severe injuries scored by the AIS system but also the likelihood of fatality from the injury site, and weights them accordingly in the calculation. It also includes the patient's age.

Injury severity score (ISS)

This is the most popular system currently used. It uses the AIS scores from the three most severe injuries and summates the squared values. The maximum core is 75 (25 + 25 + 25); any AIS score of 6 (unsurvivable) is conventionally scored as 75 regardless of other sites of injury.

The relationship between mortality rate and ISS is again non-linear, and statistical analysis non-parametric. Although in the analysis of scores of large groups of trauma patients the ISS has been validated, it is also criticised for its subjective nature.

Glasgow Coma Scale (GCS)

This system of measuring neurological status and severity of injury by Teasdale and Jennett was first employed in 1974. Three parameters are used – motor activity, eye opening and verbal response. The score ranges from 3 to 15, with 15 indicating a normal state. Patients with a GCS below 8 are usually comatose. The Glasgow Coma Scale is detailed in Chapter 16 and is an integral part of the Trauma Score and Triage Revised Trauma Score.

Trauma score

This summates five different scores obtained from respiratory rate, respiratory effort, systolic blood pressure, capillary refill and GCS.

Pre-hospital index

This is mainly used in North America and uses the same parameters as the trauma score in the pre-hospital field. It aids decisions of the crew to transport the patient to the most appropriate type of hospital facility. It is criticised for its lack of objectivity and statistical predictive value.

Triage index

This was introduced in 1980 in response to criticisms of the pre-hospital index. It combines 16 different physiological variables but some of these can only be assessed in the hospital setting. The trauma score was devised from the triage index.

Revised trauma score (RTS)

The revised trauma score was derived from work carried out in the North American Major Trauma Outcome Study (1990). This is conventionally calculated from variables measured on arrival of the patient in the A&E department. It uses respiratory rate, systolic blood pressure and GCS. From experience obtained from studies of groups of patients, each factor is multiplied by a weighting factor reflecting their predictive value in outcome. GCS is considered the most relevant, followed by systolic blood pressure and then respiratory rate.

Trauma score and injury severity score (TRISS)

This combines the RTS, ISS, age of the patient and the nature of trauma and, by applying these to an equation, the probability of survival (Ps) is obtained. It was first developed in North America, and is the current method used in the UK, and throughout Europe and Australia to audit effectiveness of system care and the management of individual patients.

Major trauma outcome study (MTOS)

This is a revised version of TRISS and is used in the UK. Values obtained are used to audit the effectiveness of trauma care and management of individual patients. It is applied to patients

admitted for more than 3 days, managed in intensive care units, referred to a specialist centre or who die in hospital. It takes into account compounding factors such as seniority of doctors present on arrival of the patient, initial management and timing of consultation and intervention.

Almost all of these systems have certain disadvantages: much of the data recorded is subjective in nature; pre-hospital interventions, such as intubation, may artificially alter the score obtained on arrival in A&E; alcohol intoxication or other substance abuse may make objective clinical evaluation difficult; and scores in the elderly may be adversely altered owing to frailness or impaired physiological response. None of the scoring systems have any predictive value concerning disability after survival from serious trauma.

CONCLUSION

Throughout this chapter, non-invasive and invasive monitoring techniques have been discussed.

It is essential that the trauma nurse is familiar with and trained in the correct usage of any equipment, and understands the indications and limitations of the devices utilised. It must be emphasised that the continuous monitoring, re-evaluation, recording and reporting of the patient's vital signs is of paramount importance in observing any deterioration, or response to treatment, in a multiply injured patient.

Technological advances in all aspects of emergency imaging, and especially in CT and MRI, have assisted all members of the multidisciplinary team in the early diagnosis and early management of potentially life-threatening problems, thus improving the quality of care given to patients suffering with multisystem trauma with a resultant reduction in morbidity and mortality.

References and further reading

Association for the Advancement of Automotive Medicine. *The Abbreviated Injury Scale, 1990 Revision*. DesPlaines, Illinois, 1990

American College of Surgeons Committee on Trauma. *Advanced trauma life support course for doctors*. Chicago: American College of Surgeons, 1997

Burdett-Smith P, Airey GM, Franks AJ. Improvement in trauma survival in Leeds. *Injury* 1995; 26 1: 51–54

Burford Nursing Development Unit. Nurses and pain. *Nursing Times* 1984; 80(19): 58

Champion HR, Copes WS, Sacco WJ, Lawnick MM, Keast SL, Bain LW, Flanagan ME, Frey CF. The Major Trauma

Outcome Study – establishing national norms for trauma care. *Journal of Trauma* 1990; 30: 1356–1365

Committee on Medical Aspects of Automotive Safety. Rating the severity of tissue damage – the abbreviated scale. *JAMA* 1971; 215: 277–280

Department of Health. *Our healthier nation – a contract for health*. London: HMSO, 1998

Department of Transport. *Valuation of road accidents highway economics note*. Number 1. London: HMSO, 1996

Diepenbrock N. *Quick reference to critical care*. Lippincott Williams & Wilkins, Philadelphia, 2004

Driscoll P, Ewinnett C, Le Duc Jimmerson C, Goodall O. *Trauma resuscitation – the team approach*. London, The Macmillan Press Ltd, 1993

Fukuda K, Ichinohe T, Kaneko Y. Is measurement of end tidal CO_2 through nasal cannulae reliable? *Anaesthesia Progress* 1997; 44: 23–26

Greaves I, Porter K, Ryan J. *Trauma care manual*. London: Arnold, 2001

Gupta K, Park C, Parnell A, Banerjee A. *Clinical radiology for accident & emergency*. Birmingham Cambridge University Press, 2000

Johnson CJH, Kerr JH. Automated blood pressure monitors – a clinical evaluation of five models in adults. *Anesthesia* 1985; 30: 471

Kirkendall WM, Feinlieb M, Freis ED, Mark AL. American Heart Association Committee Report: recommendations for human blood pressure determination by sphygmomanometers. *Circulation* 1985; 62: 1146A

McCaffrey M. *Nursing the patient in pain*. London: Harper and Row, 1983

McCaffrey M, Beebe A. Assessment. In: Latham J (ed.) *Pain management and nursing care*. London: Mosby, 1994

Miles KA, Finlay D. *Injury* 1988; 19: 177–179

Nakatani K, Yukioka H, Fujimori M, Maeda C, Noguchi H, Ishihara S, Yamanaka I, Tase C. Utility of colimetric end tidal CO_2 detector for monitoring during prehospital cardiopulmonary resuscitation. *American Journal of Emergency Medicine* 1999; 17: 203–206

National Radiation Protection Board. Protection of the patient in computerised tomography. London: HMSO, 1992

Perry NM, Lewars MD, Driscoll P. *ABC of major trauma – radiological assessment*, 2nd edn. London: BMJ, 1996

Raby N, Berman L, De Lacey G. *Accident & emergency radiology – a survival guide*. Saunders: London, 2001

Royal College of Radiologists. *Making the best use of a department of clinical radiology (guidelines for doctors)*, 4th edn. London: Royal College of Radiologists, 1998

Seldinger SI. Catheter replacement of needle in percutaneous arteriography. *Acta Radiologica* 1953; 39: 369

Smalhout B, Kalenda Z. *Atlas of capnography*. Volume 1. Amsterdam: Kerckebosch/Zeist, 1975: 28–31

Staik P. *Radiology of thoracic trauma*. Oxford: Butterworth, 1993

Teasdale G, Jennet B. Assessment of coma and impaired consciousness. *Lancet* 1974; ii: 81–84

Chapter 21

Analgesia and anaesthesia

Juergen Rayner-Klein and Catherine A. Rowe

ANALGESIA

PAIN IN RELATION TO THE TRAUMA PATIENT

According to the International Association for the Study of Pain (IASP), pain is referred to as 'an unpleasant sensory and emotional experience associated with actual or potential tissue damage, or described in terms of such damage' (Merksey, 1979).

Although the sensitivity of the human pain receptor shows little evidence of variation, its physical manifestation following trauma is a unique and individual experience, which is difficult to evaluate effectively, or to define comprehensively.

Physical trauma will result in the patient experiencing physiological and psychological discomfort. Investigations suggest that optimal pain management is rarely achieved, as it becomes a secondary consideration for the nurse confronted by the primary management of the trauma victim.

> Pain is an unpleasant sensory and emotional experience associated with actual or potential tissue damage, or described in terms of such damage

Pain may culminate in a sequence of both physiological and psychological events, resulting in an increased degree of individual morbidity and prolonged hospitalisation. Adoption of an optimal pain management strategy, therefore, may improve patient outcome and promote the restoration of an individual's functionality (Zohar et al., 2001).

PHYSIOLOGICAL AND PSYCHOLOGICAL CONSEQUENCES OF ACUTE PAIN IN THE TRAUMA VICTIM

Trauma patients will be exposed to physical and emotional pain, requiring relief for both compassionate and physiological reasons (see Case study 21.1). Suboptimal pain management evokes a reactionary stress response predominantly resulting in '...hyperglycaemia, lipolysis, protein catabolism, increased antidiuretic and catecholamine levels, immunosuppression and a hypercoagulable state' (Patel and Smith, 1999). Clinically these manifest themselves as tachycardia, hypertension, deep vein thrombosis, pulmonary embolism, hypoxia, immobility, reduced gastrointestinal motility, salt and water retention, and infection (Patel and Smith, 1999).

> Trauma patients will be exposed to physical and emotional pain, requiring relief for both compassionate and physiological reasons

Case study 21.1

A 76-year-old gentleman was admitted to hospital following an accident in which he sustained fractured ribs 6 to 10 on the left hand side. His pain was managed using the aseptic insertion of a thoracic epidural, through which he was administered both anaesthetic and opioid medication, titrated carefully according to his verbal pain report. In addition, a simple analgesic preparation of paracetamol was given orally in order to maximise effective pain management.

He had an uneventful and comfortable night where his vital signs had remained stable and during which his epidural requirements had reduced slightly. His respiratory function remained satisfactory, he was able to breathe deeply and cough effectively, and required

minimal assistance to sit out of bed and mobilise gently.

The following evening, the duty anaesthetist was contacted to assess the gentleman whose condition had 'deteriorated'. He was disorientated, hypertensive, tachycardic and tachypnoeic, with poor basal air entry and oxygen saturation levels of 88% on supplemental oxygen. Although unable to communicate his level of pain for assessment, he was clinically confused and was 'moaning'. During the day, his epidural catheter had become dislodged and because he was 'pain free' it was decided that replacement of the catheter could wait. Unfortunately, subsequent pain management had not been effective, and had resulted in the deterioration of both his physical and psychological state.

ASSESSMENT OF PAIN IN THE TRAUMA PATIENT

Effective pain management in the trauma victim is an essential component of their multiprofessional care pathway, requiring optimal resolution, if the aforementioned consequences are to be minimised. Pain transition is assumed to constitute a reliable indicator of the underlying damage; indeed, in the majority of cases, its location, characteristics and intensity will accurately reflect the extent of the insult. However, occasions arise where the extent of the trauma does not equate to the patient's pain experience and, if acute pain cannot be resolved, a missed diagnosis such as compartment syndrome should be excluded. Pain in the trauma patient is not a conclusive indicator of tissue damage and, conversely, tissue damage is not a conclusive indicator of pain (Eccleston, 2001).

For pain management to be optimised, the nurse must accept that the response will be unique to the sufferer, whose perception can be heightened by life-threatening or emotionally traumatic scenarios, the perception of an altered body image or fear of subsequent disability. Alternatively, it may be reflected inwardly and made light of beneath a stoic indifferent nature.

The most valid and reliable indicator of the patient's pain experience is their self-reporting mechanism, yet this offers a subjective basis from which the nurse must make a professional judgment concerning management. Nurses are vulnerable to intentional misrepresentation of the pain experience by the individual concerned, as this experience is beyond proof. They may even encounter times where personal prejudice has the potential to interfere with their ability to communicate or empathise compassionately. However, the gold standard in optimal pain management of the trauma victim must constitute a reflection of the patient's report and not multiprofessional opinion on what it 'should' be. Health care professionals have no right to deprive patients of clinical care irrespective of their personal bias (Pasero and McCaffery, 2001).

PAIN ASSESSMENT TOOLS

Pain is a sensation that reflects the extent to which an independent stressor affects an individual and, as such, is difficult to quantify.

The behavioural response to pain can be influenced in a number of complex ways. Social experience, culture, age or gender, fear, anxiety, previous exposure to or duration of the pain sensation and pre-emptive assumptions as to its potential consequence, may heighten or detract from the individual pain perception and expression. In addition, patients may demonstrate 'pain behaviours' as they assume the 'sick role' following traumatic injury, where those perceived to suffer believe that they will receive priority attention from the attending nurse or family, therefore affording them some secondary gain (Sarafino, 1990).

Pain assessment scales present an objective means by which to quantify pain intensity and are, therefore, recommended for use, not only to provide an initial assessment, but also to direct titration of therapy. Offering a complementary dimension to the constant surveillance that the individual trauma patient requires, the tools are less open to criticism than observer pain ratings, which are founded on both behavioural and physiological indices and considered more subjective.

The physiological indicators cited to reflect the pain experience, and most commonly interpreted by the nurse as such, include an increase in heart rate, blood pressure, respiratory rate and perspiration. Behavioural indicators likewise manifest themselves as irritability, facial expression, postural guarding and groaning (Jacobi et al., 2002), which, although considered unreliable in pain intensity prediction, are useful in the assessment process where a patient is unable to communicate effectively.

The Oucher pain rating scale

For use within the paediatric population, the Oucher scale offers a method by which children may quantify their pain, given the misconception that they do not feel it as adults do (Woodrow, 2000). It is comprised of two vertical scales, one of which depicts a score ranging from 0 to 100 and proceeds in increments of 10. The second, a pictorial scale, is comprised of six photographs illustrating a young child in varying degrees of distress, with the bottom of the scale representing 'no hurt' and the top representing 'the biggest hurt you could ever have' (Thomas, 1997).

The visual analogue and verbal rating scale

For the adult population within the acute care setting, pain assessment is easily achieved by means of simple, reproducible, unidimensional assessment tools that include both visual analogue and verbal rating scales.

The visual analogue scale is represented as a straight line, usually 10 cm in length, with each end depicting the extreme limits of the pain sensation. The patient is requested to draw a single intersecting line that describes their perception of the pain and from which quantifiable evidence can be obtained (Thomas, 1997).

Verbal rating scales likewise offer an objective means by which to assess the severity of a patient's pain and is achieved by superimposing either verbal or numerical cues on to a visual analogue scale. Using similar principles, patients are requested to define their pain as directed by the verbal cues or from 0 to 10, with an increased score representing an increase in the pain intensity.

Although simple in concept, accurate utilisation by both nurse and patient is only achievable with adequate education and support. Simple concepts can be misunderstood when patients are anxious. Explanations must, therefore, acknowledge any barriers to communication, which include hearing or visual impairment, language or learning difficulties, the nature of the trauma incurred, disorientation or neurological impairment, or a child's developmental age.

> **Key messages**
>
> - Physical trauma will result in the patient experiencing physiological and psychological discomfort
> - Suboptimal pain management evokes a reactionary stress response
> - The most valid and reliable pain indicator is the patient's self-expression
> - Pain assessment scales present an objective means by which to quantify pain intensity

PAIN MANAGEMENT IN THE TRAUMA VICTIM

As pain is usually a clinical indicator of a potentially damaging lesion, it must be treated effectively in order to prevent the development of more permanent disability or deterioration, and to address the humanitarian aspects of care.

Prevention of pain is more effective than the 'crisis' management of such; therefore, optimum pain management is best undertaken aggressively on a time-contingent basis.

The *analgesic goal* should achieve the blunting or removal of the sensation of pain (Jacobi et al., 2002), and may be achieved by adopting a combination of pharmacological, psychological and physical adjuncts, to address each dimension of the patient's pain experience. For such techniques to benefit the patient, the nurse must be familiar and confident with available methods, and identify their most appropriate and timely use in order to coordinate a holistic clinical approach.

Consideration must be given to the misconceptions that those suffering from acute head injury, thoracic trauma or abdominal pain, should be denied pharmacological relief, given the rationale that administration may mask pupillary response,

potentiate respiratory depression, may hinder diagnostic assessment or may predispose to addiction. The gold standard must dictate that appropriate titration of analgesia must be made available for all those exhibiting a clinical need.

> *Misconception*: Those suffering from acute head injury, thoracic trauma or abdominal pain, should be denied pharmacological relief, given the rationale that administration may mask pupillary response, potentiate respiratory depression, may hinder diagnostic assessment or may predispose to addiction

PAIN MANAGEMENT IN THE RESTLESS TRAUMA PATIENT

Many trauma patients exhibit signs of restlessness in response to their clinical circumstance; however, pharmacological management requires careful consideration and a comprehensive assessment must be made to determine its cause.

Restlessness may result from hypoxaemia, neurological dysfunction, the effects of alcohol or drugs, or the presence of a full bladder; therefore, analgesia should be temporarily avoided until its primary cause has been established (Greaves et al., 2001). Prolonged delay, however, is not acceptable and it should be acknowledged that effective pain management in these patients may enhance cooperation and facilitate more accurate assessment and treatment (Mackenzie, 2000).

PHARMACOLOGICAL TECHNIQUES

Pharmacological choice for effective pain management of the trauma patient depends upon the nature of injury, the severity of pain and the administration route available. The existence of allergies, current medication and potential side effects must also be considered prior to administration, in order to direct safe and effective analgesia. The routes available for analgesic drug administration are detailed below.

Oral

The oral route has limited use in the trauma victim but should not be completely excluded. During the acute management phase, the oral route may be temporarily inaccessible; prior to diagnosis, as a result of nausea and vomiting or given the nature of the injury. Although effective oral analgesics are available, reduced gastrointestinal motility and partial metabolism by the liver will make absorption rates and efficacy unpredictable.

Sublingual or rectal

Analgesic administration via the sublingual route in the trauma patient may be more accessible. Bypassing the portal circulation, drug efficacy can be more accurately predicted, rapid absorption being more readily guaranteed.

The rectal route uses the end portion of the gastrointestinal tract to secure effective drug administration. However, drug metabolism is slow and the unpredictable absorption rate achieved by this route is best suited to the ongoing maintenance of analgesia in the trauma patient rather than for acute pain management.

Intramuscular or subcutaneous

The use of intramuscular or subcutaneous analgesic agents in the trauma patient who is shocked and peripherally compromised must be judged with care. In addition to the discomfort caused by administration and the potential to bruise in the presence of coagulopathy, drug absorption may be reduced. In an attempt to achieve analgesic benefit, repeated dosage may result in a large depot of dormant drug being activated quickly once circulation is restored and may culminate in significant overdose.

Intravenous

Particularly effective in the trauma patient, the intravenous route facilitates the delivery of analgesic agents directly to their site of action in a more predictable and controllable way. Providing options to direct bolus, continuous or patient-controlled administration, peak plasma levels are rapidly attained making ongoing evaluation and further drug titration possible.

Disadvantages identified include the fact that trained personnel are required to establish venous access and, in the hypovolaemic patient, drug

action may be delayed until primary management has restored circulation.

Intraosseous

Administration via the intraosseous route secures delivery of an analgesic agent to the circulation almost as quickly as those administered through a vein. In the acute situation, and especially in small children who are hypovolaemic and where intravenous access is difficult to establish, the intraosseous route provides a temporary means by which to secure primary pain management.

Inhalation

When administered via this route, 'Entonox', a potent analgesic mix of 50% nitrous oxide and 50% oxygen, is of particular value for short-term pain relief in the trauma victim. Although dependent upon the cooperation or physical ability of the patient, it can be used as an effective adjunct to supplement other techniques, to gain rapid control of the situation, to facilitate the reduction of fractures, or to optimise splinting and the application of dressings. Therapeutic action is achieved rapidly when the patient is instructed to inhale Entonox via a tightly fitting facemask or mouthpiece. Equally, the therapeutic effect is rapidly lost if the patient does not inhale deeply and steadily. Entonox is generally well tolerated, although some trauma victims may experience nausea or light-headedness.

Not all trauma patients are suitable recipients of inhaled nitrous oxide, nitrogen decompression sickness posing an absolute contraindication. Being significantly more soluble than nitrogen in plasma, it diffuses into air-filled cavities more rapidly than nitrogen can diffuse out, therefore, increasing the net pressure or volume within the cranial vault, pleural cavity, gut and middle ear. For those patients presenting with a high index of suspicion for pneumothorax, bowel obstruction or head injury, the risks may outweigh the benefits (Case study 21.2).

Case study 21.2

A 20-year-old female was admitted to hospital with an isolated fractured shaft of femur after falling from her bicycle. She was alert, orientated and obviously distressed.

Effective pain management was initially achieved by immobilisation of the fracture using traction and a splint, a process that was facilitated carefully by administration of inhaled Entonox, which she tolerated well. Subsequent management included bolus administration of a systemic opioid, titrated carefully against its clinical effect and, finally, administration of a femoral nerve block achieved total analgesic control (Park et al., 2000).

REGIONAL ANALGESIA

Although invaluable to the management of pain within the trauma patient, the use of regional techniques including nerve blocks, intravenous regional anaesthesia (or Bier's block), and spinal and epidural blockade, are often underutilised despite the fact that they are relatively safe and may be ideal for those in a general state of ill health.

Nerve blocks

The judicious use of nerve blockade with local anaesthetic may be useful in the control of acute and severe pain within the trauma patient and has the advantage of avoiding the side effects of other analgesic agents. Common examples include infiltration of the intercostal nerve for effective management of rib fractures, blockade of the femoral nerve, obturator nerve and lateral cutaneous nerve of the thigh with a three-in-one block for a fractured midshaft of femur, and blockade of the digital nerve prior to suturing of the fingers or toes.

Intravenous regional anaesthesia (Bier's block)

The Bier's block is an effective time-limited technique that will facilitate fracture reduction or the undertaking of a short procedure on the hand or forearm, and involves intravenous injection of local anaesthetic into an exsanguinated limb. It requires the patient to be fasted, have venous access established, appropriate monitoring in

progress and the presence of two members of staff with advanced life support skills, to restore stability should toxic or hypersensitivity reactions occur (Illingworth and Simpson, 1998).

Epidural

The use of epidural analgesia within the trauma patient is especially popular in the management of thoracic pain following blunt chest injury. Its positive benefits include the restoration of effective respiratory function, thus reducing the incidence of trauma-induced atelectasis, respiratory infection and the progressive development of respiratory failure.

There are limiting factors for administration via the epidural route, which include cardiovascular instability or hypovolaemia, evidence of local infection or sepsis, anatomical abnormalities or insufficient availability of experienced staff to facilitate ongoing delivery (Patel and Smith, 1999). In the acute situation, selective placement of the catheter is not always possible and, in patients with spinal cord lesions, a neurological or sensory deficit or deranged coagulation, epidural catheterisation is contraindicated until a comprehensive neurological assessment has been made or coagulopathy controlled.

LOCAL ANAESTHETIC AGENTS

Local anaesthetic preparations as outlined in Table 21.1 include lidocaine (lignocaine), prilocaine and bupivacaine, of which bupivacaine is the most toxic. They act by temporarily blocking transmission of peripheral nerve impulses by preventing membrane depolarisation and their side effects, of which the nurse must be aware, may present progressively as visual disturbance, slurring of speech, tachycardia and hypertension, muscular twitching, bradycardia, hypotension and cardiac arrest (Greaves et al., 2001).

Contraindications include lack of patient cooperation, previous allergic reaction, evidence of infection at the proposed injection site, deranged coagulopathy and skeletal abnormalities that may make surface landmarking for placement difficult.

Table 21.1 Formulary for local anaesthetic agents for use in regional blockade in the adult trauma patient

Preparation	Dose	Potential side effects
Lidocaine (lignocaine) 0.5%, 1% and 2% solutions	3 mg/kg *Maximum 200 mg*	Confusion, complete heart block, convulsions, hypotension, bradycardia, hypersensitivity, cardiac arrest
Prilocaine hydrochloride 1% and 4% solutions	6 mg/kg *Maximum 400 mg*	Confusion, complete heart block, convulsions, hypotension, bradycardia, ocular toxicity, hypersensitivity, cardiac arrest
Bupivacaine hydrochloride (Marcain) 0.25% and 0.5%	2 mg/kg *Maximum 150 mg*	Confusion, complete heart block, convulsions, hypotension, bradycardia, hypersensitivity, cardiac arrest

Table 21.2 Analgesic formulary for mild to moderate pain management in the adult trauma patient

Preparation	Route	Dose	Potential side effects
Acetaminophen	Oral/rectal	0.5–1 g 4–6-hourly *Maximum 4 g in 24 hours*	Rash Prolonged use: acute pancreatitis, liver and renal impairment
Acetylsalicylic acid	Oral/rectal	300–900 mg 4–6-hourly *Maximum 4 g daily*	Gastrointestinal irritation, increased bleeding time, bronchospasm
Ibuprofen	Oral	300–600 mg 6–8-hourly *Maximum 2.4 g daily*	Gastrointestinal irritation, increased bleeding time, bronchospasm
Diclofenac	Oral/rectal	75–150 mg in 2–3 divided doses	Gastrointestinal irritation. Increased bleeding time, bronchospasm. Injection site reaction
	IM	75 mg once or twice daily up to 2 days	
	IV	75 mg repeated after 4–6 hours up to 2 days by infusion. *Maximum 150 mg daily*	
Ketorolac	Oral	10 mg every 4–6 hours *Maximum 40 mg daily for < 7 days*	Gastrointestinal irritation, increased bleeding time, bronchospasm, anaphylaxis, acute renal failure, convulsions, bradycardia, hypertension, palpitations, hepatic disturbances
	IM/IV	10 mg, then 10–30 mg every 4–6 hours *Maximum 90 mg daily*	

IM, intramuscular; IV, intravenous.

ANALGESIC AGENTS

Mild to moderate pain

Simple analgesic agents, as outlined in Table 21.2, including acetaminophen and non-steroidal anti-inflammatory drugs, have been shown to be effective for those trauma patients suffering from mild to moderate pain.

Common drugs available will be considered below; however, these do not represent all those presently available.

Acetaminophen
Acetaminophen, although broadly classified as a non-steroidal anti-inflammatory agent, has some important characteristics, which reduce the gastric side effects commonly associated with this group of drugs.

Available as an oral or rectal preparation, acetaminophen is believed to inhibit prostaglandin production within the central nervous system and, although widely disregarded for use within the trauma setting, has been found especially safe and effective for the first-line management of mild to moderate pain.

Non-steroidal anti-inflammatory agents
By inhibiting the effect of inflammatory mediators and reducing prostaglandin synthesis, non-steroidal anti-inflammatory drugs are rapidly absorbed following oral or rectal administration, some even being available for parenteral use.

By evoking a peripheral response at the site of trauma, they may be beneficial for treatment of mild to moderate pain and, when combined with opiate preparations, will contribute to more effective management of severe pain.

Consideration must be given prior to administration in accordance with their risks. In trauma patients with pre-existing renal impairment, who are hypoperfused or have lost more than 10% of their total blood volume, the use of non-steroidal anti-inflammatory agents prior to resuscitation may inhibit prostaglandin synthesis in the kidney and potentiate acute renal failure (Mackenzie, 2000).

Whilst the most commonly associated side effects are gastric irritation and ulceration, more insidious consequences include the precipitation of acute bronchospasm, bone marrow suppression, and their tendency to reduce platelet aggregation and prolong bleeding time.

Acetylsalicylic acid Constituting one of the oldest classes of non-steroidal anti-inflammatory agents, this salicylate may constitute the drug of choice in the management of mild musculoskeletal or arthritic pain.

Contraindicated in children under 12 years of age owing to its association with *Reye's syndrome*, its anti-inflammatory properties are limited, therefore, more modern preparations may offer an appropriate alternative and appear to be tolerated better.

Ibuprofen Ibuprofen, a propionic acid derivative, is considered the safest, most effective and most widely used preparation within this group. Although low in anti-inflammatory properties, it exhibits fewer of the potential side effects than its analogues and, when administered orally, is effective in the management of mild to moderate pain.

Alternative preparations with similar analgesic properties include *naproxen*, *fenbrufen*, *ketoprofen* and *dexketoprofen*. However, frequently reported side effects make them less popular for use in trauma patients.

Ketorolac Ketorolac is an acetic acid derivative available for oral, intramuscular and intravenous administration. Given orally or intramuscularly,

its therapeutic properties equal that of ibuprofen, whilst intravenously it equates to the analgesic effects of rectal diclofenac (Mackenzie, 2000).

Limiting factors include its prolonged analgesic onset and reports that significant numbers of patients report little or no analgesic effect (Park et al., 2000). In addition, the incidence of adverse effects have directed its use to less than 5 days, and although recognised as an effective analgesic, it is not widely recommended for use.

Diclofenac Diclofenac, an aryl acetic acid, is available as an oral, rectal and parenteral preparation that can be administered both intramuscularly or intravenously. Although injection may be painful, given parenterally, it has been used successfully to manage both renal and biliary colic (Illingworth and Simpson, 1998).

Enterally, there is evidence to prove its efficacy in the management of mild to moderate pain and, when used in conjunction with other pharmacological techniques, it can be effective in controlling even moderate to severe pain.

Severe pain

For the first-line management of severe pain in the trauma patient, intravenous analgesia and, in particular, the administration of potent opioid preparations has become the gold standard. However, less potent alternatives worth consideration are available and may minimise the incidence of unwanted side effects (Table 21.3).

Weak opioids

Weak opioid preparations include: *co-codamol*, *codeine phosphate*, which is available in both oral and intramuscular form, and *dihydrocodeine*, which can be administered orally, subcutaneously or by deep intramuscular injection. However, nausea and vomiting are common side effects, and long-term use of codeine is constipating.

Ketamine and strong opioids

Strong opioids or ketamine offer effective alternatives for the acute management of severe pain, yet their potent therapeutic action may result in the patient exhibiting a greater number of side effects, of which the nurse must be aware in order to coordinate safe administration.

Table 21.3 Analgesic formulary for moderate to severe pain management in the adult trauma patient

Preparation	Route	Dose	Potential side effects
Codeine phosphate	Oral IM	30–60 mg every 4 hours 30–60 mg every 4 hours *Maximum 240 mg daily*	Nausea, vomiting, constipation
Ketamine	IM IV	1–4 mg/kg 0.25–1 mg/kg	Hallucinations in recovery phase, hypertension, tachycardia
Morphine sulphate	IM IV	10–15 mg every 4 hours 2.5–7.5 mg slow bolus followed by further 1–2 mg increments, as titrated against pain	Respiratory depression, hypotension, sedation or drowsiness, hepatic/renal impairment, pupillary constriction, nausea, vomiting
Diamorphine	IV	2–5 mg every 4 hours by slow injection titrated against pain	Respiratory depression, hypotension, sedation or drowsiness, hepatic/renal impairment, pupillary constriction, nausea, vomiting
Naloxone (Narcan) (opioid receptor antagonist)	IV	0.1–0.2 mg. If inadequate response, increments of 0.1 mg every 2 minutes	Nausea, vomiting, tachycardia, reversal of analgesia, cardiac arrhythmias

IM, intramuscular; IV, intravenous.

Ketamine Ketamine, a non-irritant anaesthetic induction agent, which acts by blocking *N*-methyl-D-aspartate receptors, offers powerful analgesic and amnesic properties, which can be used alone or as an adjunct to opiate administration.

Its preferential qualities preserve glottic reflexes, cause less respiratory depression than opiate preparations and place the patient in a dissociated state where analgesia and amnesia are all but complete (Mackenzie, 2000). However, patients reportedly experience hallucinations in the recovery phase, and maintaining a calm and stimulus-free environment may prove beneficial. In addition, administration will result in increased sympathetic activity that will raise mean arterial pressure, heart rate and cardiac output. Therefore, for the hypertensive or head-injured patient, the use of ketamine is discouraged.

Opioids

'Opioid' refers to all opioid receptor-specific agents whose actions reduce inflammation at the site of injury and interfere with transmission of nociceptive stimuli within the dorsal horn (Mackenzie, 2000).

Several classes of opioid receptors exist, the most important for analgesic purposes being μ (mu), κ (kappa) and σ (sigma) subtypes, with available preparations acting as receptor agonists, partial agonists or antagonists to achieve their therapeutic goal.

Morphine and diamorphine As the primary active ingredient of opium, morphine exhibits pure agonist properties at μ receptors, and evokes euphoria and powerful analgesic properties. Administered intravenously within the trauma patient, its dosage must be titrated carefully in order to achieve maximum benefit and to minimise the incidence of adverse effects.

Diamorphine or heroin is a semisynthetic derivative of morphine. Being more lipophilic, it penetrates the brain tissue more readily making it an even more potent analgesic agent.

Pethidine Pethidine, a synthetic opioid agonist, is widely used in emergency care. However, there is no evidence to suggest that it offers beneficial gain even for the management of colic (McQuay, 1999). Its tendency to produce the metabolite nor-pethidine, which causes twitching, tremors and fitting, renders it an unreasonable option when other less toxic preparations exist.

Nalbuphine and tramadol Nalbuphine and tramadol offer alternative but not superior analgesic qualities to morphine, although they may potentiate fewer respiratory side effects and remain outside of controlled drug legislation.

Nalbuphine is an equally potent analgesic to morphine, its analgesic qualities being achieved by its agonist effects on κ receptors. However, in doses above 10 mg, μ receptor antagonism is reported to occur and may lead to increased morphine administration being subsequently required in order to sustain an effect (Mackenzie, 2000).

Tramadol, a synthetic opioid with the analgesic potency of pethidine, provides analgesia by inhibiting central neuronal uptake of noradrenaline and enhancing serotonin release, in addition to being an opioid receptor agonist (Park et al., 2000). Limitations for use include its inclination to cause significant nausea and vomiting, and reported seizures post administration render it contraindicated for epileptic patients.

CLINICAL CONSIDERATIONS FOR OPIOID ADMINISTRATION

Having outlined some opioid analgesia available to manage severe pain within the trauma patient, it is essential to consider their systemic effects in order to ensure safe delivery and care.

Sedation and respiratory depression

Although occasional euphoria is noted, opioid administration more commonly results in reduced consciousness or drowsiness. It may also depress respiratory function, given its tendency to suppress the respiratory centres within the medulla; therefore, in patients presenting with a reduced conscious level or in those whose respiratory rate is less than 10 per minute, administration should considered with care (Greaves et al., 2001).

Unrecognised, the symptoms above may culminate in hypercarbia, progressive coma, hypoxia and death, although risks will be minimised if the attending nurse remains vigilant to the patient's clinical signs. An alteration in the patient's respiratory rate, breathing pattern, neurological function and especially level of consciousness is of paramount importance. Any compromise must result in immediate corrective action.

Naloxone, a potent opioid antagonist, must always be available to reverse the potentially catastrophic effects of opioid administration. However, analgesic properties are also reversed, therefore, careful titration against the patient's respiratory rate and pain awareness is recommended so as to avoid exposing the patient to an acute exacerbation of their pain.

Pupillary constriction

All opioids stimulate the third cranial nerve or Edinger–Westphal nucleus, which results in pupillary constriction following administration. However, it is important for the nurse to realise that this will not prevent pupillary dilatation caused by increasing intracranial pressure, therefore clinical assessment of this will not be prevented (Mackenzie, 2000).

Nausea and vomiting

As a result of direct stimulation of the medulla and brainstem, and compounded by the fact that opioids cause contraction of smooth muscle throughout the gastrointestinal tract and delay gastric emptying, nausea and vomiting may pose a major problem. It is advisable, therefore, for an appropriate antiemetic to be administered concurrently.

Cardiovascular effects

Although bradycardia is reported to accompany the administration of morphine, adverse cardiovascular effects following opioid administration are minimal. However, the potential for histamine release and depression of the medullary vasomotor centres may result in vasodilatation and hypotension.

PHYSICAL AND PSYCHOLOGICAL ADJUNCTS TO EFFECTIVE PAIN MANAGEMENT

As previously mentioned, there are both physical and psychological adjuncts that may be adopted in order to facilitate effective pain management in the trauma patient.

Physical

Physical therapies available that may optimise pain management following trauma include:

- immobilisation
- stabilisation or elevation of the affected area or limb with splints
- slings or traction
- the application of appropriate dressings
- optimum positioning or support of the patient
- the timely reduction of fractures and early operative fixation (see Case study 21.2).

Maintaining a coordinated systematic approach to clinical care will ensure that patient disturbance and discomfort are minimised, and the localised application of warm pads may relieve aching or muscular-type spasm, whilst topical cooling may relieve pain associated with burns.

Transcutaneous electrical nerve stimulation

The use of transcutaneous electrical nerve stimulation (TENS) has been shown to alleviate pain by the non-invasive electrical stimulation of peripheral nerves. Although more effective for chronic pain, its action may be beneficial in the management of rib fractures and low back pain. As there are no apparent side effects, it can be used safely and effectively with compliant recipients in order to complement analgesic techniques.

Psychological adjuncts to effective pain management

In the acute trauma situation, it is easy to forget that pain is both a sensory and emotional experience and, in addition to physical and pharmacological management, psychological intervention is required to address this aspect of care.

Effective communication between the patient and the health care professional is essential in the management of acute pain, not only to direct appropriate assessment and therapy, but also to reduce the incidence of iatrogenic distress, which may ultimately compromise the effectiveness of pharmacological agents and heighten pain awareness (Hazinski et al., 1996).

It is essential for the trauma nurse to develop effective, compassionate and empathic communication with the individual concerned, and to ensure that sufficient detail is reiterated confidently in order for them to understand or make sense of their traumatic situation and condition (Case study 21.3).

Although not exclusively required, sedative agents as outlined in Table 21.4 may offer an appropriate adjunct within the overall pain management strategy in order to allay anxiety and mute traumatic awareness so optimising the effects of analgesic administration.

Case study 21.3

A 50-year-old male was admitted to hospital following a house fire with 15% first-degree burns to his arms. His initial pain was pharmacologically controlled with the administration of small incremental doses of intravenous opioids, carefully titrated against effect. Paraffin gauze and Lyofoam contained within a light absorbent dressing was applied to his wounds, following which his arms were elevated to reduce the presence of resultant oedema (Adam and Osbourne, 1997).

Table 21.4   Formulary for sedative agents used to relieve anxiety in the trauma patient

Preparation	Route	Dose	Potential side effects
Lorazepam	Oral IM/IV	1–4 mg daily in divided doses 25–30 µg repeated every 6 hours	Drowsiness, confusion, amnesia, muscle weakness
Diazepam	Oral IM/IV	2 mg every 8 hours 10 mg every 4 hours	Drowsiness, confusion, amnesia, muscle weakness
Midazolam	IV	2 mg bolus, then increments of 0.5–1 mg titrated against effect	Drowsiness, confusion, amnesia, muscle weakness. Profound hypotension in hypovolaemia. Slow onset, therefore, *not* a true intravenous induction agent!
Flumazenil (benzodiazepine antagonist)	IV	200 µg over 15 seconds, then 100 µg at 60-second intervals *Maximum 1 g*	Nausea, vomiting, flushing, anxiety, fear, transient hypertension/ tachycardia

IM, intramuscular; IV, intravenous.

Despite effective pharmacological management, the gentleman remained very anxious and, on further nursing enquiry, it transpired that he was concerned that his injuries would leave him permanently disabled.

The nurse was able to reassure him that, although extremely painful, permanent scarring or disfigurement from his burns would not occur. His anxiety was relieved and he consequently calmed down.

THE ACUTE PAIN SERVICE

Nursing and medical personnel have historically managed acute pain. However, vast amounts of evidence support the claim that acute pain management is poor despite advancement in available techniques (Park et al., 2000).

In order to address these inadequacies, acute pain teams have evolved nationally, and have been shown to not only improve the acute pain management of hospitalised patients but also to provide both medical and nursing colleagues with an invaluable clinical resource by which to direct their care.

Key messages

- Prevention of pain is more effective than 'crisis' management
- Restlessness in the trauma patient may be caused by factors other than pain and, therefore, requires investigation
- Regional techniques, such as nerve blockade and epidural analgesia, should be a selective option to effective pain management
- Simple, regular, analgesic administration should complement more complex analgesic techniques
- Referral to the acute pain team will facilitate optimal pain management, and provide nursing and medical staff with an invaluable clinical resource

ANAESTHESIA

The nurse caring for trauma patients requires a basic understanding of commonly used anaesthetic drugs, their indications, side effects and contraindications. Although an increasing variety of anaesthetic drugs have become available over recent years, there are a limited number of agents, which are commonly used in the UK to anaesthetise trauma patients.

A combination of drugs is administered to gain control, render the patient unconscious and abolish muscle tone. These drugs will facilitate securing a definitive airway by endotracheal intubation, and will enable the patient to tolerate an endotracheal tube and mechanical ventilation. Balanced anaesthesia utilises three groups of drugs:

1. intravenous anaesthetic induction agents – to achieve unconsciousness
2. opioid analgesic drugs – to abolish or ameliorate the stress response to intubation and for analgesia
3. muscle relaxants or neuromuscular blocking agents – to abolish or decrease any muscle tone.

It is of utmost importance that hypovolaemia is corrected prior to the use of any anaesthetic agents. All intravenous induction agents, with the exception of ketamine, cause vasodilatation to a varying degree and reduce myocardial contractility. This results in a fall in blood pressure, which is exacerbated by any coexisting hypovolaemia. Induction of anaesthesia in time-critical trauma patients with uncontrolled haemorrhage requiring immediate resuscitative surgery is particularly hazardous.

> Hypovolaemia must be corrected prior to the use of anaesthetic agents

Prior to sedating or anaesthetising a restless or combative trauma patient, it is important to seek a cause for restlessness and to treat the cause concurrently. Hypoxia, hypovolaemia, hypoglycaemia, head injury or intoxication with alcohol or drugs frequently cause agitation and render any care difficult or impossible.

INTRAVENOUS ANAESTHETIC INDUCTION AGENTS

Intravenous anaesthetic induction agents cause loss of consciousness in one arm–brain circulation time, if the patient is not severely shocked. Within a few minutes, consciousness is regained owing to redistribution of the agent, unless anaesthesia is maintained with further intravenous boluses or an infusion, or with inhalational anaesthetic agents. Dosages must be reduced in the elderly and if any degree of hypovolaemia coexists.

The safest induction agent to use in the trauma patient is *etomidate* owing to its greatest degree of cardiovascular stability. Further advantages are lack of histamine release and a low incidence of allergic reactions. Etomidate reduces cerebral oxygen requirements and cerebral blood flow, which is beneficial for control of intracranial pressure (ICP). Pain on injection, hiccoughs, a 40% incidence of nausea and vomiting, and involuntary movements are side effects the trauma team needs to be aware of. Suppression of the adrenocortical axis makes this agent unsuitable for infusions. Drug profiles of alternative intravenous anaesthetic agents are detailed in Table 21.5.

OPIOID ANALGESIC DRUGS

This group of drugs acts on opioid receptors as outlined earlier. In addition to their analgesic effects, highly potent synthetic opioid analogues, such as fentanyl and alfentanil, are more rapid in onset compared to morphine. They exhibit a greater degree of cardiovascular stability and are well suited to ameliorate the stress response to endotracheal intubation. Marked respiratory depression can occur even with small doses. However, fentanyl or alfentanil boluses or infusions facilitate tolerance of mechanical ventilation and are a valuable adjunct to maintain anaesthesia.

MUSCLE RELAXANTS (NEUROMUSCULAR BLOCKING AGENTS)

These drugs are administered to facilitate endotracheal intubation. They abolish muscle tone and protective laryngeal reflexes. They allow for laryngoscopy. It is of utmost importance for the trauma nurse to realise that, once these drugs have been administered, patients are rendered apnoeic. Patients are unable to protect their own airway, are at risk of regurgitation and aspiration of gastric contents and blood, and are unable to use their respiratory muscles to breathe for themselves. Endotracheal intubation and artificial ventilation become essential. If the trauma team is in a 'cannot intubate–cannot ventilate' situation, then death of the patient may ensue. Depending on their pharmacological action, muscle relaxants can be divided into depolarising and non-depolarising agents (Table 21.6).

Depolarising muscle relaxant: suxamethonium

Suxamethonium or 'scoline' is the muscle relaxant of choice for the trauma patient. It has the most rapid onset of action (30–45 seconds). This manifests itself with generalised twitching or

Table 21.5 Formulary of intravenous anaesthetic induction agents in the trauma patient

Preparation	Dose IV	Potential side effects	Comments
Etomidate	0.2–0.3 mg/kg	Pain on injection, hiccoughs, involuntary movements, nausea and vomiting	Cardiovascularly stable. *Not* suitable for IV infusion or repeat IV boluses
Propofol	1.5–2.5 mg/kg	Profound hypotension, if hypovolaemic	Non-cumulative. Suitable for continuous IV infusion
Thiopentone	2–7 mg/kg	Marked cardiovascular depression, particularly if hypovolaemic. Potential for severe anaphylaxis	Very effective anticonvulsant; neuroprotective
Ketamine	1–2 mg/kg	Hallucinations, emergence phenomena. Increased myocardial oxygen demand. Increased salivation, bronchial secretions	Sympathomimetic; bronchodilatation; possibly neuroprotective; potent analgesic; potent amnesia; dissociative anaesthesia state

IM, intramuscular; IV, intravenous.

Table 21.6 Formulary of depolarising and non-depolarising neuromuscular blocking agents

Preparation	Group	Dose IV	Onset	Time to recovery	Potential side effects/comments
Suxamethonium	Depolarising	1.5 mg/kg	30–45 seconds	3–5 minutes	Preferred agent for RSI. Several serious side effects: hyperkalaemia, bradycardia, malignant hyperthermia, cardiac arrhythmias, masseter spasm, suxamethonium apnoea, increased IOC and ICP
Atracurium	Non-depolarising	0.5–0.6 mg/kg	90–120 seconds	25–30 minutes	Spontaneous degradation; cutaneous histamine release
Rocuronium	Non-depolarising	0.6 mg/kg	60–120 seconds	30–45 minutes	No histamine release; mild vagolysis
Vecuronium	Non-depolarising	0.1 mg/kg	140–180 seconds	25–40 minutes	Cardiovascularly stable; needs reconstitution
Pancuronium	Non-depolarising	0.08 mg/kg	120–180 seconds	65–100 minutes	Sympathomimetic; tachycardia; cardiovascularly stable

ICP, intracranial pressure; IOC, intraocular pressure; IV, intravenous; RSI, rapid sequence induction.

fasciculations followed by profound relaxation of the vocal cords and respiratory muscles. Very importantly, recovery occurs spontaneously after 3–5 minutes owing to metabolism of the drug by plasma cholinesterase. However, there are numbers of potentially serious side effects associated with its use as listed below.

- It causes severe bradycardia with repeated doses owing to excessive vagal stimulation.
- It has the potential to increase intracranial pressure or intraocular pressure, resulting in loss of vitreous humour in penetrating eye injuries.
- It is the commonest trigger of malignant hyperpyrexia.
- It causes prolonged apnoea in patients with plasma cholinesterase deficiency.
- It has the potential to cause hyperkalaemia when administered to patients with major burns or crush injuries greater then 24 hours old, or when given to patients with massive denervation injuries or pre-existing muscular dystrophies.

To date there has been no success in producing an alternative, suitable, replacement drug with fewer side effects.

Non–depolarising muscle relaxants: atracurium, rocuronium, vecuronium, pancuronium

There are several drugs available in this group. Atracurium is often the preferred choice in the UK, as it does not require reconstitution and is non-accumulative. Its metabolism is in part independent of renal and hepatic metabolism. Atracurium takes 90–120 seconds to be fully effective and subsequently lasts for 30–40 minutes when given intravenously at a dose of 0.5–0.6 mg/kg. It is relatively cardiovascularly stable but occasionally results in hypotension owing to cutaneous histamine release. Other drugs in this group have even longer onset times, with the exception of rocuronium (60 seconds). However, these drugs last for at least 20–40 minutes depending on the initial dosage and, therefore, are potentially lethal in the 'cannot intubate–cannot ventilate' situation. Their main role is in the maintenance of muscle relaxation and facilitation of intermittent positive pressure ventilation (IPPV) after endotracheal intubation has been successfully achieved and the endotracheal tube firmly secured.

Non-depolarising muscle relaxants can be reversed with anticholinesterases, such as *neostigmine*. However, the success and time frame of successful reversal depends on the density of the neuromuscular block. The block can be assessed by monitoring the motor response following the percutaneous stimulation of a suitably accessible peripheral nerve.

Anticholinesterases act not only at the neuromuscular junction, but also on parasympathetic nerve endings. Parasympatholytic or anticholinergic drugs, such as atropine or glycopyrrolate, must be coadministered to counteract bradycardia, increase in bronchial secretions and spasm of the bladder and bowel.

RAPID SEQUENCE INDUCTION

There are essentially five indications for rapid sequence induction (RSI) in a trauma patient:

- airway protection in cases of acute or impending airway obstruction (e.g. burns, soiling, impaired gag reflex)
- failure to oxygenate adequately by other means (e.g. multiple rib fractures with flail segment and intractable hypoxia)
- control of ventilation and intracranial pressure in head-injured patients
- agitation/aggression likely to result in self-harm (severe intoxication with illicit drugs)
- pain relief in exceptional circumstances (e.g. massive burns).

The technique of rapid sequence induction

Gastric emptying is delayed in trauma patients. Therefore, the trauma team has to choose an anaesthetic technique for induction of anaesthesia that is safe for patients with full stomachs. There is an increased risk of regurgitation of stomach contents with the potential of pulmonary aspiration. This risk is further exacerbated as the patient loses his protective laryngeal reflexes with the onset of unconsciousness during induction and muscle paralysis. A rapid sequence induction is a recognised technique to safeguard against aspiration; however, this complication can still arise despite a faultless technique and best efforts.

Preparation

Preparation for anaesthesia should occur early. A check is carried out that all the equipment is working. Where anatomy or injury suggests that intubation is likely to be difficult, back-up plans must be formulated. Alternative airway adjuncts, such as the laryngeal mask airway, cricothyrotomy cannulae and the surgical airway kit should be laid out and checked before embarking on induction.

Pre-oxygenation

Patients are not 'bagged' unless their breathing is agonal or apnoeic. Bag valve mask ventilation is difficult at the best of times and spontaneous breathing through a bag valve mask device is not easy owing to high resistance. If the patient is apnoeic, a two-person technique to ventilate the patient should be used where possible. If the patient is breathing, the patient should be pre-oxygenated either with a well-fitting and working non-rebreather mask with oxygen reservoir at 12–15 litres/minute flow and an airway adjunct, preferably a nasopharyngeal airway. Alternatively 100% oxygen can be delivered via a Waters or Mapleson C-circuit primed with high flow rates of oxygen. This device gives a good 'feel' of lung compliance. It requires practice to use safely, and rebreathing of carbon dioxide occurs, particularly at low flow rates. It is essential to ensure that the reservoir is expanded by rubbing it vigorously for a few seconds to help its compliance.

Induction

Each drug is drawn up in a specific-sized syringe and labelled accordingly. Only when all tube checks have been carried out postintubation should longer-term paralysis with a non-depolarising muscle relaxant be delivered.

In patients displaying profound volume depletion, the use of an induction agent may precipitate cardiovascular collapse and cardiac arrest. In these rare situations, consideration should be given to facilitate intubation with suxamethonium only. A fluid bolus should also be delivered to minimise the effects of positive pressure ventilation. As the blood pressure rises, sedation can be addressed.

Cricoid pressure or Sellick's manoeuvre

With the onset of becoming obtunded or unconscious, patients lose their protective upper airway and laryngeal reflexes. Sellick's manoeuvre attempts to compress the oesophagus by pressing the cricoid cartilage against the cervical vertebrae and preventing regurgitation (Sellick, 1961). It is considered to be a standard component of rapid sequence induction. Pressure should be applied by a trained assistant, ideally standing at the patient's left side, as the patient begins to lose consciousness; if it is applied too early, the patient may find it uncomfortable and vomiting might ensue. There is no ultimate agreement as to the superiority of one-handed pressure on the cricothyroid membrane over two-handed cricoid pressure with one hand acting as a counterforce supporting the neck from underneath. It is paramount that the force of cricoid pressure is applied strictly in an anterior to posterior direction only, and that there is no pinching of the cricoid or displacement of the larynx. Improper techniques of applying cricoid pressure may prevent successful intubation and, at worst, result in exacerbation of cervical spine injury and contribute to death. Providers of cricoid pressure must undergo proper training and acquire a clear understanding of the procedure.

Maintenance and analgesia

In principle, there are inhalational anaesthetic agents, such as *halothane, isoflurane* or *sevoflurane* available, or intravenous anaesthetic agents, such as *propofol, midazolam* and *ketamine*, with supplementary opioids. Maintenance of anaesthesia with inhalational agents requires an anaesthetic machine. This is clearly an impractical set-up during intrahospital and interhospital transfers. Intravenous bolus techniques or, ideally, continuous intravenous infusions of anaesthetic agents are more versatile and can be administered more easily.

Irrespective of the technique used, it is important to provide a steady level of sedation and to avoid damaging hypertensive spikes owing to light anaesthesia. Where patients are haemodynamically stable, a background of incremental intravenous boluses of midazolam and morphine, carefully titrated, should be used. If there is any concern about intravascular volume depletion, a shorter-acting hypnotic, such as propofol, should be titrated against response.

Burns patients often require more sedation than the multiply injured patient. Midazolam and morphine are the maintenance agents of choice for most patients.

Intubation

Where possible, all intubations should be undertaken with the rigid collar off, or undone with manual in-line cervical stabilisation and cricoid pressure. The head and neck must be in the neutral (anatomical) position to align all seven cervical and the upper thoracic vertebrae. The 'sniffing the morning air' position with extension of the head and flexion of the neck adopted for routine endotracheal intubation is potentially dangerous in the trauma situation. It may exacerbate any coexisting spinal injury. Every effort should be made to maximise the likelihood of intubation at the first attempt. It is the authors' practice to use the McCoy® laryngoscope routinely for all trauma intubations (Gabbott, 1996; Laurent et al., 1996).

It is unwise to struggle to establish the 'best possible view'. If the person intubating can visualise the laryngeal inlet in its entirety – a grade-one Cormack–Lehane view (Cormack and Lehane, 1984), then the trachea should be directly intubated with an appropriately sized endotracheal tube. For any other views, a gum elastic bougie should be used and the endotracheal tube carefully railroaded over the bougie placed through the vocal cords down to the level of the carina. Prolonged laryngoscopy in an attempt to try to get the best possible view is unnecessary, and only potentiates the chance of cervical spine movement and hypoxia. Endotracheal intubations, which appear to be difficult from the outset or to be high risk, and those in physiologically compromised patients, should be undertaken by the most experienced operator available.

Under ideal circumstances, rapid sequence induction in trauma patients is a four-person procedure: one to intubate at the head end, one to provide in-line stabilisation working from the patient's side, one to provide cricoid pressure working from the opposite side, and one to administer drugs and intravenous fluid boluses.

Failed intubation

If there is any doubt about the placement or the position of the endotracheal tube, then it should be removed at once and the patient ventilated with the bag valve mask device using a two-person technique, ensuring a good seal around the mouth, and effective but gentle ventilations.

When the patient has been reoxygenated, a second attempt can be made. Only if reversible factors, such as waning paralysis, hamper the second attempt, should a third attempt may be made. Otherwise alternative airway techniques, e.g. the laryngeal mask airway (LMA) or the oesophageal tracheal combitube (OTC) or needle cricothyroidotomy should be considered as temporising measures. A surgical airway may be the only alternative available to create a definitive airway.

If the patient's airway anatomy suggests that oral endotracheal intubation is likely to be very difficult and the first attempt at laryngoscopy confirms this, consideration should be given to directly proceed to a surgical airway.

Familiarity with the locally adopted 'failed-intubation drill' is absolutely essential for every member of the trauma team, not just the intubator. There should be a pre-formulated consensus opinion and back-up plan of how to proceed when difficulties in airway and ventilatory management arise.

Confirmation of endotracheal intubation

The correct position of the endotracheal tube is confirmed by auscultation for air entry in both axillae and over the stomach, a visual check of the colour of skin and lips, a check of all vital signs, oxygen saturation and the presence of end-tidal carbon dioxide via direct or colorimetric ET-CO$_2$ measurements (Falk and Sayre, 1999). An oesophageal detector device may also be helpful, as it assists in detecting differences in the rigidity of oesophageal and tracheal walls. A correctly placed endotracheal tube will allow effortless, easy aspiration of air; in contrast, an endotracheal tube erroneously placed into the oesophagus will preclude any aspiration.

MINIMUM STANDARDS FOR MONITORING OF TRAUMA PATIENTS UNDERGOING TRAUMA ANAESTHESIA

These comprise a continuous display of an electrocardiogram, heart rate, pulse oximetry readings, quantitative end-tidal carbon dioxide measurement and non-invasive blood pressure readings every 2–3 minutes. Ideally, an arterial cannula should be placed expeditiously to facilitate invasive, beat-to-beat blood pressure monitoring and to allow repeat blood gas sampling. All monitor observations should be recorded or appear on a printout.

SPECIAL CONSIDERATIONS

Patients with direct trauma to the neck frequently develop massive soft tissue swelling in a short course of time similar to patients with severe facial burns. They require early securing of their airway. The chosen endotracheal tube should be used uncut, as its entire length may be required in due course.

Ketamine in anaesthetic doses may be the induction agent of choice in the following situations:

- for burns patients, where monitoring of vital signs is difficult owing to the distribution of the burns
- for combative patients, who appear to be volume depleted
- for spontaneously breathing patients, who become agitated and combative
- if severe life-threatening bronchospasm suddenly arises.

Key messages

- The trauma nurse is an integral part of the trauma team
- To offer valuable anaesthetic assistance requires an understanding of the principles of trauma anaesthesia with manual in-line stabilisation
- The trauma nurse must be trained to be able to assist with a rapid sequence induction of the trauma patient
- Incorrectly applied cricoid pressure may preclude a successful trauma intubation
- End-tidal carbon dioxide measurement is essential to confirm correct placement of the endotracheal tube in addition to clinical signs

CONCLUSION

Any trauma patient in pain deserves adequate pain relief for humanitarian reasons and to counteract any exacerbation of the stress response to trauma.

Bedside-based trauma nurses have a wide range of methods to provide analgesia at their disposal, as described in this chapter. Careful selection of the most appropriate analgesic technique, including route of application and judicious, careful administration ensures optimal results. Analgesia requirements in the trauma patient require frequent re-evaluation by the nurse. In addition, empathy and compassion are of utmost importance.

Trauma anaesthesia is potentially hazardous and requires considerable skill and experience. The trauma nurse fulfilling the role of anaesthetic assistant is essential to the success of a rapid sequence induction for a trauma victim. Such nurses require specific training for this role and a thorough knowledge of the anaesthetic agents commonly used. Furthermore they must be familiar with different techniques of managing the difficult airway. Trauma anaesthesia should only be administered by a team, including trauma nurses, which possesses an appropriate level of skill and experience.

References

Adam SK, Osbourne S. *Critical care nursing science and practice.* Oxford: Oxford University Press, 1997

Cormack RS, Lehane J. Difficult tracheal intubation in obstetrics. *Anaesthesia* 1984; 39: 1105–1111

Eccleston C. Role of psychology in pain management. *British Journal of Anaesthesiology* 2001; 87: 144–152

Falk JL, Sayre MR. Confirmation of airway placement. *Prehospital Emergency Care* 1999; 3: 273–278.

Gabbott DA. Laryngoscopy using the McCoy laryngoscope after application of a cervical collar. *Anaesthesia* 1996; 51: 812–814

Greaves I, Porter K, Ryan J. *Trauma care manual.* London: Arnold, 2001

Hazinski M F. *Nursing care of the critically ill child,* 2nd edn. St Louis: Mosby, 1996

Illingworth KA, Simpson KH. *Analgesia and anaesthesia in emergency medicine,* 2nd edn. Oxford: Oxford University Press; 1998

Jacobi J, Fraser G L, Coursin D, et al. Clinical practice guidelines for the sustained use of sedatives and analgesics in the critically ill adult. *Critical Care Medicine* 2002; 30: 119–141

Laurent SC, de Melo AE, Alexander-Williams JM. The use of the McCoy laryngoscope in patients with simulated cervical spine injuries. *Anaesthesia* 1996; 51: 74–75

Mackenzie R. Pre-hospital analgesia and sedation. *Journal of the Royal Army Medical Corps* 2000; 146: 117–127

McQuay H. Opioids in pain management. *Lancet* 1999; 353: 2229–2232

Merksey H. Pain terms: a list with definitions and notes on usage. Recommended by the IASP Subcommittee on Taxonomy. *PAIN* 1979; 6: 249

Patel N, Smith CE. Pain management in trauma. *Anesthesiology Clinics of North America* 1999; 17: 295–309

Park G, Fulton B, Senthuran S. *The management of acute pain,* 2nd edn. Oxford: Oxford University Press, 2000

Pasero C, McCaffery M. The patients report of pain: believing vs. accepting. There's a big difference. *American Journal of Nursing* 2001; 101: 73–77

Sarafino EP. *Health psychology: biopsychosocial interactions.* Chichester: Wiley, 1990: 367–372

Sellick BA. Cricoid pressure to prevent regurgitation of stomach contents during induction of anaesthesia. *Lancet* 1961; August 19: 404–406

Thomas VN. *Pain – its nature and management.* London: Baillière Tindall in association with the RCN, 1997

Woodrow P. *Intensive care nursing: a framework for practice.* London: Routledge/Taylor and Francis, 2000

Zohar Z, Eitan A, Halperin P, et al. Pain relief in major trauma patients: an Israeli perspective. *Journal of Trauma* 2001; 51: 767–772

Further reading

Greaves I, Porter K, Ryan J (eds) Analgesia and anaesthesia for the trauma patient. In: *Trauma care manual.* London: Arnold, 2001: 241–259

Gwinnutt CL, McCluskey A. Management of the upper airway. In: Driscoll P, Skinner D (eds) *Trauma care beyond the resuscitation room.* London: BMJ Publishing, 1998: 19–35

Mackenzie R. Analgesia and sedation. *Journal of the Royal Army Medical Corps* 2000; 146: 117–127

Mackenzie R, Lockey DJ. Pre-hospital anaesthesia. *Journal of the Royal Army Medical Corps* 2001; 147: 322–334

Walls RM (ed.) *Manual of emergency airway management.* Philadelphia: Lippincott/Williams & Wilkins, 2000

SECTION 4

Major trauma

Chapter **22**

Head and neck trauma

Nicholas Maartens and Graham Lethbridge

INTRODUCTION

Head injuries are a major cause of morbidity and mortality in the community. It has been estimated that each year in the UK between 200 and 300 per 100 000 of the population are admitted to a hospital with a head injury. This makes head injury one of the most common reasons for attending accident and emergency departments. Of these injuries, nine per 100 000 are fatal – approximately 5000 per year. Traumatic injury, in which severe head trauma plays a major role in over 50% of cases, remains the leading cause of death in the population below 25 years of age and, overall, the third leading cause of death, succeeded only by cardiocerebral vascular disease and cancer. As a result, craniocerebral trauma places a huge economic and psychological burden upon society. In 1985, the estimated cost to society of traumatic brain injury in the USA was $37.8 billion.

In the USA, 50% of head injuries are consequences of road traffic accidents, 21% a consequence of falls, 12% due to assaults and violence, and 10% a result of sport and recreation. Most serious head injuries and 65% of subsequent deaths are a result of road traffic accidents. The highest incidence of head injuries occurs in people 15–24 years old, with the majority being male. A second peak incidence occurs in the elderly. Excessive alcohol consumption is frequently implicated.

In 1995, a survey of 219 trauma centres in the USA was undertaken. This revealed considerable variation in the management of head injuries, with intracranial pressure monitoring being used routinely in only 28% of units. As a result, the American Association of Neurological Surgeons and the Congress of Neurological Surgeons published a document, *Guidelines for the management of severe head injury*, which has subsequently been adopted by the World Health Organisation and recommended to centres outside North America. By adopting the measures prescribed and basing acute intensive and high-dependency neurosurgical and nursing care of severely head-injured patients on scientific principles, aiming to control intracranial pressure (ICP) and maintain optimal cerebral perfusion, the outcome for severely head-injured patients has in many instances been dramatically improved. The role of the attending nursing staff in this regard is central.

PATHOPHYSIOLOGY OF HEAD INJURIES

Despite being encased in a rigid protective skull and cushioned by cerebrospinal fluid (CSF), the brain is still very vulnerable to trauma, having only the consistency of a well-set jelly. The cranial vault, formed by the skull, consists of three compartments: the anterior, middle and posterior cranial fossae, which are divided by irregular, bony buttresses. The brain is further divided into right and left hemispheres by the *falx cerebri* and the supratentorial compartment divided from the infratentorial compartment by the *tentorium cerebelli*. These dural divisions are also relatively rigid and unyielding structures. The thickness of the cranium varies and, in parts, particularly the squamous portion of the temporal bone, is very thin. This makes the underlying middle meningeal artery vulnerable to trauma, a potential cause of intracranial haematomas, as discussed subsequently. The cranium is furthermore attached to the body by a relatively mobile cervical spine. Trauma imparted to the head either takes the form of:

- *linear acceleration-deceleration forces* brought about by rapid changes in velocity along a straight line
- *rotational forces* or angular acceleration
- *deformation forces* involving direct, focal, sharp penetrating or blunt forces. These can involve scalp, skull and brain independently, or in any combination (Figure 22.1).

For both treatment and prognostic purposes, it is important to have an understanding of the mechanisms as to how the head injury occurred and how it might evolve. Abrupt deceleration of a moving head is characterised by a relatively minor injury to the brain at the site of impact (*coup injury*) and an extensive contusion of the brain remote and usually opposite to the point of impact (*contrecoup injury*) (Figure 22.2). Contusions occur where the moving brain impinges against the rough surface of the cranial base or the sharp edge of the falx cerebri. These typically occur along the undersurface of the frontal lobes, the tips of the temporal lobes, beneath the falx cerebri and in the brainstem. They are usually multiple and may occur bilaterally.

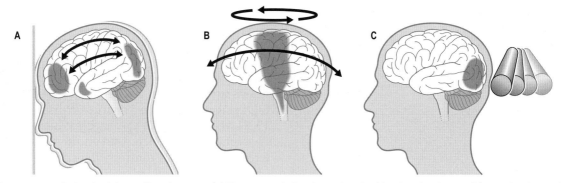

Figure 22.1 Pathophysiology of head trauma. (a) Linear translational acceleration/deceleration forces; (b) rotational angular acceleration transmitting forces down to the brainstem; (c) direct focal trauma.

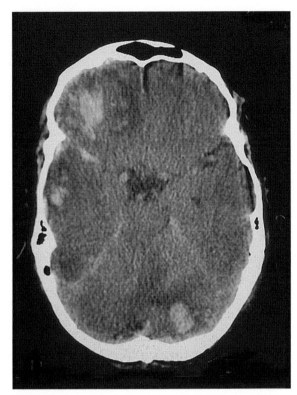

Figure 22.2 Axial computed tomography scan showing coup–contracoup contusional haematomas from an acceleration–deceleration-type injury appearing as areas of high density.

Acceleration–deceleration forces produce strains on cerebral tissue. These strains include *compression* (pushing together), *tension* (pulling apart) and *shearing* forces (tissues of different density sliding relative to each other). Abrupt acceleration of an unsupported head occurs when a moving object strikes the head. The skull accelerates against the brain, causing an extensive coup injury. The remainder of the brain may remain unchanged. When a moving object strikes a well-supported head, there is little movement of the skull and brain. Most of the force is absorbed by the skull, which will fracture. Damage to the underlying brain results from direct perforation or laceration by skull fragments. It is thus easy to understand why most cerebral contusions occur without skull fractures and why patients with spectacular fractures can often remain conscious with only minor neurological dysfunction. A classification for brain injuries is given in Box 22.1.

Box 22.1   Classification of brain injury (Glasgow Coma Scale)

Severity	GCS
Mild brain injury	13–15
Moderate brain injury	9–12
Severe brain injury	3–8

When considering the spectrum of head injury, it is useful to look at the constituents of the head, namely the scalp, skull and brain, and the ways in which they can be injured.

Scalp

The scalp is comprised of five layers (Figure 22.3). Although scalp lacerations or bruising confirm the presence of a head injury, their absence does not exclude an underlying intracranial haematoma. Hair plays a protective role and, by matting into wounds, can quite effectively assist haemostasis but likewise can effectively mask large scalp wounds. The rich vascular supply of the scalp plays an important role in healing, making the scalp very resilient to trauma.

Scalp injuries include the following:

- *Abrasion:* the top layer of the scalp is scraped away causing slight bleeding. Cleaning, debridement and dressing is all that is required.
- *Contusion:* bruising of the scalp with preservation of the skin – no specific treatment is required.

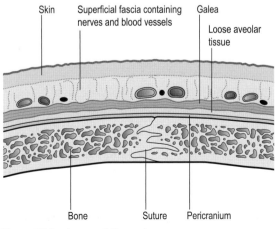

Figure 22.3 Layers of the scalp.

- *Laceration:* scalp lacerations are common and may give rise to exsanguinating haemorrhage, if not controlled. Exsanguinating haemorrhage occurs due to the blood vessels in the dense fibrous layer, superficial to the *galea aponeurotica*, being held open once transected. Lacerations should, therefore, be sutured and not bandaged. Repair should be performed in two layers, with apposition of the galea prior to closure of the skin. This should be done after shaving widely around the wound, infiltrating with local anaesthetic (0.5% Marcaine with epinephrine, being careful not to exceed the toxic dose) and then cleaning and debriding meticulously before suturing. If the scalp wound has resulted in loss of soft tissue, the wound may need to be extended to provide an extra 'flap' of healthy tissue so that the edges can be approximated without tension.
- *Subgaleal haematoma:* bleeding into the scalp usually occurs in the subgaleal areolar space that contains emissary veins emptying into the venous sinuses. It is important to exclude an underlying depressed skull fracture. The soft fluctuant centres of scalp haematomas frequently masquerade as depressed skull fractures on palpation. They are invariably associated with skull fractures in infants.

Skull

The cranium protects the brain and consists of the frontal, parietal, temporal, occipital, sphenoid and ethmoid bones. The facial bones provide a framework for the face. Different types of skull injuries may follow blunt or penetrating trauma.

Simple linear fractures

These require no specific neurosurgical management but are usually indicators of the force to which the head was subjected. They are frequently a result of blunt trauma. The bony buttresses direct the fracture towards the skull base (see 'Base of skull fractures' later). Considerable distortion of the skull, without fracturing, may occur in infants because of the elasticity of the skull. The skull sutures may also spring apart (diastasis). Patients generally require computed tomography (CT)

scanning, but should also be admitted for 48 hours observation to exclude secondary intracranial haematomas or the development of cerebral swelling. Fractures crossing the squamous portion of the temporal bone may lacerate middle meningeal vessels and cause extradural haematomas. Care must be taken to distinguish fractures from vascular markings and suture lines when evaluating skull x-rays. The latter two are usually paired structures.

Depressed skull fracture

These fractures are a result of sharper deformational trauma (Figure 22.1) – usually owing to assault trauma. The inner table of the skull is more extensively affected than the outer table. If the pericranium has been breached, the fractures are technically compound. The integrity of the dura is, however, more important. If the depressed fragments have lacerated the dura and brain (Figure 22.4), the cortical damage and subsequent risk of epilepsy are irreversible. There is also a significant risk of subsequent intracranial infection and an implantation abscess. Surgery is usually

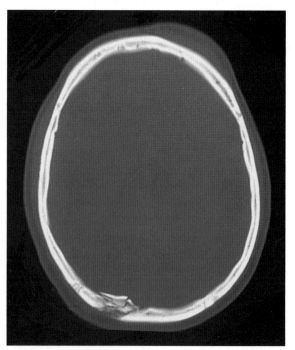

Figure 22.4 Depressed skull fracture in the right occipital region.

undertaken to prevent secondary infection, to alleviate mass effects and for cosmetic purposes. In order to preserve the option of conservative management, scalp lacerations should be cleaned, irrigated and sutured prior to transfer of head-injured patients and not simply left open beneath a compressive head dressing. Contaminated wounds require extensive debridement, irrigation and, when required, a duroplasty before closure – under general anaesthetic and in theatre. If a depressed skull fracture is compound, prophylactic antibiotics and tetanus prophylaxis should be administered and surgery under general anaesthetic performed as soon as possible. If the wound and bone fragments are heavily contaminated and there has been undue delay, the bone fragments should not be replaced and a reconstructive acrylic cranioplasty considered at a later stage.

The risk of post-traumatic epilepsy following a depressed skull fracture and cortical laceration is approximately 15%.

Base of skull fracture

These are relatively frequent fractures as already outlined – often occult radiologically but diagnosed on clinical grounds. A consequence of these fractures is the frequency with which they transverse the paranasal air sinuses, resulting in a CSF fistula. These may persist but usually seal off after 7–10 days.

Anterior fossa fractures may open into the frontal or ethmoid air sinuses, often running across the cribriform plate. They present with:

- subconjunctival haematomas extending to the posterior limits of sclera – periorbital haematomas or 'raccoon eyes' (Figure 22.5) – indicate subgaleal haemorrhage and not necessarily base of skull fracturing
- anosmia owing to injury to the olfactory nerve;
- nasal tip paraesthesiae owing to anterior ethmoidal nerve injury
- CSF rhinorrhea and/or epistaxis
- caroticocavernous fistula (Figure 22.6).

Middle fossa fractures involving the petrous temporal bone (Figure 22.7) present with:

- CSF otorrhea (or rhinorrea via the Eustachian tube) and/or bleeding from the auditory canal

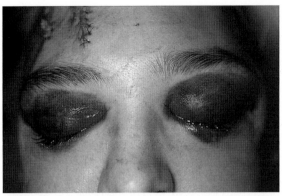

Figure 22.5 Periorbital ecchymoses ('raccoon eyes') owing to subgaleal bleeding from frontal trauma.

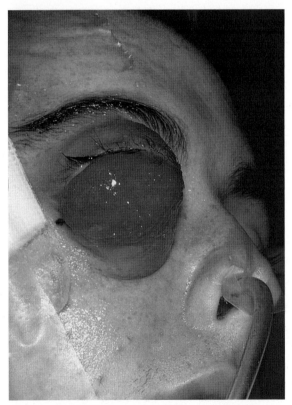

Figure 22.6 Caroticocavernous fistula, a complication developing following fracture of the petrous temporal bone with laceration of the internal carotid artery into the cavernous sinus. The pulsitile proptosis and conjunctival oedema are visible, and a bruit is audible on auscultation.

- deafness owing to disruption of the ossicular chain in the middle ear and/or VIII cranial nerve injury

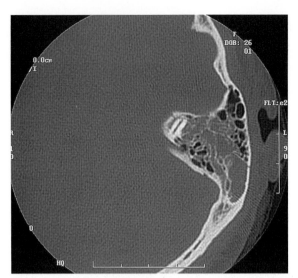

Figure 22.7 Base of skull fracture of the petrous temporal bone. The fracture line is visible and some of the mastoid air sinuses appear opacified due to bleeding

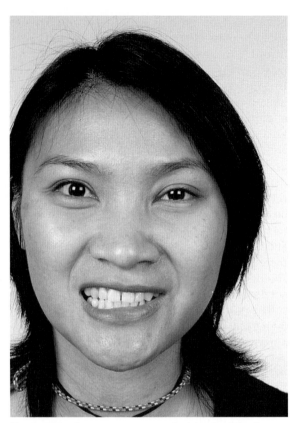

Figure 22.9 Lower motor neuron facial palsy following petrous temporal bone base of skull fracturing.

- haemotympanum
- Battle's sign – bruising over the mastoid bone (Figure 22.8)
- facial nerve palsy – often occurring in a delayed fashion (Figure 22.9).

These fractures may be visible on plain skull x-rays or on axial bone window CT scans but are usually identified radiologically by pneumocranium, sinus opacification or by air–fluid levels in the paranasal sinuses. These defects are usually plugged by brain tissue and seal, but air and bacteria can enter the intracranial compartment causing meningitis or tension pneumocranium when brain swelling resolves.

The use of prophylactic antibiotics is controversial. There is no evidence that their administration in the setting of a base of skull fracture diminishes the incidence of meningitis. Antibiotics may even act to select out more virulent organisms in those patients that develop

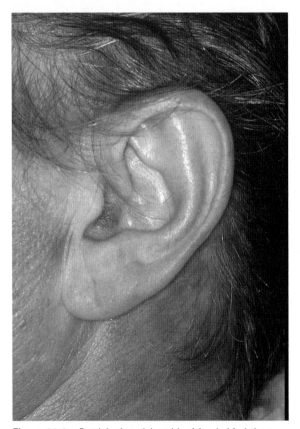

Figure 22.8 Battle's sign: delayed bruising behind the ear appearing 36 hours after a head injury with an associated petrous temporal base of skull fracture.

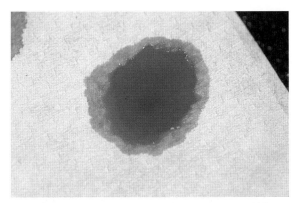

Figure 22.10 Cerebrospinal fluid rhinorrhea – the CSF component of the drop of fluid is less viscous than the blood and radiates out further, creating the characteristic halo effect of the 'target sign'.

Box 22.2   Brain injury

Primary injury
- Diffuse
  - Concussion
  - Diffuse axonal head injury
- Focal
  - Contusion
  - Laceration

Secondary injury
- Cranial
  - Intracranial haematoma
  - Cerebral swelling
  - Infection, seizures and hydrocephalus
- Systemic
  - Electrolyte disturbances
  - Neurogenic pulmonary oedema
  - Cushing's ulcers

---

meningitis, potentially increasing associated morbidity and mortality. If one is uncertain about the origin of fluid seen leaking from the nose or ear, it should be screened for β_2-transferrin ('tau' protein) to exclude the presence of CSF. CSF mixed with blood characteristically causes a *'target sign'* (Figure 22.10).

Patients with persistent CSF fistula or patients presenting with meningitis owing to an occult fistula following base of skull fracturing should undergo surgical repair. This involves initially ensuring that no hydrocephalus is present, then via a craniotomy after identifying the location of the defect, sealing the dura with autologous vascularised grafts and reinforcing the seal with fibrin glue. In the case of anterior fossa fractures, cranialisation of the frontal sinuses is usually necessary. The other complication of base of skull fracturing is an injury to the internal carotid artery where it enters the skull base causing dissection, a traumatic aneurysm or a caroticocavernous fistula.

Pond fracture
This is the cranial equivalent of a 'greenstick' fracture. It is a smooth concave depression due to blunt trauma to the cranial vault. It is usually seen in children and is also known as 'ping-pong ball' fracture.

Orbital blowout fractures
These are caused by blunt trauma to the eye. The blow transmits forces via the globe to the orbit, causing disruption of the orbital walls with herniation of the orbital contents and subsequent tethering of the orbital fat and possibly the globe within the fracture. This results in painful restricted eye movements with diplopia and requires surgical repair.

Brain injury

Primary brain injury is the injury caused at the time of impact (e.g. contusions and lacerations) and is irreversible (Box 22.2). Secondary brain injury is subsequent or progressive brain damage arising from events developing as a result of the primary brain injury or other injuries. The management of head injuries is aimed at preventing secondary injury.

Primary brain injury
Diffuse brain injury
Cerebral concussion This is a clinical diagnosis manifest by temporary cerebral dysfunction that is most severe immediately after injury and resolves after a variable period of time. The term was introduced by Pare and derives from the Latin *'concutere'* – to shake. It may be accompanied by autonomic abnormalities including bradycardia, hypotension and sweating. Loss of consciousness often, but not invariably, accompanies concussion. Amnesia for the event is common and varying

degrees of temporary lethargy, irritability and cognitive dysfunction are hallmarks. The term concussion is not strictly defined in terms of the severity of the injury; however, a minimum criterion is that the patient has a period of amnesia.

Postconcussion syndrome is a symptom complex persisting months after head injury and consists of various combinations of headache, irritability, depression, lassitude, problems with memory and concentration, and vertigo. It is frequently manifest in patients attempting returning to work or studies too quickly.

Diffuse axonal head injury This type of brain injury occurs as a result of mechanical shearing at the grey–white matter interface following severe acceleration–deceleration-type forces. This occurs as a result of the different densities of the grey and white matter, resulting in acceleration at different velocities. This disrupts and tears axons, myelin sheaths and blood capillaries. Severity can range from mild damage with confusion to coma and even death. Microscopic evidence of neuronal damage depends on the duration of survival and the severity of the injury. Axonal ballooning takes 12–24 hours to develop and may persist for some time. After a few days, microscopic *retraction balls* and *microglial clusters* are seen in the white matter. With long-term survival, weeks to months later, *Wallerian degeneration* of the long tracts and white matter appear, resulting in brain atrophy. These degenerative changes are eventually replaced by white matter *gliosis*.

Focal brain injury

Cerebral contusion Contusions can be demonstrated on CT scans as areas of haemorrhage on the surface of the brain (Figure 22.2). They usually produce focal neurological deficits that persist for longer than 24 hours. Contusions may resolve together with the accompanying deficit or they may persist. Blood–brain barrier defects and cerebral oedema are invariably associated with cerebral contusions. Their location is usually predictable with acceleration–deceleration-type injuries and they occur where the brain impacts on the bony protuberances of the skull. They are identified on CT scan and, if of sufficient size, may be accompanied by a rise in intracranial pressure.

Box 22.3 Risk of intracranial haematoma. (Reproduced from Mendelow et al. *British Medical Journal* 1983; 2: 1173–1176)	
No skull fracture – orientated	1 in 6000
No skull fracture – not orientated	1 in 120
Skull fracture – orientated	1 in 32
Skull fracture – not orientated	1 in 4

Cerebral laceration Even without a skull fracture, if sufficient force is delivered to the skull, the brain might become lacerated as a result of rapid movement and shearing of underlying brain tissue. The pia and arachnoid mater may be torn and intracerebral haemorrhage may accompany this lesion. Focal deficits are once again the rule.

Secondary brain injury

Intracranial haematomas (see Box 22.3)

Intracerebral haematoma These appear as hyperdense lesions on CT with associated mass effect (Figure 22.11). They occur as a consequence of acceleration–deceleration-type injuries in which there is shearing of cortical vessels beneath depressed fractures, and due to small punctate areas of traumatic contusion coalescing into a larger contusional haematoma. Disrupted cerebral tissue releases *thromboplastins* that potentiate haemorrhage. Fresh blood clots in coagulopathic patients may appear to have a mixed density to their haematomas on CT ('*swirl sign*'), giving the appearance of an acute on chronic haematoma. Large intracerebral haematomas should be evacuated, unless the patient's neurological state is good and is stable or improving. Small or moderate-sized intracerebral haematomas, particularly if multiple or deep in eloquent cortex, may not require removal. The attending clinician must, however, be aware that these lesions invariably expand owing to ongoing bleeding and progressive surrounding oedema, and may require subsequent evacuation or control of secondary raised intracranial pressure.

Extradural haematoma These usually occur as a result of linear squamous temporal skull fractures lacerating branches of the underlying *middle*

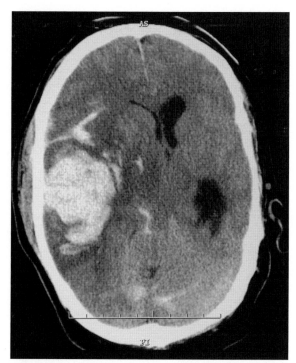

Figure 22.11 Axial CT scan showing a traumatic contusional intracerebral haematoma appearing as an area of high density with mass effect.

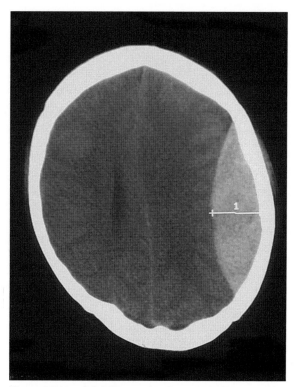

Figure 22.12 Axial CT scan showing a typical lens-shaped acute left-sided extradural haematoma owing to a squamous temporal fracture not visible on CT.

meningeal artery. They can also arise from fractured skull bone edges or rarely from laceration of the dural venous sinuses. The potential space between the dura and the inner table of the skull is developed by the expanding haematoma as it strips the densely adherent dura away, allowing it to take on the familiar convex lens configuration (Figure 22.12). The degree of trauma does not have to be severe and may in fact be trivial. There is classically a *lucid interval* following the trauma, followed by a subsequent loss of consciousness as the haematoma expands compressing the brain. They are more likely to occur in the younger age group, as the dura is less adherent and able to strip more readily off the underlying bone. Extradural haematomas, therefore, account for two-thirds of all traumatic intracranial haematomas in the under-20s age group but only 5% of haematomas in patients over 50 years.

Frequently, patients present in coma and require urgent craniotomy. An extradural haematoma is a surgical emergency that will result in death if the haematoma is not removed promptly, as the haematoma accumulates under arterial pressure. Patients should do well if delay to craniotomy and evacuation is minimised. Once again, care must be taken when assessing patients with linear fractures crossing middle meningeal artery territory.

Subdural haematomas These are the most common intracranial mass lesions resulting from head trauma. Approximately 29% of patients with post-traumatic intracranial lesions have subdural haematomas. The bleeding occurs into the space between the dura and the subarachnoid or pial layer, and thus takes up a concave configuration. They are classified into acute, subacute and chronic depending on how long they take to present clinically following the injury:

- *Acute subdural haematoma* – within 48 hours, consisting of clotted blood appearing hyperdense on CT (Figure 22.13).

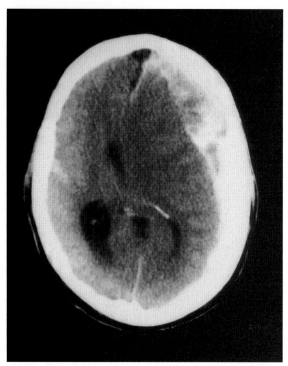

Figure 22.13 Axial CT scan showing a typical extensive concave left-sided acute subdural haematoma with midline shift.

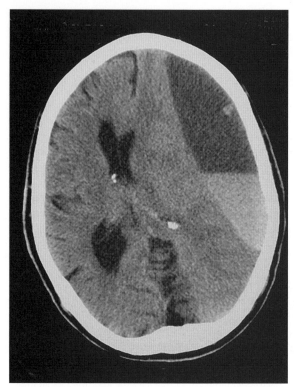

Figure 22.14 Axial CT scan showing an acute-on-chronic subdural haematoma. The fresh clotted blood appears white, while the older altered liquid blood appears black.

- *Subacute subdural haematoma* – 3–21 days, lysis of the clot has been initiated leaving blood degradation products and fluid. The blood appears isodense to brain on CT.
- *Chronic subdural haematoma* – more than 21 days, with the blood appearing hypodense on CT (Figure 22.14).

Acute subdural haematomas Most acute subdural haematomas result from torn bridging veins or from laceration of cortical vessels. They can also arise from cortical lacerations or bleeding from tears in the dural venous sinuses. They are usually associated with more severe, high-velocity trauma and are thus associated with a poorer outcome, but can be spontaneous owing to a bleeding diathesis or less frequently owing to ruptured intracranial aneurysms. '*Burst temporal lobe*' is the term sometimes used to describe the appearance of contusional intracerebral haematoma, bleeding out into the subdural space from the disrupted cortical surface. Acute subdural haematomas are

rapidly evolving lesions and early evacuation via formal craniotomy is mandatory.

Chronic subdural haematomas These haematomas are most common in infants and in adults over 60 years of age. They present with progressive neurological deficits more than 3 weeks after the trauma – typically a depressed or fluctuating level of consciousness, headache, hemiparesis, confusion and varying combinations thereof. Often the initial head injury may have been trivial and completely forgotten, and the pathology attributed to either dementia or a brain tumour until the patient is scanned (Figure 22.14). The initial haemorrhage may be relatively small, or may occur in elderly patients or alcoholics with brain atrophy, putting tension on 'stretched' bridging vessels. A subdural pseudomembrane, derived from the dura and arachnoid mater, encapsulates the haematoma, which remains clotted for 2–3 weeks then liquefies. The acute clotted blood initially appears white on a CT scan. As it liquefies it slowly becomes black (Figure 22.14). There is thus a point in time where it appears *'isodense'* with brain and all that can be seen is an apparent inexplicable shift on an otherwise normal CT. These collections may either resolve spontaneously or increase in size from repeated small bleeds. They are evacuated by drilling burrholes over the collection and then washing out the subdural space with warmed saline. If loculated or if recurrent, formal craniotomy with resection of the subdural membranes may be necessary.

Traumatic subarachnoid haemorrhage and intraventricular haemorrhage   All severe head injury is associated with some degree of traumatic subarachnoid haemorrhage. The role of calcium-channel antagonists, such as nimodipine, to protect against potential cerebral vasospasm, is still unclear. Large intraventricular bleeds may precipitate obstructive hydrocephalus.

Cerebral swelling   This occurs following trauma, either in a focal pattern around an intracerebral haematoma or contusion, or diffusely throughout the cerebrum or cerebellum. The pathological process is poorly understood, but involves a disturbance of vasomotor tone causing vasodilatation, loss of autoregulation and cerebral oedema with an increase in both intracellular and extracellular fluid volumes. In addition, cerebral contusion and petechial haemorrhages will contribute to brain swelling. It results in raised ICP and a diminished level of consciousness, and is both more common and more severe in children.

Infection, seizures and hydrocephalus   Penetrating skull trauma, depressed skull fractures and base of skull fractures all provide portals for central nervous system infection and the development of meningitis, brain abscesses or subdural empyemas. These can all exacerbate situations of raised ICP.

Hydrocephalus can develop acutely as a result of obstruction to CSF outflow owing to intraventricular blood or, more insidiously, as 'delayed post-traumatic communicating hydrocephalus' owing to impaired CSF reabsorption through the arachnoid granulations following traumatic subarachnoid haemorrhage.

Seizures can increase both cerebral metabolism ($CMRO_2$) and cerebral blood flow (CBF), therefore increasing ICP. Prophylactic anticonvulsants given acutely for the first 2 weeks post head injury are said to be of benefit. No prophylactic benefit from long-term anticonvulsant treatment has been demonstrated.

Cerebral ischaemia   This is common after severe head trauma and is caused by hypoxia, hypotension, impaired cerebral perfusion or a combination. The injured brain can lose *autoregulation* (see later) and become unable to maintain cerebral blood flow with a decreased blood pressure. *Glutamate* excess and *free radical* accumulation leads to neuronal damage. Areas of ischaemia, infarction and necrosis appear in adjacent brain tissue around contusions and lacerations. These areas are particularly vulnerable to deprivation of adequate CBF and oxygen delivery. Normally, the brain is able to maintain a constant CBF over a wide range of cerebral perfusion pressures. In the presence of a cerebral insult, such as severe head injury or subarachnoid haemorrhage, or beyond the physiological limits of normal blood pressures (see later; Figure 22.18), the CBF is no longer 'autoregulated', and is only passively and linearly related to blood pressure. Hypoxia and hypercarbia develop in the tissues causing cerebral vasodilatation. This acts to increase CBF when cerebral perfusion pressure decreases. Vasomotor tone in cerebral vessels is lost. Together with focal damage to the blood–brain barrier, this causes fluid to move out into the extracellular space causing *vasogenic oedema*.

Cerebral ischaemia has a profound effect on cerebral function. Normal CBF is about 50–55 ml/ 100 g per minute. The threshold for electrical failure and cessation of electroencephalogram (EEG) activity and synaptic transmission is about 15–20 mL/100 g per minute. Cell membrane failure occurs at 6–10 mL/100 g per minute. The hypothetical concept of an *ischaemic penumbra* (Figure 22.15), as described by Astrup, is a clinical concept that areas of destroyed cerebral tissue are surrounded by regions of compromised, electrically silent, non-functional, but still viable tissue. If properly protected and treated, these can be saved, reducing the extent of secondary brain injury.

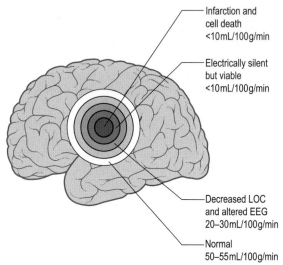

Figure 22.15 Hypothetical 'ischaemic penumbra' of Astrup. Theoretically, this is a compromised area between a region of infarction and normal brain that is at risk. Therapy is directed towards preserving this area by optimising cerebral blood flow. EEG, electroencephalogram; LOC, level of consciousness.

Electrolyte disturbances Patients with severe head injuries, particularly children, are prone to various types of electrolyte disturbances. The most common are sodium disturbances that can occur both spontaneously and as a consequence of diuretic therapy used to control raised ICP (see 'Management' later). Both hyponatraemia and hypernatraemia can further compromise consciousness, and injudicious rapid correction of sodium disturbances can cause *central pontine myelinolysis*.

Penetrating injuries

Missile injuries Although most literature on missile injuries is related to warfare, these injuries are unfortunately becoming increasingly common in civilian practice. There are three categories of missile injury as listed below.

- *Tangential* – the missile does not enter the cranium but causes a depressed skull fracture, lacerating the scalp causing an underlying cortical contusion, laceration or haematoma.
- *Penetrating* – the missile enters the cranium resulting in the deposition of metal, bone fragments and debris within the brain.

- *Through-and-through* – the missile enters and exits the cranium frequently creating more than one tract owing to fragmentation.

The cranial injury is directly related to the velocity of the missile. The energy dissipated by the missile equals MV^2, where M is the mass and V the velocity of the missile. A *'high-velocity'* injury is defined as an injury resulting from a missile traveling faster than the speed of sound (1050 ft/second). Modern ballistics has designed missiles to have maximal velocity and stability in flight with maximal dissipation of energy upon impact. The primary missile frequently fragments and can cause further secondary missiles from fragments of bone or metal (Figure 22.16). The missile causes cerebral damage via three mechanisms:

- *mechanical laceration* of brain tissue during transit
- the *shock wave* promulgated ahead of the missile
- *cavitation* in the wake of the missile.

Management of gunshot head injuries has come full circle since the Anglo-Boer War. They are treated as compound depressed skull fractures, avoiding aggressive debridement of the tract and retrieval of deep secondary missiles. High-velocity injuries, transventricular wounds and injuries resulting in a persistent low Glasgow Coma Scale following resuscitation invariably prove fatal. Care must be taken to distinguish these from the functional effect of the shock wave generated by the impact of the bullet being transmitted down to the *reticular activating system* in the brainstem causing transient unconsciousness.

Non-accidental head injuries

The infantile chronic subdural haematoma or effusion is a distinct clinical entity. Birth trauma is a frequent cause but, in many cases, a past history is inadequate to establish the nature of the injury with certainty. Chronic subdural haematomas occur in approximately 20% of *'battered children'*. The violent shaking of the immature brain might be sufficient to rupture bridging veins without evidence of external trauma. If an inadequate history is provided in such a setting, it is important to screen for a *coagulopathy*, examine the fundi for *retinal haemorrhages*, arrange a *skeletal*

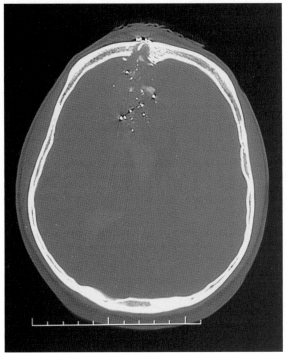
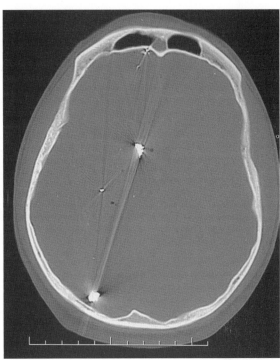

A   B

Figure 22.16 Gunshot head injury showing the secondary missiles from bone fragments and the tract of the bullet across the brain with fragments of the bullet jacket.

survey, perform a careful detailed examination and, when appropriate, involve a paediatrician and social services to ensure the patient's safety. Magnetic resonance imaging (MRI) now plays an important role in determining the chronology of cerebral injuries in infants. Collections of different chronicity or in unusual locations should alert the physician to the possibility of non-accidental injury.

BASIC CEREBRAL PHYSIOLOGY AND THE PATHOPHYSIOLOGY OF RAISED INTRACRANIAL PRESSURE

Introduction

The adult skull may be regarded as a rigid unyielding box containing brain, CSF and blood. At normal supine pressures of 5–15 mmHg (6–18 cm H_2O), measured from the level of the foramen of Munroe, these three components maintain volumetric equilibrium. An increase in the volume of any one of the components will result in an increase in ICP, unless there is a proportionate decrease in the volume of one of the other components. The pressure is also evenly distributed throughout the intracranial compartment. This has become known as the *Munro–Kellie doctrine*.

Owing to compensatory volumetric changes having physical and physiological limits, the ability to maintain a constant intracranial pressure can be exceeded by a change of volume that is too fast or too great, overwhelming compensatory measures. This intracranial pressure volume relationship is illustrated in the curve (Figure 22.17). Initially, quite large increases in volume produce only small changes in pressure. During this phase, the brain adapts by shifting CSF and moving blood from venous structures. A critical point is unfortunately reached when only a small change in volume causes an exponential rise in ICP. When patients initially present with symptoms of raised ICP, it is invariably when brain compliance has been exhausted, and small

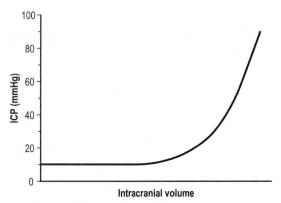

Figure 22.17   Intracranial pressure (ICP) volume relationships. Once cerebral compliance is exhausted, a small increase in volume will result in a large increase in pressure.

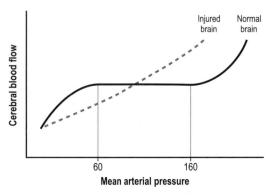

Figure 22.18   Autoregulation of cerebral blood flow. Cerebral blood flow (CBF) remains constant over a mean arterial pressure range of approximately 50–150 mmHg. The curve is shifted to the right in patients with chronic hypertension. The interrupted line indicates what happens when autoregulation is lost – the CBF becomes a linear function of the blood pressure.

intracranial volume changes have the potential to cause precipitous increases in ICP and a reduced level of consciousness.

Between physiological ranges of blood pressure, the brain is able to maintain a constant CBF. This is achieved by a process called *autoregulation* (Figure 22.18), whereby the brain adjusts the intracranial vascular resistance by altering the size and tension of the intracranial blood vessel lumens. With hypovolaemic shock, malignant hypertension, subarachnoid haemorrhage or diffuse severe head injuries, this ability is compromised and the cerebral perfusion pressure becomes virtually dependent on the mean arterial pressure.

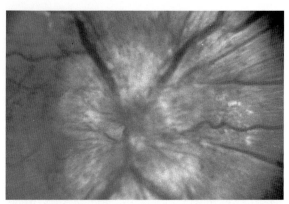

Figure 22.19   Papilloedema showing a swollen optic disc with blurred margins.

Normal cerebral blood flow is about 800 ml/minute or 20% of the total cardiac output. The blood flow is a function of the cerebral perfusion pressure (CPP) and the cerebral vascular resistance (CVR).

$$CBF = CPP/CVR$$

The *cerebral perfusion pressure* is the difference between the systemic mean arterial pressure (MAP) and the raised ICP it has to overcome.

$$CPP = MAP - ICP$$

As ICP increases, in order to maintain a constant CPP, there has to be a compensatory rise in the MAP. A systemic hypertensive response is, therefore, elicited, which classically is associated with a bradycardia. This is termed the *Cushing reflex*.

Clinical features

These are largely determined by the underlying cause. However, some of the clinical symptoms and signs of raised ICP will be the same:

- headache
- nausea and vomiting
- drowsiness
- papilloedema (Figure 22.19).

Although no randomised clinical study has ever been performed conclusively proving the value of ICP monitoring in reducing morbidity and mortality following brain injury, there is a clear relationship between raised ICP and outcome following severe head injury. The vital physiological parameter in severely head-injured patients is the CPP. This is a function of the MAP and the ICP. In order to optimise patient outcome, the CPP should be maintained above 70 mmHg while keeping all other physiological parameters and requirements as close to normal as possible. This may necessitate manipulation of the MAP using ionotropes, and requires a close working relationship between the intensive care physician, nurses and the neurosurgeon.

Cerebral herniation

Depending on the rate of increase in intracranial pressure or the position of an intracranial mass, brain herniation may occur (Figure 22.20). The three major types of herniation are:

- transtentorial
- foramen magnum
- subfalcine.

Transtentorial herniation occurs with downward displacement of the brain and herniation of the uncus of the medial temporal lobe over the sharp edge of the tentorial hiatus (Figures 22.20 and 22.22). This causes compression of the brainstem and ipsilateral *third nerve palsy*, which manifests as a dilated, sluggishly reacting pupil, looking downwards and outwards, and with ptosis (Figure 22.21). Compression of the *reticular activating system* in the brainstem further depresses the level of consciousness, leading to coma, hypertension, bradycardia, Cheyne–Stokes respiration and decerebrate posturing. When monitoring the Glasgow Coma Scale and checking the pupils, it is for the development of this process of transtentorial herniation that we are monitoring.

Compression of the ipsilateral corticospinal tracts in the brainstem causes contralateral hemiparesis (Figure 22.22). The lateral displacement of the brainstem by the herniated temporal lobe causes the contralateral corticospinal tract to impinge against the sharp, rigid opposite tentorial edge before crossing causing a 'false-localising' ipsilateral hemiparesis or *Kernohan's notch* phenomenon. This causes hemiparesis on the

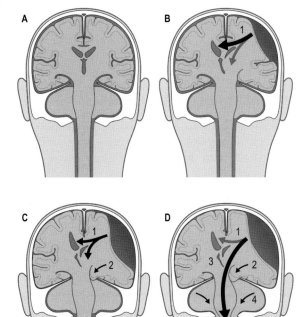

Figure 22.20 Brain herniations. A lateral supratentorial mass will sequentially cause displacement of the lateral ventricles with (1) subfalcine herniation of the cingulate gyrus below the falx cerebri; (2) herniation of the uncus or medial temporal lobe into the tentorial hiatus; (3) downward displacement of the brainstem. Raised pressure within the posterior fossa may cause herniation of the cerebellar tonsils into the foramen magnum. (4) Eventual descent of the brainstem through the foramen magnum results in coning and brain death.

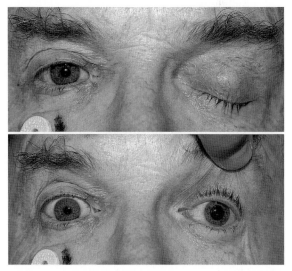

Figure 22.21 Third nerve palsy. The patient has both ptosis and a fixed dilated pupil in a downward and outward gaze position.

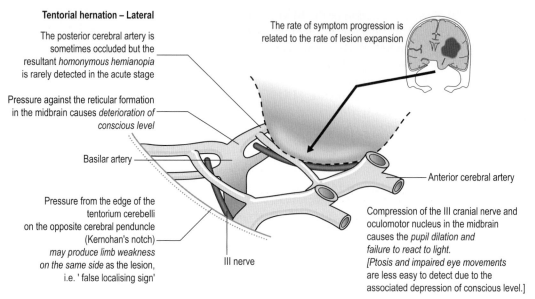

Tentorial hernation – Lateral

The posterior cerebral artery is sometimes occluded but the resultant *homonymous hemianopia* is rarely detected in the acute stage

The rate of symptom progression is related to the rate of lesion expansion

Pressure against the reticular formation in the midbrain causes *deterioration of conscious level*

Basilar artery

Anterior cerebral artery

Pressure from the edge of the tentorium cerebelli on the opposite cerebral penduncle (Kernohan's notch) *may produce limb weakness on the same side* as the lesion, i.e. ' false localising sign'

III nerve

Compression of the III cranial nerve and oculomotor nucleus in the midbrain causes the *pupil dilation and failure to react to light.* [*Ptosis and impaired eye movements are less easy to detect due to the associated depression of conscious level.*]

Figure 22.22   Transtentorial herniation. (Reproduced with permission from Lindsay K, Bone I. *Neurology and neurosurgery illustrated*, 3rd edn. New York: Churchill Livingstone, 1997)

same side as the primary pathology or the side opposite to that anticipated. Similarly, the posterior cerebral artery may be kinked causing occipital ischaemia, resulting in a homonymous hemianopia.

Increased pressure in the posterior fossa will result in herniation of the cerebellar tonsils into the foramen magnum (*tonsillar herniation*) (Figure 22.20) and compression of the medulla, causing a painful neck and possible head tilt. This can herald incipient and rapid respiratory failure, which is manifest as apnoea or abnormalities of respiratory rate and rhythm, as seen in infants with severe Chiari Type 2 malformations.

Progressive raised intracranial pressure eventually causes further downward herniation of the brainstem into the foramen magnum or 'coning'. Perforating blood vessels supplying the brainstem shear, causing haemorrhage within the brainstem known as *Duret haemorrhages*. Traction damage to the pituitary stalk with progressive brainstem herniation can result in *diabetes insipidus*. With progressive coning and brainstem damage, the pupils usually become mid-size and unreactive. These changes are invariably either very bad prognostic indicators or irreversible events leading to brainstem death.

PATHOPHYSIOLOGICAL CHANGES ASSOCIATED WITH BRAIN INJURY

The pathophysiological changes in the brain associated with severe head injury have come under extensive investigation. Although our understanding of these processes is incomplete, we now have a better understanding of the processes involved at a molecular and cellular level (Figure 22.23).

Molecular and cellular level

The initial cerebral dysfunction following head injury involves cellular energy metabolism. There is failure of anaerobic glycolysis, phosphocreatinine production and adenosine triphosphate (ATP) production. The failure of anaerobic glycolysis results in *intracellular acidosis*. Lactate accumulates and pH levels fall. As a consequence, there is failure of the sodium/potassium pump, resulting in an inability to maintain acid–base and ionic homeostasis. Potassium (K^+) leaks out of the cells, increasing the extracellular K^+. Sodium (Na^+) and calcium (Ca^{2+}) move into the cells from the extracellular space together with water, initiating *cytotoxic oedema*.

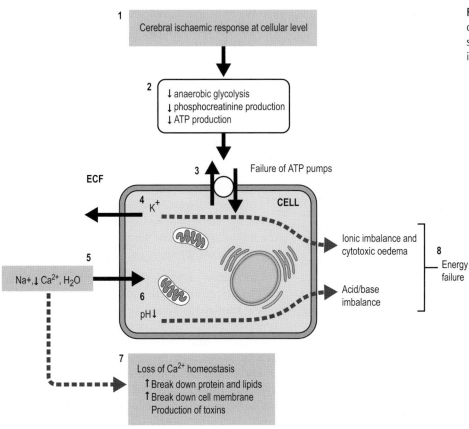

Figure 22.23 Pathway of central nervous system injury and ischaemia.

As a result of the loss of Ca^{2+} homeostasis, cellular metabolism is inhibited, resulting in the breakdown of proteins and lipids. The phospholipids in the cell membrane are broken down and the cell membrane damaged. Simultaneously, inflammatory cascades are activated, resulting in the production of toxins (eiconasoids, free radicals and platelet-activating factor). The severe cellular energy failure leads to the accumulation of the extracellular excitatory neurotransmitters: *glutamate*, *aspartate* and *acetylcholine*. The glutamate is released from depolarized neurons affected by energy depletion and stimulates receptors normally mediating excitatory synaptic transmission between neurons. This excessive stimulation opens ion channels facilitating sodium-mediated cellular swelling and calcium-mediated neuronal disintegration.

The *free radicals*, superoxide, hydroxyl and hydroperoxyl, formed by the cellular injury, further disrupt the cellular membrane. The presence of superoxide dismutase and the low tissue pH set in motion a vicious cycle, leading to further free-radical formation and cellular injury. Involvement of blood breakdown products results in another source of free radicals using free iron from haemoglobin. Cytoplasmic defences are overwhelmed and begin to oxidise cellular membranes by *lipid peroxidation*. This causes ongoing damage to the cell membrane and oxidation of membrane lipoproteins. This process spreads to adjacent cells with more cell death and swelling.

ASSESSMENT AND MANAGEMENT OF THE HEAD–INJURED PATIENT

The continuum of care begins at the trauma scene and continues until the final outcome. The key aspects in the management of patients following head injury involve:

- accurate clinical assessment of the neurological and other injuries
- determination of the pathological process involved

- prevention of secondary brain injury
- the concept that a change in the neurological signs indicates a progression or change in the pathological processes
- when faced with insufficient substrates as a result of insufficient CBF and cerebral oxygen delivery, ischaemia and hypoxia initiate the cascade of events leading to secondary brain injury.

Pre-hospital management

Initial resuscitation and stabilisation of the patient at the injury scene and en route to the trauma centre has a profound influence on outcome. Emergency treatment is directed towards maintaining cerebral metabolic needs, preventing and treating intracranial hypotension and supporting other systems following advanced trauma and life support (ATLS®) guidelines, while avoiding unnecessary delay. Simultaneously the emergency services should coordinate management so that appropriate timely transport is arranged to an appropriate referral centre, who should have been alerted as to the nature and condition of the patient about to be received, in order to mobilise the necessary resources.

Emergency department or trauma centre management

Primary and secondary survey

Assessment of head injuries must once again follow ATLS guidelines with an initial primary survey, then resuscitation, followed by a secondary survey, then definitive management; or more simply: *Airway*, *Breathing*, *Circulation*, *Disability* and *Exposure*. Care must be taken to ensure cervical spine protection at all times, as there is a 5% association of cervical spine injury (usually C1 to C3) with severe head injury.

Patient airway maintenance and breathing   Securing an adequate airway and preventing obstructive breathing or hypoventilation, as a first step, is critical in all unconscious head-injured patients. Allowing arterial PCO_2 to rise because of hypoventilation is a powerful stimulant of cerebral vasodilatation, raising intracranial pressure. This further depresses consciousness, initiating a

vicious cycle that can rapidly result in death. Under normal circumstances, ventilation is inaudible. Audible breathing is a sign of obstructed ventilation. All head trauma patients should be treated as having sustained a neck injury and care must be taken to secure the neck and spine, particularly during intubation. Endotracheal intubation may be contraindicated in cases of mid-face trauma and sometimes with base of skull fractures. Pre-intubation facemask ventilation should also be avoided to avoid potentially forcing air intracranially in patients with skull base fractures.

Once an airway is secured, appropriate measures are taken to optimise ventilation, often with the aid of a ventilator. Oxygen saturation should be continuously monitored with pulse oximetry.

Circulation   Hypotension results in reduced CPP and reduced CBF, exacerbating the effects of the primary head injury and should be treated urgently. However, fluid resuscitation should be appropriate and not excessive, as this will precipitate brain swelling. Isotonic crystalloid or colloid fluids should be utilised and Dextrose solutions avoided (see 'Management' later). Refractory hypotension may be due to occult, ongoing bleeding, lower body sympathectomy due to spinal cord injury, or hypocortisolism due to a pituitary gland injury. Resuscitation efforts should be assessed with repeated blood pressure, central venous pressure, oximetry and pulse rate measurement.

Assessment for head injuries

The mechanism of how the head trauma was sustained is important in determining both the immediate acute and future management, and for assessing likely prognostic outcome. The steps in evaluation following the resuscitation are:

- history and mechanism of injury
- vital signs
- Glasgow Coma Scale (GCS; Box 22.4)
- pupils
- external head and neck examination
- full neurological examination.

When assessing the GCS, it is the best response that must be recorded. The derivation or breakdown of the score must be specified if it is not being recorded on a formal chart (Figure 22.24). If

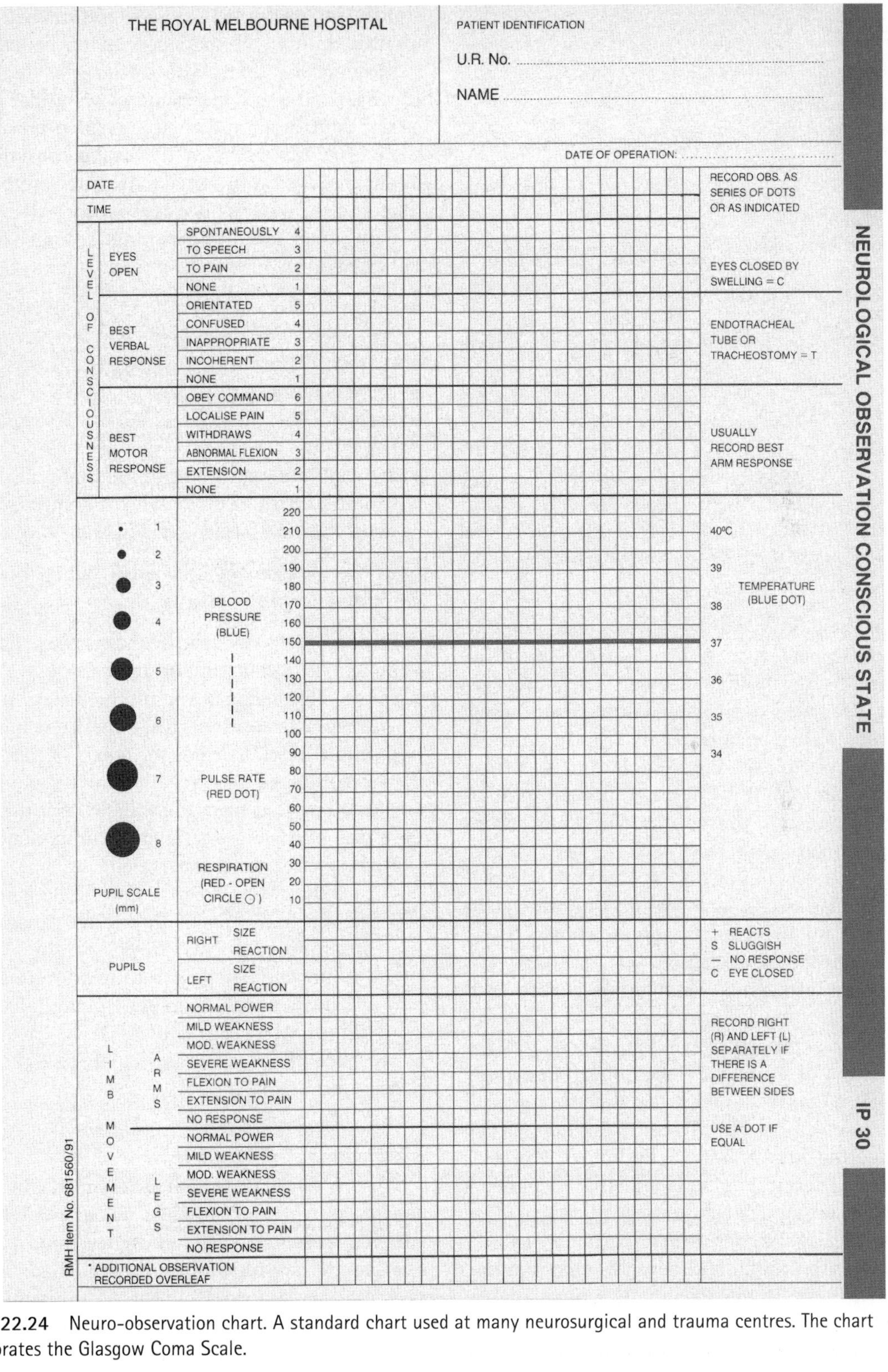

THE ROYAL MELBOURNE HOSPITAL

PATIENT IDENTIFICATION

U.R. No. ....

NAME ....

DATE OF OPERATION: ....

DATE																			**RECORD OBS. AS**			
TIME																			**SERIES OF DOTS OR AS INDICATED**			

LEVEL OF CONSCIOUSNESS

EYES OPEN	SPONTANEOUSLY	4										EYES CLOSED BY SWELLING = C
	TO SPEECH	3										
	TO PAIN	2										
	NONE	1										
BEST VERBAL RESPONSE	ORIENTATED	5										ENDOTRACHEAL TUBE OR TRACHEOSTOMY = T
	CONFUSED	4										
	INAPPROPRIATE	3										
	INCOHERENT	2										
	NONE	1										
BEST MOTOR RESPONSE	OBEY COMMAND	6										USUALLY RECORD BEST ARM RESPONSE
	LOCALISE PAIN	5										
	WITHDRAWS	4										
	ABNORMAL FLEXION	3										
	EXTENSION	2										
	NONE	1										

PUPIL SCALE (mm): 1, 2, 3, 4, 5, 6, 7, 8

BLOOD PRESSURE (BLUE): 220 210 200 190 180 170 160 150 140 130 120 110 100 90 80 70 60 50 40 30 20 10

PULSE RATE (RED DOT)

RESPIRATION (RED - OPEN CIRCLE ○)

TEMPERATURE (BLUE DOT): 40°C 39 38 37 36 35 34

PUPILS

RIGHT	SIZE											+ REACTS
	REACTION											S SLUGGISH
LEFT	SIZE											— NO RESPONSE
	REACTION											C EYE CLOSED

LIMB MOVEMENT

ARMS	NORMAL POWER											RECORD RIGHT (R) AND LEFT (L) SEPARATELY IF THERE IS A DIFFERENCE BETWEEN SIDES
	MILD WEAKNESS											
	MOD. WEAKNESS											
	SEVERE WEAKNESS											
	FLEXION TO PAIN											
	EXTENSION TO PAIN											
	NO RESPONSE											USE A DOT IF EQUAL
LEGS	NORMAL POWER											
	MILD WEAKNESS											
	MOD. WEAKNESS											
	SEVERE WEAKNESS											
	FLEXION TO PAIN											
	EXTENSION TO PAIN											
	NO RESPONSE											

* ADDITIONAL OBSERVATION RECORDED OVERLEAF

RMH Item No. 681560/91

NEUROLOGICAL OBSERVATION CONSCIOUS STATE

IP 30

Figure 22.24 Neuro-observation chart. A standard chart used at many neurosurgical and trauma centres. The chart incorporates the Glasgow Coma Scale.

Box 22.4   Glasgow coma scale

Eye opening
- Spontaneous   4
- To speech   3
- To pain   2
- Nil   1

Best motor response
- Obeys commands   6
- Localises pain   5
- Withdraws from pain   4
- Abnormal flexion (decorticate)   3
- Extension response (decerebrate)   2
- Nil   1

Verbal response
- Orientated   5
- Confused conversation   4
- Inappropriate words   3
- Incomprehensible sounds   2
- Nil   1

---

a patient cannot give a verbal response owing to an endotracheal tube being *in situ*, substitute the verbal score with the letter 'T'. If the eyes cannot be opened due to haematoma or swelling, substitute the eye opening score with the letter 'C' – in each case still scoring the total out of 15 (e.g. EcVtM4 = 4tc/15). It is important to bear in mind that the score can be compromised by small lesions causing aphasia and *inter alia* by hemiparesis, brachial plexus injuries and spinal cord injuries. Pain response assessments should thus always be performed on the cranial nerves as well if no peripheral response is elicited.

When an intracranial haematoma is suspected (Box 22.3), an early CT scan is essential. The indications for a skull x-ray have diminished since the introduction of routine CT scanning for severely head-injured patients, especially as the bony vault can be assessed by the CT scan using the survey view and the bone windows. Radiological assessment of the cervical spine is essential in patients who have sustained a severe head injury. This should ideally be performed formally by CT scanning with sagittal and coronal bone window reconstructions. If this facility is not available, antero–posterior, lateral and open-mouthed odontoid peg cervical spine films down to C7/T1

should be performed. If a significant lesion is identified and the patient cannot be assessed neurologically, then MRI scanning is indicated. Ideally, flexion and extension views under fluoroscopic control should then also be performed to exclude a dynamic lesion. If neurological symptoms or signs of a cord or nerve root injury are present, then an MRI scan is once again imperative.

Computed tomography brain scans should be performed if:

- the patient is persistently drowsy or has a more seriously depressed conscious level
- there are lateralising neurological signs
- there is neurological deterioration
- there is clinical evidence of base of skull fracturing
- associated injuries are present that will prolong ventilation, making ongoing neurological assessment difficult.

In the assessment of a head injury, points to determine from the history are:

- period of loss of consciousness
- period of post-traumatic amnesia
- cause, circumstance and mechanism of injury:
  - in vehicle accidents, this should include information, such as the speed of the involved vehicle, whether the patient had been ejected from the vehicle, or if there was intrusion of structural components into the passenger compartment
  - care should be taken to determine whether the mechanism is likely to have caused blunt injury (such as from a fall) or penetrating (such as from stab or gunshot wounds), where there may potentially be intradural foreign bodies
- presence of headache and vomiting
- seizures.

Examination of the patient

Primary survey   Head injuries must always be considered in the context of a patient who has suffered potential systemic injury and, as such, assessment should follow established trauma principles as laid down in the ATLS manual, but be individualised to the patient concerned. These principles prioritise the assessment to identify and treat the conditions that are the greatest threat to life. As with all trauma, the examination should be carried out in a focused manner, starting with a primary survey and resuscitation, then a thorough secondary examination.

In the primary survey, after management of *Airway*, *Breathing* and *Circulation*, as described previously, a rapid initial evaluation of neurological status should be carried out as part of the *Disability* assessment. This consists of assessing conscious state with the GCS (see earlier), and checking pupil size (remembering a fixed dilated pupil can be a sign of cerebral herniation, suggestive of an intracerebral haematoma requiring rapid identification and surgical intervention). Note that patients with a GCS of 8 or less will be unconscious, unable to maintain their own airway, in danger of hypoventilation or apnoea, and require intubation and ventilation (if not already performed).

Resuscitation efforts will be targeted to problems identified during the primary survey, as discussed previously. The importance of this cannot be overstated. There is good evidence that hypotension and hypoxaemia have an adverse effect on overall outcome in the head-injured patient. Of the many tubes placed to aid with resuscitation and assessment, such as intravenous cannulae, urinary catheter, arterial line and central line, a gastric catheter must be considered to reduce the risk of aspiration. If there is the possibility of a cribriform plate fracture (i.e. if there is clinical suspicion of a base of skull fracture; see earlier), this should be noted. If present, nasogastric passage of the catheter is strictly contraindicated, as the catheter may be inserted intracranially through the fracture. In this case, the gastric catheter should be inserted orally under direct vision using a laryngoscope.

Secondary survey   After the primary survey and initial resuscitation, a more thorough examination is carried out as part of the secondary survey. Vital signs measured during the primary survey should be frequently rechecked, to ensure ongoing patient stability.

The GCS should be repeated frequently and documented, to be able to assess the patient's progress over time. Deterioration of the GCS is an indication for an urgent CT scan. Pupils should also be checked frequently for size and reactivity, as this may be the only sign of impending brain herniation, if the patient has been intubated, sedated and paralysed.

Vital signs should also be continuously assessed. Apart from hypotension indicating likely continued bleeding, vital signs can suggest possible intracranial pathology, as listed below:

- Hypertension can be associated with a raised ICP.
- Hypertension combined with bradycardia (*Cushing reflex*) is a late sign, caused by brainstem herniation and an indication for urgent intervention. However, it must be remembered that many patients take beta blockers and may artificially maintain a bradycardia.
- Hypotension in a trauma victim is most commonly caused by frank or occult bleeding, when it will be associated with a tachycardia and a cool pale skin. Spinal cord injury may cause hypotension by interrupting sympathetic outflow with resultant vascular dilatation. This is associated with warm pink skin (from vasodilatation) and bradycardia (owing to loss of cardiac sympathetic supply).

Continuing the secondary survey, the head should be examined for evidence of injury. The entire scalp should be examined for lacerations or foreign bodies. Foreign bodies suspected of penetrating the skull should be left *in situ*, to await removal in theatre. Lacerations should be cleaned, debrided, closed and dressed unless the patient is proceeding immediately to theatre. The head should be felt for any scalp haematomas or evidence of skull fractures.

It is important to assess the eyes completely. Pupillary size should be assessed and documented as discussed previously (Figure 22.21). Ocular movements should be assessed, as unilateral limitation of movement may be caused by ocular muscle entrapment from a blowout fracture of the orbital margin. Bilaterally absent eye movements may be due to a brainstem injury. Conjugate eye deviation is usually due to a unilateral destructive frontal lesion or a seizure focus in the contralateral frontal lobe. If possible, acuity and visual fields should also be tested and the results documented.

A complete neurological assessment needs to be carried out. In doing so, note should be made of any sedating or paralysing agents the patient may be receiving. If the patient is awake, speech and limb power can be assessed. In all patients, peripheral and brainstem reflexes can be assessed. Breathing, corneal, pupillary and gag reflexes are particularly useful in assessing brainstem function. Limb reflexes can be absent in *spinal shock*; flaccidity, absent reflexes, loss of sweating and priapism are indicative of spinal cord injury. Again, it is of extreme importance that the neurological findings are documented and the assessments regularly repeated. A change in status is a sign of deterioration requiring urgent further investigation and management.

When completing the secondary assessment, it should be remembered that, in a trauma patient, injuries can affect any part of the body, and so a secondary survey is a complete examination looking at the entire body for evidence of any further trauma. Full body exposure, visualisation of the entire dorsal surface and performance of a rectal examination are necessary.

MANAGEMENT

The management of a patient following a severe head injury depends on the patient's neurological state and the intracranial pathology resulting from the trauma. Following primary assessment and resuscitation, the following then generally applies:

- The patient undergoes a secondary survey and CT scanning.
- If the CT scan shows an intracranial haematoma with mass effect, then this should be evacuated immediately.
- If surgery is not indicated, or postoperatively, the management is as follows.

Intensive care

The patient is admitted to an *intensive care unit* for ventilation, monitoring and neurological observation using a chart with the GCS (Figure 22.24 and Box 22.4). In these patients, an *intracranial pressure*

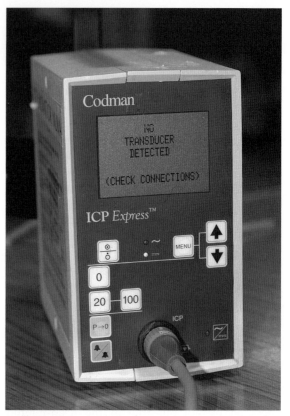

Figure 22.25 A Codman Microsensor® intracranial pressure monitor and the transducer.

monitor (such as a Camino® or Codman® transducer) (Figure 22.25) should be inserted to assess the intracranial pressure as accurately as possible. Usually, the transducers are placed intraparenchymally via a twistdrill craniostomy. A simple catheter placed into the ventricle will give both an accurate reading of the intracranial pressure and allow CSF to be drained to help control the ICP. However, the disadvantages of an intraventricular catheter include difficulty with placement, if the ventricles are small, possible injury to the brain during placement and infection resulting in meningitis following prolonged monitoring.

An intracranial pressure monitor will also be useful in patients requiring prolonged sedation and ventilation as a result of other injuries, particularly if they have to be taken to theatre, making repeat CT scanning impossible. Measurement of the ICP provides an essential monitoring parameter to optimise CPP. Any sustained rise in

ICP will be an indication for careful reassessment and, if necessary, repeat CT scanning. Following the insertion of the ICP monitor, the patient must be transferred to the intensive care unit.

Brain swelling and control of ICP

Measures to diminish brain swelling and control ICP are instituted as follows:

Management of the airway
There must be careful management of the airway to ensure adequate oxygenation and ventilation. Hypercapnia will cause cerebral vasodilation, increase CBF and so exacerbate brain swelling.

Elevation of the bed
The head of the bed should be elevated 20–30°, ensuring that the neck is in a neutral position with no constrictive taping. Clearance of both the cervical and lower spine should be undertaken early to facilitate this. If this is not performed early, preferably in the emergency room, a window of opportunity can often be missed before brain swelling and ICP become exacerbated, preventing the patient from being moved at all.

Fluid and electrolyte balance
Fluid restriction is no longer practised. Maintenance isotonic fluid requirements, avoiding dextrose solutions and following resuscitation, should be administered until the patient is able to commence nasogastric feeding. With ischaemia and brain injury, plasma glucose is metabolised to lactic acid, thereby lowering tissue pH and causing acidosis. An elevated serum glucose may thus aggravate ischaemic insult in head-injured patients. Likewise, hypotonic solutions should be avoided because these solutions will lower the plasma osmolality and drive water across the blood–brain barrier into the swollen brain, increasing ICP. Blood loss from other injuries should be replaced with colloid or blood, and not with crystalloid solutions. Care should be taken to avoid overhydration or over-resuscitation, as this will increase cerebral oedema.

Following general injury there is *retention of salt and water*, and excretion of potassium. The reten-

tion of water is usually greater than the retention of sodium, resulting in mild hyponatraemia. Following a severe head injury, fluid and electrolyte abnormalities may occur for a variety of reasons. Severe hyponatraemia (sodium of less than 130 mmol/l) may be due to excessive fluid intake or, occasionally, because of *syndrome of inappropriate antidiuretic hormone secretion* (SIADH) or *cerebral salt wasting*. The urine is usually hypertonic with a high sodium level, probably as a result of suppression of aldosterone secretion occurring as a response to overhydration and expansion of the circulating volume. Serum sodium of less than 125 mmol/l may produce neurological impairment with depression of conscious state. If due to SIADH, the usual treatment is to restrict the fluid intake to 800 ml per day or less. In the case of cerebral salt wasting, the patient is both volume and salt depleted, and requires an opposite management, emphasising the importance of the correct diagnosis.

Hypernatraemia is usually associated with hyperosmolality and often results from inadequate fluid intake. Other causes are *diabetes insipidus*, as a result of hypothalamic injury or pituitary stalk traction owing to raised ICP and excessive use of osmotic agents for control of intracranial pressure. Excessive administration of some feeding mixtures may lead to electrolyte abnormalities, particularly when complicated by diarrhoea.

Temperature control

Pyrexia may be due to *hypothalamic damage* or traumatic subarachnoid haemorrhage. However, infection as a cause of the fever must be excluded. The most common sites of infection after a head injury are the respiratory and urinary tracts, particularly if a urinary catheter has been inserted. If the injury is compound, and especially if there has been a CSF leak, intracranial infection should be suspected. The temperature can usually be controlled using tepid sponges, and rectal paracetamol or aspirin. Chlorpromazine, to abolish the shivering response, should be administered, if a cooling blanket is required. Every attempt should be made to control the temperature because hyperthermia can elevate the ICP, will increase the cerebral metabolic rate of oxygen consumption

(CMRO$_2$) and body metabolism, and will predispose to seizure activity. Each degree Celsius above 37°C increases CMRO$_2$ and maintenance fluid requirements by 10%. Although hypothermia down to 35°C has been advocated in the management of a severe head injury, no clear benefit has yet been demonstrated in the literature. Hypothermia in the management of severe head trauma is currently still under investigation

Nutrition

Proper nutritional support should be commenced as soon as possible as 'feeding the gut' has been shown to improve outcome and prevent complications. Care must be taken to ensure that the patient does not chronically aspirate past the endotracheal tube cuff. Feeding is best done by intragastric administration – usually by a *nasogastric* or ideally a nasojejunal tube – unless this is precluded by other injuries. The nasogastric feeding should supply 2500–3000 calories per day with a calorie:nitrogen ratio of 180:1. The feeding should commence slowly, with dilute mixtures, and the stomach should be *aspirated regularly* to assess absorption, and prevent regurgitation and pulmonary aspiration. If feeding cannot be commenced within 3–4 days, then intravenous hyperalimentation should be commenced.

Gut protection

Head injury increases the risk of gastric irritation, ulceration and haemorrhage – *Cushing's ulcer*. H$_2$ receptor antagonists such as ranitidine (Zantac®, 150 mg bd po or 50 mg tds iv), proton pump inhibitors such as omeprazole (Losec® 40 mg po or iv daily) or gastric coating agents such as Sucralfate®, should be administered appropriately – intravenously or via a nasogatric tube. Cimetidine (Tagamet®) in combination with phenytoin should be avoided.

Nursing

Nursing care of the unconscious patient including bowel, bladder, airway toiletry and pressure care should be undertaken. A silastic urinary catheter should be inserted under aseptic conditions and the urinary cell count regularly checked. Bowel movements should be monitored, stool softeners given and patients should be turned and suctioned regularly, ensuring that they are adequately sedated and paralysed before any external manipulations. Pressure sores or chest infections can be a cause of serious morbidity and mortality in head-injured patients. Once the patient is no longer in danger of haemorrhagic extension of intracerebral haematomas or contusions, or increasing ICP, prophylactic subcutaneous heparin should be administered to diminish the incidence of deep vein thrombosis and pulmonary emboli.

More aggressive methods to control intracranial pressure are advisable if:

- the patient's neurological state continues to deteriorate and the CT scan shows evidence of cerebral swelling without an intracranial haematoma
- there is a posturing (decerebrate) response to stimuli
- the Glasgow Coma Score is less than 8
- ICP monitoring shows a sustained ICP of greater than 20–25 mmHg.

Controlled ventilation, maintaining PaCO$_2$ at 30–35 mmHg (4–4.5 kPa) will reduce cerebral vasodilatation and consequently decrease the intracranial pressure.

Sedation, analgesics and neuromuscular blockade

Sedation
This should be maintained to prevent raised intracranial pressure related to agitation, posturing, reaction to manipulations such as turning and suctioning, and struggling against the mechanical ventilator. If sedation is going to be long term, then *midazolam* is used, as it is inexpensive, effective and does not influence ICP or CBF. If short-term ventilation is required or if the intention is to waken a patient, then sedation should be maintained with *propofol* (Diprivan®). This has the advantage of being very short acting and, furthermore, decreases ICP, CMRO$_2$, CBF and CPP, and prevents seizures. It is, however, considerably more expensive and induces hypotension in high doses.

Analgesia

Analgesia should be administered in addition to sedatives, as pain leads to increased agitation and raised ICP. Parenteral narcotics such as *morphine* or *fentanyl*, intramuscular codeine compounds (*codeine phosphate* or *dihydrocodeine*). and oral, nasogastric or rectal *paracetamol* can be used.

Neuromuscular blockade

This must always be used in combination with sedation. It helps prevent reactions to suctioning and can assist in enabling easier ventilation, helping control raised ICP. Drugs used include *atracurium, pancuronium* and *vecuronium*.

If the pressure remains elevated despite hyperventilation, CSF can be drained from a *ventriculostomy* catheter, if this has been inserted. The pressure at which the drain opens can be set by adjusting the height of the burette relative to the head. The aim is to keep the intracranial pressure below 20 mmHg. Care must be taken at all times to avoid potential bacterial contamination of the ventriculostomy causing meningitis. Where possible, the drain should be left as a closed system after catheter placement.

Cerebral perfusion pressure is a vital physiological parameter in the management of severely head-injured patients. The cerebral perfusion pressure (i.e. mean arterial blood pressure minus the ICP) should be maintained above 70 mmHg. Consequently, head injury management involves ensuring that the arterial blood pressure and optimal CPP is maintained whilst the intracranial pressure is reduced. This often involves close cooperation between the neurosurgeon and the intensive care physician, and may require the use of ionotropic agents.

For *diuretic therapy*, intermittent administration of mannitol or furosemide (frusemide) (20–40 mg tds) can be used, if the preceding techniques have failed to control the intracranial pressure. *Mannitol* is an osmotic diuretic and may also exert its effect by increasing serum osmolality and drawing water out of the brain. The usual dose is 0.5–1.0 g/kg. Mannitol must be used in caution in patients with large areas of blood–brain barrier breakdown, such as contusions. While mannitol reduces normal surrounding brain volume, it can leach out into the area of contusion, increasing the mass effect. This can decrease ICP overall but simultaneously increase midline shift causing more brainstem compression. Administration of mannitol should thus be performed in consultation with the attending neurosurgeon. The serum osmolality should not be allowed to exceed 320 mosmol/kg. A recent trend is to administer hypertonic saline solution (3.0%). This acts in a similar capacity, altering osmotic gradients and driving the serum sodium towards the upper limit of normal decreasing brain water and hence ICP. It also temporarily increases cardiac output and systolic blood pressure.

Barbiturate therapy can also be considered, if the intracranial pressure is resistant to treatment with the above techniques. Given as a bolus *thiopentone* (Pentothal® 3–5 mg/kg) provides brain protection by reducing $CMRO_2$ and, therefore, ICP. EEG monitoring is necessary to titrate the required maintenance dose to control *burst suppression*. The disadvantages of barbiturate therapy are hypotension, paradoxical ('pseudo') hypokalaemia and its extremely prolonged effect on consciousness owing to its fat absorption.

Although *steroids* dramatically reduce the vasogenic oedema around cerebral tumours, they have little effect in controlling brain swelling, predominantly due to loss of autoregulation and cytotoxic oedema, following a head injury. Numerous complications, *inter alia*, gastrointestinal bleeding, poor wound healing and infection, may result from their administration. A study re-evaluating the role of steroids in severe head and spinal trauma is currently underway.

In some centers, *hypothermia* (to reduce $CMRO_2$ and ICP) has been advocated – cooling patients down to 34°C. However, there is not yet any clear evidence that it is beneficial, and it may result in increased infection and postoperative haematomas owing to coagulopathy. Trials reassessing the role of hypothermia in severe head injury and subarachnoid haemorrhage are also currently under way.

Hyperbaric oxygen has been used in the past, but without any proven benefit.

Decompressive craniotomies should be considered *early*, if cerebral swelling and problems controlling ICP are anticipated. A large hemicraniotomy or bifrontal craniotomy together with temporal region decompression should be performed inserting artificial gusset grafts in the dura, if the brain is already swollen.

Post-traumatic *seizures* are classified according to their relationship to the time of injury:

- immediate – within 24 hours of trauma
- early – 24 hours to 7 days
- late – more than one week after the injury.

Immediate or early seizures are usually reactions to the injury and do not usually herald post-traumatic epilepsy as such. Seizures greatly increase $CMRO_2$ and hence ICP and, therefore, all efforts should be made to prevent them during the critical period of brain swelling. Meta-analysis of studies has, however, indicated that prophylactic anticonvulsants may only have a role in preventing seizures in the first 2 weeks after the injury. Beyond this period, they do not influence the incidence of post-traumatic epilepsy. If a patient actually develops epilepsy, then there is a clear role for instituting anticonvulsant therapy. Seizure prophylaxis or treatment is usually undertaken using phenytoin (loading dose 17 mg/kg, then maintenance at 4 mg/kg and by monitoring levels). It can be administered via a nasogastric tube or slow intravenous infusion. Care should be taken, as it is intensely thrombophlebitic, and may induce cardiac arrhythmias and hypotension.

Patients fully sedated, paralysed and analgesed may develop subclinical seizures or even status epilepticus without any motor activity. This may present as idiopathic periods of increased ICP or prevent a patient from 'waking up' or surfacing from sedation as well as anticipated. EEG monitoring needs to be performed to exclude this possibility.

There is some controversy concerning the effectiveness of the more aggressive techniques to treat patients with severe head injuries. If a patient has suffered a profound brain injury and the neurological examination shows little or no remaining brainstem function, when on little or no sedation or paralysis, then it is obvious that the aggressive techniques will provide no benefit and only delay the inevitable. Similarly, there are some patients who have suffered a severe head injury and whose intracranial pressure continues to rise despite all the above strategies. Other patients can have a fatal brain injury without any substantial rise in ICP, usually when the brainstem has been the primary site of injury. However, about 30% of patients who have suffered a severe brain injury will obtain substantial benefit from control of the ICP.

No clinical studies have, as yet, conclusively proven a benefit to ICP monitoring (ICPM) in reducing morbidity and mortality following a brain injury. It is thought that the reason for this is that patients in early studies may have been overventilated, as was the trend at the time, and their CBF was compromised as a result, causing ischaemia. There is consensus nowadays that using ICPM to control raised ICP will not only decrease mortality in severe head injury but will improve the quality of the patient's outcome. Therefore, it is, unlikely that, ethically, any future randomised trials investigating ICPM would ever be sanctioned.

Other monitoring techniques

Jugular venous oxygen saturation

The aim of treatment for a severe head injury is to maintain a continuous and adequate oxygen supply to the brain in order to meet metabolic demands. In order to monitor the oxygen extraction by the brain, the oxygen saturation of the arterial and the jugular venous blood uncontaminated by extracranial sources, is measured. This requires the retrograde placement of a catheter into the jugular venous bulb via the internal jugular vein and measurement of the arterial–jugular oxygen difference, allowing early identification of cerebral ischaemia or hyperaemia. Oxygen utilisation by the brain is determined in three ways: calculating cerebral oxygen extraction, calculating arteriovenous oxygen difference, or by monitoring jugular venous oxygen saturation ($SjvO_2$). Normal $SjvO_2$ levels are approximately 60–80%. The limitation of this modality is that it gives a global and not a more focal assessment of intracranial pathophysiology.

Transcranial Doppler

This is a non-invasive technique for assessing blood flow – usually of the middle cerebral artery.

It determines flow velocities and provides a pulse index enabling one to anticipate the development of cerebral vasospasm, facilitating proactive management. Its drawback is that it does not easily discriminate between the development of changes such as vasospasm and haemodynamic changes owing to alterations in the cardiac output.

Electroencephalogram

An electroencephalogram can, in some instances, recognise distinctive electrical characteristics of coma due to certain aetiologies (e.g. subacute sclerosing panencephalitis). To a limited extent, it can also prognosticate for outcome in coma. Its main role in head trauma is for excluding subclinical status as a cause of decreased consciousness and for monitoring burst suppression therapy in barbiturate coma.

Near-infrared spectroscopy and microdialysis

New monitoring modalities have been introduced, such as transcranial near-infrared spectroscopy (NIRS) and intracerebral microdialysis. NIRS measures the changes in the concentration of oxygenated and deoxygenated hemoglobin in the tissue by the amount of infrared light absorbed. This is a new technique to provide non-invasive monitoring for tissue oxygenation and hemodynamics of the brain. Especially it reflects the temporal change of cerebral blood volume (CBV).

Microdialysis is a technique to monitor the chemistry of the extracellular space in living tissue. Microdialysis gives a 'preview' of what goes on in the tissue – before any chemical events are reflected in changes of systemic blood levels. When a physiological salt solution is slowly pumped through the microdialysis probe, the solution equilibrates with the surrounding extracellular tissue fluid. After a while, it will then contain a representative proportion of the tissue fluid's molecules. Instead of inserting an 'analysis instrument' into the tissue (e.g. a biosensor), microdialysate is extracted and later analysed in the laboratory or by the bedside (for clinical microdialysis).

These modalities are, as yet, of limited clinical value and their potential role is still under investigation. Up to this date, they have been used mainly in research for brain pathophysiology.

Multimodality monitors

New multimodality intracranial monitors have been introduced allowing simultaneous measurement of brain O_2, CO_2, pH, temperature and ICP monitoring (e.g. Neurotrend®).

Associated pathology of head injury

Victims of severe head injury are prone to developing dysfunction of any organ system. This may be because of associated damage to other organ systems suffered during the initial trauma, or it may be as a result of prolonged immobility and invasive procedures required in the management of a comatose patient. It is, therefore, important in the management of such a patient that consideration is paid to identifying risk areas, in order to treat or prevent associated pathology.

Respiratory system

The comatose intubated patient is at high risk of developing respiratory complications related to ventilation, immobility, airway protection and trauma. It is vital that care is taken to maintain respiratory function, as it is the lung's ventilation and gas exchange that maintains blood oxygenation – a significant factor in determining prognostic outcome and preventing hypercapnia that contributes significantly to raised ICP.

The trauma patient may have sustained chest trauma and suffered pulmonary contusion, pneumothorax, haemothorax, flail ribs or diaphragmatic rupture. Whilst these may have been diagnosed in the initial assessment, there is the potential for problems to progress (e.g. contusions can extend and pneumothoraces can enlarge). Therefore, the trauma patient needs regular clinical assessment and repeated chest x-ray examinations when pathology is suspected, while oxygen saturation and ventilation indices are being continuously monitored.

Those patients who are ventilated face several challenges. Vigilance needs to be taken with equipment; endotracheal tube position, cuff inflation pressures and ventilator settings need to be regularly checked. Ventilators use positive-pressure ventilation, so there is always risk of causing or exacerbating an existing pneumothorax. The ventilated patient has an absent cough reflex, so tracheal suctioning is required, remembering to limit time off the ventilator to prevent a rise in ICP owing to elevated CO_2 and to increase sedation beforehand to prevent gagging.

An immobile patient is at an increased risk of developing atelectasis (a condition of basal lung collapse associated with hypoventilation). Steps to prevent atelectasis include turning the patient, chest physiotherapy, encouraging deep breathing, where possible, and positive pressure end-expiratory ventilation. These strategies have to be balanced against the slight increase in ICP that they cause. The immobile patient with multiple 'lines' is also at increased risk of developing pneumonia. Aspiration can occur at the time of the insult, which frequently happens when patients have a full stomach and are also intoxicated, or subsequently in hospital. The organisms responsible are often anaerobic. Hospital-acquired pneumonia is a concern, as the ventilated patient has compromised defences against lung infection. This may be due to the endotracheal tube and also due to immunosuppression associated with severe illness. Prevention includes those steps employed to prevent atelectasis and aspiration, and maintaining an aseptic environment. Again, regular examination, monitoring and investigation are required to identify the onset of pulmonary complications.

Cardiovascular system

The cardiovascular system is obviously at risk in the trauma patient. Volume loss from bleeding needs fluid replacement as described previously. The heart may be compromised by contusion from direct trauma. This may cause cardiac arrhythmias and evidence of cardiac damage with ECG changes and elevated cardiac enzymes. Manipulation of cardiac function to optimise CPP can impact on the heart. Adrenergic drugs given to increase mean arterial pressure can increase cardiac afterload, which increases the heart's oxygen consumption, placing it at risk of ischaemic damage. Confusingly, brain injury can be associated with primary pulmonary oedema (so-called *neurogenic oedema*) and ST segment changes on the ECG. Again the importance of regular examination (vital signs and chest examination), monitoring and investigation as required (chest x-ray, cardiac enzymes, ECG) should be stressed.

Fluid derangements should be considered as part of the cardiovascular assessment. As previously discussed, the aim is to maintain normovolaemia. Electrolytes should be maintained within normal limits. It is especially important to avoid hyponatraemia as this will increase cerebral oedema and thus ICP. Hyponatraemia may be secondary to SIADH. This can occur secondary to head injury, and results in water retention and thus hyponatraemia. The reverse, diabetes insipidus, can also occur where damage to the pituitary axis causes failure of antidiuretic hormone production, loss of fluid through production of dilute urine, and thus hypernatraemia and dehydration.

The haematological system should also be considered. Aggressive *cooling* as a means of controlling ICP is now used less commonly than previously, so coagulopathy associated with hypothermia is uncommon. However, as in all patients with systemic derangements, clotting abnormalities can still develop. This can include coagulopathy associated with large blood transfusions or *disseminated intravascular coagulation* (DIC). This is a condition in which there is widespread activation of the coagulation cascades throughout the blood vessels, with subsequent thrombosis of blood vessels and a paradoxical *coagulopathy* caused by consumption of available clotting factors and platelets. It can be caused by systemic disturbances, including sepsis. DIC can rapidly cause multiorgan failure and death. Treatment involves replacing deficient factors and treating any underlying systemic pathology, while supporting other organ systems. Management of the haematological system involves examination (looking for excessive bruising, blood in the tracheal aspirates or haematuria) and regular checks of clotting. More specific tests for DIC include evaluating D-dimers and fibrin degradation products.

Skin

Skin care is important, as with all bedridden patients. This includes regular turning and inspection of pressure areas to prevent development of pressure sores. Special care must be taken when patients are required to wear cervical collars. These frequently cause occipital pressure sores, increasing the risk of infection if cranial surgery is to be contemplated.

The head-injured patient, because of factors unique to head trauma, and because of associated body trauma, is vulnerable to dysfunction of any organ system and a management approach must address all areas, with an emphasis on regular examination and investigation of the patient.

REHABILITATION

Those patients who survive an acute admission for a severe head injury are likely to suffer some degree of brain dysfunction following discharge from hospital that affects their level of functioning. Some patients will not be capable of returning to independent living. These patients need the early involvement of a coordinated *multidisciplinary team*, to assess their physical and cognitive functioning, and to plan support and rehabilitation to maximise function.

It can be useful to predict, as early as possible in an admission, the likely prognosis and level of functioning. This can be measured with tools such as the *Glasgow Outcome Scale* (Box 22.5). Age (younger people do better), GCS and CT features have all been shown to be predictive of outcome. In a meta-analysis of available papers, the *Brain Trauma Foundation* determined that those patients grouped into the lowest GCS category (i.e. severe head injury) had an 80% mortality rate, and only 8–10% had an eventual Glasgow Outcome Score of 4 or above. It was commented that GCS was only useful when accurately assessed and when performed in the absence of sedating drugs. The ultimate outcome of any severe head injury can really only be determined after approximately 18 months have elapsed. Likewise, the sequelae of any brain injury need not only be acute but delayed (Box 22.6).

THE FUTURE

Our improved understanding of the pathophysiology of head injury, particularly at a neurochemical level, has led to the possibility of developing neuroprotective agents. Although most are still being trialled, they should become available for use in the near future. Free radical scavengers, antioxidants and *N*-methyl-D-aspartate (NMDA) receptor antagonists to block the effects of

Box 22.5	Glasgow Outcome Scale
5	Good outcome, no neurological deficit, independent and working
4	Moderate disability, independent but cannot return to work
3	Severe disability, dependent on others for activities of daily living
2	Persistent vegetative state
1	Dead

Box 22.6 Delayed effects of head injury

- Post-traumatic epilepsy
- Cerebrospinal fluid fistula
- Postconcussional symptoms
- Cumulative brain damage ('punch drunk syndrome')
- Neurological deficits

glutamate are all on the horizon. Another line of research is looking at cytokines responsible for cerebral oedema, namely interleukins 1, 6 and 8, and tumour necrosis factor, with the possibility of developing pharmacological interventions. The other major trend is the increasing use of routine ICP monitoring, early decompressive craniotomies, the use of MRI and CT scanning in diagnosis and prognosticating for head injury, and the adoption of evidence-based practice. Despite all these advances, the role of the neurosurgical nurse remains central to patient outcome.

SUMMARY

In managing head-injured patients, it is important to understand that the brain cannot be managed in isolation. A good outcome depends on normal functioning of all body systems to maintain vital parameters at an optimum level to prevent secondary injuries. From the initial assessment and resuscitation, the emphasis is primarily on ensuring respiratory and cardiovascular function, so that brain oxygenation and perfusion can be maintained. Only once this has been achieved can more specific management be directed at brain parameters, such as ICP and CPP. Ongoing care must also encompass all systems, as the nature of the head-injured patient means that they are more vulnerable to compromise. It should be stressed that this ongoing care needs regular monitoring, examination and investigation, so that any deterioration can be identified and treated appropriately.

The psychological and socioeconomic sequelae of a severe head injury are devastating for both the family and society. While the medical management of severe head injury has undergone considerable improvement, ongoing preventative measures to avoid or minimise head trauma should not be neglected.

Further reading

Hickey JV. *Neurological and neurosurgical nursing*, 4th edn. Philadelphia: Lippincott, 1997

Jennet WB, Teasdale G. *Management of head injuries*. Philadelphia: Davis, 1981

Kaye AH. *Essential neurosurgery*, 3rd edn, New York: Churchill Livingstone, 2004

Lindsey KW, Bone I. *Neurology and neurosurgery illustrated*, 3rd edn. New York: Churchill Livingstone, 1997

Chapter **23**

Cardiothoracic trauma

Tessa Sharpe and Richard S. Steyn

INTRODUCTION

Injuries to the chest wall and its underlying structures are sustained largely by road traffic accidents, falls from heights, falls on to objects or by direct compression of the chest. In the UK, the majority of trauma to the chest is blunt, although the incidence of penetrating injuries from stab wounds and gunshot wounds, while still uncommon, is increasing. Outcome measures reveal thoracic trauma as causing one in four trauma deaths and contributing to another 25% (Driscoll et al., 1993). Central to the management of such patients are the prevention of hypoxia, the provision of adequate pain relief and ventilatory support. This group of patients represents a particularly rewarding challenge to trauma nurses using a team approach to care with many improvements in the patient's condition rapidly following interventions. The majority of injuries are treated by intercostal chest drainage, while emergency thoracotomy is indicated for less than 10% of patients. Knowledge of the types of injuries sustained and the associated mechanism of injury play a vital role in their assessment and treatment.

This chapter will focus on enabling trauma nurses to apply their knowledge of anatomy and physiology to the possible underlying injuries in patients who have sustained chest trauma, and to apply their knowledge of blunt and penetrating trauma and the mechanisms of injury involved to their care of such patients. The use of a structured multidisciplinary approach to patient assessment and clinical examination, as outlined in the primary and secondary survey, will be advocated, and the signs, symptoms and types of injuries that warrant immediate treatment addressed. The importance of patient education and the provision of support will be emphasised as an ongoing part of patient care, and the relevance of radiology and scanning in confirming a diagnosis in the patient who has sustained chest trauma made apparent.

> Injuries to the thorax are responsible for 25% of all trauma deaths and contribute to a further 25%

ANATOMY AND PHYSIOLOGY

The chest can be divided into two parts: the thoracic cage, which involves bones and supporting muscles, and the thoracic cavity, which refers to the underlying organs and structures.

The thoracic cage is a bony framework that is supported by muscles and cartilage. It consists of 12 pairs of ribs, which are attached to the 12 thoracic vertebrae posteriorly, and to the sternum and costal cartilage anteriorly. Ribs one to seven are attached to the sternum by their costal cartilages, while ribs eight to ten do not attach directly to the sternum but have their costal cartilage fused with the cartilage in the seventh rib. Commonly referred to as floating ribs, ribs 11–12 attach at the thoracic vertebra only and are shorter in length. The ribs are supported by the intercostal muscles, vital for respiration, which pass above and below each rib. Muscles of particular importance include the pectoralis major, a large muscle on the upper anterior part of the chest, and the pectoralis minor, a small muscle lying deep to the pectoralis major. The chest wall also comprises the latissimus dorsi, the main muscle on the side, and the trapezius at the back. A dome-shaped elastic sheet of muscle comprises the diaphragm, which separates the thoracic cavity from the abdominal cavity.

The thoracic cavity contains the trachea, right and left bronchi, left and right lungs, pulmonary arteries, pulmonary veins, pleura, pleural cavity and the diaphragm. In its middle is the mediastinum containing the heart, thoracic aorta, superior vena cava, inferior vena cava, oesophagus, trachea, many other blood vessels, nerves and lymph glands.

The lungs, which are separated by the mediastinum form a large part of the thoracic cavity and are surrounded by a serous membrane, the pleura. Each lung is divided into lobes with the right lung having three lobes (i.e. upper, middle and lower) and the left lung having two (i.e. upper and lower). Each lobe is comprised of alveoli and bronchioles which join with each other to form the larger bronchi surrounded by a framework of fibrous and interstitial tissue containing blood and lymphatic vessels. The pulmonary artery supplies the lungs with deoxygenated blood while the pulmonary vein circulates oxygenated blood away from them. The pleura consists of two layers: the visceral layer, which forms the outer covering of the lungs, and the parietal layer, which lines the interior of the chest wall (ribs) and the upper surface of the diaphragm. These two layers are moistened by a small amount of serous fluid, which acts as a lubricant so that the two surfaces can glide over each other without friction during respiration.

Positioned between the two lungs is the heart, two-thirds of which lies on the left hand side of the chest with the remaining third on the right. The heart is covered by a strong fibrous sac, the pericardium, which is made up of two layers, the outer parietal pericardium and the inner layer, the visceral pericardium. Pericardial fluid present between the two layers prevents friction during contraction of the heart.

GAS DIFFUSION

The normal process and function of the lungs is to replenish the oxygen in the blood, thereby delivering oxygen to the tissues and removing carbon dioxide from the blood. The mechanism of respiration has three phases: inspiration where air is taken into the lungs, expiration where air is expelled from the lungs, and a short pause in between. This process occurs approximately 15 times each minute. Respiration is controlled by the respiratory center situated in the medulla oblongata, which responds to nerve impulses and the chemical composition of the blood. Carbon dioxide is excreted from the blood via the lungs in response to chemotaxic receptor stimulation. The respiratory center is highly sensitive to the level of carbon dioxide (carbonic acid) in the blood. If the levels become excessively high, nerve impulses stimulate the diaphragm to increase respirations to rapidly excrete it, lowering the level in the blood to normal. If the levels become excessively low, respiratory stimulation is temporarily depressed until the carbon dioxide level in the blood has built back to its original level.

Ventilation of the lungs allows air to move freely in and out. The alveoli are richly supplied with blood vessels and exchange of gases takes place here by diffusion. This process enables oxygen to diffuse into the pulmonary capillaries and carbon dioxide out of the capillaries, and depends on an intact alveolar surface and a normal circulating blood volume. Oxygen utilisation is dependent on haemoglobin to transport oxygen to the tissues. In hypovolaemia this is reduced and, if pulmonary ventilation is also compromised, blood and haemoglobin in the pulmonary circulation cannot be saturated with oxygen. This results in blood leaving the lungs having a low oxygen saturation potentially resulting in reduced oxygen delivery to the tissues.

Impairment of gas exchange

Major impairment of gas exchange may result from diffuse interstitial and alveolar haemorrhage as seen after pulmonary contusion, a major factor in the morbidity and mortality associated with chest trauma. This progressive condition involves initial haemorrhage and oedema, which are followed by interstitial fluid accumulation and decreased alveolar membrane diffusion. These changes in turn produce relative hypoxaemia, increased pulmonary vascular resistance, decreased pulmonary vascular flow and reduced lung compliance. Other causes of pulmonary injury may also result in impaired ventilation and impaired gas exchange. Poor oxygen saturation can occur if, following injury, there are areas of the lung that receive a good blood supply but poor ventilation. This is termed *ventilation perfusion mismatch*. The poor ventilation may be due to bruising, contusion, haemorrhage or obstruction.

> Pulmonary contusion is a progressive condition that is a major factor in the morbidity and mortality associated with chest trauma

TYPES OF INJURY

Injuries to the chest can be classified into two types: penetrating and blunt.

Penetrating trauma

Penetrating injuries may be caused by objects entering and potentially crossing the chest wall. These may occur, for example, as a consequence of impalement, e.g. falling on to a spiked fence or, less commonly in the UK, by knives or bullets. When assessing the mechanism of injury, the energy and force of the object entering the chest provides vital information as to the possible underlying injuries. In gunshot wounds, the entry sites may be small and insignificant, while simultaneously causing catastrophic underlying damage. Exit wounds should also be actively sought. This will, however, only provide a guide to the direction of the projectile, as bullets can bounce off ribs and other structures and not follow a straight line.

> The mechanism of injury, energy and force of the object penetrating the chest may provide vital information regarding possible underlying injuries

Occasionally, patients will arrive in the resuscitation room with an impaled object still *in situ* in the chest. No attempt should be made to remove this, as the knife or object may be arresting haemorrhage from a vessel or underlying structure. Removal should be undertaken in the controlled environment of the operating theatre.

> Penetrating objects should only be removed in the operating theatre

Blunt trauma

Blunt trauma to the chest may cause injury by one or a combination of three mechanisms namely deceleration, direct impact and compression. Motor vehicles, motorbike accidents and falls from heights may cause deceleration-type injuries. The speed or velocity of the body coming to a stop causes a rapid deceleration, which in turn creates a shearing force and tears organs and blood vessels. Direct impact injuries are caused by blows or by objects striking the chest, such as car steering wheels. These can result in fractures to the ribs or sternum and may cause damage to underlying structures. Compression injuries are caused through a crushing mechanism. Blunt injuries are often a combination of all three types of injuries, particularly when the injuries are severe.

ASSESSMENT AND PRIMARY SURVEY

Nursing assessment of the patient who has sustained trauma to the chest requires a systematic team approach dealing with life-threatening conditions first, in accordance with advanced trauma life support guidance (American College of Surgeons, 1997).

> Nursing assessment of the patient who has sustained trauma to the chest requires a systematic team approach

Trauma to the chest wall is rarely isolated and more commonly occurs in patients who have sustained multiple trauma. Other potentially significant injuries to the chest that may compromise the airway and/or cause hypovolaemia should also be considered. Assessment should be based on the ABC approach focusing on the patient's airway, breathing and circulation, with the history of the incident providing valuable information about the mechanism of injury sustained. Information from paramedics and other pre-hospital providers can also yield valuable information regarding any treatment given and its associated response, which may serve as a guide to the severity of the injuries.

> Information from paramedics and other pre-hospital providers can yield valuable information

History

A history of the event must always be obtained from ambulance staff or other pre-hospital team members as well as the patient and his/her friends or relatives. This often provides vital information relating to the mechanism of the injuries sustained, and yields vital clues for diagnosis and the potential for further injuries. Documentation of these findings, in addition to all vital signs obtained at scene and en route to hospital, and any interventions carried out is an essential part of the trauma patient's care.

Airway

The initial assessment of the airway should focus on its patency, actual and potential risks of obstruction, and any interventions that are required. Foreign bodies or the tongue falling back in the unconscious patient may, for example, occlude the airway. For patients who have difficulty in maintaining their airway, a definitive airway will be required (i.e. intubation). All airway interventions should be undertaken whilst remembering cervical spine immobilisation. If the history, clinical picture and mechanism of injury suggest possible cervical injury, this consideration must be borne in mind until cervical injury is excluded. If the patient can speak, it can be assumed that their airway is intact. In such circumstances, supplementary oxygen should be administered via an oxygen mask with a non-rebreathing reservoir bag.

If the patient has vomited, it is possible that they may also have aspirated. Such patients may require physiotherapy and possibly bronchoscopy during later stages of their care. Measures to prevent further aspiration are key considerations in treatment. Patients must, therefore, be closely monitored as aspiration pneumonia can rapidly develop. Patients who are at particular risk of aspiration and airway obstruction due to injury are those with raised intracranial pressure, those who are intoxicated or who have consumed/abused substances, and those who require ventilatory support. This group of patients often require endotracheal intubation and mechanical ventilation.

A summary of airway interventions is provided in Box 23.1.

Breathing

The chest should be exposed and the rate, depth and adequacy of respirations assessed. Rapid respirations may be suggestive of significant underlying injury. Measurement of respiratory rate is a frequently missed observation that may provide vital clues to the extent of the underlying injury. Chest wall movements should be observed for equality and symmetry, noting any evidence of splinting and paradoxical movements, which may be indicative of a *flail chest*. Bruising to the chest wall should also be noted, including the presence of abrasions, seat belt markings or wounds. Whether wounds are penetrating or sucking must be determined at an early stage. The chest should also be examined for subcutaneous crepitus from surgical emphysema.

An open pneumothorax is an immediately life-threatening condition that must be dealt with instantly. In an open pneumothorax where the wound is large, air entering the chest takes the path of least resistance entering through the wound and rapidly collapsing the lung, allowing the mediastinum to move to the opposite side, which may partially collapse the other lung. This is termed a *tension pneumothorax* which requires immediate intervention. In the event that a tension pneumothorax is detected in an un-controlled environment (e.g. out of hospital) or where immediate access to an intercostal drain is not available, then a *needle thoracocentesis* may be required until such interventions are available.

An open pneumothorax is an immediately life threatening condition that must be dealt with instantly

Ongoing measurement of physiological observations is essential in these patients. These must include respiratory rate and depth, use of accessory muscles of respiration, adequacy of respiration and oxygen saturation. Caution should be exercised in the cold, hypovolaemic, shivering patients or those covered in dirt, as pulse oximetry readings may be misleading.

Circulation

All patients who have suffered chest trauma must be connected to a cardiac monitor immediately. Ongoing assessment of heart rate, rhythm, quality and regularity must be undertaken, and an observation of skin colour and temperature maintained. Cool pale extremities may be indicative of circulatory compromise. Capillary refill time should be assessed by pressing on the nailbed for 5 seconds and the pressure released; this will cause the nailbed to blanch. If the time taken for the circulation to return is longer than 2 seconds, this may also be indicative of circulatory compromise. Caution should be exercised with regard to the hostile or external environment where the patient may be cold or hypothermic, as this measurement can be misleading. Where blood pressure cannot be recorded normally, an estimation can be obtained by palpating pulses at key anatomical points. A palpable radial pulse is suggestive of a systolic blood pressure of at least 80 mmHg; if only a carotid pulse can be palpated, the blood pressure is estimated to be at least 60 mmHg; if a femoral pulse but not radial pulse can be palpated, the systolic blood pressure can be estimated at 70 mmHg. Blood pressure can be measured in the normal way, if time allows, and more emergent interventions are not required. The first blood pressure to be recorded manually should allow the presence of pulsus paradoxus to be assessed. This is a reduction of more than 10 mmHg in systolic pressure during inspiration indicating cardiac tamponade.

Two large-bore intravenous lines should be inserted into both antecubital fossae, and blood samples taken for measurements of haemoglobin, cross-match, urea and electrolytes, and glucose. Arterial blood samples should also be obtained for blood gas analysis. A delay of approximately 45 minutes in obtaining cross-matched blood is not uncommon while a delay of 10 minutes is typical for type-specific blood. If blood is required more urgently, O-negative blood, the universal donor, should be used. All fluids given should be warmed and care taken not to overload patients as this may result in secondary complications. The intention is to administer fluids in order to achieve and maintain a systolic blood pressure of 90 mmHg, an approach often referred to as permissive hypotension. Where underlying injury to the great vessels is suspected, this approach is particularly advocated to maintain blood pressure slightly lower than normal to prevent movement of blood clots or haematomas, which may have formed around injuries, hence minimising bleeding. Fluid management should thus take into account the patient's condition and other injuries sustained.

> Fluids are administered to achieve and maintain a systolic blood pressure of 90 mmHg

CLINICAL EXAMINATION

Using a team approach, clinical examination takes place alongside the nursing assessment. The tracheal position should be determined as part of the initial airway and breathing assessment, noting any deviation indicative of tension pneumothorax or injury to the trachea. Neck veins should similarly be assessed, noting whether they are 'flat' or distended; distended neck veins being suggestive of *cardiac tamponade*. Caution must be taken when interpreting this finding, owing to its potential for unreliability, as patients may have accompanying hypovolaemia with 'flat' neck veins. Compression or crush injury to the chest may also cause distension of neck veins as well as petechial haemorrhages to the upper chest, neck and face.

Inspection and observation of the chest will reveal any deformities, bruising, wounds, lacerations or other defects. *Palpation* of the chest will enable any crepitus, surgical emphysema or bony tenderness to be identified. *Percussion* of the chest

will reveal areas of dullness, indicative of possible underlying haemothorax or pulmonary contusion, or areas of hyper-resonance (drum-like sounds) indicative of possible tension pneumothorax. *Auscultation* of the chest will determine bilateral air entry or detect any underlying problems, such as reduced or absent air entry, and the presence of any crackles or wheezes, the latter suggestive of possible aspiration pneumonia or underlying disease processes, such as asthma. The heart sounds will be listened to, noting whether they are normal or muffled, an indication of cardiac compromise or tamponade. It must be remembered that, in a noisy environment, these signs can be difficult to ascertain.

Hyper-resonance and reduction or absence of breath sounds on the affected side are indicative of tension pneumothorax, a life-threatening condition that requires immediate intervention, namely needle decompression of the affected lung or lungs, followed by intercostal chest drain insertion (*tube thoracostomy*). If the chest is dull to percussion and breath sounds are diminished, this may be suggestive of a haemothorax or pulmonary contusion. Massive haemothorax is a life-threatening condition; however, tube thoracostomy should not take place until intravenous access has been established. Cardiac tamponade is more common in penetrating injuries and frequently not all the signs are present. If the patient is not compromised, it is safer to wait for further investigation and evaluation rather than intervening immediately; if compromised, urgent thoracotomy will be required. Needle decompression of the pericardium may be attempted, provided it does not cause delay, leaving the cannula and three-way tap *in situ* in the event that further aspiration is required. All patients who have a positive 'tap' (i.e. positive *pericardiocentesis*) will require urgent thoracotomy. Patients should also be log-rolled prior to transfer to theatre to check for the presence of injuries to the posterior chest wall.

During the primary survey, six life-threatening conditions may be detected that directly affect the chest: airway obstruction, tension pneumothorax, open pneumothorax, massive haemothorax, flail chest and cardiac tamponade (Box 23.2). The primary survey resuscitation of the trauma patient

Box 23.2   Life-threatening conditions that may directly affect the chest (primary survey)

A	Airway obstruction
T	Tension pneumothorax
O	Open pneumothorax
M	Massive haemothorax
F	Flail chest
C	Cardiac tamponade

Box 23.3   Life-threatening conditions that may directly affect the chest (secondary survey)

- Simple pneumothorax
- Haemothorax
- Pulmonary contusions
- Tracheobronchial tree injuries
- Blunt cardiac injury
- Traumatic aortic rupture
- Traumatic diaphragm rupture
- Mediastinal traversing wounds

is rapid, often with multiple procedures being performed simultaneously. Preparation for these enables the rapid response required to optimise the patient's chances of survival.

The more detailed secondary assessment takes place after the primary survey and life-saving interventions, with ongoing assessment of the airway, breathing and circulation. Patients must be fully undressed to enable a top to toe examination, assessing all injuries. Further tests, investigations and interventions can then be carried out. Eight life-threatening conditions that may directly affect the chest in the secondary survey have been identified: simple pneumothorax, haemothorax, pulmonary contusions, tracheobronchial tree injuries, blunt cardiac injury, traumatic aortic rupture, traumatic diaphragm rupture and mediastinal traversing wounds (Box 23.3).

All patients must have their cardiac rhythm, heart rate, blood pressure and oxygen saturation continuously monitored and documented at regular intervals, their frequency determined by the patient's condition. A record of all drugs given, fluid input, urinary output and all interventions must also be maintained.

Rib fractures

Rib fractures can range from very simple to more complex injuries, such as flail segment, which require more complex interventions and management. In all presentations, whatever the classification, the initial assessment should follow the same pattern.

Rib fractures can be classified as follows:

- simple rib fractures
- complex rib fractures

- first rib fractures
- rib fractures in children
- sternal fractures
- flail chest.

Simple rib fractures

The classical presentation of patients who have sustained rib fractures includes pain on inspiration and expiration, crepitus and bony tenderness. Dependent upon the mechanism of injury, bruising to the chest, seat belt markings and dyspnoea may also be present. Splinting of chest wall movements and reduced expansion of the lungs are often caused by pain. Respirations may be increased or decreased, with patients sometimes exhibiting acute pain and tenderness over the site of the injury, causing them to avoid moving the chest wall and resulting in shallow respirations.

The diagnosis of simple rib fractures relies upon an understanding of the mechanism of injury and follows the initial ABC assessment, excluding life-threatening conditions first followed by a more detailed secondary assessment. Diagnosis is often made on clinical examination alone, sometimes confirmed by chest x-ray; however, not all rib fractures can be identified on x-ray, particularly those that separate the sternum from the costal cartilage.

Simple rib fractures are the most common form of blunt trauma sustained to the chest and, in the majority of cases, require no therapeutic intervention other than effective pain relief and advice regarding breathing exercises to prevent secondary chest infection. Education is the most important issue in this group of patients; nurses have a key role in ensuring that patients are given verbal

Box 23.4   Chest injury instructions provided to patients by the Accident and Emergency Department, Addenbrooke's Hospital, Cambridge. (Reproduced with permission of BOE Publishing Ltd, Blackpool.)

You have either bruised or broken your ribs. If they are bruised the pain you feel when breathing, coughing or sneezing may last up to two to four weeks. If the ribs are broken (cracked, fractured) the pain may last for up to six to eight weeks. It may increase in severity for the first two weeks, then gradually subside over the following four weeks. A fractured sternum may be painful for up to two months. The pain is very uncomfortable and the painkillers may only be able to soothe it a little, but it is important to use them and follow the instructions below.

You must return to your nearest A&E immediately:
- If you develop sudden shortness of breath, as this may be due to a collapsed lung

You must see you GP the same day or, if unavailable, go to your nearest A&E department:
- If you develop a fever, cough, shortness of breath or change in your usual sputum, as this may be due to a chest infection.

To prevent problems such as chest infection it is important to:
- Take your painkillers regularly as prescribed by the doctor:

  ....
  ....

- If you are going to cough press your hand against the painful area to provide counter pressure, this makes it less painful and lets you clear your chest
- Every hour when awake carry out a breathing exercise, take a breath as deeply as possible, hold it, and then let the breath out as far as possible. Repeat this five times. It may cause a bout of coughing but will keep your lungs clear. If coughing occurs provide the counter pressure with your hand or a warm towel.
- If you are a smoker try to stop smoking. This will be helpful in the long term. However, initially it may result in you producing more and coughing up thicker sputum. Remember to take your painkillers regularly and support the painful area with your hand.

If you need further advice, please contact the nursing staff of the Accident and Emergency Department on ....

advice and written information (Box 23.4). Adequate analgesia and a supply of oral analgesic agents should be given prior to discharge.

Elderly patients characteristically have reduced vital capacity of their lungs as a consequence of the ageing process. This is also a common presentation of a number of chronic medical conditions, which are likely to have a significant impact on injuries sustained to the chest wall.

All patients with rib fractures worsen after the initial injury, as the pain and bruising of the chest wall and underlying lung contusion reduce both ventilation and compliance of the lungs. Even seemingly minor injuries, such as chest wall contusion with haemorrhage or fractured ribs, can lead to life-threatening complications (Maberry and Trunkey, 1997). The elderly and patients with poor pulmonary reserve are particularly at risk. Effective analgesia and breathing exercises profile

highly in patient education and treatment. In elderly patients with two or more fractured ribs, admission to hospital is recommended to ensure adequate physiotherapy and pain relief to prevent secondary complications. Follow-up in the community by the primary health care team is also strongly recommended for this group of patients.

Complex rib fractures

The clinical features most commonly associated with complex rib fractures include pain on inspiration and expiration, dyspnoea, crepitus, subcutaneous emphysema, bony tenderness and, dependent upon the mechanism of injury, bruising and seat belt markings. Respirations may be increased or decreased with splinting of chest wall movements. Assessment follows the ABC approach excluding life-threatening conditions first followed by a more detailed secondary assessment. Diagnosis can be made clinically or by chest x-ray. When assessing rib fractures, it is vital to give consideration to the underlying organs and structures that may be damaged as a consequence of the injury.

Rib fractures occur most commonly in the fourth to tenth ribs. All patients who sustain fractures to four or more ribs must be admitted for observation, pain relief and physiotherapy to assist in the movement of bronchial secretions and prevention of secondary chest infections. Fractures to the lower ribs are commonly associated with splenic or hepatic injury. It is, therefore, necessary to monitor vital signs regularly to detect any underlying compromise and, if indicated, to intervene surgically to repair any injuries sustained.

Fractures to the lower ribs are commonly associated with splenic or hepatic injury

First rib fractures

Of particular importance in assessing these patients is the degree of force involved. Clinical features of fractures to the first rib typically include pain on inspiration and expiration, dyspnoea, crepitus, subcutaneous emphysema, bony tenderness and bruising. As before, initial assessment and diagnosis follows the primary survey excluding life-threatening injuries followed by a more detailed secondary assessment. Diagnosis can be made on clinical examination and chest x-ray findings. The first and second ribs are protected by the clavicles and scapulae, and the surrounding muscles. Fractures to the first rib, therefore, require a great deal of force. This should give rise to a high index of suspicion for potential underlying injury to the lungs, great vessels, head, cervical spine and spinal cord, all of which carry a high mortality rate. Treatment consists of the provision of adequate pain relief, the prevention of hypoxia, respiratory support, and careful monitoring to detect and treat underlying injuries.

Rib fractures in children

As with fractures to the first rib, the key consideration in rib fractures in children is the massive force involved and the potential for significant underlying injury. Clinical features characteristically include pain on inspiration and expiration, dyspnoea, crepitus, subcutaneous emphysema, bony tenderness and bruising. As with adults life-threatening injuries are excluded and more detailed secondary assessment is performed. Diagnosis can be made on clinical examination and later confirmed by a chest x-ray or computed tomography scan.

Rib fractures in children are rare as the rib cage is extremely resilient and elastic. Significant underlying trauma may be experienced in the absence of fractures; indeed, pulmonary contusions are common findings. Where rib fractures are present, it must be assumed that considerable force has been exerted and associated injuries are common. Children most commonly sustain ruptures to the bronchus and diaphragm. Treatment consists of adequate analgesia, respiratory support, the prevention of hypoxia, close monitoring of vital signs and surgical repair of associated injuries where indicated. All patients should receive regular physiotherapy to assist in the movement of bronchial secretions and prevention of secondary chest infection.

Significant underlying trauma may be present in the absence of fractures

Sternal fractures

Key considerations when dealing with sternal fractures are the degree of pain experienced and associated underlying injuries, such as cardiac contusion and great vessel injury. The characteristic clinical presentation comprises sternal pain, dyspnoea and seat belt markings. Upon completion of the pulmonary survey and a detailed clinical examination, a lateral chest x-ray may confirm the diagnosis. The chest x-ray is also key to excluding a widened mediastinum, while an electrocardiograph will eliminate signs of cardiac contusion and form a baseline, should myocardial status deteriorate. Sternal fractures require a high degree of force to the chest wall and commonly occur with seat belt and steering wheel injuries, although the latter is less common owing to seat belt legislation in the UK. Such legislation has significantly increased the number of sternal fractures seen in this country. In the absence of evidence of cardiac contusion and a relatively stable fracture, patients may be discharged home with effective analgesia and advice regarding breathing techniques; otherwise they should be admitted for pain relief and monitoring of vital signs. Elderly patients should always be admitted for the above.

> Legislation has significantly increased the number of sternal fractures seen in UK

Flail chest

The patient with a flail chest often presents a challenge to the trauma team, the key considerations being adequate pain relief, the prevention of hypoxia and the provision of ventilatory support. Clinical features typically include pain, paradoxical movement of the chest wall, respiratory distress, hypoxia, splinting of chest wall movements, subcutaneous emphysema, bony tenderness, bruising and seat belt markings. Assessment of airway, breathing and circulation, excluding life-threatening injuries followed by a secondary survey is the bedrock of assessment. Diagnosis can be made on the basis of clinical examination and confirmed by chest x-ray.

A flail chest occurs when three or more ribs are fractured in two or more places, which results in a loose or flailing segment of the rib cage that moves independently from it. On inspiration, it moves inwards instead of outwards, and on expiration it moves outwards instead of inwards, a process referred to as *paradoxical breathing*. Paradoxical breathing impairs normal ventilation of the lung, while pain from the injury causes splinting. Considerable trauma will have been sustained to cause a flail chest, with certain underlying pulmonary contusions impairing ventilation further. Posterior flail segments are particularly difficult to diagnose as the muscles of the scapulae and back support the chest wall, reducing paradoxical movements. A flail chest/flail segment may become more obvious as the patient tires and when splinting becomes reduced.

Treatment is based on effective pain relief to support adequate breathing. Epidural analgesia may be required in addition to intravenous analgesia. Alternatively intercostal nerve blocks may be suitable for a small group of patients, their main disadvantages being their duration of action

of only 6 hours and the need for multiple injection sites. Patients must receive regular physiotherapy to assist in the movement of bronchial secretions and the prevention of secondary chest infection. Blood gas analysis must be undertaken on a regular basis to monitor respiratory status closely; this is particularly crucial should the patient tire, respiratory status deteriorate and mechanical ventilation be required. Surgical intervention to fix fractures is rare. It should be noted that all patients who sustain rib and sternal fractures may experience pain for up to 6 months after the injury.

Pneumothoraces

A *pneumothorax* can be defined as a collection of air in the pleural cavity and commonly occurs owing to a rupture within the lung or a fractured rib lacerating the pleura. This type of injury is classified as a closed injury as air (and often blood) enters the pleura from the lungs, while the chest wall remains intact. In the case of an open pneumothorax, air enters the pleural cavity from an open wound. Intrathoracic pressure is normally negative, which is the basis for the regulation of normal lung expansion; when air or blood enters the pleural cavity, this negative pressure diminishes, thereby causing collapse of the lung or lungs. This collapse can be rapid requiring immediate life-saving intervention. Initial assessment and treatment follow the same pattern outlined in the primary and secondary surveys.

Pneumothoraces can be classified as follows:

- pneumothorax
- open pneumothorax
- tension pneumothorax
- haemothorax
- massive haemothorax
- haemopneumothorax.

Pneumothorax

Of significance is the fact that a simple pneumothorax can develop into a life-threatening tension pneumothorax, if left untreated, or if the patient requires mechanical ventilation. As the pneumothorax develops, clinical features include an increased respiratory rate, diminished or absent breath sounds, hyper-resonance of the chest, and pain on expiration and inspiration. Diagnosis can be made following clinical examination and an erect chest x-ray, assuming clearance of the cervical spine. A pneumothorax is most commonly caused by laceration of the lung or fractures, although some invasive procedures can also be causative, for example, insertion of central venous lines.

Treatment consists of tube thoracostomy attached to an underwater-seal drain followed by clinical examination of the chest and a chest x-ray to confirm tube placement and re-expansion of the lungs. It should be noted that, in circumstances where air leakage may be large, suction can be added to the underwater-seal drain to assist with lung re-expansion. Large air leakages may be indicative of bronchial rupture, highlighted by continuous bubbling of the underwater chest drain. Should a patient deteriorate after connection of suction, the suction should be disconnected and the patient reassessed, as suction may occasionally increase the air leak or block the drainage of air through the chest drain system.

Open pneumothorax

Wounds or defects to the chest wall, often described as 'sucking chest wounds', are highly suggestive of an open pneumothorax. Early clinical features include a rapid respiratory rate, altered conscious level, and agitation and combativeness due to hypoxia. The trachea may be deviated to the side opposite from the injury, neck veins may be raised, air entry may be diminished or absent, and the chest may be hyper-resonant. Tachycardia and hypotension may also be present.

An open pneumothorax develops as a chest wound communicates with the underlying pleural cavity. Where the wound is large, air enters it with each respiration as air follows the path of least resistance; it cannot, however, escape to the same extent, resulting in the potential for a tension pneumothorax to develop. To prevent further air entry from the defect, the wound should be covered with a sterile occlusive dressing taped on three sides to create a one-way valve effect. This prevents further air entry through the wound with each respiration and allows air to escape via the wound and the taped dressing. If the wound were covered completely, air would rapidly build up in the pleural cavity causing a tension pneumothorax. An Ashermann chest seal could, alternatively, be used. Definitive treatment in the form of a tube thoracostomy attached to an underwater-seal drain should be performed as soon as possible to relieve the pneumothorax. The chest should be clinically re-examined to evaluate the effectiveness of treatment, and a chest x-ray taken to confirm tube placement and re-expansion of the lung. Wounds may require surgical exploration and closure.

Tension pneumothorax

A tension pneumothorax develops when air enters the pleural cavity, rapidly causing a build up of air. This in turn causes the affected lung to collapse, pushing the mediastinum to the opposite side and causing compression of the vena cava; this reduces ventricular flow, causing a drop in blood pressure. The trachea then deviates away from the side of the injury, the jugular veins may distend and cyanosis may become apparent if the affected lung is not rapidly decompressed. Cardiac arrest may rapidly ensue. If the patient is ventilated, the positive pressure of mechanical ventilation will rapidly increase the pleural air volume and a simple pneumothorax may be converted to a tension pneumothorax. Bag-mask ventilation may then be difficult to achieve, with loss of lung compliance and increased airway pressures.

A tension pneumothorax presents a life-threatening situation and requires immediate intervention. Clinical features include tachypnoea, altered conscious level, agitation, combativeness due to hypoxia or patients may be rendered unconscious. Tracheal deviation away from the side of the injury is a late sign; distended neck veins may be present but are unreliable, as the patient may be hypovolaemic. Breath sounds are reduced or absent on the affected side, chest sounds are hyper-resonant to percussion, and tachycardia and hypotension may be present. This condition can be confused with a cardiac tamponade; in such situations, percussion of the chest helps to confirm the diagnosis. Diagnosis should be made on clinical examination alone; chest x-ray should never be used to confirm the diagnosis, as this delays treatment and may prove fatal.

Treatment consists of rapid decompression by *needle thoracocentesis* followed by chest drain insertion (tube thoracostomy) attaching the tube to underwater-seal drainage. The chest is reassessed by clinical examination while chest x-ray examination confirms tube placement and re-expansion of the lung.

Haemothorax

Key considerations in the management of patients who have suffered haemothoraces include blood loss and the prevention of a clotted haemothorax. Clinical features generally include tachypnoea, diminished breath sounds, dullness to percussion, and pain on expiration and inspiration. Diagnosis can be made on clinical examination and later confirmed by chest x-ray; once again, an erect chest film is preferred, assuming that the cervical spine has been cleared. Defined as a collection of blood in the pleural cavity, a haemothorax is commonly caused by rupture of the internal mammary or intercostal arteries, or occasionally by lung lacerations.

Treatment consists of intravenous access and fluid replacement followed by tube thoracostomy attached to an underwater-seal drain. Blood loss and vital signs should be measured frequently, with particular vigilance to detect continued blood loss; loss in excess of 200 ml/hour over the first 4 hours and any deterioration in the patient's vital signs all indicate a need for further clinical evaluation. All haemothoraces should be drained to prevent a clotted haemothorax, a problem that requires surgical intervention.

Massive haemothorax

Key considerations in the management of the patient with a massive haemothorax are the likely damage to underlying structures and potential hypovolaemia. Clinical features typically include a rapid respiratory rate, agitation, combativeness due to hypoxia and hypovolaemia, diminished or absent breath sounds, dullness of the chest to percussion and pallor, tachycardia and hypotension. Diagnosis can be made based on clinical examination and confirmation obtained on chest x-ray. An erect chest film is preferred, providing that the spine has first been cleared. A massive haemothorax results from a rapid accumulation

of blood in the thoracic cavity, usually in excess of 1500 ml of blood. Penetrating chest wounds or damage to major blood vessels are the most common causes.

Intravenous access and fluid replacement, preferably blood, should be established prior to drainage of the haemothorax by tube thoracostomy attached to an underwater-seal drain. Continued blood loss should be measured frequently in association with the patient's vital signs. Deterioration in the vital signs associated with continued blood loss is an indication for further investigation and probable surgical intervention.

Haemopneumothorax

A haemopneumothorax is a combination of blood and air in the pleural space. The clinical features, diagnosis and treatment are the same as for pneumothorax and haemothorax. Clinical procedures must be performed immediately and efficiently in order to optimise the chance of a successful outcome. Treatment consists of needle thoracocentesis followed by tube thoracostomy, fluid replacement and ongoing assessment to detect early signs of clinical deterioration.

Related clinical procedures

Needle thoracocentesis

This involves the placement of a large-gauge cannula (14 gauge minimum) in the second intercostal space in the mid-clavicular line. Communication should be maintained with conscious patients and their consent obtained, if possible. Key anatomical landmarks should be identified: the second intercostal space in the mid-clavicular line. After cleansing the area, the cannula should be inserted *over* the rib into the second intercostal space thereby puncturing the parietal pleura. The needle should be withdrawn and a hiss of air may be heard, indicating a release of pressure. The cannula should be left open *in situ* and secured with tape or an intravenous dressing. As this procedure is not definitive only partially expanding the lungs, and the aim is to expand the lungs fully, a tube thoracostomy must be performed as soon as possible. If no air is heard upon aspiration, it is possible that a simple pneumothorax may have been created. This will also require treatment by tube thoracostomy and re-examination of the chest to gauge the efficiency of the procedure.

Tube thoracostomy (intercostal chest drain insertion)

In preparation for this definitive treatment of many conditions identified earlier, intravenous access must be established, ideally at two sites using wide-bore cannulae. Communication should be maintained with conscious patients and their consent obtained, if possible. Key anatomical landmarks should be identified, namely the fifth or sixth intercostal space between the anterior and mid-axillary lines. After preparing the skin with antiseptic solution, local anaesthetic is administered, if required (approximately 20 ml lignocaine 1%) and time given to achieve its effect. A 3 cm horizontal incision is then made into the skin, the subcutaneous tissues bluntly dissected down to and *over* the top of the rib, the parietal pleural punctured with a clamp and a gloved finger inserted into the wound to identify any underlying organs and free any clots or adhesions. The thoracostomy tube is clamped at one end and advanced into the pleural space; the tube should mist up during the expiratory phase of respiration, often referred to as *'fogging'*. The tube is then connected to an underwater-seal drain and secured by suturing the tube in place and dressing the drain site.

The water level in the tubing inside the underwater seal drain should rise and fall with the patient's respirations; this is commonly referred to as *'swinging'*. Air will also bubble in the drain. A large air leak that bubbles continuously should be addressed immediately; this is suggestive of a possible ruptured bronchus and indicates the need for immediate clinical assessment and evaluation. The use of low-pressure suction may be required, if the air leakage is large. Chest drains should never be clamped, except when changing the bottle; the practice of clamping chest drains when moving patients is a dangerous one which should never be undertaken owing to its potential for creating a tension pneumothorax and causing further underlying lung damage. Drainage from the thoracostomy tube should be monitored

regularly and recorded in the patient's notes. Excessive blood loss must be reported immediately to determine the need for further clinical evaluation and possible intervention. Tube placement should be checked by clinical examination and confirmed by chest x-ray.

> Chest drains should never be clamped other than when changing the bottle

Pericardiocentesis

Pericardiocentesis is the term given to emergency decompression of the pericardial sac surrounding the heart, as is required in aspiration of a haemopericardium, which is causing cardiac tamponade. Communication should be maintained with conscious patients and their consent obtained, if possible. Monitoring of vital signs and cardiac rhythm must be maintained before, during and after the procedure; continuous monitoring during the procedure is of particular importance to detect and treat any abnormalities that may arise as a consequence. Key anatomical landmarks should be identified, namely the xiphoid and subxiphoid areas of the chest. If the patient is conscious and if time allows, local anaesthetic (lignocaine 1%) may be administered in preparation for the procedure. The angle between the xiphisternum and the left costal margin should be located and the area cleansed. The needle, with 30 ml syringe attached, is advanced into the chest pointing upwards towards the tip of the left scapula at an angle of 45°. If the needle is advanced too far into the ventricular muscle, the cardiac rhythm will change, demonstrating extreme ST wave changes or a widened QRS complex; if this occurs, the needle should be withdrawn slightly until the electrocardiogram (ECG) returns to normal. As the needle tip enters the pericardial sac, non-clotted blood is aspirated; after aspiration is completed, the syringe is removed and a three-way tap attached to the catheter, which is then secured by an intravenous dressing or tape to allow for further aspiration, if required. If the patient continues to demonstrate ECG changes, the catheter must be withdrawn completely. If the needle has entered the heart, it will be felt to move with the pulsations; if the syringe is removed from the needle, blood will pulsate from this end. All patients who undergo this procedure should also undergo urgent thoracotomy.

Thoracotomy in the resuscitation room

Thoracotomy within the resuscitation room is indicated for a small group of patients only. Closed heart massage for pulseless electrical activity is not effective for hypovolaemic patients, where the hypovolaemia is due to cardiac tamponade. Patients with exsanguinating or penetrating injuries, who are pulseless but have evidence of electrical activity, may undergo emergency thoracotomy in the resuscitation room by a doctor qualified to do so. If no electrical activity is demonstrated, this procedure will be unsuccessful.

Cardiac contusions

Cardiac contusions can be subtle in presentation. Clinical features include chest pain similar to angina, ECG changes: such as sinus tachycardia, atrial fibrillation, atrial flutter, premature ventricular contractions, and changes suggestive of ischaemia. They may be considered as bruises to the heart and, like any bruise, have the potential to expand and develop. Diagnosis is based on a high index of suspicion, particularly if there are ECG changes, the heart is enlarged and the mechanism suggests injury to the chest. Signs can be subtle and not all cardiac contusions are readily apparent; a mild injury can have ECG changes but no evidence on echocardiogram, while an extensive injury can be demonstrated by a 12-lead ECG and echocardiogram. Cardiac enzymes should also be measured, although changes may take some time to develop.

Treatment involves monitoring the patient's cardiac rhythm for 24 hours and recording of serial 12-lead ECGs, treating symptoms conservatively as they arise. If the ECGs remain normal after 24 hours, the patient may be discharged. Should extensive injury have been demonstrated on the echocardiogram, for example, valvular rupture, this will need to be treated appropriately.

Cardiac rupture

Cardiac rupture is a life-threatening event that may present with the following clinical features: chest pain similar to angina, bruising to the chest wall, severe unexplained shock, distended neck veins and muffled heart sounds. It occurs most commonly following penetrating injury to the heart and can involve any part of its structure. It is less commonly encountered with blunt injuries. Most patients with cardiac rupture die on scene; when alive at presentation, they are indistinguishable from those with cardiac tamponade. The diagnosis of cardiac rupture can be made by the presence of unexplained shock, changes in cardiac rhythm, muffled heart sounds. The presence of penetrating wounds that yield a high index of suspicion, a widened mediastinum and an enlarged heart on chest x-ray. Distended neck veins may be present but are not always a reliable sign, as patients may have accompanying hypovolaemia. An echocardiogram may identify the injury and can be undertaken at the patient's bedside.

Treatment may consist of urgent intervention, such as aspiration of pericardial blood, if cardiac tamponade is present, followed by urgent thoracotomy.

Pain relief

The provision of adequate and effective pain relief is central to the management of all patients. For relatively minor injuries, non-steroidal anti-inflammatory drugs may be given, providing that there are no contraindications to their use. Where the parenteral route is indicated, the intravenous route should be selected over the intramuscular route; in shocked patients or in those who are cold or shut down, absorption can be delayed, resulting in potentially dangerous effects when the patient starts to recover or warms up. Opiates such as morphine can be given intravenously with the amount titrated to the patient's response; patient-controlled analgesia is also effective, enabling patients to retain control of their pain relief. Epidural analgesia should be considered for more complex injuries to the chest wall to facilitate effective breathing. Intercostal nerve blocks are indicated for a small group of patients but their drawbacks must be considered, most notably the need for multiple injection sites and a duration of action of around 6 hours.

Diagnostic evaluation

A supine x-ray of the chest may be taken during the initial primary survey and resuscitation of the patient to determine the presence of rib fractures, pneumothoraces, haemothoraces, pulmonary contusions, a widened mediastinum and the heart size. Only some rib fractures can be identified on chest x-ray and pulmonary contusions usually develop later. Ideally, an erect film of the chest gives a more detailed picture and enables a raised hemidiaphragm to be observed more readily. This is indicated in all trauma patients, but may have to be delayed in those who have sustained trauma to the neck or back or where the spine has not been cleared from injury.

Blood gas analysis should be taken at the earliest opportunity to provide a baseline of the patient's respiratory status and to determine the need for initiating further respiratory support. Blood samples should also be sent for analysis of urea and electrolyte levels, full blood count, blood glucose, cardiac enzymes and other parameters as required. Twelve-lead ECGs should be carried out on all patients who have sustained trauma to the chest to detect any abnormalities and to provide a baseline should the patient's cardiac status deteriorate.

Computed tomography (CT) scans are often of diagnostic value. CT scanning of the thorax may reveal pulmonary contusions, pneumothoraces, pleural effusions and rupture of the aorta. With conventional CT scans, a failure rate of 10% regarding ruptured aortas has been noted. Greater reliability has been found with the spiral volumetric helical CT, which provides a more reliable view of the aorta. This can differentiate between initial findings suggestive of aortic injury and mediastinal haematoma. Diagnostic difficulties can arise when one considers that fractures of the ribs, sternum and vertebrae are also associated with mediastinal haematoma. CT scanning can also reveal other vessel injuries and may yield false-positive results with pre-existing vessel disease. The finding of mediastinal haematoma via spiral CT previously indicated the need to proceed with angiography; however, given the accuracy of this technique, angiography is now rarely performed. The spiral CT scan has been shown to identify other injuries accurately and

provide specific information on pulmonary contusions, pneumothoraces and haemothoraces. The CT scan yields four times more information than a conventional chest x-ray. It should be noted, however, that the CT scanner is not a place for the unstable patient other than in exceptional circumstances.

> The CT scanner is not a place for the unstable patient other than in exceptional circumstances

Angiography remains the gold standard for detecting aortic rupture and injuries to the great vessels. This procedure involves injecting radio-opaque dye into the heart and great vessels. Its advantages include clear definition of anatomy, precise location of aortic tears and blood supply to the coronary arteries. Its main disadvantages relate to the duration of the procedure, taking on average approximately 90 minutes to complete; moving unstable patients for this length of time carries considerable clinical risks, and lack of availability during the out-of-hours period causes problems. It may be necessary to delay the procedure, if other life-threatening injuries require more immediate intervention.

Transoesophageal echocardiography (TEE) has the advantage that it can be performed at the patient's bedside. This procedure provides detailed pictures of the descending aorta, but does not require an injection of contrast medium and is much faster than conventional angiography. Its main disadvantages are the level of skill required to undertake the procedure, inability to visualise the aortic arch due to it being a 'blind spot' for TEE, and contraindications to the procedure in patients with cervical spine and oesophageal injury.

Newer techniques are increasingly being reported. These include the use of three-dimensional CT angiography for detecting aortic injury, as reported by Richard Wolfe. Here, multiple thin 'slices' are taken through the aorta during the injection of iodinated contrast. Early reports state a good correlation between CT angiography and conventional angiography. Intra-vascular ultrasound is another new technique that utilises an intra-arterial transducer for detecting aortic injury; relatively few centres are performing this at present and few reports have been published. It is usually undertaken in the operating theatre in patients who are already undergoing surgery or in intensive care units where patients are too unstable to move.

Echocardiography in the relatively stable patient has the advantage of being able to be carried out at the patient's bedside. This gives a detailed picture of the heart, its chambers and yields valuable information on cardiac function.

SUMMARY

Chest injuries may present as immediately life-threatening problems or as minor injuries. Firm adherence to a structured assessment of the ABC parameters will enable nurses to diagnose most serious problems. Life-threatening problems must be dealt with immediately as they are found. Pain relief is an important part of the treatment and should not be underestimated. A high index of suspicion must be maintained, particularly if the mechanism of injury is suggestive of chest injuries. Vigilance will save lives.

References and further reading

American College of Surgeons Committee on Trauma. Thoracic trauma. In: *Advanced trauma life support programme for physicians*. Chicago: American College of Surgeons, 1993

American College of Surgeons. *Advanced trauma life support student course manual*, 6th edn. Chicago: American College of Surgeons, 1997

Bavaria JE, Edmonds LH. Traumatic aortic rupture. In: Edmonds LR (ed.) *Cardiac surgery in the adult*. New York: McGraw-Hill, 1997: 1245–1670

Blaisdell FW, Trunkey DD, *Cervicothoracic trauma*. Stuttgart: Thieme, 1994

Demetriades D. Penetrating injuries to the thoracic great vessels. *Journal of Cardiac Surgery* 1997; 12(Suppl.): 173–180

Driscoll P, Gwinnutt C, Le Duc C, Goodall O. *Trauma resuscitation: the team approach*. London: Macmillan, 1993: 67

Kirklin JW, Barratt Boyes VG. Cardiac trauma. In: *Cardiac surgery*, 2nd edn. Edinburgh: Churchill Livingstone, 1993: 1627–1634

Maberry JC, Trunkey D. The fractured rib in chest wall trauma. *Chest Surgery Clinics of North America* 1997; 7(2): 239

Mansour KA. Trauma of the chest. *Chest Surgery Clinics of North America* 1997; 7(2)

McLaughlin JS. Seminars in thoracic and cardiovascular surgery. *Thoracic and Cardiovascular Trauma* 1992; 4(3)

McLaughlin JS, Ficco M. *Blunt penetrating trauma to the heart and great vessels*. New York: McGraw Hill, 1997

Pearson FG et al. Trauma. In: *Thoracic surgery*. Section VIII. Edinburgh: Churchill Livingstone, 1995: 1523–1642

Rooney S et al. Chest injuries. In: Skinner D et al. (eds) *ABC of major trauma*. London: BMJ Publishing Group, 1994

Von Segesser LK et al. Diagnosis and mangement of blunt great vessel trauma. *Journal of Cardiac Surgery* 1997; 12(Suppl.): 181–192

Westaby S, Odell JA. *Cardiothoracic trauma*. London: Arnold, 1999

Chapter **24**

Orthopaedic trauma

Mike Smith

CHAPTER CONTENTS

INTRODUCTION

The term orthopaedics gained popularity towards the end of the last century in describing management of the child with physical deformity and is derived from the Greek language, literally meaning 'straight' (*orthos*) and 'child' (*paedios*). It may seem somewhat ironic, therefore, that a significant number of those sustaining orthopaedic trauma at the beginning of this century are the increasing elderly population. This chapter describes the physical assessment and initial intervention of those sustaining injuries that come under the broad definition of orthopaedic trauma.

GENERAL DIAGNOSTIC TESTS AND MEDICAL INVESTIGATIONS

Physical examination

Physical examination of the affected area(s) is a fundamental part of orthopaedic assessment. It is vital for the nurse in a trauma situation to be aware of a joint's particular range of movement, the signs and symptoms of specific orthopaedic injuries or conditions, and the symptoms of common associated complications, such as compartment syndrome. Not only is this essential when reaching a diagnosis but, also as important, is the awareness of the possibility of a changing situation, particularly in patients with multitrauma and those with neurological or neurovascular involvement. Additionally, there is a need to avoid worsening a condition through inappropriate management; for example, attempting to take an injured joint through its normal range of movement too soon may affect healing, increase patient pain or cause further damage to the affected part. More importantly, there are situations that potentially are life threatening, such as moving patients with unstable vertebral fractures, resulting in irreversible damage to delicate structures with potentially life-changing consequences.

There are many 'named' tests for particular orthopaedic conditions. Table 24.1 below provides some examples of these, although it is worth noting that these comprise only some of the more commonly used tests. There are, of course, many more physical testing methodologies in patients with musculoskeletal conditions of non-traumatic origin, but these are beyond the scope of this chapter. Reference to relevant tests will be made in the sections detailing specific orthopaedic conditions as appropriate. Further specific information relating to physical assessment is provided under individual fractures, emergency orthopaedics and neurovascular complications.

Common diagnostic radiological tests following orthopaedic trauma

In the initial hours following orthopaedic injury, the use of x-ray, computerised tomography (CT) and magnetic resonance imaging (MRI) scanning are commonplace. These are discussed individually later and detailed within specific sections in the chapter as relevant. There are cautions (i.e. worthy of informing the radiologist) and contraindications to these diagnostic procedures (Table 24.2), and it is the responsibility of those performing the physical assessment to ascertain the potential presence of these prior to ordering such tests.

There are many other tests (e.g. ultrasound, isotope bone scan) that may be of subsequent use;

Table 24.1 Common physical examination and diagnostic tests	
Test	**Procedure and possible diagnosis**
Anterior drawer	The knee is flexed to approximately 90° and the proximal tibia is pulled forward. Excessive movement is indicative of an anterior cruciate ligament tear
Apley test	Whilst in a prone position, the knee is flexed 90°. While compressing the knee, the lower leg is rotated in both directions. Pain during this procedure is indicative of a meniscal tear
Apprehension test	The shoulder is forcefully abducted and externally rotated. Patients who have experienced either dislocation or subluxation of the shoulder will become extremely apprehensive and attempt to stop the examination
Impingement test	The shoulder is forcefully abducted, or abducted and internally rotated, causing the greater tuberosity to press against the undersurface of the acromion. A positive test indicates an impingement syndrome
Lachman test	The knee is flexed to approximately 20° and the proximal tibia is pulled forward. Excessive motion of the tibia anteriorly is indicative of an anterior cruciate ligament tear
McMurray's test	The patient lies supine with knee fully flexed. The foot is rotated fully outward and the knee is slowly extended. If a painful 'click' results, this indicates a medial meniscus tear. Inward rotation of the foot with pain indicates a lateral meniscus tear
Patellar apprehension test	With the knee slightly flexed, the patella is pushed in a lateral direction. Patients with a patellar subluxation/dislocation will become very apprehensive and attempt to stop the test
Posterior drawer	The knee is flexed to 90° and the proximal tibia is pushed posteriorly. Excessive movement is indicative of a posterior cruciate ligament tear
Straight leg raising	With the knee extended and the patient supine or seated, the hip is flexed (with the leg straight). A positive test results in pain in the sciatic nerve distribution and suggests a disc herniation
Supraspinatus isolation	The supraspinous muscle is isolated through abducting and forward flexing the arm with the forearms in internal rotation. If there is weakness present, it is suggestive of a rotator cuff tear
Trendelenburg test	The patient stands erect facing away and is instructed to lift one leg and then the other. When weight is supported by the affected limb, the pelvis on the healthy side falls instead of rising. This indicates either gluteus medius weakness or a dislocated hip

Table 24.2   Cautions and contraindications of common radiological investigations

Investigation	Cautions	Contraindications
Magnetic resonance imaging	Prosthetic joint replacements Metallic implants, e.g. internal fixation of fracture previously Injury involving metallic objects, e.g. shrapnel Claustrophobia	Pacemaker Neurostimulator for pain or spasticity control Aneurysm clips
Computerised tomography scan	Previous reaction to injection of contrast medium (if required)	Claustrophobia
X-ray	Possibility of pregnancy	

discussion of these is beyond the scope of this chapter, however reference is made to them, where appropriate, in later sections.

X-rays

Plain x-rays are vital parts of the diagnostic armoury

The plain x-ray or radiograph is a vital part of the diagnostic armoury. Prior to any surgical intervention, after any actual or suspected injury and at regular intervals during a patient's health care episode, the x-ray remains a key tool. Densities, relationships between different bones, continuity of bone, and bone contour are all key features that may indicate the presence of an orthopaedic condition. In trauma, the use of x-rays can be invaluable (Box 24.1). They are often used to recognise the presence and severity of fractures, determine the accuracy of closed reduction, assess the degree of comminution, view articular surfaces, identify the presence of concomitant and predisposing bone disease such as pathological fractures that may occur in osteoporosis or with bone tumours, and identify the presence of foreign and loose bodies.

Generally speaking, the interpretation of x-rays is a relatively simple and straightforward procedure. However, failure to identify abnormal findings is not uncommon and may result in patients experiencing significant disability or compromise. To minimise such consequences, it is recommended that a structured approach be used when interpreting such 'films', following a logical and systematic format. The general rules that should be followed are outlined in Box 24.2. Some

---

Box 24.1   Use of x-rays in trauma

- Fracture recognition and severity
- Accuracy of closed reduction
- Ascertain degree of comminution
- Viewing of articular surfaces
- Identification of concomitant and predisposing bone disease
- Identification of foreign and loose bodies

Box 24.2   General rules for the interpretation of x-rays

- Ensure that the correct x-ray is ordered – be specific regarding suspected injury and views required
- Views must be taken in at least two planes, e.g. anteroposterior (AP) and lateral
- X-rays are usually at right angles – exceptions are the hands and feet, where overlap may obscure constructive views. In such cases, oblique views may be necessary
- A combination of x-rays and other radiological techniques may often be beneficial
- Absence of obvious radiological problems may not necessarily signify no fractures

---

may seem straightforward and even common sense; however, their importance should not be underestimated.

X-ray interpretation is a systematic process and should follow the approved sequence, as outlined in Boxes 24.3 and 24.4.

The interpretation of x-rays becomes easier with practice. An increasing number of internet sites are becoming available, each offering online

---

Box 24.3   Systematic approach to the interpretation of x–rays

- Ensure the name of patient matches that on the x-rays
- Ensure a good knowledge of normal anatomy
- Ensure the date of the investigation is current
- Ensure the appropriate films have been obtained, e.g. AP and lateral views of the right knee
- Ensure the ABC sequence is followed (see Box 24.4)

Box 24.4   The ABC sequence

A   *Adequacy*: ensure that the joints above and below the injury are visible
Alignment: ensure that the x-ray is a true lateral view (direction of beam)

B   *Bone*: assess the quality of the films and look for the presence of fractures, the alignment and relationship with other bones, and the deformity and contour of bones when compared with normal anatomy

C   *Cartilage and soft tissues*: look for ectopic calcification, wounds or discs

---

practice in this area; an increasing range of practical clinically focused courses aimed at facilitating learning in this field are similarly available. It is recommended that experience is gained not only through direct patient contact and examination, but also through initiatives such as these.

There is a strong argument in favour of nurses working in the trauma environment to have at least a basic knowledge of x-ray interpretation, if only to be able to educate patients regarding their injuries. Clearly those progressing to nurse practitioner or consultant nurse level may well require a much more in-depth knowledge dependent on the clinical setting and the responsibilities associated with such posts.

Absence of obvious radiological abnormality may not necessarily indicate the absence of fractures

---

Computed tomography scans
X-ray beams pass through body parts at different angles of rotation. This information is transformed into cross-sectional images after the application of complex mathematical algorithms. Significantly more information can be gained via CT scanning than with traditional x-rays, although not to the same degree as that which can be obtained through MRI scans.

In some circumstances, intravenous contrast may be given to outline vascular structures and to assess the characteristics of pathological processes. This is of particular use when there is actual or suspected associated vascular injury (e.g. in supracondylar fractures of the humerus). No special physical preparation is normally required for CT scanning with the exception of abdomino-pelvic scans, where contrast media may be used. As with other procedures and investigations, it is beneficial to explain to patients what will happen to them to facilitate their compliance during the procedure, and to allay their fear and anxiety.

Magnetic resonance imaging scans
Magnetic resonance imaging is based on the interaction between nuclei of hydrogen atoms, which are present in abundance in all biological tissues, and the magnetic fields generated and controlled by the MRI system's instrumentation. The images produced provide detailed information regarding the majority of body tissues and are of increasing diagnostic benefit.

The main indications for MRI examinations are in neurological and musculoskeletal conditions where the observation of soft tissues as well as bone is advantageous, not only when making a diagnosis but also when planning medical intervention. The main contraindications to their use are cardiac pacemakers, cochlear implants, epidural electrodes and ferromagnetic aneurysm clips. Relative contraindications include the first trimester of pregnancy and claustrophobia. Psychological preparation, as well as the identification of any physical contraindications, is vital prior to the procedure.

FRACTURES – AN OVERVIEW

Fractures are commonly defined as disruptions to the continuity of bones. They may occur across the lifespan, although their aetiology will differ dependent upon age and lifestyle. Causes include trauma, pathological events such as tumours, osteoporosis, infections such as osteomyelitis and tuberculosis, and stress, resulting, for example, in 'repetitive strain injuries'. Generally speaking, fractures may be broadly classified into two main groups: compound or open fractures, where wounds allow communication with the air, or simple or closed fractures, where the integrity of the skin is not broken.

The aetiology of fractures varies according to age and lifestyle

Although it is well established that the aetiology of fractures varies across the lifespan, their associated signs and symptoms apply more generally. Those most commonly identified include (Box 24.5): pain and point tenderness over the affected area; deformity such as shortening, dislocation or rotation, particularly in relation to limb fractures (Figure 24.1); local swelling; reduced range of movement; joint dysfunction; crepitus; and signs of shock, which may present in fractures to the long bones and pelvis, and vertebral fractures involving damage to the underlying spinal cord.

Fracture patterns

Fracture patterns may be visible on x-ray and are useful both in assessing the severity of fractures and in determining optimal management strategies. Their causes, implications for management and clinical sequelae are outlined later. Fractures may be considered under ten main patterns: spiral, oblique, transverse, comminuted, greenstick, complicated, avulsion, impacted, wedge and depressed (Figure 24.2 and Box 24.6).

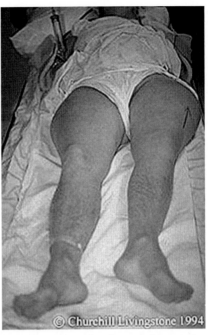

Figure 24.1   Leg adducted and externally rotated, indicative of a trochanteric fracture of the hip.

Box 24.6   Fracture patterns

Spiral	Classically involve rotational forces
Oblique	Fracture lines run at an angle of < 90° to the long axis of the bone
Transverse	Fracture lines run at an angle of 90° to the long axis of the bone
Comminuted	More than two fragments of bone are present
Greenstick	Classically occur in children
Complicated	Neighbouring structures are involved
Avulsion	Fragments of bone are removed by ligaments or muscles
Impacted	One fragment of bone is driven into the other
Wedge/burst/ compression	Bones are compressed beyond their tolerance limits, e.g. vertebrae
Depressed	Segments of bone are depressed below the level of the surrounding bone, e.g. skull

Spiral fractures often result when rotational forces are involved in the mechanism of injury and may be sustained by indirect violence. The classic picture in such injuries is one of the fractures curving in a spiral fashion around the bone.

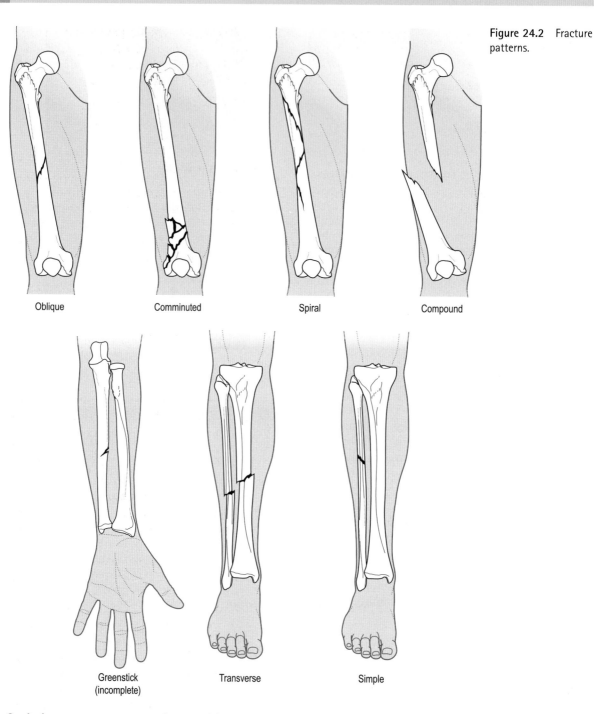

Figure 24.2 Fracture patterns.

Such fractures are commonly unstable in nature and will require early surgical intervention.

In *oblique fractures*, the fracture lines run at an angle of less than 90° to the long axis of the bone and, like spiral fractures, may be caused by indirect violence.

Transverse fractures classically run at right angles to the long axis of a bone and, unlike spiral and oblique fractures, are usually caused by direct violence. Such patients often have associated soft tissue damage around the fracture site, necessitating close observation of neurovascular status.

In *comminuted fractures*, more than two fragments of bone are present, ranging from slight to highly comminuted, depending on the number and size of fragments involved; are unstable. Marked comminution is indicative of severe violence and is associated with an increased risk of nerve, muscle, tendon and skin damage.

Greenstick fractures classically occur in children, although not all children's fractures are of this type. In these injuries, the less brittle bones of children tend to buckle on the side opposite to the force applied, and there is no loss of bony contact. Tearing of the surrounding soft tissues is often minimal and healing is usually rapid.

Fractures may be described as complicated or uncomplicated, with *complicated fractures* occurring when other neighbouring structures are involved.

Avulsion fractures are relatively common and occur when fragments of bone are removed by ligaments or muscles, for example, as a consequence of momentary subluxation or dislocation.

Impacted fractures are also relatively common and occur when one fragment is driven into the other. Classic examples include fractures of the neck of femur and fractures of the proximal humerus. These are generally managed with surgical intervention and have associated risks of long-term problems, such as avascular necrosis (osteonecrosis).

Compression fractures, also referred to as *wedge* or *burst fractures*, occur in cancellous bone, which is compressed beyond its limits of tolerance. Common sites for such fractures include the vertebrae, as a result of flexion injuries, and the heels, following falls from a height. In the former, if there is an associated instability of the vertebral column, there is a risk of damage to the delicate spinal cord or spinal nerves that comprise the cauda equina, either immediately as a direct consequence of the injury or subsequently, if incorrectly moved.

The last fracture pattern to consider is that of *depressed fractures*, which are most commonly associated with the skull, and occur when sharply localised blows depress a segment of cortical bone below the level of the surrounding bone. In such cases, neurological assessment is vital, as there may be a degree of traumatic brain injury in some patients, if the causative forces were severe.

From the above, it should be clear that identification of fracture patterns is not only vital in determining potential mechanism and management of the bony injury itself, but will also be indicative of potential associated complications that should be observed for, both in the initial and subsequent physical assessment of the patient.

Fracture management

Central to the management of fractures is the concept of rehabilitation, in that all interventions involving the restoration of movement and function must be viewed within the context of ultimately achieving optimal patient outcomes. Such functional outcomes may only be achieved if the mechanical integrity is restored to the affected area and secondary complications are avoided.

Considerations influencing this management include the type, location and severity of fractures, the presence of concomitant injuries or disease processes, delay in diagnosis or treatment, and the available resources and facilities.

Open fractures necessitate early surgery for debridement as well as reduction of the fracture and are associated with more potential complications than those that are closed. The pattern and severity of fractures may limit surgical options, particularly those that are severe, and are more likely to lead to the need for prosthetic replacements. Where other concomitant injuries are also present, priorities in the overall clinical management of the patient may change, which may impact upon the early management of fractures. Pre-existing medical conditions or underlying orthopaedic pathology, such as osteoporosis, may impact on the ability to perform some types of fixation techniques and may limit the range of treatment options available. However, it is worthy of note that developments in surgical technology and surgical expertise have increased such options, and the presence of osteoporosis may not mean that conservative management is indicated (Cornell et al., 2003). Any delay in diagnosis will inevitably affect eventual outcome, hence the need for early diagnostic intervention. Similarly, the availability of theatre time will clearly influence the process and even outcome of treatment and must be considered within the overall management plan; for example, early surgery for long bone fractures is associated with a reduction in the incidence of fat embolism and subsequent pain. Other related considerations include the pre-morbid function of the affected area, and the post-injury patient's and/or the individual surgeon's expectations.

The nature and availability of resources and facilities are also key to the patient's rehabilitation and follow-up. For example, patients may live and work in rural areas, and equipment may be limited; in such circumstances, early discharge from hospital may not be appropriate, even in patients with uncomplicated closed fractures should the social situation be inhibitory. Lastly, culture plays an important part in any treatment plan and should not be underestimated, for example, in relation to the need for fluid replacement in patients who are practising Jehovah's witnesses.

Finally, orthopaedic trauma is obviously not restricted to adults and is common in children. Although it is beyond the scope of this chapter to detail paediatric orthopaedic trauma specifically, it is noteworthy that, as well as the considerations outlined earlier, which are still applicable, the additional issues relating to the immature musculoskeletal system of children, including that of anticipating bone growth and minimising physeal injury, must be considered in assessment and management strategies (Musgrave and Mendelson, 2002). This is, of course, combined with other general paediatric issues regarding potential difficulties in physical and radiological examination, and the impact on parents and caregivers (Norris, 2001).

> The type, location and severity of fractures, presence of concomitant injuries or disease processes, delay in diagnosis or treatment, and available resources and facilities, all affect fracture management

Fracture healing

The healing of fractures may be associated with a number of potential problems and complications, hence the need for regular monitoring and follow-up. Key problems fall into three main categories:

non-union, where no uniting of the fracture takes place; mal-union, where healing takes place, but there is malalignment or incorrect positioning of bones; and delayed union, where union may take up to 8 weeks.

As a general rule of thumb, union of fractures managed conservatively should take 8 weeks. In children, this timeframe may be halved and doubled for lower limb injuries. A fractured shaft of femur may take up to 12 weeks to heal in an adult but 6 weeks in the child.

Factors that may influence delayed union are numerous (Box 24.7), including local blood supply, infection, individual characteristics of bone, severity of the fracture (e.g. joint involvement), success of intervention, compliance with prescribed treatment regime, nutritional factors with regard to bone remodelling, pre-existing hormonal influences, medications taken (e.g. steroids), environmental issues, pre-existing medical and/ or orthopaedic conditions, a history of substance abuse and further injuries being sustained. A prime example of this would be in the case of a patient with diabetes mellitus. Injuries around the ankle are susceptible to delayed healing because of a diminished blood supply. In a patient with diabetes mellitus, this will be exacerbated, making surgical intervention much more likely to produce a desired outcome than conservative management (Bibbo et al., 2001).

Box 24.7   Factors affecting fracture healing

- Age
- Local blood supply
- Infection
- Individual bone characteristics
- Severity of fracture
- Success of intervention
- Compliance with prescribed treatment regime
- Nutritional factors
- Hormonal influences
- Medications
- Environmental factors
- Past medical history
- Substance abuse
- Further injury of affected part

All of these factors must be considered from the beginning of a management regime and may influence strategies adopted.

Complications of fractures

Complications of fractures may occur at various stages throughout the healing process and may be considered as immediate, early or those that occur in the medium to long term. They are summarised in Table 24.3, and are covered in greater detail in later sections on orthopaedic emergencies and neurovascular complications.

Immediate complications are those that are associated with potential loss of life or function including hypovolaemic shock due to potentially life-threatening haemorrhage, and damage to other tissues and/or organs. Such major haemorrhage may, for example, be sustained from pelvic fractures (where more than 3 litres of blood may be lost), from femoral fractures (where between 1 and 1.5 litres may be lost) and from tibial fractures (where 0.5 litres may be lost). Damage to other tissues or organs may be considerable, and includes traumatic brain injury in association with skull fractures, lung injury in association with rib fractures, spinal cord injury in association with spinal fractures, aortic damage associated with sternal fractures, splenic injury such as that sustained in association with fractures of the tenth and eleventh ribs on the left, and liver injury such as that sustained in association with fractures of the 10th–12th ribs on the right.

Early complications tend to occur later in the healing and recovery process, and include fat embolism (in fractures of long bones), compartment syndrome (particularly prevalent in those with associated soft tissue damage, notably fractures of the tibia), 'fracture blisters' and infection, particularly in relation to patients who have sustained compound fractures. These are discussed in detail later in the chapter as they form a key component of the assessment and management of those with orthopaedic trauma in the initial stage following injury.

Other complications may also occur later in the recovery phase and may arise in the medium to long term. These include: avascular necrosis; the complications of reduced mobility, such as deep vein thrombosis (DVT) and pulmonary embolism in lower limb trauma (Wang et al., 2002), pressure areas and chest infections; soft tissue infections or osteomyelitis as a consequence of open fractures; delayed union, slow union or non-union (Figure 24.3); post-traumatic arthritis or joint stiffness; myositis ossificans; and neurological and vascular complications.

UPPER LIMB TRAUMA

Upper arm/shoulder fractures

Fractures of the clavicle and scapula, shoulder and elbow dislocations, and fractures of the proximal humerus and shaft and head of humerus are the most common upper arm and shoulder fractures.

Table 24.3   Complications associated with fractures

Immediate	Early (within hours or days)	Late (within weeks and long term)
Haemorrhage and hypovolaemic shock, e.g. pelvic fractures	Fat embolism	Post-traumatic osteoarthritis
Damage to other organs, e.g. head or spinal injury, abdominal and thoracic organs in rib fracture (especially multiple fractures)	Wound infection – acute osteomyelitis in compound fracture	Deformity
	'Fracture blisters'	Chronic pain
	Deep vein thrombois, pressure ulcer and other complications of prolonged immobility	Delayed/non-union/mal-union of fracture
	Neurovascular compromise to limbs, including compartment syndrome	Myositis ossificans
		Chronic osteomyelitis
		Reduced functional ability (often due to reduced range of movement and/or pain)

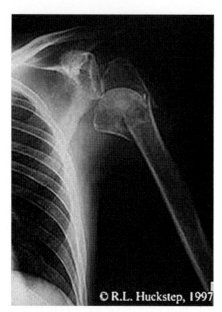

Figure 24.3 Malunion of a humeral head fracture.

These will be considered in addition to supra-condylar, olecranon fractures and fractures to the radial head. Although upper limb fractures may be considered by some to be 'less serious' than those of lower limbs, and indeed are invariably not as life threatening in nature, the effects can be immense to the patient's short- or long-term quality of life in those with complications or residual disability once the fracture has healed (Altizer, 2003). It goes without saying, therefore, that the need for comprehensive physical (on an ongoing basis) and radiological assessment is not only vital for detecting the presence of bony injury, but also for associated complications (Blake and Hoffman, 1999). Complex joints, such as the elbow, necessitate a knowledge of normal and postinjury anatomy to alert the team to the potential for these complications (Kuntz and Baratz, 1999).

Fractures of the clavicle
Clavicular fractures are generally caused by direct trauma or falls on to the outstretched hand, with the force being transmitted up the arm to the clavicle. They may also be caused by blows on the point of the shoulder and by direct violence. Most occur at the junction of the middle and outer thirds of the clavicle, but they are also

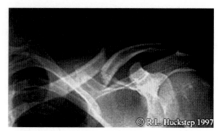

Figure 24.4 Fractured clavicle.

common throughout the middle third, and to a lesser extent, the outer third (Figure 24.4). Patients classically present with visible slumping of the shoulder on the affected side as a consequence of the weight of the arm, reduced range of movement, and localised pain and swelling at the fracture site. Local bruising is also a striking feature in cases seen some days after the injury.

Appropriate x-rays may confirm the diagnosis; a single AP view of the shoulder is usually adequate in the adult. Although there is a paucity of evidence in relation to the optimal management of clavicular fractures, most are successfully managed with a broad arm sling or collar and cuff for 2 weeks, and appropriate analgesia where required. These provide support for the weight of the arm, which has lost its clavicular tie (McCoy et al., 2000). Patients are then instructed to commence active exercises when the pain subsides and to continue these until full mobility is restored. In those who have sustained compound fractures with associated soft tissue injury, have non-union following conservative management or present with instability, treatment may progress to surgery, where an *open reduction with internal fixation* (ORIF) of various types may be performed (Anderson, 2003). Patients should also be advised that a residual palpable or visible deformity at the fracture site may be present after healing has occurred (Figure 24.5).

Fractures of the scapula
Scapular fractures are uncommon injuries and are usually due to direct trauma, often associated with an assault. Even when comminuted and angulated, healing is usually extremely rapid and most have a positive outcome.

On presentation, patients classically complain of severe pain around the fracture site with

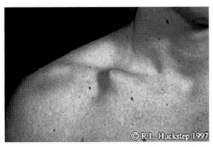

Figure 24.5   Deformity post healing of fractured clavicle.

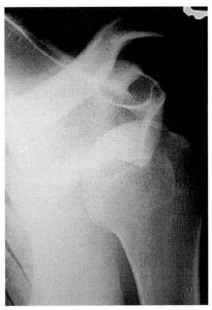

Figure 24.6   Anterior shoulder dislocation.

obvious bruising and swelling. Common fracture sites include the neck and body of the scapula, the acromion process and the coracoid process. Management of these fractures is dependent on their location, although most can be conservatively managed with a broad arm sling and analgesia, with patients instructed to perform early active exercise as pain allows.

Shoulder dislocations

Anterior shoulder dislocations account for around 95% of shoulder dislocations and typically occur as a consequence of falls onto the fixed hand, leading to external rotation of the shoulder and the humerus being driven forward with subsequent tearing of the joint capsule (Figure 24.6). Damage to the anterior structures is not uncommon, including damage to the axillary artery and brachial plexus. Shoulder dislocations most commonly occur in adults aged between 18 and 25 years, commonly due to motorcycle and sports injuries, and are rare in children. They are also relatively common in the elderly, where the stability of the shoulder may be impaired by muscle degeneration and where falls are common.

Patients characteristically present physically supporting the arm on the affected side, with a flattened lateral outline when compared to the unaffected side, and complain of localised pain and tenderness, and a strong resistance to movement. Often the arm does not lie into the side, appearing to be in slight abduction; the outer contour of the shoulder may appear to be slightly kinked owing to displacement of the humeral head. *Axillary nerve palsy* is the most common neurological complication; integrity of this nerve should, therefore, be assessed in all patients.

Diagnosis may be confirmed by physical examination and by comparing both sides. Standard AP x-rays of the shoulder may also be helpful; here, the humeral head will be seen to be displaced anteriorly and medially, and loss of congruity with the glenoid noted. In some cases, additional views may be required, particularly where the diagnosis is in doubt. Most patients can be managed with closed reduction of the dislocation using one of Kocher's methods or an alternative method of reduction, and the application of a sling with instructions to mobilise after 2 weeks. Repeat x-rays are important to confirm the position post reduction. In some patients, a body bandage may also be applied to prevent external rotation.

In younger patients, there is a relatively high incidence of recurrence within 2 years, occurring in approximately 50%. For these patients, the limb may be supported for a longer period of time to give the torn tissues time to heal. Patients who have suffered repeated dislocations on four or more occasions should be considered to be suffering from recurrent dislocation and assessed for reconstructive surgery. In the elderly, the risk of recurrent dislocation is minimal but the risks of stiffness are great. For this reason, referral for physiotherapy is advisable in these patients. Similarly, physiotherapy is indicated in cases of axillary nerve palsy with loss of deltoid function.

Posterior dislocations of the shoulder are usually associated with fractures and most require referral to the orthopaedic trauma team for possible surgical intervention. They may result from falls on the outstretched, internally rotated hand or from a direct blow on the front of the shoulder. Here, the head of the humerus is displaced directly backwards; because of this, a single AP view on x-ray may show little or no abnormality. The characteristic clinical presentation is that of pain, deformity and local tenderness.

Fractures of the proximal humerus

These fractures are most commonly sustained as a result of falls onto the outstretched hand and are commonly experienced in the elderly population. They may also be caused by falls on to the side, often leading to impacted, minimally displaced fractures, or by direct violence. Fractures of the 'surgical neck' are the most common, with a degree of impaction often visible on x-ray. These may present with involvement of the humeral head, displacement of greater/lesser tuberosities or associated anterior dislocation of the shoulder. The 'Neer' classification may be used (Neer, 2002). In essence, this classification examines the involvement of four anatomical structures, namely:

1. anatomical neck
2. surgical neck
3. greater tuberosity segment
4. lesser tuberosity segment.

Each structure is examined for the presence of a displacement of > 5 mm or angulation of 45°. It is then classified as one, two, three or four part with/without head splitting and associated dislocation.

Patients often present with major bruising over the shoulder and upper arm, pain on movement and obvious swelling. Many present supporting the arm with the other hand. Tenderness over the proximal humerus is likely and, in severely angulated or displaced fractures, there may be obvious deformity. Later, significant bruising gravitating down the arm may be noted. Diagnosis is established by x-ray investigation; more than one

view is required for confirmation. Management of these fractures is dependent on their severity. A large number can be managed conservatively, with mild displacements often corrected by the weight of the arm in collar and cuff alone. Mobilisation may be commenced after the acute symptoms have resolved. The presence of severe displacement with involvement of the humeral head may necessitate further intervention in the form of internal fixation (Figure 24.7), excisional arthroplasty, hemiarthroplasty or joint replacement (Hoffmeyer, 2002). In such cases, the risks of avascular necrosis with persistent pain and stiffness are high. Although there seems little doubt that complex proximal humerus fractures are best managed through surgery to achieve optimum outcome, there is currently little definite evidence in systematic reviews to differentiate in outcome between fixation and arthroplasty (Misra et al., 2001).

Patients may be instructed to use 'pendulum exercises' as soon as pain tolerance allows, with instructions given either from the emergency department, fracture clinic or ward, as appropriate. Although there will be some local idiosyncrasies, pendulum exercises generally involve the patient placing the arm down by the side, then gently swinging the hand forward and backward, then side to side, and then clockwise and anticlockwise.

Axillary nerve damage is a potential initial complication that must be tested for, particularly in those with associated anterior dislocation. Such

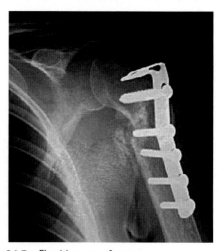

Figure 24.7 Fixed humerus fracture.

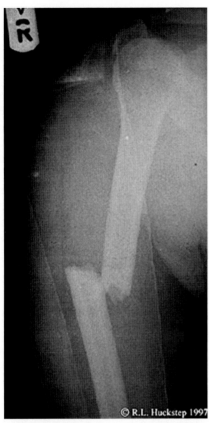

Figure 24.8   Fractured shaft of humerus.

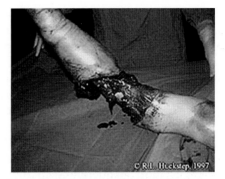

Figure 24.9   Severe compound humerus fracture.

patients will present with an inability to raise the arm and elbow flexion is likely to be reduced. In the long term, such injuries are often associated with stiffness, malunion or non-union and avascular necrosis, hence arrangement of follow-up is vital.

Fractures of the shaft of humerus

Fractures of the humeral shaft represent about 1% of all fractures (Figure 24.8). Fracture types vary dependent on the mechanism of injury and include spiral fractures, transverse and oblique fractures, and transverse or comminuted fractures. Spiral fractures are typically caused by falls onto the outstretched hand with a twist, while transverse and oblique fractures tend to occur as a result of falls onto the elbow with the arm abducted. Transverse or comminuted fractures are most commonly sustained as a consequence of a direct blow. In fractures involving the upper third of the humeral shaft, the proximal fragment tends to be pulled into adduction by the unopposed action of the pectoralis major. In those involving the middle third, the proximal fragment tends to be abducted owing to deltoid pull. Radial nerve palsy, non-union and compounding of fractures are most common in this patient group (Figure 24.9).

Presenting symptoms typically include pain, reduced range of movement, and bruising and swelling with deformity when compared to the unaffected side. The arm is usually flail and is supported by the other hand. Obvious mobility at the fracture site may be noted and may help to confirm the diagnosis. Diagnosis is confirmed by x-ray investigation. Although a relatively uncommon complication, radial nerve palsy should be looked for in all patients, as evidenced by drop wrist and sensory impairment of the dorsum of the hand.

Conservative management is dependent on individual clinician choice and the severity of the fracture. Options include a collar and cuff, hanging cast and a U-slab. Simple single fractures may be treated by the application of a U-slab, while hanging casts offer an alternative for ambulant patients. Evidence suggests that the optimal treatment method is lacking, although patients who are judged potentially to have difficulty in complying with 'resting' the affected side, may be managed using a cast.

With more complicated fractures, patients may progress to *open reduction with internal fixation* – plate fixation most commonly with occasional intramedullary nailing – if a satisfactory reduction is not maintained, or in those who have open, bilateral or pathological fractures. Potential complications include radial nerve damage, which is estimated to occur in 6–17% of patients with displaced fractures, vascular damage, delayed union or non-union, and stiffness in the long term. Recovery from radial nerve palsy generally commences 6–8 weeks after the initial injury, if there is no indication for exploration. Recovery may be assisted by the use of a drop-wrist splint and physiotherapy. If there is no recovery after 8 weeks, an electromyogram (EMG) may be indicated and exploration of the radial nerve considered. Non-union is most frequently seen in middle third fractures, especially in obese patients, where support of the fracture may be difficult or where gravitational distraction of the fracture occurs.

Supracondylar fractures

The typical history associated with these injuries is patients having fallen on outstretched, often rotated hands. Supracondylar fractures of the humerus are fractures that occur in the distal third of the bone and most commonly occur in children, peaking at around 8 years of age, although they do occur in adults with a comminuted pattern. Such fractures may be classified as extension, flexion, transcondylar or intercondylar, each of which may influence their management. Patients characteristically present with swollen painful elbows, deformity, tenderness over the distal humerus, and an equilateral triangle and 'fat pad' signs on x-ray are reported as being typical. Children will typically be more challenging to examine, and more vague as regards symptoms, hence early x-ray may be the optimum use of time and least distressing for the injured child, if such an injury is suspected.

X-ray diagnosis is mandatory, although interpretation can be difficult. Vascular complications may occur where there is appreciable displacement and where the proximal fragment may affect the brachial artery. Circulation should be assessed in every patient and recorded prior to any manipulation. Absence of the radial pulse should be looked for in addition to other evidence of arterial obstruction, including pallor and coldness of the limb, pain and paraesthesia in the forearm, progressive weakness and paralysis of the forearm muscles. Evidence of excessive swelling and bruising around the elbow should similarly be looked for. Reduction of the fracture is indicated where there is evidence of arterial obstruction, and the fracture is displaced or angulated.

Most children are treated conservatively with closed reduction, and the application of a collar and cuff, which is then strapped with the elbow flexed. In adults and adolescents, a plaster of Paris (POP) backslab will be applied as a general rule. Neurovascular assessment is vital as compromise is not uncommon; Volkmann's ischaemia with associated contractures may also occur (neurovascular complications section). In the long term, weakness, avascular necrosis, deformity and ongoing pain are all potential complications associated with this injury. Physiotherapy is indicated if there is still significant restriction in movement after 2 weeks.

Elbow dislocations

These are particularly complex injuries in the sphere of orthopaedic trauma not only in the challenges relating to obtaining satisfactory postinjury outcomes but also in the high risk of associated secondary complications (Figures 24.10 and 24.11).

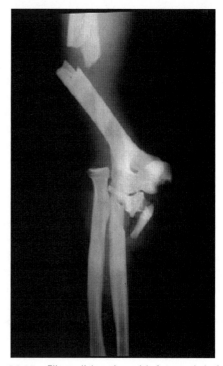

Figure 24.10 Elbow dislocation with fractured shaft of humerus.

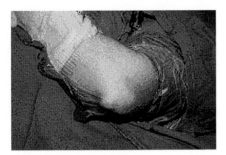

Figure 24.11   Elbow dislocation.

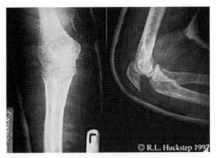

Figure 24.12   Fractured olecranon.

Vigilant and comprehensive assessment are therefore essential (Ring and Jupiter, 2002).

Posterior dislocations account for the vast majority of these injuries, which are commonly caused by falls onto the outstretched hand or by direct trauma. They are common in both children and adults, and may sometimes be confused with supracondylar fractures. Clinical distinction may be made based on x-ray examination and by searching for the equilateral triangle formed by the olecranon and epicondyles. In elbow dislocations, this is typically disturbed but is intact with supracondylar fractures. Additional symptoms and signs found with elbow dislocations include a prominent olecranon, flexed forearm, obvious deformity and pain. Damage to the ulnar nerve, median nerve or brachial artery are uncommon, but should always be looked for, and function assessed. The ulnar nerve may be assessed by noting the ability to grip a sheet of paper between the ring and little finger, ensuring that the fingers are not flexed at the metacarpal pharyngeal joints. In the case of the median nerve, contraction and power may be assessed by feeling the muscle while the patient attempts to resist the thumb being pressed from a vertical position into the plane of the hand. Sensory function in the areas supplied by the median and ulnar nerves should also be quickly tested. Lastly, the brachial artery can most easily be assessed by identification of the radial pulse.

Anterior dislocations are invariably due to a blow to the elbow whilst the arm is flexed. Signs and symptoms are the same and, similarly, early reduction whilst avoiding potential neurovascular complications is the treatment goal.

Diagnosis is usually confirmed by x-ray investigation with treatment generally carried out under general anaesthetic. Repeat x-rays should also always be taken after the procedure. Management involves closed reduction of the fracture, the application of a collar and cuff, and an exercise regime which should be commenced after a period of 2 weeks. Mobilisation too early or that is too vigorous runs the risk of myositis ossificans, and passive movements must be avoided in the early postreduction period.

Surgical intervention is commonplace owing to the severity of many of these injuries. Surgical goals aim to restore the articular surfaces and stabilise the structures around the joint (Lee, 2001).

Fractures of the olecranon

Fractures of the olecranon are usually caused either by a fall onto the point of the elbow, a direct blow or by a fall onto an outstretched hand while using the triceps (Figure 24.12). They may also occur as a direct result of triceps contraction.

Patients commonly present with pain and swelling around the olecranon. Diagnosis is usually straightforward and is confirmed by x-ray examination. Management of these fractures is surgical through tension band wiring. Initial complications are rare, unless combined with other injuries. Long-term complications may include elbow stiffness, osteoarthritis and myositis ossificans.

Myositis ossificans will normally become observable on x-ray 10 days after the initial injury, and will appear as a peripheral rim of calcification, which will become more apparent with time as the bone formation matures (Figure 24.13). As this

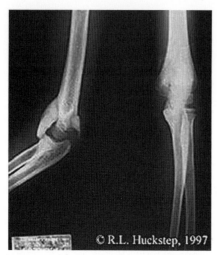

Figure 24.13 Myositis ossificans at the front and back of the elbow.

bone formation has rough edges, similar to the idea of a small cactus, the muscle becomes easily irritated with even small contractions. Typically rest is the first order of treatment, followed by gradual strengthening and return to activity, often over a period of months. Surgery is rarely required for this secondary complication.

Fractures of the radial head
Radial head fractures again commonly result from indirect violence, such as that caused by falling onto an outstretched hand, transmitting force up the radius and pushing the radial head against the capitulum. Consequently, the radial head may be split or broken. They may also be caused by direct violence, such as falls or blows on the side of the elbow. The mechanism of injury causes fracture of the radial head but may also damage the articular surface of the capitulum, prolonging recovery. Patients typically present with painful swollen elbows, often with local bruising. Underlying haemarthrosis may also be present. In minor fractures, tenderness may not be apparent until the damaged portion of the head is rotated under the examining thumb (i.e. gentle pronation and supination while palpating the radial head). The range of pronation and supination is often full, but elbow extension is usually restricted.

Diagnosis is usually confirmed on standard x-ray examination; however, if there is clinical

evidence of a fracture and x-rays are negative, additional AP views are required to visualise all portions of the radial head. Where fractures are undisplaced, patients may be discharged home from the emergency department with a collar and cuff or broad arm sling, and fracture clinic follow up. Mobilisation may be commenced after a period of 2–3 weeks, and an excellent clinical outcome can be expected, although many months may elapse before full extension is regained. In severe cases, open reduction with internal fixation or excision of the radial head may be required. The arm will then be rested in a sling for 2–3 weeks before mobilisation is commenced.

Forearm fractures

Fractures of the radius, ulna and scaphoid occur with considerable frequency, and will be reviewed along with Monteggia and Galeazzi fracture–dislocations.

Fractures of the radius and ulna
Patients presenting with fractures of the radius and ulna commonly describe a history of a fall with a twisting injury or sustaining a direct blow to the affected area (Figures 24.14 and 24.15). Pain, swelling and obvious deformity of the forearm are the usual presenting features. Displacement,

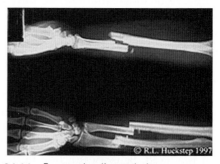

Figure 24.14 Fractured radius and ulna.

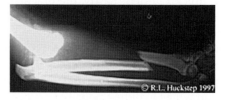

Figure 24.15 Fractured radius and elbow dislocation.

which will be revealed on x-ray examination, is often marked and rotational deformities frequent, making reduction difficult. Late recurrence of deformity is common, if treated in plaster.

Surgical intervention is required for the majority of these injuries, with open reduction and internal fixation with compression plating now almost routine. Postoperatively, plaster fixation is usually maintained until union occurs. This will usually be *in situ* for at least 6 weeks with regular fracture clinic follow-up to ascertain progress prior to removal. This is one of the more common causes of compartment syndrome, hence assessment of neurovascular function is vital. In adults, it is reasonable to treat fractures of the forearm bones conservatively. This is particularly the case if the fractures are undisplaced, in the elderly or in those suffering from multiple injuries, where the duration of anaesthesia required for open reduction and internal fixation is considered hazardous. In those circumstances where internal fixation is not employed, careful monitoring is required to ensure the early identification and treatment of problems.

In children, fractures of the radius and ulna are usually greenstick in pattern. In the undisplaced angulated greenstick fracture, a general anaesthetic should be given and the angulation corrected. In the undisplaced greenstick fracture with no axial rotation of any of the fragments, the position of the forearm is important in preventing re-angulation while in plaster. Where fractures are displaced, the application of traction and apposition of bony edges may restore anatomical positioning, while the application of a plaster of Paris cast and broad arm sling may provide immobilisation and promote recovery. Open reduction and internal fixation are rarely indicated.

Monteggia fracture–dislocations

Severe angulation of the forearm bone is usually accompanied by fracture or dislocation of the other forearm bone. In the Monteggia fracture–dislocation, fracture of the upper third of the ulnar shaft is associated with dislocation of the radial head (Figure 24.16). The most easily understood mechanism is when a violent fall or blow on the arm fractures the ulna and displaces the radial head anteriorly. Most commonly, the injury results

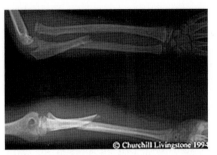

Figure 24.16   Monteggia fracture.

from forced pronation, such as that caused by a fall on the outstretched fully pronated arm when the trunk continues to turn over the fixed hand and the radius is forced against the ulna fracturing it, and in turn is levered away from the capitellum. Greenstick fractures of the ulna are often difficult to detect, which partly accounts for the fact that Monteggia fractures are frequently overlooked in children.

Patients typically present with severe pain, loss of movement and will be supporting the arm on presentation to the emergency department. The key to successful management of this potentially difficult injury is accurate reduction of the ulnar fracture. As a standard, it is imperative that, in all cases of visible fracture of the ulna, the trauma team check the radial head (Perron et al., 2001). In adults, most will be managed with open reduction and internal fixation, whereas closed reduction and a plaster of Paris cast extending above the elbow is preferred in children. Physiotherapy is often required in these patients.

Galeazzi fracture–dislocations

These are almost mirror images of the Monteggia fracture–dislocations, albeit more common, presenting as a fracture of the distal third of the radial shaft with dislocation/subluxation of the inferior radioulnar joint (Figure 24.17). As above, it is vital that the radioulnar joint is checked in all radial shaft fractures (Perron et al., 2001). Patients characteristically present with swelling, pain and a prominent ulna. In adults, such patients are almost always managed with open reduction and internal fixation, where it is essential that full reduction is achieved, as there may otherwise be impairment of pronation and supination in the long term. In children, these injuries should be

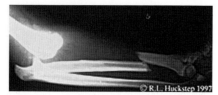

Figure 24.17 Galeazzi fracture.

manipulated and put in plaster in supination; open reduction is seldom required.

Fractures of the wrist and hand

Fractures of the wrist and hand are sustained by increasing numbers of the population across the age span and will be considered in this section. In particular, Colles' fractures and scaphoid fractures will be reviewed in addition to Smith's and Bennett's fractures and fractures of the phalanges. There are other fractures and fracture–dislocations involving the carpal and metacarpals, but these present less commonly, hence readers are guided to other specialist texts relating to wrist and hand injuries.

Colles' fractures

Colles' fractures are commonly presenting injuries, which comprise transverse fractures of the distal radius (3 cm) with dorsal angulation of the distal fragments, characteristically caused by falling on to the outstretched hand. Radial deviation is present as well as swelling and pain. The altered contour of the wrist in a badly displaced Colles' fracture is striking and is referred to as a classic 'dinner-fork deformity' (Figure 24.18). The most common of all fractures in this area, it is mainly seen in middle-aged and elderly women, with osteoporosis frequently cited as a contributory factor. Impaction is not uncommon and occurs when the shaft of the radius is driven into the distal fragment.

Where wrist pain and tenderness over the distal end of the radius are experienced after a fall, x-rays should be taken in every case. The site of maximum tenderness will help to differentiate this injury from a fracture of the scaphoid bone. Where there is marked displacement, the clinical appearance is so characteristic that diagnosis presents no difficulty. Where there is no such

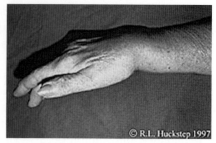

Figure 24.18 Classic 'dinner-fork deformity with Colles' fracture.

marked displacement, diagnosis may be confirmed by x-ray examination; in the majority of cases the fracture is easily identified, only being missed where impaction has rendered the fracture line inconspicuous.

Where fractures are grossly displaced, they should be manipulated and reduced; where they are undisplaced, no manipulation is required. Anaesthesia is necessary for the reduction of this fracture, and either a general anaesthetic or intravenous regional anaesthetic (Bier's block) may be used with success. Repeat x-rays should be taken after the procedure to check positioning and alignment of bones. After treatment through closed reduction, commonly a below-elbow plaster of Paris backslab is applied for 10 days and then replaced by a full plaster of Paris for 6 weeks.

There is much debate regarding optimum management of distal radius fractures, primarily owing to the potential for the common long-term complications. These include stiffness and *carpal tunnel syndrome* (median nerve compression). There is some evidence that surgery will provide optimum functional outcomes of displaced fractures rather than the current practice of closed reduction in emergency departments. Additionally, in some centres, the approach is to apply a full POP immediately following reduction rather than the backslab. The backslab approach has traditionally been popular owing to the risk of compartment syndrome due to initial swelling around the fracture site, but there are those who doubt the efficacy of the backslab as regards maintaining the support of the fracture itself. Much more research is required to ascertain not only the optimum conservative technique (Krishnan, 2002) but also whether these displaced fractures should be treated

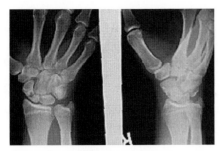

Figure 24.19   Scaphoid fracture.

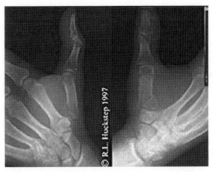

Figure 24.20   Bennett's fracture with dislocation.

conservatively at all. Irrespective of management choice, there is a great need to instruct patients in suitable mobilisation regimes prior to discharge from the trauma area and at follow up, with the involvement of physiotherapy in most cases.

Smith's fractures

This type of fracture may be thought of as a 'reversed Colles' fracture', where there is anterior displacement of the distal fragment visible on x-ray. Patients typically present describing the cause as a fall on a dorsiflexed, supinated hand, and complain of pain, deformity and loss of function. As with Colles' fractures, most may be managed through closed reduction and the application of a long-arm plaster of Paris. Physiotherapy is usually required after removal of the plaster.

Scaphoid fractures

Scaphoid fractures account for 75% of all carpal fractures and frequently result from falling on to the outstretched hand with the wrist dorsiflexed (Figure 24.19). Suspicion should be raised when there is a complaint of pain on the lateral aspect of the wrist following any injury. The typical presentation is of reduced wrist movement, a painful or tender 'anatomical snuffbox' and pain over the scaphoid itself. In true scaphoid fractures, tenderness will also be elicited on the application of pressure over the dorsal aspect of the scaphoid, and also on pressure over the palmar aspect. Tenderness in these additional sites very seldom occurs in other injuries in this area, no matter how severe.

X-rays are required in all suspicious cases. Fractures of the scaphoid are often not seen initially on x-ray, hence patients presenting with the above history and symptoms will be managed as though a fracture were present. In all suspi-

cious but unconfirmed cases, x-rays should be repeated 10–14 days after the injury. Those with confirmed fractures at this stage may be treated conservatively and should have a full plaster of Paris cast applied for 6 weeks (Krasin et al., 2001). If non-union has occurred after more than 12 weeks, open reduction with internal fixation with bone grafting may be performed. Current thinking is suggestive of better outcomes with surgical intervention in those with displaced or intra-articular involvement (Cole, 2002). Long-term complications include avascular necrosis, non-union and osteoarthritis in the wrist.

Bennett's fractures

The most common injuries involving the base of the thumb are Bennett's fractures, fractures of the thumb metacarpal and carpometacarpal dislocation of the thumb (Figure 24.20). Injuries of the thumb base usually result from force being applied along the long axis of the thumb (e.g. from a fall or blow on the clenched fist) or from forced abduction of the thumb. Bennett's fractures, the most common of this group of injuries, can be identified by fracture of the base of the first metacarpal involving the carpometacarpal joint, which is often caused by punching. Management may be through open reduction and internal fixation, commonly with a percutaneus pin and application of a plaster of Paris cast for up to 6 weeks, dependent on the surgeon's preference and severity of injury.

Phalangeal fractures

Phalangeal fractures constitute the most common upper limb injury. Undisplaced simple fractures of the proximal and middle phalanges seldom present problems. Patients typically present with swelling, pain and potential deformity of the affected area.

Treatment with closed reduction and the application of 'neighbour strapping' or 'buddy splinting' is usually adequate, although open reduction and internal fixation may be required where there is joint involvement. Where symptoms are marked, neighbour strapping may be supplemented by the use of a volar or dorsal plaster of Paris slab with finger extension. Various methods of fixation may be used depending on the severity of the injury and preference of individual clinicians including: foam-plastic-covered malleable aluminium splints, rolled bandages, volar POP slabs and intramedullary wires. In all cases, uninjured fingers should be left free and exercised, and rigid fixation should be discarded as soon as possible. Finger stiffness is the most common and most disabling complication, caused by joint adhesions, fibrosis in the adjacent flexor tendon sheaths and collateral ligament shortening. Infection in open fractures may also be a major contributory factor. Stiffness may be minimised by elevation, correct splinting, early mobilisation, and intensive physiotherapy and occupational therapy. Early mobilisation is, therefore, indicated in all patients for optimum long-term function.

Fractures of the terminal phalanges are painful but relatively unimportant injuries. Treatment of any associated soft tissue injuries takes precedence (e.g. debridement and suture of pulp lacerations). Nevertheless, the use of plastic finger splints may relieve pain and prevent any painful stubbing incidents.

Finally, phalangeal injuries that are a result of a crush necessitate vigilant assessment of vascular integrity and neurological function. Comprised blood supply, movement or sensation necessitates early intervention by a hand surgical team, should there be a chance of functional recovery (Reagan et al., 2002).

Mallet fingers

'Mallet fingers' are caused by forced finger flexion from an extended position with either resultant tearing of long extensor tendons from their attachment to the phalanges or avulsion of bone fragments. Patients are unable to extend the distal interphalangeal joints fully, causing drooping of the distal phalanges, which may be slight or severe (Wang and Johnston, 2001). In late cases, there may also be hyperextension of the proximal interphalangeal joints. Patients present with a reduction in movement in the affected finger. Treatment with immobilisation in a 'mallet splint' is adequate in most cases.

> Assessment of neurovascular function is essential in all patients who have sustained fractures

PELVIC FRACTURES

Pelvic anatomy

The anatomy of the pelvis comprises a number of bones and ligaments configured so as to provide support to the pelvic organs. These consist of two fused coxae, ischium, ileum, pubis, coccyx and sacrum. The two halves of the pelvis are joined to the sacrum by the immensely strong sacroiliac ligaments. In front, they are united by the symphysis pubis, an arrangement which forms a cylinder of bone known as the pelvic ring, which protects the pelvic organs. Differences in shape are found between the genders to facilitate childbirth in females.

Generally speaking, the pelvis has three main functions: it transmits weight through the axial skeleton; provides attachment for muscles and ligaments; and, importantly from a trauma perspective, houses terminal parts of reproductive, genitourinary systems and the gastrointestinal tract.

Pelvic fractures account for 3–6% of all fractures and occur in 20% of polytrauma cases, usually occurring as a result of high-velocity blunt trauma from motor vehicle accidents, crush injuries and falls. Mortality is relatively high – 10% in adults and 5% in children – and constitutes one of the few potentially life-threatening orthopaedic injuries. Death from pelvic fractures is the third leading cause of death following motor vehicle accidents, with open fractures being associated with a 30% mortality rate. Associated injuries to the abdomen and chest are indicative of potential high mortality risk.

The complications tend to be more life threatening than the fractures themselves and include haemorrhage, damage to vessels (common and internal and external iliac arteries, lumbar and sacral arteries), bladder, lower lumbar and sacral spinal nerves, terminal ends of the urinary and gastro-intestinal tracts and reproductive systems.

Classification of pelvic fractures

Several classifications of pelvic fractures (Figure 24.21) are used, some of which involve acetabular fractures (Kane type IV). Often, the terms stable and unstable are used to refer to pelvic fractures, and in particular, to pelvic ring stability.

Those fractures involving a stable pelvic ring, which account for 55% of pelvic fractures, usually affect the anterior pelvic or iliac rim. These may be termed Kane type I and II injuries (i.e. there is no interruption or single break to the ring respectively). Unstable injuries, Kane Type III injuries, may be divided into three groups:

1. *lateral compression fractures* – which involve transverse fractures of the pubic rami ipsilateral or contralateral to posterior injury.
2. *anterior-posterior compression fractures* – which involve longitudinal pubic rami fractures and involvement of the sacroiliac joints.

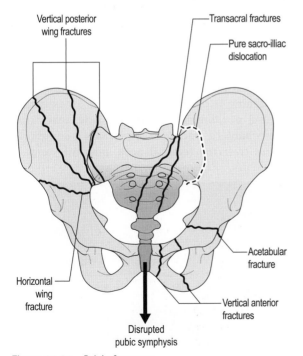

Figure 24.21   Pelvic fractures.

Labels on figure:
Vertical posterior wing fractures
Transacral fractures
Pure sacro-illiac dislocation
Horizontal wing fracture
Acetabular fracture
Vertical anterior fractures
Disrupted pubic symphysis

3. *vertical shear* – often involving vertical displacement through the sacroiliac joints and associated with major complications.

Physical examination

Upon questioning patients typically reveal a history of blunt trauma, and present with tenderness, pain and/or palpable instability over the pelvis on gentle compression and distraction over the iliac wings. Although symptoms are dependent on the severity of fractures, all patients present with reduced mobility. Those with unstable fractures will generally present with an inability to walk. Other symptoms are associated primarily with Type III injuries, resulting from high impact trauma, are worst with vertical shear and may include: rectal, urethral or vaginal bleeding; haematuria; neurological deficit; and haemodynamic instability due to hypovolaemic shock (Routt et al., 2002).

Management of pelvic fractures

Substantial internal haemorrhage commonly occurs with pelvic fractures, particularly where there is disruption of the pelvic ring. The potential for shock must be anticipated in all but the most minor of fractures by: routine blood grouping and cross-matching; establishing good intravenous access; and ongoing monitoring of haemodynamic status, including urinary output where applicable. Replacement requirements are frequently substantial and additional measures for monitoring response may be required. The effect of massive transfusion must be borne in mind and appropriate precautions taken, such as blood warming. Bruising appearing in the scrotum or buttocks, or spreading diffusely along the line of the inguinal ligament is indicative of major internal haemorrhage. In the abdomen, a large peritoneal haemorrhage may be felt as a discrete mass on palpation. Where the peritoneum has been broached, blood may escape into the abdominal cavity. In rare cases, intraperitoneal haemorrhage may result from the tearing of mesenteric vessels.

The complexity of pelvic fractures means that, as a minimum, as well as good plain x-rays, a CT scan should be a standard diagnostic investigation to ascertain the optimum course of management

(Theumann et al., 2002). Arteriograms, urethrogram, diagnostic peritoneal lavage (DPL) and abdominal ultrasound may also be used dependent upon symptoms. In all patients with pelvic fractures, urinalysis should be performed to determine the presence of blood, and a suprapubic catheter passed where urethral injury is suspected. Stable injuries should be treated with rest and appropriate analgesia. Type II injuries may rarely be associated with gastrointestinal and urinary tract injuries; these should be addressed accordingly. In those patients with Type III injuries, priorities for management are the control of haemorrhage, fluid replacement, provision of adequate appropriate analgesia, internal–external fixation and treatment of associated injuries. Where open fractures with gastrointestinal involvement have been sustained, a temporary colostomy may be indicated. Where neurological deficit has been sustained, bladder and bowel management are necessitated. The need for anticoagulation therapy may also be indicated in some patients.

Complications of pelvic fractures are numerous and may occur at any stage in the patient's recovery. Ischaemia in one leg is of grave significance and may be due to rupture or damage of an iliac artery. In addition to those mentioned above, complications include paralytic ileus, rupture of the diaphragm, limb shortening, neurological damage, obstetric difficulties, persistent sacroiliac joint pain, persistent symphyseal instability and osteoarthritis of the hip.

> Haemodynamic status should be closely monitored in all patients with pelvic fractures

TRAUMA TO THE LOWER LIMB

Lower limb fractures

Classification of hip fractures

Hip fractures are classified according to their specific location. Common broad classifications comprise three types: fractures of the femoral head and neck, often referred to as intracapsular fractures, which account for 53%; intertrochanteric fractures; and subtrochanteric fractures – 5 cm below. The latter two groups are often referred to as extracapsular fractures and account for 47% of hip fractures. Many more classifications exist (e.g.

Garden, Lavarde) that aim to allow comparisons between populations, and provide education with regard to surgical techniques and prognosis.

Patients generally fall into one of two distinct groups: falls in the elderly, often associated with older, postmenopausal women with osteoporosis (Figure 24.22); and, less commonly, younger patients who sustain their injury through high-velocity trauma. Motor vehicle accidents account for up to 75% of these. Consequently there is a 3:1 female to male ratio. Other documented risk factors have been outlined including dementia, institutional living, previous fractures, low body weight, alcohol abuse and impaired vision. As 50% of these fractures occur in those aged over 80 years, there will often be additional pathology present that in some cases may have resulted in a fall. As well as the potential for increased preoperative and postoperative problems in the long term, displaced fractures of femoral neck and femoral head fractures can often lead to avascular necrosis (Bachiller et al., 2002). Other secondary complications such as DVT, fat emboli, pressure ulcers, chest infection and non-union or malunion have all been reported in the literature with frequency (Webb, 2002).

Assessment of hip fractures

In most cases, there is a history of falling or major trauma, often with associated risk factors. Patients generally present with pain and an inability to move the hip or to bear weight. Evidence of limb shortening is present in most, as is an externally rotated position in the affected side, other than in trochanteric fractures. Tenderness is commonly found over the femoral neck anteriorly and, in

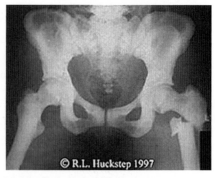

© R.L. Huckstep 1997

Figure 24.22 Pathological hip fracture.

extracapsular fractures, over the greater trochanter. Bruising is a late sign in extracapsular fractures, but is absent in acute injuries and in intracapsular fractures.

Anteroposterior and lateral x-rays confirm the site and severity of most fractures. MRI scanning is usually necessary only where the fracture is not obvious or has major soft tissue involvement. As with all patients who have sustained fractures, ongoing neurovascular assessment is vital. Management includes immobilisation of the affected limb, intravenous access and fluid replacement, blood samples taken for grouping and cross-match, effective analgesia usually given via the intravenous route, and pre-operative siting of an indwelling urethral catheter. A full medical assessment to determine fitness for anaesthesia is also essential.

Fractures of the neck of femur

Fractures of the femoral neck are generally classed according to their level. The AO classification or the 'Garden' classifications (Box 24.8) are the most commonly used international classifications. With Garden type I fractures there is an incomplete fracture through the femoral neck, whereas in the Garden type II category, the fracture is complete. Both types I and II are associated with no obvious displacement of the fragments relative to each other. Type III fractures are associated with complete fractures and a degree of impaction and displacement. Garden type IV fractures may be identified by superior migration of the femoral neck relative to the femoral head, and have the highest risk of avascular necrosis. Types III and IV carry the worst prognosis.

Box 24.8   Garden classification of neck of femur fractures

Garden type I	Incomplete fracture through the femoral neck
Garden type II	Complete fracture through the femoral neck
Garden type III	Complete fracture associated with impaction
Garden type IV	Femoral neck is superiorly migrated relative to the femoral head

---

Although most authors agree that early surgery is indicated, it has been suggested that up to 20% may wait for longer than 72 hours (Scottish Intercollegiate Group Network, 2000). The advent of 'fast-tracking' systems for this patient population has potentially improved this situation. Management is by surgical reduction as soon as theatre time allows. If the fracture is undisplaced, then internal fixation with screws is the most common procedure. If the fracture is displaced, although internal fixation may be possible, many progress to prosthetic replacement; this will usually be the first choice if other orthopaedic pathology exists, e.g. Paget's disease or rheumatoid arthritis, in the affected joint. Mobilisation should be commenced as soon as possible after the procedure, often including physiotherapy. This is particularly important in the elderly owing to the well-documented dangers associated with prolonged bed rest.

Femoral head fractures

Fractures of the femoral head most commonly occur as a consequence of anterior hip dislocation. Consequently, closed or open reduction and internal fixation with screws are often indicated. Where larger fragments are present, prosthetic replacement may be considered. The main postoperative aim is to restore patients to full weight-bearing capacity by the fifth day, with restrictions on the range of movement that can be undertaken for the following 3 months.

Intertrochanteric fractures

Fractures of this type occurring at the base of the neck have a number of points in their favour. As this is a well-vascularised area compared to the femoral neck and head, the longer-term complications of avascular necrosis and non-union are rare. This does, however, mean that haemorrhage and consequent hypovolaemia are possible in these patients, and must be borne in mind with this patient group. Also, owing to the size of the neck and head fragments, good internal fixation can usually be achieved, and early weight bearing after this is usually possible.

Most patients progress to surgery for fixation with a dynamic hip screw or intramedullary nails/ rods. On the rare occasions that a non-surgical management strategy is followed, patients will usually be in traction for 6–12 weeks dependent on surgeon preference and the rate of healing.

Subtrochanteric fractures

Subtrochanteric fractures constitute the most common site of pathological fractures. As this area is well vascularised, haemorrhage may again pose a problem. Where the patient's general condition is very poor, pain relief may be obtained by applying traction via a Thomas splint. In all other cases, surgical fixation will be undertaken where possible, and intramedullary nails/rods inserted as the most common surgical technique (Sims, 2002). Prosthetic devices are not usually an option owing to the anchoring limitations, resulting from the underlying pathology, e.g. osteoporosis.

Femoral shaft fractures

Fractures of the femoral shaft comprise three main types, namely spiral or transverse (most common), comminuted (Figure 24.23) or compound (Figure 24.24). Associated injuries are common, as the mechanism of injury is often high-impact trauma from a direct blow or indirect force transmitted from the knee. Considerable force is usually required to fracture the femur, the most common causes being road traffic accidents, falls from a height and crush injuries. Pathological fractures owing to osteoporosis are common in the elderly, where there is an associated mortality rate of approximately 15%.

Patients commonly present with visible deformity, tenderness ranging to severe pain dependent on the severity of the injury, limb shortening and crepitus. Blood loss of more than 1.5 litres is common from the fracture itself, and is more in open fractures (may be doubled) or where there are other associated injuries. Hypovolaemic shock is, therefore, commonplace in this patient group. Neurovascular assessment is essential in all cases. Immediate management consists of fluid replacement, haemodynamic monitoring, intravenous pain relief and immobilisation of the affected limb (Russell et al., 2002). Prophylactic intravenous antibiotics should be administered in those with open fractures and blood taken for group and cross-matching. Traction may be applied in an attempt to reduce the fracture to a near normal alignment and reduce local bleeding and shock, particularly in the out-of-hospital setting, although most will progress to surgery rapidly, particularly those with open fractures or other tissue involvement. Adults are generally surgically managed with internal fixation using intramedullary nailing. Children, on the other hand, may be treated with traction for a period of 4 weeks, followed by a body spica. Significantly, femoral shaft fractures comprise the major risk for *fat embolism syndrome*, which may ensue as early as 12 hours following injury.

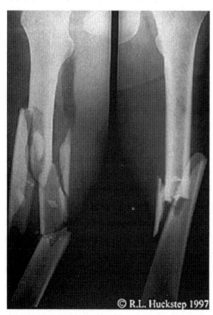

Figure 24.23 Bilateral comminuted femoral shaft fractures.

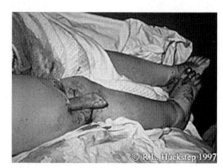

Figure 24.24 Compound femur fracture with early gangrene.

Knee fractures

Fractures of the knee include fractures of the patella, femoral condyles, tibial tuberosities and tibial plateau, and can be caused by direct and indirect forces. Trauma, both direct and indirect, may be the causes as well as chronic stress and pathologic conditions. Patients may present with oedema, crepitus, pain, limb shortening or rotation, and will have the potential for compromised neurovascular status. Popliteal artery injury may result from a displaced distal femur or from tibial plateau fractures, while peroneal nerve injury may occur as a consequence of a fracture of the proximal fibula. AP, lateral and oblique x-ray views are required to confirm the diagnosis and to determine the severity of the injury. Other complications include compartment syndrome, fat embolism syndrome and, in the long term, delayed union or non-union, post-traumatic arthritis, knee stiffness and chondromalacia patella.

The relatively abundant cartilage around the paediatric knee may make diagnosis more difficult on x-ray and so merit MRI scanning for all those injuries that are clinically suspicious in the child (Zionts, 2002).

Fractures of the patella

Patellar fractures are invariably caused by a direct blow to the front of the knee. Other causes include road traffic accidents in which the knee strikes the fascia, falls against hard surfaces such as the edge of a step, and by heavy objects falling across the knee. Symptoms include an inability to extend the knee, bruising and abrasions, any palpable gap above or below the patella, and obvious proximal displacement of the patella. In all cases, x-rays are required to confirm the diagnosis; AP and lateral views will normally suffice (Figures 24.25 and 24.26). Non-displaced patellar fractures may be treated conservatively with knee immobilisers, with patients partially weight bearing for up to 6 weeks. In some patients, a similar time in a cylinder plaster of Paris cast may be preferred. Displaced fractures, or fractures associated with a disrupted extensor mechanism, require exploration and possibly open reduction and internal fixation. Open fractures will progress to surgery quickly for debridement and irrigation. Physiotherapy and instructions regarding appropriate exercise regimens may prove to be useful.

Patellar fractures are commonly associated with ligament damage notably the anterior cruciate

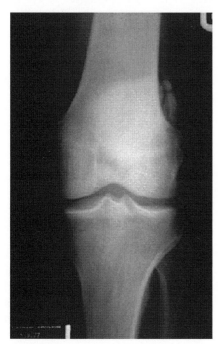

Figure 24.25 Patella fracture (AP view).

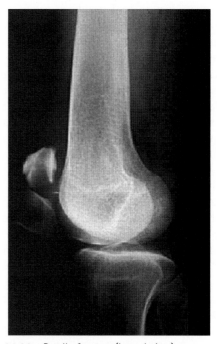

Figure 24.26 Patella fracture (lateral view).

ligament. Less commonly the posterior cruciate ligament and menisci may also be damaged. Management of these is covered in detail within the sports injury chapter.

Femoral condyle fractures

Femoral condyle fractures may be classed as supracondylar, intercondylar, or condylar, and occur in patients across the age span. These are usually associated with a fall from a height or direct trauma. Patients will commonly present with point tenderness, swelling and potential joint instability around the knee. Diagnosis will be confirmed with x-ray, although some patients should progress to CT or MRI if there is some evidence of displacement.

In children, fractures of the distal third of the femur are frequently only minimally displaced and may be successfully treated by the application of a cylinder plaster of Paris cast. Weight bearing should not be permitted until there is x-ray evidence of early union; however, mobilisation with crutches may be permitted during this period. In adults, supracondylar fractures have a tendency for the distal fragment to rotate due in part to the pull of the gastrocnemius. Where fractures are undisplaced, mobilisation should be started as soon as possible to avoid the not inconsiderable risk of knee stiffness. Where fractures are displaced or where a good reduction cannot be maintained by conservative methods, surgical intervention in the form of internal fixation is likely. Undisplaced tibial plateau fractures should similarly be immobilised and treated conservatively, whereas displaced or depressed fractures are likely to require open reduction and internal fixation (Figure 24.27).

Fractures of the tibia and fibula

Fractures of the tibia are the most common of long bone fractures and are usually transverse or oblique, although spiral fractures may be sustained following twisting injuries (Figures 24.28 and 24.29). Isolated fibular fractures may occur as a result of a direct blow, but are rare. Open fractures are common, and loss of limb may occur as a consequence of severe soft tissue trauma, compartment syndrome or infection, hence the importance of ongoing neurovascular

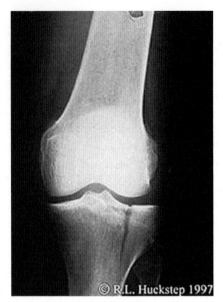

Figure 24.27 Tibial plateau fracture.

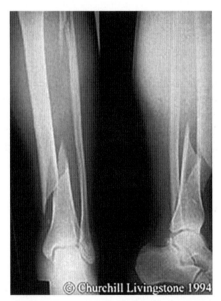

Figure 24.28 Tibia and fibula fracture.

assessment. Fractures of the tibia and fibula are the most common site of delayed or non-union in long bones and, as such, may be associated with an increased incidence of complications. Peroneal nerve injury may also occur, manifesting as foot drop, often associated with fractures of the fibular neck.

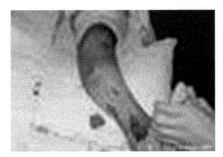

Figure 24.29 Tibial fracture.

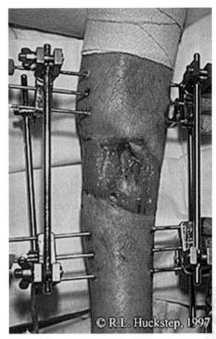

Figure 24.30 Osteomyelitis following tibial fracture with external fixator.

Assessment and management of tibial and fibular fractures Most patients present with a history of direct trauma, such as that occurring in a motor vehicle accident, from a direct blow or fall from a height, or indirect trauma, such as that sustained through twisting. As the tibia is vulnerable to torsional stresses, for example, in sporting injuries, and force transmitted through the feet, the incidence of injury is high. Patients with tibial fractures tend to present with pain, swelling and an inability to walk. Deformity and crepitus are also often present.

Diagnosis is confirmed by x-ray examination with AP and lateral x-ray views normally undertaken. Intravenous analgesia will enhance patient comfort and enable a full assessment to be undertaken. Open fractures require immediate surgery for debridement, in addition to tetanus prophylaxis and intravenous antibiotics as a standard intervention. Stable undisplaced closed fractures are generally managed by reduction and immobilisation in a plaster of Paris cast, whereas unstable oblique and spiral fractures generally require reduction and fixation, traditionally internally. Unstable transverse and comminuted fractures require 'blind' intramedullary nailing from the upper end of the tibia. Ilizarov frames are commonly used, particularly in those with associated soft tissue injury (Figure 24.30). The correction of angulation in this weight-bearing bone is particularly important as, unlike angulation in femoral shaft fractures, which can be compensated at the hip, residual angulation in tibial fractures may create stress at the ankle and/or the knee, leading to pain and secondary osteoarthritis.

Neurovascular assessment on initial presentation and on an ongoing basis is absolutely vital for the early detection of problems and early intervention. Tibial fractures are the most common site for compartment syndrome, particularly in those with open and/or comminuted fractures (see neurovascular complications section). Major associated soft tissue injury may necessitate discussion relating to the viability of the limb. Although this falls outside the scope of this chapter, there is much debate within the orthopaedic community regarding the merits of limb salvage versus amputation in severe cases (Tomaino, 2001).

Toddler's fracture is a distal spiral fracture of the tibia, and is most common in children aged between 9 months and 3 years. Sudden twisting of the tibia following a fall, slip or trip comprise the main causes. Often this is unwitnessed by parents/guardians, so an exact history may not be possible.

The child will present with minor swelling, may be reluctant to bear weight comfortably on the affected leg and will have pain. Detection may be difficult, as fractures are not easily visible on x-ray initially and CT scan may aid confirmation of diagnosis. Management is usually in a cast with the usual instructions given to parents.

Relating the presenting injury to the mechanism of injury is vital as with all fractures in children. Child abuse may be suspected in mid-shaft fractures of the tibia that appear unrelated to significant trauma. Standard interventions in relation to potential non-accidental injury should be implemented in such cases.

Isolated fibular fractures present less of a management challenge in that the associated symptoms and potential complications are significantly less than in tibial fractures. Immediate ambulation is often possible with isolated fractures of the fibula. In patients with isolated mid-shaft or proximal fibular fractures, immobilisation is not usually required. Such patients can usually be discharged from the emergency department with analgesia and instructed to bear weight as tolerated. Standard practice dictates that such patients are reviewed in the fracture clinic, hence a follow-up appointment should be made.

Ankle fractures and dislocation

Fractures of the ankle are common and can result from eversion, inversion, external rotation and vertical compression injuries (e.g. following falls from a height). Many occur during the course of walking or running, where additional forces are transmitted through the ankle joint. Haemarthrosis, changes in the foot relative to the ankle, deformity, swelling, bruising, point tenderness, discoloration, temperature changes (especially cold), and an inability to bear weight are all indicative of a fracture. Open fractures are associated with a high risk of infection; intravenous antibiotic therapy is, therefore, always indicated. Where fractures are associated with a dislocation, neurovascular compromise inevitably results, necessitating immediate reduction. AP, lateral and mortise x-ray views are required to obtain a full radiological picture of the extent and type of fracture.

As ankle injuries comprise a major musculoskeletal trauma group, there have been attempts to limit the number of unnecessary x-rays in light of the fact that the majority of these will be soft tissue rather than bony injury. Evidence seems to support the use of the 'Ottawa rules' as an accurate instrument for excluding ankle fracture and reduces the number of ankle x-rays by up to 40% (Bachmann et al., 2003). In brief, the assessment comprises observation of the patient's ability to walk four steps and assessment of six potential points of tenderness (Figure 24.31). An inability to walk or tenderness over the points necessitates further assessment through x-ray.

As the ankle is a complicated joint, many attempts to classify ankle fractures have been made. The term Potts fracture, once commonly used to describe the more severe ankle fractures, has now essentially been superseded by other classifications (e.g. Weber), which provide more information as to potential management strategies.

Injuries to the ankle are, in essence, at one or more of three points, namely the medial malleolus of the tibia, the lower end of the fibula involving the lateral malleolus, and the posterior margin of the tibia (posterior malleolus). Fractures of one (single malleolar fracture), or more than one (bimalleolar, trimalleolar fractures) together with potential damage to the three key ligaments and the inferior tibiofibular syndesmosis, determine the severity and management of the injury.

Diagnosis of the type and severity of fracture will be ascertained through x-ray as previously described, and potentially CT or MRI scan, particularly in those that will progress to surgical intervention.

Management strategies depend on the severity of the injury. Undisplaced single malleolar fractures can be managed in below-knee plaster of Paris casts for around 6 weeks. Patients may be discharged home from the emergency department, if appropriate, with plaster instructions, crutches, and instructions to remain non-weight bearing for 2 weeks, with follow-up review in the fracture clinic. Generally, patients will be allowed to bear weight for the remaining 4 weeks, if the follow-up x-ray views are satisfactory. Avulsion fractures (Weber A) may not require casting; patients may be discharged with mild analgesia and a follow-up fracture clinic appointment. Bimalleolar and trimalleolar fractures will almost certainly require surgical management with plates, wires or screws dependent on the type and extent of fracture and ligament damage.

More so than most injuries, ankle fractures are often responsible for secondary complications

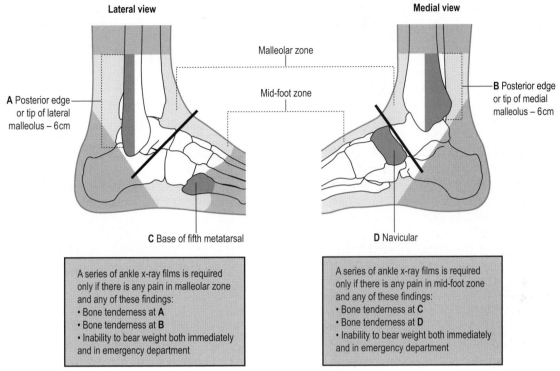

Figure 24.31   Ottawa rules assessment.

(Leyes et al., 2003). The ankle is a complex joint and surgical intervention to restore pre-injury function is often difficult, hence inadequate fixation or intra-articular penetration of hardware are risks. Pre-operatively and postoperatively, compartment syndrome and infection comprise the major secondary complications for the first few days and late complications, such as joint stiffness and osteoarthritis, have also been reported.

Ankle dislocations occur as a result of high-impact trauma and are associated with both fracture and significant soft-tissue damage with neurovascular compromise (Figure 24.32). The management of these injuries is difficult and remains controversial. Reduction of the dislocation should be attempted at the earliest opportunity. Internal fixation with or without external fixation in combination with aggressive soft tissue management is thought, in severe cases, to provide an opportunity for healing of the joint capsule and associated structures, and to facilitate good long-term outcome (Pearse et al., 1995).

Injuries to the foot

This section will briefly outline fractures to the talus, calcaneum, tarsus and phalanges. The foot is in a vulnerable position and bears the weight of the body, hence is often subject to forces resulting in injury. As well as fractures, severe forces may result in fracture dislocation (Figure 24.33).

Fractured talus

This injury is usually as a result of twisting forces to the foot or sudden dorsiflexion with force, and may be fractured through the body, neck or lower, resulting in osteochondral fracture. The patient will present with pain, swelling and reduced mobility. These fractures are notoriously problematic from a long-term perspective. Osteoarthritis, avascular necrosis and non-union are all reported. Fractures of the neck must be managed surgically and internally fixed. Other injuries may be managed conservatively through early mobilisation, as pain allows, unless there is major displacement (often associated with other severe injuries).

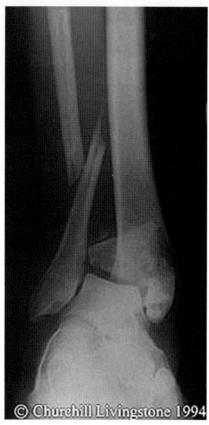

Figure 24.32   Ankle dislocation.

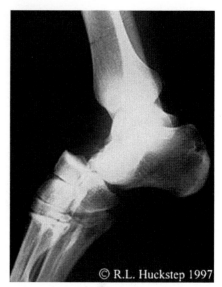

Figure 24.33   Mid-foot dislocation.

Fractured calcaneum

The usual injury history of fractured calcaneum involves a fall from a height on to the heel. It is often a difficult fracture to see on x-ray. The classic symptoms are severe pain around the heel, an inability to put the foot on the ground and, if presentation to accident and emergency is a few hours postinjury, there may be a 'horseshoe-shaped' bruise starting to appear around the heel.

Management depends on severity. If the fracture is undisplaced or a mild displacement is present only, it will be treated conservatively with a period of non-weight-bearing of up to 6 weeks. Major displacement usually merits surgical intervention with open reduction and bone grafting.

Fractured tarsus

These are rarely injured and any fracture will be associated with a dislocation. Again these are difficult for all but the experienced eye to see on x-ray. Diagnosis and management with open reduction and internal fixation is required to prevent long-term deformity.

Metatarsal fractures

These are commonly caused by a direct blow from a falling object. There will be swelling, pain and point tenderness directly over the fracture. Undisplaced fractures should not require any more intervention than a firm crepe bandage. A cast is usually not indicated and, indeed, may adversely influence mobility in the medium term owing to developing stiffness. Multiple displaced fractures are usually associated with a crush-type injury and may involve a degree of dislocation of the tarsometatarsal joints. Such cases often require immobilisation with percutaneous pins.

Fractures of the phalanges

These are common injuries again due to a blow from a falling object. Patients will present with pain and swelling. Such injuries rarely require any intervention apart from elevation of the foot until swelling subsides and pain relief. Toes may be 'buddy-splinted' for comfort or following reduction of any rotational deformity.

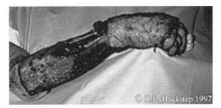

Figure 24.35 Upper limb degloving injury.

This should be gently irrigated with Hartmann's solution or normal saline, wrapped in a wet swab and finally, placed in a plastic bag and the bag then placed in ice (*but not directly on the ice*). Surgical intervention is then required. Firstly, the bone is shortened and fixed. The nerves are then repaired prior to anastomosing the arteries, then the veins. Finally, the flexor and extensor tendons are repaired and skin coverage performed.

Degloving injuries

The term 'degloving injury' refers to the skin being peeled back over the bones usually due to the limb being caught and pulled violently. Common sites include forearm, hands and fractures of the tibia and fibula (Figure 24.35). Referral for plastic surgery to replace the affected area with a skin graft should be actioned. Further discussion of major soft tissue damage associated with tibia fractures is discussed within that section.

EMERGENCIES AS A CONSEQUENCE OF ORTHOPAEDIC CONDITIONS

Acute compartment syndrome

The arterial blood flow distal to a fracture is occasionally interrupted; assessment of the circulation in fractured limbs, therefore, forms an essential part of the examination. Such interruption of arterial blood flow may result in loss of distal pulses, pallor and coldness of the skin, loss of capillary responses, severe pain in the limb, paraesthesia and eventually muscle paralysis. Within individual muscle compartments, deep fascia envelops the limbs. Other fascial planes divide the limbs into compartments. Fascia itself is tough inelastic connective tissue, the purpose of which is to maintain the muscle compartments with their respective vessels and nerves, and to

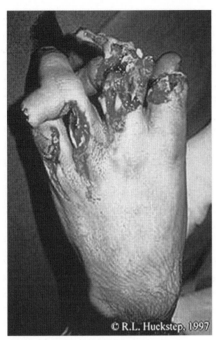

Figure 24.34 Crush injury to fingers.

EXTREMITY TRAUMA

Traumatic amputation

Traumatic amputation accounts for approximately 10% of all amputations. Road traffic accidents and industrial injuries are the major modes of injury. Re-implantation is indicated in thumb amputations, multiple digit amputations, metacarpal amputations, almost any body part in a child, and in wrist or forearm amputations. In some instances, reimplantation is contraindicated, particularly for severely crushed or mangled parts (see MESS score in soft tissue injury chapter), where there are amputations at multiple levels, amputations in patients with other serious injuries or diseases, and where the vessels are arteriosclerotic.

In those with severe injury owing to 'crushing' of limbs and digits (Figure 24.34), although the injured part may not have been amputated at time of injury, extensive vascular and soft tissue damage may result in surgical amputation being indicated.

Digital reimplantation
Success of reimplantation is dependent on appropriate care of the affected part being provided.

enhance the power of the muscle during contraction. Limbs have a variable number of compartments; the forearm has two, the thigh has three and the lower leg has four.

In trauma, the major fractures that result in compartment syndrome are tibial fractures, especially comminuted fractures and fractures of the forearm. Additionally, traumatic crush injuries, which can be thought of as a multicompartment syndrome, burns and prolonged limb compression, are among the commonest causes. The normal lower limb venous pressure is a few millimeters of mercury, creating normal intracompartmental pressures within the range 0–10 mmHg. This level of pressure neither interferes with blood flow nor the transmission of nerve impulses. In *acute compartment syndrome* (ACS), as the name suggests, there is an alteration of this normal level. This occurs as a result of an increase in this pressure as a consequence of either an increase in compartment contents, such as haemorrhage, oedema from injury, or a decrease in compartment size (e.g. as a result of external pressure from a tight bandage or plaster cast).

This increased pressure results in initial venous compromise and may progress to reduced capillary flow, which exacerbates the ischaemic insult and further increases pressure. A vicious cycle of increasing pressures may, therefore, be initiated, ultimately resulting in permanent damage. Arterial inflow is rarely reduced unless pressure exceeds systolic blood pressures.

A history of injury or the presence of a cast or compression bandage should alert the nurse to the potential for compartment syndrome. Signs and symptoms of neurovascular compromise are often referred to as the five 'Ps': pain, pallor, paraesthesia, paralysis and pulselessness. However, in acute compartment syndrome, these are not clinically reliable because they are frequently late signs. Pain that is disproportionate to the original injury or precipitating factor is the earliest and most significant symptom of compartment syndrome in alerting the nurse to the possibility of ACS. This is caused by increasing pressure on the nerve endings. Classically, the pain is described as severe and unrelenting, unrelieved by opiate medication, and a sign of muscle ischemia. Pain from ACS is progressive and will intensify with passive stretching of the digits of the affected extremity sometimes referred to as stretch pain. Paraesthesia, such as numbness or a burning sensation, is indicative of increased oedema and tissue pressure. Pallor reflects decreased oxygen delivery to the tissues. Muscle weakness may occur, and progress to paresis and paralysis of the affected extremity, indicating tissue necrosis, while pulselessness is a late and ominous sign.

Table 24.4 indicates the compartments and their respective nerves. This may give an indication of the affected compartment during the physical assessment of the patient with suspected ACS, and hence guide intervention.

Pressure monitoring

Intracompartmental pressure can be measured by several means including: wick catheter, simple needle manometry, infusion techniques, pressure transducers and side-ported needles. Despite various suggestions, there is presently no consensus agreement on the absolute critical pressure for diagnosing compartment syndrome requiring surgical intervention. Three methods and parameters may be considered:

- an absolute intracompartmental pressure greater than 30 mmHg
- a difference between diastolic pressure and intracompartmental pressure of greater than 30 mmHg
- a difference between mean arterial pressure and intracompartmental pressure of greater than 40 mmHg.

Where the cause is external, for example, constricting casts or splints, or these are contributory factors, it should be removed. If there is no improvement, prompt fasciotomy is required. The skin and deep fascia should be divided along the length of the compartment, and the wound left open. This may ultimately require closure or skin grafting days later. Timely surgery produces a positive functional outcome, however, delay may result in muscle ischaemia and necrosis.

Crush syndrome

Crush syndrome, or traumatic rhabdomyolysis, occurs as a consequence of major trauma and

Table 24.4   Muscle compartments

	Compartment	Muscle type	Nerve	Muscles
Brachium	Anterior	Flexor muscles	Musculocutaneous nerve	Coracobrachialis, biceps brachii, brachialis
	Posterior	Extensor muscles	Radial nerve	Triceps brachii
Antebrachium	Anterior	Flexor muscles (plus pronator)	Median and ulnar nerves	Pronator teres, flexor carpi radialis, palmaris longus, flexor carpi ulnaris, flexor digitorum superficialis, flexor digitorum profundum
	Posterior	Extensor muscles (plus supinator)	Radial nerve	Brachioradialis, extensor carpi radialis longus, extensor digitorum, extensor carpi ulnaris supinator
Thigh	Anterior	Flexor muscles at the hip	Femoral nerve	Quadriceps femoris sartorius
	Anteromedial	Adductor muscles	Obturator nerve	Adductor longus, adductor brevis, adductor magnus, anterior portion gracilus
	Posterior	Extensor muscles at the hip, flexors at the knee	Sciatic nerve	Hamstrings
Lower leg	Anterior	Dorsiflexors of the foot	Deep peroneal nerve	Tibialis anterior, extensor digitorum longus
	Lateral	Evertors of the foot (from fibula)	Superficial peroneal nerve	Peroneus longus, peroneus brevis
	Posterior	Plantar flexors of the foot	Tibial nerve	Gastrocnemius, soleus posterior, flexor digitorum longus, tibialis

results when there are prolonged compression forces to the limbs. It is common in patients who are involved in major disasters, such as building collapse, train accidents and bombings. Crush syndrome may start to develop after 1 hour in a severe crush; however, 4–6 hours of compression are commonly required for the processes that cause crush syndrome to occur. The associated effects of this muscle injury are the release of toxins, which in large quantities will cause systemic symptoms, and may be fatal. The full effect of crush injury may not be clear at the time of injury (i.e. when the limb remains crushed). However, when the injured parts are freed, the disintegration of the muscle tissue has the effect of releasing myoglobin, potassium and phosphorus into the circulation. This release of substances from the ischaemic muscle causes a wide variety of systemic issues, summarised in Table 24.5. These should form the basis for a battery of tests to determine the severity of the syndrome and potential interventions required to minimise the risk of mortality. Additionally, an accurate history, including an estimate of compression time and

length of time since extraction, may indicate potential severity as well as the progression of symptoms.

As well as the complex set of variables outlined above, the majority of patients will be in hypovolaemic shock, as well as exhibiting signs of compartment syndrome in the affected compartments, and may soon show evidence of hyperkalaemia with ECG changes. Initial management follows that of any multitrauma patient. With regard to the specifics of crush syndrome, aggressive fluid management is vital not only to manage the hypovolaemia but also to correct the electrolyte imbalance. Sodium bicarbonate is thought to be useful both in reversing the acidosis and in increasing the pH of the urine, and is thought to decrease the precipitation of myoglobin in the kidneys. With reference to hyperkalaemia, other drugs may also be given dependent on the severity of the injury (e.g. insulin, furosemide, and calcium), depending on local regimes. Mannitol has also traditionally been prescribed to offer renal protection and to increase cardiac contractility. Urine output must be monitored closely, the

Table 24.5 Substances released as a result of muscle disintegration following crush injury

Substance	Effect
Amino acids and other organic acids	Contribute to acidosis, aciduria and dysrhythmia
Creatine phosphokinase (CPK) and other intracellular enzymes	Serve as laboratory markers for crush injury
Free radicals, superoxides, peroxides	Formed when oxygen is reintroduced into ischaemic tissue, causing further tissue damage
Histamine	Vasodilation, bronchoconstriction
Lactic acid	Major contributor to acidosis and dysrhythmias
Leukotrienes	Lung (ARDS) and hepatic injury
Lysozymes	Cell-digesting enzymes that cause further cellular injury
Myoglobin	Precipitates in kidney tubules, especially in the setting of acidosis with low urine pH; leads to renal failure
Nitric oxide	Causes vasodilation, which worsens haemodynamic shock
Phosphate	Hyperphosphataemia causes precipitation of serum calcium, leading to hypocalcaemia and dysrhythmias
Potassium	Hyperkalaemia causes dysrhythmias, especially when associated with acidosis and hypocalcaemia
Prostaglandins	Vasodilation, lung injury
Purines (uric acid)	May cause further renal damage (nephrotoxic)
Thromboplastin	Disseminated intravascular coagulation (DIC)

ARDS, acute respiratory distress syndrome.

aim being to maintain a urine output of at least 200 ml/hour and a pH higher than 6.5. Prophylactic intravenous antibiotics, analgesia, appropriate wound management and tetanus prophylaxis are all standard interventions. Studies have been shown to suggest the benefits of hyperbaric chambers; however, access remains a key issue.

Fat embolism syndrome

Fat embolism syndrome (FES) is associated with fractures to the long bones and pelvis, the incidence increasing in those with multiple skeletal fractures. Two theories related to the development of FES have been proposed. Firstly, bone marrow fat globules from the fracture site are released into damaged vessels and the systemic circulation. These may be large enough to interfere with blood flow within the pulmonary microcirculation. Secondly, abnormal amounts of free fatty acids are released as part of the body's metabolic response to stress following a fracture. Again the result is the potential for large globules to block capillaries. It is also thought that this latter mechanism may be exacerbated by the presence of shock.

Only a small proportion of patients (1–3%) develop the classical fat embolism syndrome characterised by three classical symptoms. These are *respiratory distress*, *mental disturbances* and a *petechial skin rash* occurring within 72 hours of the injury on the upper, anterior part of the body (e.g. upper arm, chest and neck). Patients will also present with the non-specific symptoms of tachycardia, elevated temperature, hypoxaemia, and occasionally mild neurological symptoms (Parisi et al., 2002).

Chest x-ray will often demonstrate a 'snow-storm' appearance with evenly distributed, fleck-like pulmonary shadows as well as increased pulmonary markings. Other diagnostic tests tend to be unhelpful as a general rule. Although blood can be tested for serum lipase, haematocrit and cytology for fat globules, these tests will not necessarily indicate the presence of FES. There is sufficient evidence to suggest that reduction of long bone fractures as soon as possible after the injury is the most effective preventative measure, hence many are taken to theatre as soon as possible. Attempts to reverse any deficit in circulating volume are vital to minimise the exacerbating effect of hypovolaemia. It has been suggested that a proportion of the replacement fluids should be albumin, as this may bind to circulating fatty acids. Obviously, any respiratory problems require to be managed with appropriate oxygenation and potentially ventilatory support in severe cases. An increasing body of support is developing for the administration of high-dose corticosteroids in preventing the development of FES, but to date this is not an established treatment.

Neurovascular injury

Peripheral nerve injury

Peripheral nerve injuries may be broadly classified as being 'open', whereby there is an open wound (e.g. from gunshot, stabbing or compound fracture), or 'closed' in which case there is no obvious external connection to the air. Such closed injuries may be caused by the following.

- In a closed fracture, nerves could be damaged by direct injury by the fracture ends (e.g. radial nerve palsy in a mid-shaft fracture of the humerus).
- In dislocations, the nerve could be damaged by stretching of the nerve by the displaced bone end (e.g. sciatic nerve palsy in dislocated hip).
- Traction of the nerve, as in falls from a height or road traffic accidents (e.g. brachial plexus paralysis).
- Compression due to external pressure on the nerve (e.g. wrist drop as in crutch palsy owing to compression in the axilla, or foot drop owing to lateral popliteal nerve palsy as a complication of a below-knee cast or pressure from a 'Thomas splint').

Seddon's classification of nerve injury, based on the basis of structural changes in the cut nerves, is commonly used and comprises the following.

- *Neurotmesis*: complete anatomic division of the nerve fibres with obvious discontinuity of the nerve sheath.
- *Axonotmesis*: microscopic division of nerve fibres (axons) without obvious discontinuity of the nerve sheath.
- *Neuropraxia*: injury without any anatomical discontinuity but resulting in functional disruption (nerve concussion).

Physical assessment for nerve injuries

Clearly the history of injury, particularly in violent trauma, may be indicative of nerve injury and merits a full examination for peripheral nerve injury. More specifically, particular fracture locations carry a risk of associated nerve injury and form part of the assessment regime for that particular fracture. These are summarised in Tables 24.6 and 24.7.

Comprehensive assessment and documentation of nerve involvement following fracture is vital not only to offer guidance as to appropriate management but also to utilise as a baseline to determine potential worsening of an injury. This assessment should include the following components:

- Motor power in relevant myotomes to be assessed using the Medical Research Council muscle grading score:
  0 – nil (no power at all)
  1 – muscle flicker only present (no power to move the joint)
  2 – power to move a joint but only when gravity is eliminated
  3 – power to move a joint against gravity
  4 – power to move a joint against gravity and resistance
  5 – normal power.
- Sensory function in relevant dermatomes to be assessed through objective testing to touch and pin prick as well as noting any subjective reports of burning, tingling or paraesthesia.
- Presence of any other motor signs notably anhidrosis (an area of dry skin due to absence of sweating).
- Tropic changes in the skin, for example, skin smoothness and shiny areas, ulceration and subcutaneous tissue atrophy.
- Reflex testing.
- Tinel's sign – an indication of recovery whereby the injured nerve is trapped and the point at which sensation and motor function are reported.
- Neurophysiological testing will offer objective measurement in those with confirmed nerve injury and include electromyelogram and nerve conduction studies.

Table 24.6 Upper limb nerve injuries

Nerve	Level	Cause	Clinical signs
Radial	Axilla	Compression, e.g. by inappropriate crutch use	– For axilla only: no active extension at the elbow – For all: inability to dorsiflex wrist (wrist drop), extend fingers (finger drop) and thumb (thumb drop)
	Humerus	'Saturday night palsy'	– Sensory loss in dorsum of hand and over metacarpal of thumb and index finger
	Elbow	Dislocation of radial head	
Median	Elbow ('high median nerve injury')	Supracondylar fracture of humerus or anterior elbow dislocation	– 'Pointing index finger' when hands clasped – Inability to flex thumb – 'Ape thumb deformity' and inability to abduct thumb – 'Opponens palsy', i.e. inability to touch thumb with other tips of fingers
	Wrist	Laceration to wrist	– Sensory loss in thumb, index, middle and radial half of ring finger.
	Carpal tunnel	Dislocated lunate or chronic carpel tunnel syndrome	
Ulnar	Elbow	Traction injuries due to avulsion fracture at medial condyle and lateral elbow dislocation. Also in supracondylar fracture of humerus	Deformity of the ring and little fingers, 'ulnar claw hand'. Inability to adduct the fingers – tested by asking patient to grip paper between fingers. Unable to abduct little finger against resistance Loss of power at the wrist when the patient is asked to flex with adduction
	Wrist	Laceration	Sensory loss at the medial half of the index and little fingers, and the ulnar border of the hand

Table 24.7 Lower limb nerve injury

Nerve	Level	Cause	Clinical signs
Sciatic	Gluteal	Posterior hip dislocation	Paralysis of all muscles below injury and sensory loss corresponding to L4–S3 nerve roots
	Thigh	Laceration	Hamstrings preserved in thigh injuries
Lateral popliteal nerve	Around the neck of fibula	Lacerations and fracture fibula neck.	– 'Foot drop'. Inability to dorsiflex ankle and extend the toes.
		Abduction and adduction knee injuries associated with fractures to lateral and medial condyles, respectively	– Loss of sensation around outer aspect of affected leg and dorsum of the foot

Specific nerve injuries

Upper limb The radial, median and ulnar nerves originate from the cords of the brachial plexus, and may be injured at various levels along their length depending on the mechanism and type of trauma sustained (Figure 24.36).

Table 24.6 briefly outlines the aetiology and physical assessment parameters. Clearly there are other texts that cover this topic in greater detail (see Further reading). Brachial plexus injury is also briefly explored later, although again readers are encouraged to read further texts on the subject for more detailed information.

Brachial plexus injury The brachial plexus has roots, trunks, divisions and three cords. Injuries to this structure can be devastating to the individual owing to the commonly associated poor prognosis for neurological recovery in many cases. Although commonly associated with birth trauma, this

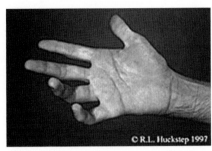

Figure 24.36 Ulnar nerve palsy.

section focuses on those occurring through accident.

Brachial plexus injuries may be classified in a number of ways. Injuries may be described as open, for example, in contact with the open air (e.g. due to major laceration), or closed, for example, due to motorcycle accident or fall.

Supraclavicular injuries tend to damage the upper part of the brachial plexus with a forced lateral flexion of the cervical neck with depression of the shoulder. If the arm is violently abducted in falls (often associated with anterior shoulder dislocation), the injury is described as being infraclavicular. These injuries damage the lower portion of the brachial plexus and have a better prognosis than those at a higher level.

A comprehensive neurological assessment of the affected side is vital to gain an accurate anatomy of the injury. As well as a physical examination of sensory and motor function, an EMG may be performed to identify the roots involved.

The location of the injury in relation to the dorsal root ganglion is the key prognostic indicator. Pre-ganglionic lesions will not recover, whereas post-ganglionic lesions may respond to microsurgical repair or grafting. Rarely reconstructive procedures, such as triceps transfer to allow some limb function, may be performed. Early referral to a specialist centre is indicated.

The author would recommend further study in more detailed texts for those interested in gaining more than this brief overview.

Lower limb Lower limb nerve injuries are less common than in the arm. Again aetiology and a brief description of clinical signs is outlined in Table 24.7. Other entrapment nerve injuries exist but relate to chronic compression associated with old fractures, and fall beyond the scope of this chapter.

Vascular injury

Major vascular injury including open arterial injury may, of course, be present in the patient with orthopaedic trauma. These are covered in other chapters and, as part of the primary survey, have a greater management priority than any fractures that may have been sustained. Therefore, this section will focus on closed vascular injuries associated with 1% of all fractures, particularly occurring in patients with major injuries around the pelvis, knee, shoulder and elbow (Ashwood and Challanor, 2003).

Acute traumatic ischaemia can result externally, for example, in compression from a tight cast or subfascial haematoma, resulting in compartment syndrome, or from direct pressure from the fractured ends of a bone, or internally following injury to the arterial wall. Early detection and prompt intervention are necessary, as much of the initial damage is irreversible: delays may result in necrosis and contracture development with associated long-term disability (Bollinger, 1998).

Muscle infarction (commencing within 6 hours following injury) will lead to areas of necrosis and subsequent fibrosis. This leads to shortening of the muscle and a contracture will develop, causing joint deformity and decreased function. Both nervous and skin tissue will also develop necrosis should ischaemic changes be prolonged, leading to decrease in motor and sensory function in the affected body part and the potential for gangrene, respectively.

Specific arterial injuries

Three specific arterial injuries merit further brief exploration, namely injuries to the brachial, popliteal and tibial arteries (Table 24.8). Emergency management of these involves prompt restoration of blood flow, decompressing the affected artery through manipulation. Obvious division of the artery or unsuccessful closed manipulation necessitate surgery as soon as is possible for repair. Fasciotomy is occasionally required in such cases.

In tibial artery ischaemia, fasciotomy over the anterior, superficial and deep posterior compart-

Table 24.8   Injuries to the brachial, popliteal and tibial arteries

Artery	Causes	Clinical symptoms
Brachial	– Supracondylar fracture of humerus – Comminuted fracture of distal humerus – Elbow dislocation	– Gross swelling around elbow – Absent /diminished radial pulse – Poor capillary perfusion in nail bed – Cramping pain – Limb cold on palpation – Reduced sensation – Results in 'Volkmans ischaemic contracture', if delay in treatment. Resulting in long-term contracted forearm and clawed fingers with ulnar and medial nerve palsy
Popliteal	Supracondylar, intercondylar or comminuted distal femur fractures	– Tense swelling around and just above the knee – Limb cold on palpation – Dorsalis pedis and posterior tibial pulses absent
Tibial	Proximal tibial shaft fracture	– Serious risk of compartment syndrome

ments may well be indicated to decrease the risk of long-term disability and potential amputation owing to gangrene from necrosis of ischaemic tissue (Figure 24.37)

EDUCATION OF THE PATIENT FOLLOWING ORTHOPAEDIC TRAUMA

As many patients with minor orthopaedic injuries such as strains, sprains and simple fractures, will be discharged home with follow-up as appropriate, patient education is fundamental not only in optimising function but also in the prevention of secondary complications. It is commonplace that crutches will be prescribed and administered to the patient, and dressings/bandages or plastering of the affected part will have taken place. It is insufficient to provide written instructions and expect patients to be in a position to comply fully with what is optimal self-care.

The patient with crutches

When issuing crutches, patients should be instructed to adhere to the following instructions:

- wear well-fitting, low-heeled shoes with non-slip soles
- support body weight on the handgrips with the elbows slightly bent
- 'squeeze' axillary pads between the upper arms and ribcage

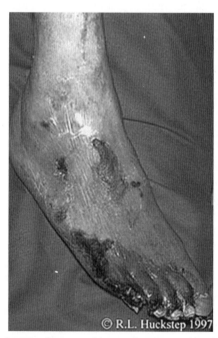

Figure 24.37   Gangrene from popliteal artery impairment.

- move the crutches and injured/weaker leg 12–15 inches ahead of the unaffected leg
- swing the unaffected limb about 12–15 inches ahead of the crutches
- move the crutches to the first position with the weight on the unaffected leg
- place weight on the handgrips when going upstairs, while the good leg is moved up one step

- place body weight on the stronger leg while the crutches and the weaker leg are moved up to the same step
- use handrail, where available, for safer support instead of one of the crutches when going up stairs
- sit down or lean against a wall rather than shifting the weight on to the axilla should tiredness occur.

When going through doors, patients should face them turning the body at a slight angle to clear them of the feet as it opens. The doorknob should then be turned with one hand while supporting the body weight on the crutch with the other hand. As the door opens, the crutch tip should be placed against the door to keep it open.

The patient in a plaster of Paris cast

Plaster of Paris takes a minimum of 24 hours to attain its full strength. Casts should be supported by a soft surface, such as pillows, throughout this period, as hard surfaces may result in pressure problems underneath the cast. Artificial heating to facilitate drying should be avoided, as the cast is likely to become brittle. During this drying period, the extremities of the relevant limb should be inspected on a 2-hourly basis, testing each digit for temperature, colour, sensation and mobility. As previously outlined, acute compartment syndrome may be caused through the application of a cast that is applied too tightly; it must, therefore, be ensured that casts impair neither circulation nor neurological conduction. Any adverse observation should be immediately reported and patients instructed to return for review. Once the cast has dried, the frequency of such observations may be reduced to a twice-daily basis.

Complaints of pain by patients from beneath casts should always be acted upon, and potential causes of pain determined. These may relate to the initial injury or the site of surgical intervention in which case the appropriate prescribed analgesia should be administered. However, pain may also be the result of a developing sore underneath the plaster, as a consequence of swelling of the affected limb or the application of a cast that is too tight (potentially highlighting the need for increased frequency of neurovascular observations in the limb). Such a situation merits immediate consultation with the plaster team or clinical staff. It is worth noting that casts on paralysed limbs (e.g. in clients as a result of stroke or spinal cord injury) should always be bivalved (split into two), and kept in place with a crepe bandage wrapped around the cast. Patients (or carers) must be instructed to remove this on a daily basis to inspect the skin, as the major symptom of pain indicative of a developing sore or a tight cast will be absent.

Casts should be kept dry even during meeting hygiene needs. Casts that become wet may become soft thereby potentially reducing their effectiveness. During bathing or any activity that may potentially put casts in the presence of water, they may be temporarily covered with a plastic bag. Patients should be strongly discouraged from putting items down the side of the cast to relieve the symptom of itching. The potential resulting trauma to the skin from such activity may initiate development of a sore or crease the lining of the plaster, resulting in increased pressure over that area. It is worth noting that severe irritation may occur as an adverse reaction to the material in the cast or lining and, if suspected, should be reported. A rise in temperature, or offensive smell may also be indicative of sore development and should be investigated. Windows may be cut in the plaster to facilitate changing of dressings or to check for potential sore development. Exercising the affected limb should be commenced only after the cast is completely dry. Casts that have become loose will be ineffective and should be renewed.

SUMMARY

This patient population comprises a major part of the business of any trauma service. Although most orthopaedic trauma is not initially life threatening, with the exception of major pelvic and femur fractures, unless associated with other injuries, the clinical implications for the patient from health, functional and social perspectives may be profound. Minimising the risk of potential complications to neural and vascular tissues in the early stage of management and providing comprehensive, accurate diagnostic information is fundamental in producing optimum patient outcomes.

A knowledge of normal musculoskeletal and peripheral nerve and vascular anatomy, pathophysiological processes resulting from orthopaedic trauma, and an ability to perform a thorough physical assessment and appropriate interventions to detect, reduce the incidence of and manage secondary complications are vital for the trauma nurse.

Additionally, as many of these patients will be discharged from accident and emergency, the nurse must perform well in the role of educator, as the potential effects of non-compliance owing to lack of knowledge may cause patient problems for months and years to come as well as use valuable health care resources. We must ensure that patients leave with education related to their condition and are not simply given a set of plaster or crutch instructions.

Developments over recent years in the role of the emergency nurse practitioner (ENP) have added value to the management of these patients. As for the future, perhaps a more focused orthopaedic ENP may yet add more to the service in producing the patient outcomes we desire.

References

Altizer L. Hand and wrist fractures. *Orthopaedic Nursing* 2003; 22: 232–239

Anderson K. Evaluation and treatment of distal clavicle fractures. *Clinics in Sports Medicine* 2003; 22: 319–326

Ashwood N, Challanor E. Managing vascular impairment following orthopaedic injury. *Hospital Medicine (London)* 2003; 64: 530–534

Bachmann LM, Kolb E, Koller MT, Steurer J, Rietter G. Accuracy of Ottawa ankle rules to exclude fractures of the ankle and mid-foot: systematic review. *British Medical Journal* 2003; 326: 405–406

Bachiller FG, Caballer AP, Portal LF. Avascular necrosis of the femoral head after femoral neck fracture. *Clinical Orthopaedics and Related Research* 2002; 399: 87–109

Bibbo C, Lin SS, Beam HA, Behrens FF. Complications of ankle fractures in diabetic patients. *Orthopedic Clinics of North America* 2001; 32: 113–133

Blake R, Hoffman J. Emergency department evaluation and treatment of the shoulder and humerus. *Emergency Medicine Clinics of North America* 1999; 17: 859–876

Bollinger WS. Vascular injuries associated with orthopedic trauma. *Topics in Emergency Medicine* 1998; 20: 39–45

Cole PA. Scapula fractures. *Orthopedic Clinics of North America* 2002; 33: 1–18

Cornell CN, Lane JM, Poynton AR. Orthopedic management of vertebral and long bone fractures in patients with osteoporosis. *Clinics in Geriatric Medicine* 19: 433–455

Hoffmeyer P. The operative management of displaced fractures of the proximal humerus. *Journal of Bone and Joint Surgery (Brit)* 2002; 84: 469–480

Krasin E, Goldwirth M, Gold A, Goodwin DR. Review of the current methods in the diagnosis and treatment of scaphoid fractures. *Postgraduate Medical Journal* 2001; 77: 235–237

Krishnan J. Trauma update. Distal radius fractures in adults. *Orthopedics* 2002; 25: 175–180

Kuntz DG Jr, Baratz ME. Fractures of the elbow. *Orthopedic Clinics of North America* 30: 37–61

Lee DH. Treatment options for complex elbow fracture dislocations. *Injury* 32 (Suppl 4): SD41–69

Leyes M, Torres R, Guillen P. Complications of open reduction and internal fixation of ankle fractures. *Foot and Ankle Clinics* 2003; 8: 131–147

McKoy BE, Bensen CV, Hartsock LA. Fractures about the shoulder: conservative management. *Orthopedic Clinics of North America* 2000; 31: 205–216

Misra A, Kapur R, Maffulli N. Complex proximal humeral fractures in adults – a systematic review of management. *Injury* 2001; 32: 363–372

Musgrave DS, Mendelson SA. Pediatric orthopedic trauma: principles in management. *Critical Care Medicine* 2002; 30(11 Suppl): S431–433

Neer CS. Four-segment classification of proximal humeral fractures: purpose and reliable use. *Journal of Shoulder and Elbow Surgery* 2002; 11: 389–400.

Norris TG. Pediatric skeletal trauma. *Radiologic Technology* 2001; 72: 345–373

Parisi DM, Koval K, Egol K. Fat embolism syndrome. *American Journal of Orthopedics* 2002; 31: 507–512

Pearse MF, Iero JJ, Morandi M. Severe fracture dislocations of the ankle joint: a management protocol. *Journal of Orthopaedic Techniques* 1995; 3: 164–168

Perron AD, Hersh RE, Brady WJ, Keats TE. Orthopedic pitfalls in the ED: Galeazzi and Monteggia fracture–dislocation. *American Journal of Emergency Medicine* 2001; 19: 225–228

Reagan DS, Grundberg AB, Reagan JM. Digital artery damage associated with closed crush injuries. *Journal of Hand Surgery (Brit.)* 2002; 27: 374–377

Ring D, Jupiter JB. Fracture-dislocation of the elbow. *Hand Clinics* 2002; 18: 55–63

Routt ML Jr, Nork SE, Mills WJ. High-energy pelvic ring disruptions. *Orthopedic Clinics of North America* 2002; 33: 59–72

Russell GV Jr, Kregor PJ, Jarrett CA, Zlowodzki M. Complicated femoral shaft fractures. *Orthopedic Clinics of North America* 2002; 33: 127–142

Scottish Intercollegiate Group Network 2000 – see website below

Sims SH. Subtrochanteric femur fractures. *Orthopedic Clinics of North America* 2002; 33: 113–126

Theumann NH, Verdon JP, Mouhsine E, Denys A, Schnyder P, Portier F. Traumatic injuries: imaging of pelvic fractures. *European Radiology* 2002; 12: 1312–1330

Tomaino MM. Amputation or salvage of type 3B/3C tibial fractures: What the literature says about outcomes. *American Journal of Orthopedics* 2001; 30: 380–385

Wang F, Wera G, Knoblich GO, Chou LB. Pulmonary embolism following operative treatment of ankle fractures: a report of three cases and review of the literature. *Foot and Ankle International* 2002; 23: 406–410.

Wang QC, Johnson BA. Fingertip injuries. *American Family Physician* 2001; 63: 1961–1966

Webb LX. Proximal femoral fractures. *Journal of the Southern Orthopaedic Association* 2002; 11: 203–212

Zionts LE. Fractures around the knee in children. *Journal of the American Academy of Orthopaedic Surgeons* 2002; 10: 345–355

Further reading

Berger RA, Arnold-Peter CW. *Hand surgery*. Philadelphia: Lippincott, Williams and Wilkins, 2003

Dandy DJ, Edwards DJ. *Essential orthopaedics and trauma*, 4th edn. Edinburgh: Churchill Livingstone, 2003

Magee D. *Orthopaedic physical assessment*, 4th edn. Philadelphia: WB Saunders, 2002

McCrae R, Esser M. *Practical fracture treatment*, 4th edn. Edinburgh: Churchill Livingstone, 2002

Simon R, Koenigsknecht SJ. *Emergency orthopaedics*, 4th edn. New York: McGraw-Hill Professional, 2000

X-ray websites

http://www.mc.vanderbilt.edu/vumcdept/emergency/xrhome.html

http://rad.usuhs.mil/medpix/medpix.html

http://www.swsahs.nsw.gov.au/livtrauma/education/xray.asp

http://www.nyerrn.com/x/xray.htm

Orthopaedic/trauma websites

http://www.orthopaedic.ed.ac.uk/trauma.htm – general trauma protocols.

http://www.emedicine.com/emerg/TRAUMA_AND_ORTHOPEDICS.htm – web guide to emergency orthopaedics.

http://www.east.org/tpg.html – trauma practice guidelines.

www.trauma.org – *the* trauma site.

http://www.show.scot.nhs.uk/sign/guidelines/fulltext/56/index.html – clinical guideline for fractured hip.

http://www.orthoteers.co.uk – for all things orthopaedic.

http://www.ortho-u.net/med.htm – site of Wheeler's textbook of orthopaedics – most comprehensive orthopaedic site on the web.

Chapter **25**

Spinal trauma

Sheenagh M. Gallagher

INTRODUCTION

Spinal cord injury (SCI) is a catastrophic outcome of injury in any person's life. It is usually of sudden onset, as the result of a traumatic injury and, depending on the level of injury, its effects potentially impact on all the body's systems and functions to some extent.

There is an annual incidence of spinal cord injury within the UK of 10–15 per million of the population. There appears to be an increasing rate of admissions with cervical injuries, which now seem to be the most common indication for admission to a spinal injuries unit.

CAUSE OF SPINAL INJURY

Causes of spinal cord injury are often collated into the following groups.

- Road traffic crash:
  - car, van, or lorry
  - motorcycle
  - cycle
  - pedestrian
- Domestic or industrial injury:
  - falling down stairs
  - falling from scaffolding or ladders
- Sporting injuries:
  - rugby
  - horse riding
  - diving into shallow water
  - motocross
- Self-harm or criminal assault.

Spinal injuries are often associated with other injuries, such as head injury, chest injury and multiple skeletal injuries.

Causes of spinal injury taken from one hospital over a 28-month period are listed in Table 25.1. Box 25.1 shows the distribution of cause from another data source.

There is considerable public awareness of the main outcomes of spinal cord injury – paralysis and loss of skin sensation below the level of injury, and the subsequent need for a wheelchair. However, what is not commonly appreciated is the possibility of severe difficulties with all the body's systems and functions, such as elimination, cardiovascular system, respiratory system, gastrointestinal system and mobility; nor is it widely noted that the resultant outcomes of two people with the same level injury will be different. Each person has a unique presentation of outcomes.

ASSESSMENT AND CLINICAL EXAMINATION

At the scene of the accident

The care the patient receives at the scene of the accident is of paramount importance in the case of a spinally injured patient. Whilst ensuring a clear airway, controlling serious external bleeding and removing the patient from immediate danger are the main priorities, it should always be considered that the patient might have sustained a spinal cord injury.

> It should always be assumed that an unconscious patient has a spinal cord injury until proven otherwise

It should be remembered that a spinal cord injury can mask other injuries and prevent their being easily noted. Likewise, other injuries (e.g. a head injury) may prevent a spinal injury being noted.

If it is necessary to move the patient at the scene of an incident, spinal alignment must be maintained at all times. In the event that the patient is wearing a crash helmet, it should not be removed without appropriate assistance unless the airway is at immediate risk.

Removal and transport of the patient from the scene should be on a long board (commonly referred to as a spinal board). The patient must be securely immobilised on the board with straps across the body and the head. In-line manual immobilisation must be maintained until the patient is secured on the board

> When applying long board straps always secure the body before the head

If the patient is conscious, a brief history can be taken; this may help identify other injuries that may alter the patient's condition and may allow the paramedic to determine the level of spinal injury. A short examination, including a baseline neurological assessment, can be made by simply asking the patient what they can feel and move.

One should always remember that the patient's condition could deteriorate without warning. This is especially true of the respiratory system should the level of lesion rise. Continuous monitoring of the patient for neurological changes in the patient is required en route to hospital. Ensure hard objects have been removed from the patient's pockets (e.g. coins and keys) and anaesthetic areas of the body are protected to prevent pressure sore formation.

Table 25.1 Causes of spinal injury (Addenbrooke's Hospital, Cambridge, February 1989–May 1991)

Mechanism of injury	Number of patients
Car driver	27
Car passenger	10
Motorcycle	11
Simple fall	10
Fall from a height	27
Horse riding	6
Cycling	3
Other sports	5

Box 25.1 Incidence of spinal injury (Duke of Cornwall Spinal Treatment Centre, 1993–1995)

Road traffic accidents	36%
Domestic and industrial accidents	37%
Injuries at sport	20.5%
Self-harm and criminal assault	6.5%

The destination accident and emergency unit (A&E) should be alerted so that they can prepare to accept the patient.

In the accident and emergency department

When the patient arrives at hospital, a full detailed history must be taken, and a full general and neurological examination is required. A thorough examination is required to ensure all other injuries are noted.

Caution is required to ensure that other injuries are not missed. For example, in patients with injuries above T7, it may be difficult to diagnose intra-abdominal injuries during the phase of spinal shock, as abdominal sensation is impaired and, with flaccid paralysis, the typical signs of an intra-abdominal emergency – distension and paralytic ileus – may well be absent.

The neurological assessment of patients with spinal cord injury must include:

- tone and power of all muscle groups;
- sensation to pinprick;
- sensation to fine touch;
- proprioception (joint position sense);
- reflexes;
- cranial nerve function.

It is by examining dermatomes and myotomes in this way that the level of neurological damage is decided.

The lowest level of normal spinal cord function determined by the above examination is referred to as the level of lesion. This does not, however, always equate with the level of bony injury. The neurological and the bony levels should both be recorded in the patient's notes.

The trolley on to which the patient is placed in the A&E department should allow radiological examination, thus preventing further unnecessary movement between surfaces. A full radiological examination in all planes prevents missing multiple fractures or dislocations. The fractures to the odontoid peg and C7 are commonly missed, if this approach is not taken.

The main aim of care at this stage is to stabilise the patient's condition and to detect any life-threatening changes that occur as the extent of the lesion develops.

> If a patient is inexpertly handled, injury to the spinal cord leading to paralysis could occur

One should always remember that, until proven otherwise by specialist medical opinion supported by radiological and other examinations, the future of patients who have sustained a spinal injury depends entirely upon careful handling by the nursing staff caring for them.

SIGNS AND SYMPTOMS OF SPINAL INJURY

Motor signs

Motor signs include weakness or flaccid paralysis of the limbs and/or the trunk muscles.

Sensory signs

Sensory signs include absence or alteration in the feeling of the limbs and/or of the trunk.

Pain

Midline pain or tenderness on palpation of the spine or neck is a common symptom in spinal injury. Radiating pain suggests nerve root compression irritation.

Superficial signs

Abrasions, lacerations or deformities of the spine, neck or head region should alert carers to the possibility of underlying bony disruption.

Incontinence

Loss of bladder or bowel control may be indicative of spinal injury.

Hypotension

In injury above T6, hypotension owing to impairment of the sympathetic outflow can occur; however, hypovolaemia must be excluded first in the hypotensive spinally injured patient.

Bradycardia

In high-level injuries, bradycardia can accompany hypotension owing to the loss of sympathetic innervation.

Poikilothermia

Patients are unable to control their own temperature and so they assume the temperature of the environment.

Neurogenic shock

Spinal shock describes the collective physiological abnormalities that may occur following injury to the spinal cord. It occurs in lesions between T1 and L2, where the thoracolumbar sympathetic outflow is interrupted leaving vagal tone unopposed.

> Neurogenic shock is characterised by hypotension, bradycardia and vasodilation with warm dry skin

Spinal shock

This condition is often confused with neurogenic shock; however, it is a transient condition following an initial injury where a complete loss of all sensation below the level of injury occurs along with a flaccid paralysis. It is a poorly understood phenomenon that is thought to occur as a result of the massive swelling that occurs within the cord following an injury. It is akin to 'concussion' of the spinal cord.

Spinal shock may last from a few hours to several weeks. The return of reflex activity is usually heralded by the return of the anal and bulbocavernosus reflexes, when the lesion is above the sacral segments.

NEUROLOGICAL AND NEUROVASCULAR ASSESSMENT

Assessment of the level and completeness of the injury determines the management and the prognosis that can be made.

If the lesion is complete from the outset, that is to say there is no sign of spinal cord activity below the level of lesion, then recovery is far less likely than in an incomplete lesion. There are some recognised patterns of abnormality associated with incomplete lesions, but neurological signs and symptoms that do not fit a classic pattern must not be dismissed.

Anterior cord syndrome

The anterior part of the cord is usually injured by a flexion–rotation force to the spine, producing an anterior dislocation, or by a compression fracture of the vertebral body with bony encroachment upon the vertebral canal. Anterior spinal artery compression often occurs so that the corticospinal and spinothalamic tracts are damaged by a combination of direct trauma and ischaemia. The result is loss of power, reduced pain and loss of temperature sensation below the lesion.

Central cord syndrome

This is usually seen in older patients with cervical spondylosis. It is the result of a hyperextension injury, often as a result of relatively minor trauma that compresses the spinal cord between the irregular osteophytic vertebral body and the intervertebral disc anteriorly and the thickened ligamentum flavum posteriorly. The injury affects the more centrally situated cervical tracts, which supply the arms, so there is flaccid weakness of the upper arms (lower motor neuron) and relatively strong but spastic leg function (upper motor neuron). Sacral sensation and bladder and bowel function are often partially spared.

Posterior cord syndrome

This is seen most often in hyperextension injuries with fractures of the posterior elements of the vertebrae. There is contusion of the posterior columns, which means that the patient may have good power and pain and temperature sensation but, owing to the loss of proprioception, a profound ataxia may occur making walking difficult.

Brown–Sequard syndrome

Classically, this results from stab injuries but they are also common in lateral mass fractures of the vertebrae. The signs of the Brown–Sequard syndrome are those of a hemisection of the cord. There is reduced or even absent power, but a relatively normal pain and temperature sensation on the side of the injury. This is because the spinothalamic tract crosses over to the opposite side of the cord. The uninjured side, therefore, has good power, but reduced or absent sensation to pinprick and temperature.

LEVELS OF MOTOR AND SENSORY FUNCTION

It is important in the understanding of spinal injury that carers are familiar with a basic assessment of motor and sensory function. This will help in the diagnosis of the level of injury and whether the lesion is complete or partial. The various levels and functions are summarised in Table 25.2.

TRAUMA AFFECTING THE SPINAL COLUMN/CORD

The mechanisms of injury are usually a combination of several of the following:

- flexion
- extension
- compression
- rotation
- distraction
- avulsion.

It is necessary to consider the mechanisms that produced the injury in order to understand how fractures are classified (Box 25.2), and whether or not they are stable. The common fractures are described below.

Box 25.2   Classification of spinal injuries

- Wedge compression
- Stable burst fractures
- Unstable burst fractures
- Flexion distraction (seat belt)
- Fracture dislocation/subluxation

N.B. C1 and C2 are atypical vertebra and have specific types of injury.

Table 25.2   Levels of motor and sensory function in the spine

Level	Motor function	Sensory function	Reflexes
C2–C3	Neck muscles	Neck	
C3, 4, 5	Diaphragm		
C4		Clavicle	
C5	Shoulder abductors	Lateral arm	
C5, 6	Elbow flexors		Biceps jerk
C6	Supinators/pronators	Radial forearm	Supinator jerk
	Wrist extensors	Thumb	
C7	Wrist flexors	Middle finger	Triceps jerk
	Elbow extensors		
	Finger extensors		
C8	Finger flexors	Ulnar border of hand	
T1	Intrinsic hand muscles	Ulnar forearm	
T2		Medial arm/axilla	
T7	Intercostals	Xiphoid	
T10	Intercostals	Umbilicus	
T12	Intercostals	Inguinal	
L1, 2	Hip flexors	Upper thigh	
L2, 3	Hip abductors	Mid-thigh	
L3, 4	Knee extensors	Knee	Knee jerk
L4, 5	Ankle dorsiflexors	Medial shin	
L5	Toe extensors	Lateral calf, dorsum foot	
L4, 5 and S1	Knee flexors		
	Ankle plantar flexors	Lateral foot	Ankle jerk
	Toe flexors	Posterior leg/thigh	
S2, 3,4	Anal sphincter	Perianal	Bulbocavernosus reflex
			Anal reflex
			Plantar reflex

Ninety-five per cent of spinal fractures occur in flexion (forward movement). The majority of these occur in the thoracic and lumbar regions of the spine. The percentage of fractures occurring solely as a result of extension is extremely low. When describing a spinal cord injury, the vertebral column can be divided into three: the anterior column, the medial column and the posterior column. With every spinal fracture there is an axis of flexion. This axis does not move.

Wedge compression fracture (crush fracture)

Type 1 – stable
This involves a simple crush injury to part of the vertebral body of the affected vertebra. It is treated conservatively with pain relief, bedrest and discharge home.

Type 2 (if compression > 50%) – unstable
This injury includes damage to the spinal ligaments and, therefore, has the potential to cause chronic instability. The patient requires admission.

Burst fracture

During the impact, the vertebra 'explodes' backwards into the spinal canal. If the pedicles remain intact, then the fracture is known as a *stable burst fracture*. The patient requires admission and analgesia. There is a risk of neurological damage from this type of injury but it is rare. Patients can be discharged wearing a three-point brace.

Unstable burst fracture

If the pedicles do not remain intact, then the fracture is described as an *unstable burst fracture*. The patient may or may not have neurological deficit. If *no deficit* is present, the patient is admitted, given analgesia and fitted with a hyperextension plaster of Paris jacket (be aware of cast syndrome) and can then be discharged home. As the fracture heals, the patient can be fitted with a three-point brace after 1 month. The fracture site becomes more stable as it heals.

Flexion distraction injury (seat belt injury)

With this form of fracture there is little chance of any neurological deficit, but it is often accompanied by abdominal injuries, especially a duodenal tear. If there is ligament and disc damage, the fracture in known as a Kalfer fracture. Treatment involves immobilisation in a plaster jacket or surgery.

Fracture dislocation

This occurs if the axis of the injury is not located in the midline, and flexion along with rotation leads to fracture dislocation. The incidence of neurological deficit in this instance is 75%. If no neurological deficit has occurred, then this unstable type of fracture has the potential to cause further injury. Acute instability occurs at the time of impact; chronic instability can occur at any time.

> The spinal cord stops at L1; a spinal cord injury cannot be sustained at L2 or below

MANAGEMENT OF THE PATIENT WITH NEUROLOGICAL DEFICIT

Paraplegia or quadriplegia may be motor or sensory, and it may be complete or incomplete. In complete paralysis, *nothing* can be felt below the level of the injury. If this is still the case 48 hours after injury, then it *never* recovers. *Any* form of feeling or flicker of movement indicates incomplete paralysis. In this instance, the extent of recovery will only be decided 2 years after injury.

> Increasing neurological deficit is an indication of an epidural haematoma and surgery is necessary

Patients with neurological deficit will be admitted and treated according to a set spinal protocol as outlined below.

The patient will be assessed and the degree of loss of muscle power will be noted. The level of sensory loss will be established with the use of sharp and blunt instruments. Once both motor and sensory levels have been established, then a decision as to whether the paralysis is complete or incomplete must be made.

If the deficit is incomplete, the medical staff have two options:

- surgical intervention;
- conservative management.

If surgery is the chosen option, the approach is usually anterior. This is major surgery and can only be performed once the patient is ready to undergo such extensive treatment. This may be days or weeks following the injury, as all other life-threatening injuries must be addressed first.

COMMON TYPES OF INJURIES

C1 (atlas)

This is a burst fracture (Jefferson fracture).

C2 (axis)

This is odontoid peg (dens) fracture and dislocation. It may cause sudden death, although minimal displacement does not often cause neurological deficit.

C2 on C3 (hangman's) fracture

This is caused by severe hyperextension forces giving rise to fracture across the posterior arch of the axis with or without subluxation of C2 on C3.

Lower cervical vertebra (C3–C7)

A variety of dislocations and subluxations can occur with flexion–rotation injuries.

Thoracic vertebrae

These are usually fractures or fracture dislocations where the mechanism includes axial loading and flexion forces with a rotational element.

Thoracolumbar injuries

These are usually compression fractures associated with flexion and rotational forces.

Lumbar and sacral injuries

These have a similar pattern to thoracolumbar injuries.

Chance fracture

This is a seat-belt injury that is unique to the lumbar spine. It is due to severe flexion and rotation at a fixed axis, namely the pelvis, which has been secured by a lap belt. It results in bony and ligamentous disruption to the lumbar spine. It is commonly associated with intra-abdominal injuries.

USE OF RADIOLOGY/SCANNING IN DIAGNOSIS AND TREATMENT

If a correct diagnosis is to be made, then any radiography must be of a high standard. Ideally, the patient will be on a trolley that allows radiography to take place without further transferring the patient on to an x-ray table. However, as any x-rays obtained whilst the patient is on this surface will be from portable machines, the quality of the x-ray films will be invariably inferior. Staff should also remember that not all sandbags and collars are radiolucent, and clearer films may be obtained if they are removed, but that manual in-line immobilisation of the head and neck must be maintained, if these devices are removed.

The first and most important film to be taken on any patient with a suspected cervical spinal injury is the lateral view, and this can be taken without moving the supine patient. For a complete set of cervical films to be taken, an anteroposterior radiograph and an open-mouth view of the odontoid process must be taken as well. Within the views it must be possible to see C1–T1 in order that both the odontoid peg and C7 are visualised. If this is not the case, the lateral view must be repeated. C7 is often missed because it is obscured by the shoulders.

Two methods can be used to ensure C7 is captured on x-rays:

1. traction on both arms – but this must be stopped, if it produces pain in the neck;
2. swimmer's view – one arm down by the side and the other placed up and over the head.

Bony definition is best demonstrated by computed tomography (CT) scan. This will show accurate detail of the bony injury and show the extent of encroachment within the spinal canal by vertebral displacement or bone fragments. Magnetic resonance imaging (MRI) is excellent at showing the extent of cord damage and oedema. MRI can be used to show ligamentous injury; this is useful in deciding upon spine stability.

PROTOCOL OF CARE

The Spinal Injury Association believes that all hospitals in the National Health Service (NHS) should have a common protocol to ensure that all people with definite or suspected spinal cord injury have access to staff with the knowledge and level of practice to manage spinal injury effectively.

Ideally, patients should be admitted immediately to a recognised spinal injury unit. There are 11 spinal injury units within the UK (Figure 25.1) and, because there are so few, they are responsible for very large catchment areas. Because they treat only spinal-injured patients, the staff within these units have a high level of knowledge and experience in this field. It is recognised this is an area of expertise where colleagues

throughout the country may be apprehensive in caring for such patients and the units, therefore, welcome and actively encourage contact advice.

With so few spinal injury units, the probability of being admitted directly to a specialist unit is fairly small. However, a simple protocol, summarised in Box 25.3, can outline the care required to stabilise the patient initially and prepare them for transfer to a recognised specialist unit where rehabilitation can be commenced in the acute phase of injury. Any local protocol should ideally be drawn up in consultation between both the general hospital and the regional unit.

Contact telephone numbers should be available for staff to use *at any time*, if problems of any sort arise, staff should know that they can use these numbers without reproach. A good liaison between both the general hospital and the spinal injury unit should be fostered, and continuous links between them should be maintained. This

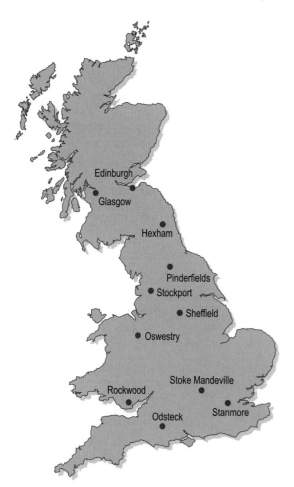

Figure 25.1 Location of spinal injury units in the UK.

Box 25.3   Areas of care that should be included in a spinal injury protocol

- Specific statements of care, which *must* be adhered to
- Complications that can arise and their signs/symptoms
- Which staff can undertake which aspects of care
- A named person responsible for the competencies of staff
- Where such patients can be admitted
- Checklists of equipment
- Communications – who has been informed and at what stage
- Aspects of care:
    - moving and handling
    - admission procedure
    - preparation of bed area and documentation
    - analgesia
    - observations
    - x-rays and scans
    - diet and fluids
    - anticoagulation
    - H_2 receptor antagonists
    - steroid therapy
    - bladder care
    - bowel care
    - multidisciplinary team
    - transfer to spinal injury unit

ensures that there is both support for the general hospital from the specialist unit and that the patient receives the best possible care until their transfer to the unit. General hospital staff should not see this as undermining their ability to care for these patients but rather as enhancing the care they give by utilising their best possible resource of care – the specialist units.

CONCLUSION

Spinal injury is always an emotive problem to handle in the A&E department. Whilst it is true that the damage is usually done before the patient arrives and that the care is designed to give comfort to the patient before rehabilitation begins, it is essential that all those nursing patients within A&E are fully aware of the possibility of other injuries being present and of the need for careful handling of such patients. There are few worse disasters than to see a partial cord injury become a full cord injury because of careless handling. By strictly following the guidelines in this chapter, the nurse will be able to give optimum care to those patients in their care who have suffered a spinal injury.

Further reading

Coleman M, Matthewson M, Shewring D. *Spinal injuries – the Cambridge experience*. Cambridge: Addenbrookes Hospital, 1991

Gallagher SM, Matthewson M. *Protocol to admit spinal injured patient to the trauma and orthopaedic unit*. Cambridge: Addenbrookes NHS Trust, 1998 (in conjunction with The Princess Royal Spinal Injuries Unit, Northern General Hospital, Sheffield)

Green Barth A, Eismont F, O'Heir J. Pre-hospital management of spinal injuries. *Paraplegia* 1997; 25: 229–238

Grundy D, Swain A. *ABC spinal cord injury*, 3rd edn. London: BMJ Books, 1996

Harrison AP. *Information for acute care sector staff*. Sheffield: Northern General Hospital NHS Trust, 1989

Keene G, Robinson A, Bowditch M, Edwards D. *Key topics in orthopaedic trauma surgery*. 1999

Matthewson M. *Overview spinal injuries*. Spinal Injuries Association, 1997

Spinal Injuries Association. *Moving forward after paralysis – a charter for support*. Spinal Injuries Association, 1997

Swain A, Dove J, Baker H. *ABC of major trauma*, 2nd edn. London: BMJ Books, 1996

Chapter 26

Multiple trauma

Tim Kilner

INTRODUCTION

In a literal sense, the term 'multiple injuries' refers to the coexistence of two or more injuries. However, this definition does little to convey a sense of the complexity and severity of multiple injury. Patients with multiple injuries often have injuries that involve a number of anatomical areas or body systems, hence the term multisystem trauma. It may, therefore, be useful to regard the term multiple injuries as the coexistence of injuries involving two or more anatomical areas or body systems. It is this interplay between physiological responses from each of the involved body systems that creates many of the difficulties in the assessment and management of the patient with multiple injuries.

> Multiple injuries refers to the coexistence of two or more injuries

The care of the patient with multiple injuries starts long before the patient arrives at the hospital. The assessment and management of the patient starts in the pre-hospital environment, at the scene of the incident and en route to the hospital. This phase of care for the patient with multiple injuries may be just as important in influencing the outcome as the care provided in the hospital. Nurses are becoming increasingly more involved in the provision of pre-hospital emergency care, from within the ambulance service (Walsh and Little, 2001), as part of a hospital-based mobile medical and nursing team, or as part of specialist immediate care medical and nursing teams. It is precisely these types of patients that such individuals and teams will be tasked to, the patient who may be difficult to extricate from the incident, where rapid evacuation to hospital is not an option and where the management of the patient is complex. The role of pre-hospital care is covered in detail in Chapter 4, but the specific issues associated with the assessment and management of the multiply injured patient in the pre-hospital environment will be discussed within this chapter.

ASSESSMENT AND MANAGEMENT OF THE PATIENT WITH MULTIPLE TRAUMA

As with the management of the multiply injured patient in the pre-hospital environment, a team approach is also adopted in the hospital phase of care. The availability of senior specialist clinicians, certainly within the early hospital management of the patient, is a double-edged sword. Speciality opinion and management within the team may mean the patient receives best care for a specific injury; this may be at the expense of taking a broader view of the patient and considering the relationship of competing patient needs. Thus each injury assumes its own importance with each potentially given a high priority. If all are regarded as high priority, then there is no prioritisation. The difficulties of patient assessment and management of patients with multiple injuries and, therefore, competing needs, within the hospital setting will be considered in detail.

Complexities of multisystem involvement

Most texts, and many educational programmes aimed at trauma care, consider serious trauma system by system, with specific sections relating to chest trauma, abdominal trauma, extremity trauma and neurological trauma, for example. Whilst it is true that many patients have life-threatening conditions resulting from an isolated injury, in clinical practice, many more patients have actual or potential injuries involving more than one body system or anatomical region. For example, following either blunt or penetrating trauma to the chest there may be considerable potential for a coexisting intra-abdominal injury with the involvement of the respiratory and cardiovascular systems.

The extent to which other systems or anatomical areas are involved is determined by the mechanism of injury. Where an incident has involved sufficient force to produce a potentially life-threatening condition in a single system, it is highly likely that other systems have been exposed to similar forces, potentially producing life-threatening conditions in those systems. Where only a single injury is immediately apparent, yet the patient was exposed to multiple forces, the search for occult injury must be fastidious. The effects of multiple forces can be illustrated in the road traffic collision, which may produce flexion, extension and rotational forces, direct trauma from intrusion of the engine or the vehicle's body work, the individual colliding with structures within the vehicle such as the steering wheel, and deceleration forces sheering the viscera. The potential for such forces to cause injury involving more than one system is high, yet only a single injury may be immediately apparent.

Isolated injuries may or may not be potentially life threatening; in the case of multiple injuries, the cumulative effects increase that risk of life threat. Where a single closed femoral shaft fracture or two fractured ribs may pose a relatively low life threat risk, the combination of two fractured ribs and bilateral femoral shaft fractures significantly increases that risk. In much the same way, a haemothorax in isolation may be potentially life threatening as a single entity, but in the presence of other visceral injuries the life threat from hypovolaemia increases further.

The involvement of a number of systems may also serve to produce a confusing clinical picture and, if the health care professional is not cognisant of this, it may have disastrous consequences. An important indicator of hypoxia and hypovolaemia is tachypnoea but, in the clinical scenario, both conditions may coexist, making it difficult to determine what extent each condition is having on the respiratory rate. Where there is a combination of apparent and covert injuries, there is a risk that clinical signs are attributed to the apparent and not identifying the covert. This situation often arises when the patient has a reduced level of consciousness following trauma; immediate thoughts turn to a closed head injury, yet the reduction in consciousness may be a result of hypovolaemia. Collecting a breadth of appropriate clinical data may help build up a clearer clinical picture of the patient but, where multiple systems are involved, many of the differences may be extremely subtle.

THE PRE-HOSPITAL PHASE

Immediate care of the multiply injured patient – the problems

The provision of pre-hospital trauma care is predominated by the ambulance service, with care being delivered by ambulance technicians and paramedics. The involvement of other health professionals within the pre-hospital arena is inconsistent, with little uniformity in terms of structure, organisation, availability and level of expertise.

It is believed that, on average, each ambulance paramedic will provide care for one case of serious trauma each month (Nicholl et al., 1998). The emergency nurse or emergency physician manages serious trauma much more frequently, but generally has little experience of working in the pre-hospital environment. There are examples of emergency nurses or emergency physicians with expertise in the pre-hospital arena providing care to patients in the pre-hospital arena (Walsh and Little, 2001; BASICS website). There are also a number of projects currently under way exploring the possibilities of rotating emergency nurses and paramedics through roles in both the pre-hospital arena and the emergency department, with the aim of exposing each professional group to the management of trauma on a more regular basis in order to enhance the care of the trauma patient in the pre-hospital arena.

The environment often conspires against the emergency care provider in caring for the multiply injured patient out of hospital. Assessment of the multiply injured can be difficult at the best of times but, in a potentially hostile environment with poor lighting and access, limited equipment and human resources, these difficulties may become extreme. There are occasions when the emergency care provider is faced with a number of potentially injured individuals at a single incident and where additional skilled personnel may initially be scarce. In such circumstances, the emergency care provider must not only establish priorities within the patient but also between patients. Whilst this type of situation can occur in the hospital environment, generally some prioritisation has already taken place, availability of personnel is likely to be less critical, patients may arrive at different times and multiply injured individuals may have been dispersed to more than one receiving facility.

It is rare for the patient with multisystem trauma not to have at least one component that is time critical. That is where a significant factor in determining the patient's survival is the time delay from incident to definitive care, which in most cases would be surgery. This means that the time available for assessment and initial management of the patient on scene is limited. In relation to time-critical trauma, many emergency care providers aim for an on-scene time of no more than 10 minutes. In practical terms, the on-scene time may be prolonged beyond this but should be kept to an absolute minimum. A recent study in the USA concluded that advanced life support procedures at the scene following major trauma did not significantly prolong on-scene times beyond those where only basic interventions were applied. The mean on-scene times were 12.8 minutes and 11.0 minutes, respectively (Eckstein et al., 2000).

> It is rare for the patient with multisystem trauma not to have at least one component that is time critical

Identification of the patient with multiple injuries

Because of the time-critical nature of multisystem trauma, the pre-hospital emergency care provider must be able to rapidly identify those patients with life-threatening injuries that are potentially survivable. In order for the assessment to be rapid and appropriately detailed, the approach must be systematic and rehearsed, but with a sufficient degree of flexibility to allow response to the environment and the clinical condition of the patient.

In some cases, the multiple injuries may be immediately apparent at the first contact with the patient. This initial impression of the patient is likely to be based upon obvious anatomical injury (e.g. the patient with an open head injury, facial injury and long bone fractures). However, time-critical trauma may be occult and difficult to detect on first impressions (e.g. insidious blood loss from a visceral injury). It is often possible to detect these injuries during a more detailed assessment of the patient and the measurement of vital signs. Mechanism of injury is taught widely in many courses aimed at both hospital and pre-hospital providers. The concept of interpreting the mechanism of injury in the context of trauma scoring may help identify more accurately those with serious trauma (Bond et al., 1997) but lack the specificity to allow the identification of specific injuries.

Obvious anatomical injury is, by definition, generally easier to detect than occult injury. Consequently, where multiple injuries are of an obvious anatomical nature, pre-hospital emergency care providers are likely to identify the potential threat to life rapidly. Where injuries are covert, the risk of failing to identify the life threat is greater. For many patients with multiple injuries, the life threat results from a combination of these factors, both obvious and occult injury. The danger here is that the pre-hospital care provider identifies the obvious, engages in the treatment of those injuries and fails to recognise the occult injury; consequently, the patient may not be seen as having multiple injuries but merely an isolated long bone fracture, for example. In order to minimise this type of risk, each patient is assessed and managed in a structured way that reflects clinical priorities.

Initial assessment

The framework generally accepted in the UK for initial assessment and treatment of identified life-threatening conditions is the AcBCDE approach, collectively known as the primary survey (Box 26.1). Early work on this framework was outlined by the American College of Surgeons in their 'Advanced trauma life support course', but the

Box 26.1	The primary survey
Ac	Airway with consideration of the cervical spine
B	Breathing and ventilation
C	Circulation and haemorrhage control
D	Disability
E	Exposure, environmental control and evacuation

concept has been adapted for the pre-hospital phase of care by other agencies, such as the National Association of Emergency Medical Technicians in Pre-Hospital Trauma Life Support.

The aim of the primary survey is to identify and initiate treatment of immediately life-threatening conditions sequentially based upon clinical priority. Thus the airway is considered first, with appropriate regard to the cervical spine, followed by an assessment of breathing with management of ventilation and so forth. By adopting a systematic approach to the assessment of the patient, potentially life-threatening conditions are identified in priority order, there is less risk of focusing upon one injury at the expense of others and the cumulative effects of multiple injuries are identified.

By the end of the primary survey, the pre-hospital emergency care provider should have a sense of the stability or instability of the patient, the combination of injuries and the extent to which these injuries pose an actual or potential life threat. This information is the basis for decision-making regarding the priority for evacuation to hospital, the receiving facility to which the patient should go and the means of transportation to hospital. In the case of entrapment, this information should inform the decision to call for additional expertise, such as an immediate care doctor or mobile surgical team.

A number of pre-hospital emergency care agencies utilise a system of trauma scoring, which enables patients to be prioritised based on a number of clinical parameters. The use of trauma scoring in this way is of value to the management of the patient with multiple injuries in that each parameter is influenced by the cumulative effects of multiple injuries. A system commonly utilised in the UK is the Triage Revised Trauma Score

Table 26.1 The Triage Revised Trauma Score (TRTS)	
Parameter	TRTS points
Respiratory rate	
0	0
1–5	1
6–9	2
>9	3
10–29	4
Systolic blood pressure	
0	0
1–49	1
50–75	2
76–89	3
≥90	4
Glasgow Coma Score total	
3	0
4–5	1
6–8	2
9–12	3
13–15	4

(TRTS). The TRTS is the sum of the coded score of three parameters: respiratory rate, systolic blood pressure and Glasgow Coma Score (Table 26.1). Therefore, even if the specific nature of the injury is not known, the clinical priority can be established. For example, where hypoxia and hypovolaemia coexist, the combined effect on the respiratory system and on the level of consciousness will be detected by the TRTS.

Assessment difficulties in the pre-hospital phase

Given that the multiply injured patient is likely to have some occult injuries, be they actual or potential, adequate assessment is essential to identify those with life-threatening multisystem trauma. The nature of the pre-hospital environment presents a number of unique difficulties in the assessment of the multiply injured patient. The environment frequently conspires against the pre-hospital emergency care provider, making assessment difficult – poor lighting, confined spaces, difficult access, low or high ambient temperatures, wind, rain, snow and noise often make patient assessment difficult.

Clinical signs are often subtle and equivocal in a number of patients with multiple injuries, particularly when physiological compensatory mechanisms are active and the manifestation of clinical signs delayed. Whilst this is not unique to the pre-hospital phase, they are compounded by the environmental difficulties, the availability of monitoring equipment, the limited numbers of personnel on scene and the availability of a range of expert help on scene.

The assessment of the multiply injured patient in the pre-hospital environment has its own difficulties, but pre-hospital providers are often faced with an additional dimension, that of several multiply injured individuals at the same incident. Not only does the pre-hospital care provider have to identify priorities within each individual but also to establish priorities between individuals.

In accepting that these difficulties in assessment exist, it is important for the hospital team to understand that a definitive clinical picture of the patient cannot be established on scene. The identification of the patient with multiple injuries may, therefore, be a result of a degree of suspicion about the patient's risk of multiple injuries and the inability to exclude those injuries positively. Consequently, the clinical picture communicated to the hospital staff may be incomplete or have some inaccuracies. However, it is essential that the pre-hospital provider is able to 'flag up' those areas of uncertainty during the assessment as well as any positive findings.

Pre-hospital management of the multiply injured patient

It is well established that multiple injuries are commonly time-critical injuries and that definitive care cannot be provided for these individuals at the scene of the incident. It is, therefore, reasonable to view the pre-hospital phase as being time limited and that patient care should be restricted to an absolute minimum of essential interventions. Depending upon the location of the incident and its distance to an appropriate receiving facility, management may be merely an initial assessment, essential airway care, oxygenation and rapid evacuation. For others, further interventions may be necessary; for example, when the patient is trapped and rapid evacuation is not possible, or when transport distances to an appropriate facility are considerable.

The philosophy for the on-scene management of the multiply injured individual and en route to hospital should be essential priority-based care. However, the interpretation of essential information is dynamic and does not necessarily mean simple or basic. With the need for increasingly complex interventions, there is a need for care providers with more sophisticated skills. Pre-hospital care providers must be cognisant of this in the context of their own limitations. For example, the trapped patient who is combative following a closed head injury needs the care of an individual skilled in rapid sequence induction (RSI) of anaesthesia. This type of intervention could in no way be regarded as basic care but it may nevertheless be essential care.

The key to the pre-hospital management of the patient with time-critical multiple injuries is to identify the patient with multiple injuries rapidly, make essential interventions and minimise delay prior to transporting the patient to an appropriate facility. Overtreatment, the provision of non-essential interventions and delay in on scene times is not desirable, as this merely serves to erode the envelope beyond which survival is unlikely.

Communication and evacuation

The ability to transport the patient in a timely manner to an appropriate facility is an important factor in the management of the multiply injured patient. The benefits and limitations of trauma centres within the UK is as yet unproven, but it seems reasonable and in the patients' best interest to deliver them to a facility that has clinical services appropriate to the patients' needs. For example, those patients with significant chest injuries may benefit from being managed in a facility that has cardiothoracic services in addition to other trauma services. However, a balance has to be achieved between the clinical need and the time it will take to reach that facility. In recent years, in an attempt to overcome this difficulty, there has been a proliferation of air ambulance services. The transportation of patients from scene by air has opened up opportunities to transport patients greater distances in relatively short time

frames. This has had the effect of bringing a wider range of receiving facilities within the time envelope. Whilst this type of service offers a number of advantages, it is not the complete solution, with factors such as current restrictions in the UK on night flying militating against a seamless 24-hour provision. The very nature of multiple injuries often means that patients have diverse clinical needs and the specialist services for each are in different locations. For example, neurosurgical services are at one facility and cardiothoracic at another. The dilemma for the aircrew is where to transport the patient with significant head and chest injuries.

Current practice in the UK means that the majority of injured patients are taken by road to the closest hospital with an A&E department. This may not be the most desirable way of managing those patients with complex needs, and where clinical specialities beyond A&E are limited either by their existence or by lack of senior clinician cover out of hours. The policy of transporting the patient to the nearest A&E department is in part driven by the expectation that pre-hospital providers will make the decisions regarding destination in isolation and without clinician support. Direct communication and consultation between the pre-hospital provider and senior clinicians may result in an informed decision regarding the most appropriate destination of the patient with multiple injuries.

Pre-arrival information from the scene to the receiving facility is important in order for decisions to be made regarding the composition of the receiving team, the need to alert staff in supporting roles and to make ready equipment. The quality of that information is important; it should be concise, relevant and structured. A more detailed verbal report must be provided when handing the patient over to the receiving facility.

The verbal report at the receiving facility should also be concise, relevant and structured, but may be more detailed than the initial report from en route to the facility. The report should also be a two-way interaction between the pre-hospital provider and the hospital trauma team. The report should outline findings and treatment, but should also relate instances where the pre-hospital provider is suspicious of injury but has been unable to positively exclude the possibility of injury.

THE INITIAL HOSPITAL PHASE

The trauma team

The success of the management of the patient with multiple injuries is dependent upon a team approach to care. No individual or single professional group is able to deliver the total package of care required by the patient. However, the activities of the team must be coordinated and directed. Priority for activity must be established by an individual who is able to appreciate the overall needs of the patient and not just the isolated system or injury. Whilst this is important for all seriously injured patients, it is crucial for those patients with multiple injuries, whereas an isolated injury may be serious but may not pose the same degree of life-threat as other injuries. Given the clinical complexity of the patient with multiple injuries, it is important that the coordinator or team leader is an appropriately senior and experienced clinician. A team with no leader or with many leaders often results in unmitigated disaster, where activity takes place simultaneously, without regard for priority, and planning of ongoing management of the patient is confused. In a further attempt to ensure a coordinated response to the management of the injured patient, specific roles for team members should be defined and allocated prior to the arrival of the patient.

Many hospitals now operate a trauma team to provide the initial assessment and management of the seriously injured. Activation of the team is generally based upon information received from the pre-hospital care providers. Clearly patients with obvious and severe multiple injuries will result in the activation of the trauma team before the patient arrives. However, it may be necessary to alert the team after the patient arrives, if their life-threatening problems are not immediately apparent and are only identified following their initial assessment.

The initial hospital response will generally be based upon:

- information on the pre-hospital phase of care:
  - prior to arrival at hospital
  - on arrival at hospital;
- assessment:
  - primary survey
  - secondary survey
  - monitoring, investigations, imaging;
- initial and immediately necessary treatment;
- forecasting and planning:
  - definitive care
  - referral
  - transfer.

Information from the pre-hospital phase

The hospital team at the receiving facility is likely to have the advantage of advanced warning of the patient's arrival in addition to some basic clinical information. It may also be possible to gain some sense of the severity of the patient's condition based upon the pre-hospital provider's perception, which may or may not be based on objective data. Those patients with obvious multiple injuries or with occult injuries identified in the field are likely to be identified by the pre-hospital provider. Adopting an approach of exclusion where injuries are regarded as being present until proven otherwise will result in a number of patients who were initially regarded as having serious multiple injuries, after further assessment, actually having minor injuries. Whilst these false positives may be a drain on resources, it is a safe approach for the patient. The hospital team must be cognisant that there may be a number of patients brought to the receiving facility with as yet unidentified multiple injuries and who may potentially bypass the trauma team. Pre-arrival information may also allow for appropriate additions to be made to the team. For example, if the patient is identified as having facial injuries, including the eye, the team may wish to alert the maxillofacial team and the ophthamologists, who would not routinely form part of the team.

As in the pre-hospital phase of care, due regard should be paid to the mechanism of injury as this may be the first indication, or the only initial indication, that the patient may have received potentially life-threatening multiple injuries. The most reliable source of information regarding the mechanism of injury will be provided by the pre-hospital team, who have seen the physical evidence at first hand and have had the opportunity to talk to witnesses about the incident. The trauma team may be able to gain some additional subjective information if the patient is able to provide it. The use of instant photographs and video at scene may help convey the mechanism of injury to the trauma team. With future development of telemedicine techniques, real-time images from the scene to the hospital prior to the arrival of the patient may become widespread. The team leader is crucial in this interface between the pre-hospital team and the trauma team in collecting and collating information regarding possible mechanisms of injury. It is this initial contact that is the start of the in-hospital assessment of the patient and the identification of those patients with potentially life-threatening multiple injuries. A number of factors have been identified as predictors of serious injury (Greaves, 2001) such as:

- a fall of greater than 6 metres;
- a pedestrian or cyclist struck by car;
- the death of other occupant in same vehicle;
- ejection from a vehicle or bike;
- major vehicular deformity or significant intrusion into the passenger space;
- an extrication time of more than 20 minutes;
- vehicular roll-over.

Many if not all of these mechanisms are highly suggestive that the patient may have sustained multiple injuries. The particular injury pattern is likely to be determined by the type of incident. With this information, the trauma team, under the direction of the team leader, are able to seek out likely injuries based upon suspicion, working to the principle that the injury is present until positively excluded.

Further evidence of mechanism of injury may be identified during the inspection of the patient system by system. This will be conducted in more detail during the primary and secondary survey along with palpation, percussion and auscultation. However, wounds and pattern bruising may be evident during the transfer of the patient from the ambulance trolley to the hospital trolley. If identified in the field, the pre-hospital team presents this evidence during their report to the trauma team; this is particularly important where bruising and wounds may be obscured by the

position of the patient. For example, reports of pattern bruising to the patient's loins may prompt the trauma team to log roll the patient from the spinal board earlier than they would routinely, in order to examine the patient's back. However, this decision will be taken in the context of the primary survey with the airway, breathing and circulation assuming appropriate priority.

This information will be used by the team leader in the formulation of a plan for the assessment and management of the patient, as well as providing an initial impression of the likelihood of important multiple injuries. The team leader will also liaise with the pre-hospital team to establish the findings from their assessment, serial clinical parameters such as vital signs, treatments initiated in the field and *en route* to hospital and the results of those interventions. This activity will take place simultaneously with the hospital initial assessment of the patient.

The primary survey

In the words of the American College of Surgeons 'Patient management must consist of a rapid primary evaluation, resuscitation of vital functions, a more detailed secondary assessment, and finally, the initiation of definitive care'. During the past two decades, this philosophy has become widely adopted within hospital emergency practice in the UK. This system provides the trauma team with a structured approach to the assessment of systems reducing the risk of life-threatening conditions not being identified.

> Patient management must consist of rapid primary evaluation, resuscitation of vital functions, more detailed secondary assessment and the initiation of definitive care

The initial phase of the assessment process is the primary survey (see Box 26.1), which is aimed at identifying life-threatening conditions and the simultaneous initiation of management interventions. Clinical examination of the patient continues to be based upon a systematic approach of inspection, palpation, auscultation and percussion. These basic clinical skills remain invaluable in the identification of multisystem trauma.

Airway with cervical spine control

As with all seriously injured patients, scrupulous attention must be paid to the airway. The patient with multiple injuries is no different. Regardless of distracting and apparently serious injuries, the assessment and appropriate management of the airway must take priority. Assessment of the effectiveness of pre-hospital airway interventions is appropriate. Due consideration must be given to the cervical spine when undertaking airway interventions.

Whilst unconsciousness is a common cause of airway obstruction, in the seriously injured patient and, in particular, in those with multiple injuries, attention should also be given to other possible modalities of airway obstruction, such as, facial injury, laryngeal trauma, wounds and oedema. The airway must be rapidly assessed and definitive airway management in place at the earliest appropriate opportunity.

The trauma team must consider the risk to the cervical spine and take appropriate action to immobilise the cervical spine until injury has been excluded clinically and radiologically. The patient is likely to have been presented to the hospital on a spinal board with a semirigid cervical collar, head blocks and body straps. Whilst the use of cervical collar, blocks (or sand bags) and tapes should remain in place until the cervical spine is 'cleared', the spinal board should be removed as soon as the primary survey is completed.

Breathing and ventilation

Often patients with multiple injuries manifest problems associated with breathing. Assessment of breathing is important but the interpretation of findings may be difficult. Crude assessment to identify the presence or absence of breathing is important, but must be followed by an assessment of the adequacy of ventilation. Absent or inadequate ventilation must be remedied immediately by means of assisted ventilation with high concentrations of supplemental oxygen. For all other patients with serious trauma and multiple injuries who currently have adequate ventilation, high-concentration oxygen administered through a close-fitting mask with a reservoir bag is a minimum intervention.

Consideration should be given to the underlying cause of abnormal respiratory signs. Possible mechanisms include injury interfering with the mechanics of respiration (mechanical or neurological), injury to the lungs or damage to major airways. However, signs may not necessarily relate directly to the respiratory system, such as head injury or hypovolaemia. A confusing picture may emerge in the patient with multiple injuries, who may have a combination of these features. An examination of the thorax is important and may lead to the identification of some possible causes of abnormal respiratory signs but other systems must also be considered to exclude their possible implication.

It is also essential that an examination of the neck is conducted either as part of the airway assessment or the breathing assessment. The five cardinal features in the neck which should be identified, if present, and which relate to airway and breathing are:

- tracheal deviation – tension pneumothorax, although a late sign
- wounds
- surgical emphysema – indicative of major airway disruption
- laryngeal crepitus – indicative of laryngeal disruption
- distension or flattening of the neck veins – cardiac tamponade, hypovolaemia (often equivocal).

Circulation and haemorrhage control

Whilst the assessment of the respiratory system may benefit from additional monitoring and investigations, assessment of circulation often depends more upon monitoring and investigative techniques in order to detect covert conditions with equivocal signs. However, the basic clinical assessment techniques, such as pulse rate, rhythm, volume and location, blood pressure and appearance, will doubtless be of value.

In terms of management, haemorrhage should be considered in relation to two types: compressible and non-compressible. Compressible haemorrhage is external blood loss, which can be controlled by either direct or indirect pressure. This type of haemorrhage is generally evident, but not always, and can be underestimated. For example, a scalp laceration can result in insidious but nonetheless severe hypovolaemia. Non-compressible haemorrhage is that which cannot be controlled by either direct or indirect pressure and is generally internal. This type of haemorrhage is less immediately apparent and is more likely not to be recognised than compressible external haemorrhage. The patient with multiple injuries may have both types of haemorrhage coexisting. Whilst the presentation of compressible and non-compressible haemorrhage is different, their management is also contrasted. External compressible haemorrhage, at least in the short term, may be managed by direct or indirect pressure; non-compressible haemorrhage will require surgery to control the haemorrhage.

Disability

Formalised neurological assessment is reserved for the secondary survey; however, Glasgow Coma Scale and papillary reaction are likely to be conducted. Again, it is important to recognise that a reduced level of consciousness may not be attributed to a head injury but may be associated with hypovolaemia.

Exposure and environmental control

Exposure of the patient to facilitate the secondary survey is necessary, but due consideration must be given to the dignity and privacy of the patient. Furthermore, the patient must be protected from reduced body temperature as hypothermia may result in clotting disorders, potentially compounding hypovolaemia.

The secondary survey

On completion of the primary survey and any immediately necessary interventions, a secondary survey will be conducted. In general, this is a more detailed head to toe assessment, but may be abridged in those patients who have unresolved circulatory problems requiring immediate surgical intervention.

Potential conditions are detailed in the relevant chapters relating to each system or anatomical region; however, it is again important to recognise that the complexity of the clinical picture in the multiply injured patient results from the impact of one injury or physiological process on another.

MONITORING, INVESTIGATION AND IMAGING

A range of monitoring options are available to the trauma team in order to assess the patient with multiple injuries and to help in the identification of the underlying processes producing similar clinical features. The basic range of monitoring available to the trauma team includes cardiac monitoring, non-invasive blood pressure measurement and pulse oximetry. More sophisticated monitoring is available as the patient's management continues and may include end-tidal carbon dioxide monitoring, invasive blood pressure monitoring and central venous pressure monitoring. Crucial to the value of any of the monitoring techniques is the interpretation of trend data. A single measurement of heart rate or blood pressure is of little value; an emerging pattern of changing physiology is much more important and should be interpreted in the context of other clinical findings.

Clinical monitoring should be appropriate and, as far as possible, near patient testing should take place. This is particularly important where findings have influence over patient management, for example, arterial blood gas analysis.

Advances in imaging are of immense value to the trauma team when managing the patient with multiple injuries. Plain x-rays of the chest, pelvis and cervical spine remain valid and important early investigations, which are often used as a means of exclusion (i.e. exclusion in conjunction with clinical examination for significant cervical spine injury, or serious chest and pelvic injury). These techniques are not infallible and are supplemented by more sophisticated imaging techniques. However, more sophisticated techniques are more time consuming and it may not be possible to perform them in the resuscitation room. Consequently, they are unlikely to be carried out in the early stages of assessment.

Computed tomography (CT) scanning is relatively commonplace in the assessment of head-injured patients but also has a place in the assessment of the cervical spine where the plain x-ray proves inadequate. Spiral CT enables the whole cervical spine to be rapidly imaged. Additionally, spiral CT also allows complete imaging of the chest, abdomen and pelvis. Magnetic resonance imaging (MRI) is also an option in trauma but the environment in which imaging takes place may not be the most appropriate for seriously injured patients. Contrast studies of the patient may be of value in some patients but are unlikely to feature in the early stages of assessment and resuscitation.

Bedside abdominal ultrasound is increasingly becoming available and is of value in detecting covert intra-abdominal haemorrhage. It has a number of advantages over diagnostic peritoneal lavage, in that it is faster and cheaper, whilst producing similar results in detecting free fluid in the abdomen.

INITIAL AND IMMEDIATELY NECESSARY TREATMENT

Initial treatment is aimed at managing immediately life-threatening conditions; some interventions may be definitive and others buy time whilst arranging definitive treatment. For life-threatening non-compressible haemorrhage, immediate treatment is likely to be surgery.

Airway interventions assume the highest priority, using simple manoeuvres with airway adjuncts. The gold standard for the unconscious patient is endotracheal intubation, performed with due consideration to the cervical spine or, in some circumstances, the surgical airway. The conscious patient who has an airway problem, or who is hypoxic and combative, may need advanced airway interventions facilitated by rapid sequence induction of anaesthesia. Consequently, there is a need for an anaesthetist on the trauma team; however, a recent report suggests that non-anaesthetist emergency physicians can safely perform this procedure providing they have a clearly defined course of action in the event of a failed intubation (Carley et al., 2002).

Basic interventions relating to breathing should include the administration of high-concentration oxygen administered via a well-fitting mask with reservoir bag. Assisted ventilation is appropriate for those patients with absence of or inadequate ventilation. Should mechanical ventilation be necessary, then rapid sequence induction (RSI) may need to be considered. In the presence of pneumothorax or haemothorax, chest drainage forms part of the initial resuscitation and, in the case of a tension peneumothorax, may be preceded by needle decompression or thoracocentesis.

Part of the initial resuscitation will involve gaining vascular access, drawing blood for investigations and intravenous volume replacement. Current practice leans towards permissive hypotension, where volume replacement is titrated to a systolic blood pressure of 80–90 mmHg in respect of non-compressible haemorrhage. The fluid of choice in the initial resuscitation of the trauma patient remains controversial. The control of compressible haemorrhage by direct or indirect pressure is a minimum standard, which may be all that is required in some circumstances, whilst in other cases it may be an intervention that buys time until definitive repair can be arranged. The use of large temporary sutures may be considered in conjunction with direct pressure and may have a role in preliminary haemostasis of large wounds.

Those patients with multiple injuries are likely to have a significant degree of pain. Adequate pain control and analgesia are essential in the management of these patients, and should be considered early. Arguments about analgesia masking symptoms are redundant in light of modern diagnostic and imaging techniques.

FORECASTING AND PLANNING

Establishing clinical priorities and planning the ongoing care are essential roles for the trauma team leader. Taking advice from appropriate specialists from members of the trauma team, the team leader needs to plan the programme of investigations and ultimate referral of the patient. This role requires the ability to identify the priorities between competing clinical needs to optimise the management of the patient seeking specialist referrals as necessary. Early decision-making regarding investigations and transfer of the patient are essential in order that other services are alerted early and can prepare for the arrival of the patient. This ultimately reduces the number of unnecessary delays. This process is sometimes facilitated by a trauma coordinator who, as part of their role, facilitates the smooth flow of the patient to the appropriate services.

CONCLUSION

The management of the patient with multiple injuries follows well-established principles in the management of the seriously injured patient. However, these patients often have time-critical covert injuries, of which the pre-hospital and in-hospital teams must be suspicious and actively seek out. The teams must also be aware of the confusing clinical picture presented by the coexistence of a range of pathophysiological processes.

References

BASICS (British Association for Immediate Care) website: http://www.basics.org.uk/data/index.htm

Bond RJ, Kortbeek JB, Preshaw RM. Field trauma triage: combining mechanism of injury with the pre-hospital index for improved trauma triage tool. *Journal of Trauma* 1997; 43: 283–287

Carley SD, Gwinnutt C, Butter J, Sammy I, Driscol P. Rapid sequence induction in the emergency department: a strategy for failure. *Emergency Medicine Journal* 2002; 19: 109–113

Eckstein M, Chan L, Schneir A, Palmer R. Effects of prehospital advanced life support on outcomes of major trauma patients. *Journal of Trauma* 2000; 48: 643–648

Greaves I, Porter K, Ryan J. *Trauma care manual*. London: Arnold, 2001

Nicholl J, Hughes S, Dixon S, Turner J, Yates D. The costs and benefits of paramedic skills in pre-hospital trauma care. *Health Technology Assessment* 1998; 2: 1–7

Walsh M, Little S. Study of a nurse practitioner working in a paramedic role. *Emergency Nurse* 2001; 9: 11–14

Chapter 27

Abdominal trauma

Adam Brooks, Ann Paynter and Emyr Phillips

CHAPTER CONTENTS

INTRODUCTION

Abdominal injury is a significant source of morbidity and mortality in the trauma patient. Blunt abdominal trauma frequently occurs as part of multisystem injury as a result of high-speed road traffic collisions. The diagnosis of abdominal trauma in this situation is often challenging and may cause the trauma team management difficulties in prioritisation of the injuries. Penetrating injury, although less common in the UK, is increasingly frequent in inner-city hospitals. Although the initial presentation of these injuries may be more straightforward, there is a high incidence of intra-abdominal injury. The rapid investigation and diagnosis of abdominal injury is vital to reduce the associated morbidity. Recent advances in technology have led to changes in the investigation of abdominal injury whilst an increased understanding of the physiological derangement associated with severe abdominal injury has altered the resuscitation and surgical management of abdominal trauma (Johnson et al., 2001). The priority remains to transfer the unstable patient with abdominal injuries to theatre under the care of an experienced surgeon as soon as possible.

This chapter is aimed at addressing issues relating to the epidemiology and common mechanisms of abdominal injury, the assessment and resuscitation of patients with abdominal trauma, reviewing the investigation of patients with suspected abdominal injuries and considering abdominal injuries in specific population groups.

EPIDEMIOLOGY OF ABDOMINAL INJURY

Abdominal injury is a significant contributing factor in 20% of the 12 000 trauma deaths in the UK per annum and a major factor in the 10 000 patients sustaining multiple injuries (Anderson et al., 1989; Burdett-Smith et al., 1995; Office for National Statistics, 1997). Mortality from abdominal injury occurs in two main peaks. Early deaths arise as a result of massive haemorrhage from abdominal vascular injuries or trauma to the solid organs – liver, spleen and kidneys. Urgent surgery is vital to control bleeding in these patients. A second peak of deaths occurs later from the development of sepsis leading to the systemic inflammatory response syndrome and ultimately multiple organ failure. The cause of this sequence of events is multifactorial, but delayed or missed diagnosis of bowel injury and gross abdominal contamination from faeces are significant contributing factors to the development of the inflammatory response.

In the UK and most European countries, the majority of abdominal injuries occur as a result of blunt trauma; however, in the USA and South Africa, penetrating injury is far more common both from stab wounds and gunshot wounds (Buckman, 1999). Whilst stab wounds of the abdomen result in gastrointestinal injury in only 50% of cases, the incidence from gunshot wounds is far greater at 90%.

Anatomy

External anatomy

The full extent of the abdominal cavity is frequently not recognised. On full expiration, the abdomen extends from the fifth intercostal space (nipple level in the male), to the inguinal ligaments and pubic symphysis inferiorly. Some of the abdominal organs are, therefore, concealed from clinical appraisal by the bony protection of the lower ribs; therefore, abdominal injury should be suspected in all cases of lower chest trauma. The pelvic bowl also conceals the abdominal viscera from assessment. In addition, it is vital that the abdominal evaluation includes the flanks and back, since wounds can classically be concealed in these regions. The flank encompasses the area between the anterior and posterior axillary lines, whilst the back is posterior to this, and its thick musculature may offer some partial protection to stab wounds.

Internal anatomy

The abdomen is divided into the peritoneal cavity, retroperitoneum and the pelvis.

Peritoneal cavity The peritoneal cavity contains the majority of the abdominal organs including the liver, spleen, stomach, small bowel, parts of the duodenum and parts of the large bowel. The ribs and pelvis may offer some partial protection from injury.

Retroperitoneum The retroperitoneum is the posterior part of the abdomen and contains the posterior organs and major blood vessels. It can be divided into central, lateral and pelvic zones to facilitate surgical decision-making at operation. The central zone contains the major vessels (aorta and inferior vena cava), and haematomas should be explored surgically in both blunt and penetrating trauma. The lateral zones contain the kidneys, ureters and colon. Most blunt injuries in this region can be managed conservatively. The retroperitoneal pelvis is the third zone and, in pelvic fracture, may contain a huge haematoma. Surgical exploration of this is dangerous and difficult. Observation, packing and interventional radiology techniques are more appropriate.

Pelvis The pelvic cavity is formed by the pelvic bones and contains the bladder, rectum and the internal genitalia in females.

Mechanism of injury

Blunt trauma

Blunt trauma is by far the commonest cause of abdominal injury in the UK. High-speed road traffic collisions, including motorcyclists and the interaction of pedestrians with vehicles, lead to devastating multisystem injury. Abdominal evaluation is extremely difficult in these situations and prioritisation of investigation and management is vital. Abdominal injuries are created by direct impact and crushing of organs between the striking object and bony structures, or by deceleration and rotational forces that impinge on the intra-abdominal organs, especially at the interface between mobile and fixed structures. The solid organs, especially the liver and spleen, are the most commonly injured in blunt trauma by impact and deceleration, and devastating haemorrhage can follow. Bowel injury occurs either through an acute increase in intraluminal pressure on impact or by shearing at points of transition from fixed to mobile areas.

Penetrating trauma

Stab wounds Stab wounds are more common in the UK than gunshot injuries. Injuries from a stab wound are confined to the track of the wounding implement; however, stab wounds are frequently multiple and may involve the limbs and hands, injured whilst attempting to provide protection, as well as the chest, abdomen and the back. Occasionally it may be useful to have information on the length or type of weapon; however, this is frequently inaccurate, and each situation must be managed on the clinical picture and signs. Little information is also available on the depth or direction of the wound, and full assessment of the patient is essential. It is also important that a thorough inspection is made for multiple knife wounds, as significant wounds can occasionally be hidden in the axilla, natal cleft or back.

Gunshot wounds Gunshot injuries are classified according to the amount of energy transferred to the tissues. The amount of energy transferred depends on the kinetic energy of the bullet and the retardation of the bullet as it passes through the body. Rounds from handguns typically produce low-energy transfer that inflicts injury along the path of the bullet, but little collateral damage. The tissue damage associated with the high-velocity bullets fired from military rifles is far greater. They typically produce high-energy transfer wounds with an associated cavitation effect, wide destruction of surrounding tissue and gross contamination (Cooper and Ryan, 1990). Abdominal gunshot wounds have a 90% incidence of organ damage, and associated cavitation may injure organs distant to the missile track as well drag dirt and debris into the wound.

$$\text{Kinetic energy} = \frac{1}{2}\,mv^2$$

where m is the mass of the missile and v^2 is its velocity.

A shotgun blast at a range less than 5 metres is fatal in 90% of cases (Ordog, 1988). The multiple lead shot acts as a single mass on impact with a large surface area. The individual shot then spreads out, leading to massive transfer of energy to the tissues. Each piece of shot can cause multiple bowel and vessel perforation.

Fragment wounds Patients injured from fragmentation devices are fortunately a rare occurrence in civilian emergency departments. Modern military fragmentation devices are designed to deliver hundreds of fragments. These armaments are intended to mutilate and maim, but not necessarily kill the victim. It is important to assess all patients exposed to these weapons thoroughly for discrete penetrating wounds and to have a low threshold for abdominal investigation. Terrorist bombs utilise pre-formed fragments such as nails, bolts and nuts around the charge, which can lead to widespread devastation and horrific abdominal injuries (Ryan et al., 1997).

Blast injury Blast injuries tend to be multisystem and can lead to significant injury; it is important that the victim is examined thoroughly as part of the secondary survey. The auditory system is especially susceptible to blast injury, and even subtle changes in hearing are an important indication of exposure to blast and should raise the index of suspicion for the development of pulmonary sequelae. Hearing changes may range from mild ringing in the ears to deafness from haemorrhage and perforation of the tympanic membrane.

Blast can cause abdominal injury through a number of mechanisms. The blast wave, a dynamic pressure wave, can lead to compression, organ contusion and disturbance at tissue interfaces leading to haemorrhage. The blast wind can be sufficiently powerful to throw the victim, resulting in further blunt injury. Secondary injuries can arise from fragments from the bomb or surrounding area and can cause penetrating abdominal wounds, which may be multiple. The victim may also be at risk from flash burns, fire and collapsing buildings.

THE ABDOMINAL TRAUMA PATIENT IN THE EMERGENCY DEPARTMENT

Triage

Patients with suspected abdominal injury either from the mechanism of injury, physical signs or associated injuries should be triaged to the highest priority and received in the resuscitation room by a waiting trauma team.

> Patients with suspected abdominal injury either from the mechanism of injury, physical signs or associated injuries should be triaged to the highest priority and received in the resuscitation room by a waiting trauma team

Clinical presentation

Abdominal trauma occurs either in isolation from penetrating injury or beatings or, more frequently, as part of multisystem injury from road trauma. It can present with obvious eviscerated bowel or massive abdominal distension or, more subtly, with few clinical signs in early intra-abdominal bleeding. The mechanism of injury is very important and will provide information on the likely forces involved and potential injuries. However, there must be a high index of suspicion at all times, and a low threshold for investigation and referral to general surgeons.

Immediate assessment

The assessment of all trauma patients must take place in accordance to the Advanced Trauma Life Support (ATLS)® principles of airway, breathing and circulation (American College of Surgeons, 1997). The initial evaluation of the abdomen takes place during the circulation assessment of the primary survey. This clinical assessment must take into account the mechanism of injury, and pre-hospital information provided by the paramedics and ambulance personnel. A few patients will have clinically obvious abdominal injury, protruding weapons, evisceration of bowel, etc. However, in many patients, the earliest findings are more subtle and, therefore, early referral to a general surgeon is vital in all patients with suspected abdominal injury. The purpose of the initial clinical assessment is to confirm or exclude the abdomen as a source of concealed bleeding that requires immediate surgery in the unstable patient.

Resuscitation

In the face of massive or ongoing abdominal haemorrhage, the priority of the resuscitation effort is to transfer the patient to the operating theatre where the bleeding can be stopped at laparotomy by an experienced surgeon. An organised and coordinated team approach is vital to achieve this. Other patients with less catastrophic injuries may respond rapidly to the initial fluid resuscitation and allow time for more detailed investigation; however, subsequent cardiovascular deterioration in the light of suspected abdominal injuries requires rapid surgery.

Fluid management – hypotensive resuscitation

A limited amount of clinical research has suggested that, in patients with penetrating injury, limiting fluid resuscitation to a systolic blood pressure of 90 mmHg may confer a survival advantage (Bickell et al., 1994). There is a theoretical basis for applying this principle to all trauma victims (with the exception of head injuries, where it may have a detrimental effect) and resuscitating patients to a blood pressure sufficient to maintain perfusion of vital organs, without disruption of established clot or precipitation of coagulation abnormalities. Some institutions, therefore, apply a policy of judicious warmed fluid administration just sufficient to maintain perfusion of the vital organs. The administration of intravenous fluids is never an alternative to the rapid transfer of the patient to theatre, laparotomy and the control of bleeding by a surgeon.

ADJUNCTS TO THE MANAGEMENT OF ABDOMINAL INJURY

Nasogastric tube

Although it can be distressing to the patient, a nasogastric tube is an essential part of the management of abdominal trauma. Occasionally, gastric distension will occur, especially in distressed children and infants who can swallow a lot of air. The nasogastric tube will reduce this distension and, therefore, decrease the risk of aspiration; however, thick food matter will not pass up the tube and its placement can in certain circumstances induce vomiting. Blood in the tube contents can provide some indication of injury to the upper gastrointestinal tract but may represent swallowed blood. A correctly positioned, functioning nasogastric tube is essential before commencing diagnostic peritoneal lavage (DPL). Caution must be exercised in patients who have sustained facial trauma or where mid-face fractures are suspected. In these patients, an orogastric tube should be placed in lieu of a nasogastric tube to avoid the potential for intracranial passage.

Urinary catheter

A urethral urinary catheter is required in all major trauma patients except where urethral injury is suspected, as the urine output reflects renal perfusion and hence the state of ongoing resuscitation of the patient. Bloodstained urine may also provide evidence of injury to the urinary tract. Catheterisation, where urethral injury is suspected (pelvic fracture, high-riding prostate on rectal examination, perineal or scrotal bruising or blood at the penile meatus), is contentious and should be discussed with a urologist. It is essential that rectal and genital examination is performed before any attempt at urethral catheterisation. Although some experts suggest a single gentle attempt at catheterisation when injury is suspected, others recommend a contrast urethrogram and formal suprapubic cystostomy, if there is urethral injury. The safe approach is not to attempt catheterisation where injury is suspected but to proceed to suprapubic catheterisation. A urinary catheter must always be placed before DPL is attempted.

Investigation

The importance of rapid and accurate abdominal investigation has been shown by a number of important studies looking at missed injuries at post mortem. As early as 1979, Trunkey reported on a series of preventable deaths in Orange County,

USA (Bickell et al., 1979). All but one of the deaths was attributed to shock from inadequate recognition of intra-abdominal bleeding. In 1988, Anderson et al. reviewed 1000 trauma deaths in the UK. One-third of the deaths occurring after major injury were found to be preventable and unrecognised or inadequately treated haemorrhage was a major factor in these deaths. The introduction of new technology and techniques in the assessment of the abdomen has allowed rapid and accurate diagnosis of injury.

> One-third of the deaths occurring after major injury were found to be preventable, and unrecognised or inadequately treated haemorrhage was a major factor in these deaths

Clinical assessment

The initial clinical examination of the abdomen in trauma can be misleading, as blood in the abdominal cavity may initially cause few physical signs. In addition, the effect of drugs, alcohol, head injury, spinal trauma and other distracting injuries may mask abdominal signs, making the clinical examination alone little better than guesswork in this group of patients.

> The initial clinical examination of the abdomen in trauma can be misleading, as blood in the abdominal cavity may initially cause few physical signs

A small group of patients will have distended or rigid abdomens on examination and require immediate surgery; however, where the abdominal assessment is equivocal, clinical examination should be augmented by another investigation. In resource-constrained environments, physical assessment may be the only available diagnostic tool available. In this situation, serial clinical examinations will detect progression of abdominal signs and studies have shown this approach to be a sensitive means of investigation. There is no role for sequential girth measurements in the evaluation of abdominal trauma. Markers of injury, such as seat-belt pattern bruising, must be recognised, as they are associated with a high incidence of intra-abdominal injury.

Diagnostic peritoneal lavage

Diagnostic peritoneal lavage has been the gold standard for the investigation of blunt abdominal trauma in the multiply injured patient for over 30 years (Root et al., 1965). This simple technique involves the instillation of 10 ml/kg of warmed Hartmann's solution into the patient's abdominal cavity. After a short while, the fluid is drained and the effluent assessed either macroscopically or microscopically for the presence of red blood cells, white blood cells or vegetable matter. In trained hands, the technique is reliable and simple. It is associated with a 1% complication rate (Powell et al., 1982) and 10–15% non-therapeutic laparotomy (Wherry and Punzalan, 2000), when surgery is undertaken based on the findings of 100 000 red cells or 500 white cells per ml. Although often practised, assessment of the lavage fluid by eye directly or the ability to read newsprint through the fluid is notoriously inaccurate and should not be used. A nasogastric tube and urinary catheter are prerequisites for DPL to avoid gastric or bladder penetration. The same technique has been validated for the evaluation of potential penetrating injuries using cell counts of 10 000 red cells and 50 white cells per millilitre as the cut-off for surgery.

Focused assessment with sonar for trauma (FAST)

Ultrasound has been employed in medicine for many years; however, it is only during the last 10 years that it has gradually become accepted in the evaluation of the acute abdomen in trauma (Rozycki and Shackford, 1996, 1997). FAST is an acronym first used in the 1990s to describe the simple ultrasound technique that is performed either by a trained accident or emergency physician or surgeon in the resuscitation room (Scalea et al., 1999). In Europe and the USA, FAST is progressively becoming the initial investigation of choice in suspected abdominal injury. The procedure involves the assessment of four distinct regions of the torso with ultrasound to detect fluid (blood). The four regions are perihepatic, perisplenic, pericardial and pelvis (Rozycki et al., 1993; Figures 27.1 and 27.2).

If blood is detected, then the patient goes to theatre, if cardiovascularly unstable, or for further imaging using computed tomography (CT). The

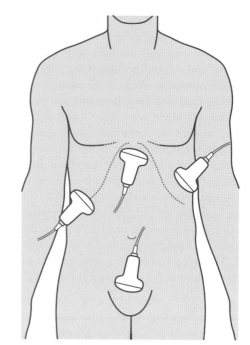

Figure 27.1   The four regions assessed by FAST: pericardial, perihepatic, perisplenic, pelvis.

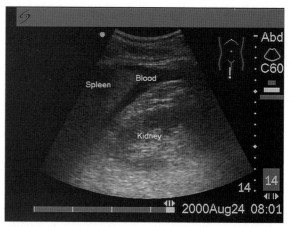

Figure 27.2   Positive FAST; blood is visible between the spleen and kidney.

negative predictive value of FAST is less reliable and a negative examination requires further imaging, either with CT or a repeat ultrasound after a delay of a few hours. The use of this technique to detect free fluid has recently been increased in some centres to include the detection of haemothorax and haemopericardium (cardiac tamponade) in chest injury.

One of the key advantages of FAST is that non-radiologists can be trained in a short amount of time to perform FAST as reliably as radiologists (Buzzas et al., 1998). Therefore, with the advent of small portable ultrasound machines in the resuscitation room, trained accident and emergency physicians can accurately locate abdominal bleeding as part of the initial circulation assessment, allowing the resuscitation to be rapidly focused and reducing the time to surgical intervention.

Computerised tomography

The CT scan is the investigation of choice for the assessment of abdominal injury in stable patients; however, the CT scanner is unsuitable for unstable patients, as rapid catastrophic deterioration can occur whilst monitoring and access to the patient is difficult. The CT scan not only shows abdominal bleeding, but also provides information on specific organ injury and may allow a non-operative management protocol to be followed for some injuries to the liver or spleen. However, CT is less reliable in diagnosing injuries to the small bowel and may miss pancreatic injuries (Sherck and Oates, 1990). Intravenous contrast should be used in all trauma scans. CT is also the investigation of choice in stab wounds to the back where intravenous, oral and (if large bowel injury is suspected) rectal contrast is required to delineate injury to the posterior retroperitoneal structures.

Laparoscopy

Laparoscopy has very limited application in the diagnosis of blunt abdominal injury, as the technique is expensive, requires a general anaesthetic and may not provide sufficient information to confidently exclude all injuries, especially small bowel perforation (Brooks and Boffard, 1999). The only appropriate indication in blunt trauma is for the diagnosis of diaphragm rupture in patients where it is suspected but other methods have failed to provide a diagnosis. In penetrating trauma, diagnostic laparoscopy is the most sensitive technique in the evaluation of abdominal and thoracoabdominal stab wounds in stable patients. The technique has been shown to have 100% sensitivity in determining peritoneal breach and, therefore, is the investigation of choice for these

injuries (Leppaniemi and Elliot, 1996; Zantut et al., 1997). Confirmation of penetration at laparoscopy should be followed by a laparotomy for formal evaluation of the injuries. In some institutions where there is significant experience of gunshot wounds, laparoscopy has been used to evaluate tangential gunshot wounds for potential penetration. This practice is not recommended where the experience of firearm injuries is limited.

Wounds

All penetrating wounds of the abdomen need to be clearly documented in the notes. They may be associated with protrusion of omentum or even organ evisceration. Wounds apparently distant to the abdomen need to be thoroughly evaluated for possible communication with the abdomen. Buttock wounds especially have a high incidence of communication with the peritoneum and its contents.

Wound exploration

Wound probing in the emergency department should be actively discouraged. Unless the patient is in the position in which they were injured, the tract will be difficult to find and dislodgment of an underlying blood clot may have devastating consequences. In addition, the negative predictive value (i.e. the ability to rule out abdominal penetration definitively) has been shown to be extremely poor. Where it has to be performed, wound exploration should be undertaken as a surgical procedure in theatre with a cooperative patient under local anaesthesia or general anaesthetic, with the patient's consent to proceed to immediate laparotomy.

DIAGNOSIS OF BLUNT ABDOMINAL TRAUMA

FAST is the ideal screening investigation for all trauma patients and should be integrated into the initial assessment of circulation during the primary survey of resuscitation. With horizontal organisation of the trauma team, this preliminary investigation can be performed within minutes of the patient's arrival and can detect the presence of intra-abdominal bleeding within seconds. The results will direct the further investigation and management.

Table 27.1	Diagnosis of penetrating trauma	
Wound	Condition	Investigation
Gunshot wound	Stable	Laparotomy
Stab wound – anterior/ thoracoabdominal	Stable	Laparoscopy
Stab wound – back	Stable	Triple-contrast computed tomography

DIAGNOSIS OF PENETRATING TRAUMA

Unstable patients with penetrating abdominal or thoracoabdominal injuries need urgent surgical intervention; however, further imaging may be appropriate in stable patients with certain penetrating injuries (Table 27.1). FAST is less sensitive in penetrating trauma, as the volume of blood in the abdomen that requires surgery is very small. However, FAST can be used to screen for abdominal bleeding and, if positive, a laparotomy should be performed. Directed investigation can be applied when the initial ultrasound is negative.

GENITOURINARY TRAUMA

Trauma to the kidneys, ureters, bladder or urethra needs special investigation and attention. A urine dipstick for haematuria should be undertaken in all trauma patients as a screening investigation. Classically, macroscopic haematuria should be investigated in blunt injury and both microscopic or macroscopic haematuria investigated in penetrating trauma; however, the situation may be more complicated as complete disruption of the renovascular pedicle may lead to clear urine in penetrating injuries. In stable patients, an abdominal CT scan with intravenous contrast is the appropriate investigation for evaluation of renal and ureteric injuries, as it provides structural as well as functional information (Figure 27.3).

In unstable patients, the injuries are likely to be discovered at laparotomy; however, a one-shot intravenous urogram in theatre will provide valuable information on the function of the contralateral kidney before nephrectomy is performed. If bladder disruption is suspected from the mechanism of injury or associated injuries, then a contrast cystogram with full,

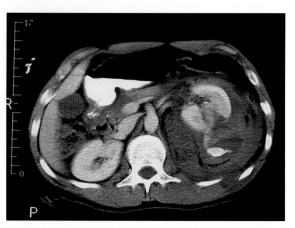

Figure 27.3 Abdominal computed tomography scan of a left kidney injury and perirenal haematoma following a stab wound.

oblique and postmicturition films is required to detect a leak. Alternatively, this can be performed at CT. Where urethral injury is suspected, a gentle urethrogram may provide evidence of full or partial disruption of the urethra. However, investigation and further management of these injuries should be under the direction of a specialist urologist.

SPECIAL TECHNIQUES

Interventional radiology

Interventional radiology (IR) techniques have developed an increasing role in the management of abdominal trauma in recent years. IR can be used as an adjunct to the non-operative management of solid organ injury in the abdomen (Sclafani et al., 1995). The technique involves percutaneous access to the vessels, usually in the groin, and a catheter is then introduced under radiological screening. Contrast medium is injected whilst imaging continues and extravasation of the contrast determines the site and degree of injury. Various techniques can be attempted to control or stop the bleeding. Embolisation involves the deployment of multiple metallic coils through the catheter into the vessels supplying the injured organ. These act as scaffolding for clot formation, which then leads to occlusion of the damaged vessels. Alternatively, balloon catheters can be passed either side of a bleeding point in a vessel and inflated to occlude flow to provide temporary control until surgical access is gained.

Interventional radiology techniques may be employed in a number of situations. The presence of a contrast blush in the spleen on abdominal CT suggests ongoing bleeding – arteriography and coil embolisation can be used to stop the bleeding and avoid surgery. Interventional radiology can be used as an adjunct to the packing of major liver injuries; therefore, all patients who have liver packing for injuries should proceed directly to the angiography suite following surgery for imaging and embolisation of bleeding vessels. It is also valuable in the management of pelvic bleeding in pelvic fractures.

SPECIAL SITUATIONS

Weapons in situ

All weapons should be left *in situ* during resuscitation and only removed in the more controlled environment of the operating theatre. This may produce logistic dilemmas and problems; however, impalement injuries and retained weapons may be providing tamponade of potential vessels, which can bleed catastrophically if removed in uncontrolled environments.

Evisceration

Penetrating abdominal injuries can occasionally lead to protrusion of the omentum or bowel through the wound. Although there are reports, from countries where there is tremendous experience of penetrating trauma, of the omentum being returned to the abdomen after ligation of bleeding vessels, and the patient managed expectantly, this would not be recommended in UK practice. The viscera should be covered with saline-soaked gauze and provision made to proceed to formal exploration at laparotomy.

ABDOMINAL TRAUMA AT THE EXTREMES OF AGE

Trauma in the older patient

Attempting to define the older age group for medical purposes in terms of age alone remains a difficult task. While socioeconomic and legal definitions exist, there is a broad spectrum of those affected at different ages from the effects of the ageing process; for example, chronic illness and disability may affect those before the age of 65, while those in their 70s or 80s may enjoy full and active lifestyles.

Owing to improved health, lifestyle changes and medical interventions, changing demographics show that the older age group is set to increase in both numbers and as a percentage of the population.

Injury mechanisms are broadly similar to those already described, with blunt trauma the most common form, particularly from falls, road traffic collisions (especially as pedestrians) and, unfortunately, assaults. As with other trauma patients, the possibility of abuse and neglect should be borne in mind, although it may be more difficult to elicit in the older patient.

A key component of caring for the older trauma patient is an understanding of the effects of the ageing process, coexisting medical conditions and medication history. Whether the older patient has an isolated abdominal injury or multiple trauma, these factors can further complicate the clinical picture for the older patient with abdominal trauma, owing to a variety of multisystem conditions. For example, the older patient is susceptible to constipation, which could affect the abdominal examination.

The ageing process affects all body systems, physical appearance and mental state. Sensory impairment may hamper effective communication with the patient and hence affect the physical assessment. Communication methods should be modified accordingly to elicit as much information as possible.

The clinical features of hypovolaemia may not be so readily recognisable in the older patient, which can lead to an underestimation of the amount of blood loss. The older patient compensates poorly for blood loss: a relatively small blood loss can result in hypotension owing to a reduced sympathetic nervous system response. Similarly, those taking beta-blocker medication will not exhibit tachycardia owing to inhibition of the positive inotropic response of the sympathetic nervous system. Those with pacemakers may also not exhibit a tachycardia in response to hypovolaemia, as the rate may be pre-set within particular parameters. Hypotension will, however, be evident.

Urinary output as an indicator of perfusion may not be reliable in the older patient owing to renal changes and reduced total body water content, affecting the ability of the kidneys to concentrate urine.

> The clinical features of hypovolaemia may not be so readily recognisable in the older patient, which can lead to an underestimation of the amount of blood loss

The older patient is particularly susceptible to hypothermia, which results in hypotension, bradycardia and reduced respiratory rate, which in turn can affect the clinical picture presented, and the management of abdominal injury.

The initial assessment and management of the older trauma patient should follow the ATLS® principles of airway, breathing, and circulation with consideration of physiological changes due to the ageing process, pre-existing medical conditions and medication history (American College of Surgeons, 1997).

ABDOMINAL TRAUMA IN CHILDREN

Injury is the commonest cause of death in childhood and blood loss is frequently a major contributing factor. The abdomen can be a significant site of concealed haemorrhage and, therefore, must be assessed early in the child's resuscitation. Although the priorities in the assessment and management of injured children are the same as the adult, the anatomical and physiological differences require specialist consideration.

> Injury is the commonest cause of death in childhood and blood loss is frequently a major contributing factor

Most abdominal injuries that occur in children in the UK are the result of blunt trauma; most frequently motor vehicle collisions. Penetrating trauma requires immediate surgical involvement.

Certain abdominal injuries are more common in children than their adult counterparts as a result of the anatomical differences and differing activities. Bicycle handlebars can cause duodenal haematomas or pancreatic injuries; bladder injuries may occur, as the pelvis is more shallow and the solid organs (liver, spleen, kidney) are frequently injured. The assessment of the injured child can be difficult and it is important that the resuscitation is carried out in a calm and reassuring manner. Air swallowed when the child is crying can cause discomfort, and decompression of the stomach may be required. The severely injured child needs urinary catheterisation. Abdominal examination in the conscious child should avoid undue distress and painful palpation should be deferred to the end of the examination.

The management of abdominal injury in children differs markedly from adult practice. DPL is not recommended in children, as it is invasive. FAST can provide an initial screening of the abdomen; however, CT with its ability to provide more organ-specific information is the preferred investigation in injured children who are cardiovascularly stable. Non-operative management of solid organ injury in children has been the approved standard for the vast majority of these injuries for a number of years (Smith et al., 1992; Losty et al., 1997) and was the forerunner of this approach in adults (Carillo et al., 1998). Bleeding from the liver, kidney and spleen is generally self-limiting and can usually, unless there is gross haemodynamic instability, be managed non-operatively. The decision to follow this approach should be made by the surgeons and close observation in a high dependency or intensive care area is necessary, and frequent re-evaluation of the child is required, as deterioration may require urgent surgery.

TRAUMA IN PREGNANCY

The challenge for the trauma team is that, in pregnancy, trauma may affect both the mother and the fetus. Successful resuscitation and management of the mother will determine the outcome for the fetus. Like the non-pregnant woman, trauma in pregnancy may be blunt or penetrating, but is more commonly blunt. This may be the result of road traffic collisions, falls and direct blows to the abdomen. Awareness of the possibility of domestic violence in some cases should always be borne in mind.

Epidemiology

In the UK between 1991 and 1993, 7% of maternal deaths were due to trauma. Approximately 8% of even minor trauma admissions have been seen to result in complications that include premature labour, placental abruption and fetal injury (Goodwin and Breen, 1990).

Anatomical changes in pregnancy

The uterus remains within the pelvis during the first trimester of pregnancy. At this stage, it is a thick-walled organ protected by a bony pelvis. As the pregnancy progresses, the uterus rises out of the pelvis and becomes an intra-abdominal organ. By the 20th week, it has reached the umbilicus. As the fetus develops, the uterus displaces the abdominal viscera upwards toward the diaphragm. By the third trimester, the uterus is large and thin walled, amniotic fluid volume is decreased and exposure to the risk of trauma is augmented.

The inelastic placenta is usually attached to the uterine wall anteriorly. Its lack of elasticity renders it vulnerable to shearing forces associated with blunt trauma. On examination, the pregnant trauma victim may present with concealed or vaginal bleeding.

Physiological changes during pregnancy

Airway
- Risk of aspiration is greater owing to the tendency for gastric reflux.
- Oedema of neck or epiglottis can make endotracheal intubation difficult.

Breathing/ventilation
- Increased oxygen requirements result in hyperventilation.
- Tidal volume is increased by up to 40%.
- Forced vital capacity is reduced (hypocapnoea) – 4.0 kPa ($PaCO_2$ 30 mmHg).

Circulation
- Plasma volume increases by up to 50%, leading to a relative haemodilution.
- Haemoglobin increases slightly but, as there is a greater increase in plasma volume, the haematocrit is decreased (physiological anaemia of pregnancy).
- Cardiac output increases by 1–1.5 litres/minute owing to the increase in plasma volume.
- Heart rate increases 5–15 beats per minute.
- Blood pressure decreases 5–15 mmHg during the second trimester, returning to normal by term.
- In a supine position, the gravid uterus may press on the inferior vena cava, reducing the venous return by up to 30%, therefore, reducing cardiac output (supine maternal hypotension).

Mechanisms of injury

Mechanisms of injury are similar to those of the non-pregnant woman.

Blunt trauma
Shearing forces and direct blows to the abdomen can result in placental abruption or traumatic uterine rupture. The fetus may also sustain direct injury as a result of blunt trauma. If the mother sustains a fractured pelvis, the engaged head of the fetus may sustain a skull fracture.

In road traffic collisions, seat belts have been shown to reduce maternal mortality (Schonfield et al., 1987) and, if correctly fitted, they have been seen to improve fetal outcome (Pearse, 1992). The use of seat belts also prevents ejection of the pregnant woman from the vehicle.

Penetrating trauma
In later pregnancy, the uterus acts as a shield for the mother in penetrating trauma with the incidence of maternal organ damage being quite low (Lavin and Scott Polsky, 1983); however, the uterus and fetus are at high risk of injury from stab wounds, firearm injuries or penetrating objects.

Initial assessment and management
Initial assessment and management of the pregnant trauma victim should follow the ATLS®

(American College of Surgeons, 1997) principles of airway, breathing, and circulation with the following considerations.

- Early consultation with an obstetrician is essential for the outcome of both mother and fetus.
- There is an increased risk of aspiration owing to gastric reflux and so vigilant airway management is crucial. Decompression of the stomach with a nasogastric tube will reduce the risk of aspiration.
- Elevation of the right hip using a wedge will prevent supine hypotension.
- Owing to an increased circulatory volume, the mother may compensate for a long period of time before signs of hypovolaemia become apparent.
- During this time, the fetal circulation will be reduced and may result in a poor fetal outcome.
- Early intravenous access and volume replacement are essential, and systolic blood pressure should be as near to normal as possible; but none of these procedures should delay the need for early surgical intervention

involving laparotomy or early Caesarian section.

> Owing to an increased circulatory volume, the mother may compensate for a long period of time before signs of hypovolaemia become apparent

CONCLUSION

The trauma patient with suspected abdominal injury should be managed in accordance with the ATLS® principles by the trauma team. The rapid and accurate diagnosis of abdominal trauma is vital in the management of the trauma patient to reduce the morbidity and mortality associated with abdominal injury. The introduction of FAST ultrasound is a valuable advance in the resuscitation room and should be used early in the primary survey to direct the search for bleeding. CT scan in stable patients allows more accurate diagnosis of injury and may allow a non-operative approach to be pursued.

> Unstable patients who have intra-abdominal bleeding need rapid resuscitation and urgent transfer to theatre for surgery

References

American College of Surgeons. *Advanced trauma life support student course manual.* Chicago: American College of Surgeons, 1997

Anderson ID, Woodford M, Conbal FT, Irving M. Retrospective study of 1000 trauma deaths from injury in England and Wales. *British Medical Journal* 1988. 296: 1305–1308

Bickell WH, Wall MJ, Pepe PE, Martin RR, Ginger VF, Allen MK, Mattox KL. Immediate versus delayed fluid resuscitation for hypotensive patients with penetrating torso injuries. *New England Journal of Medicine* 1994; 331: 1105–1109

Brooks A, Boffard K. Current technology – laparoscopic surgery in trauma. *Trauma* 1999; 1: 53–60

Buckman RF, Scalea TM (eds). International approaches to trauma care. *Trauma Quarterly* 1999; 14

Burdett-Smith P, Airey GM, Franks AJ. Improvement in trauma survival in Leeds. *Injury* 1995; 26: 45–48

Buzzas GR, Kern SJ, Smith SR, Harrison PB, Helmer SD, Reed JA. A comparison of sonographic examinations for trauma performed by surgeons and radiologists. *Journal of Trauma* 1998; 44: 604–608

Carrillo EH, Platz A, Miller FB, Richardson JD, Polk HC Jr. Non operative management of blunt hepatic trauma. *British Journal of Surgery* 1998; 85: 461–468

Cooper GJ, Ryan JM. Interaction of penetrating missiles with tissues: some common misapprehensions and implications for wound management. *British Journal of Surgery* 1990; 77: 606–610

Goodwin TM, Breen MT. Pregnancy outcome and fetal maternal hemorrhage after non-catastrophic trauma. *American Journal of Obstetrics and Gynecology* 1990; 162: 665–671

Johnson JW, Gracias VH, Schwab CW, Reilly PM, Kauder DR, Shapiro MB, Dabrowski GP, Rotondo MF. Evolution in damage control for exsanguinating penetrating abdominal injury. *Journal of Trauma* 2001; 51: 261–271

Lavin JP, Scott Polsky S. Abdominal trauma during pregnancy. *Clinical Perinatology* 1983; 10: 423–427

Leppaniemi AK, Elliot DC. The role of laparoscopy in blunt abdominal trauma. *Annals of Medicine* 1996; 28: 483–489

Losty PD, Okoye BO, Walter DP, Turncock RR, Lloyd DA. Management of blunt liver trauma in children. *British Journal of Surgery* 1997; 84: 1006–1008

Office for National Statistics. *Mortality statistics. Injury and poisoning 1993 and 1994*. Series DH4, no. 19. London: HMSO, 1997

Ordog GJ (ed.). *Management of gunshot wounds*. New York: Elsevier, 1988

Pearse M. Seat belts in pregnancy. *British Medical Journal* 1992; 304: 586–587

Powell DC, Bivins BA, Bell RM. Diagnostic peritoneal lavage. *Surgery, Gynecology and Obstetrics* 1982; 155: 257–264

Root HD, Hauser CW, McKinley CR, Lafave JW, Mendiola RP. Diagnostic peritoneal lavage. *Surgery* 1965. 57: 633–637

Rozycki GS, Oschner MG, Jaffin JH, Champion HR. Prospective evaluation of surgeons' use of ultrasound in the evaluation of trauma patients. *Journal of Trauma* 1993; 34: 516–526

Rozycki GS, Shackford SR. Ultrasound, what every trauma surgeon should know. *Journal of Trauma* 1996; 640: 1–4

Rozycki GS, Shackford SR. Trauma ultrasound for surgeons. In: Staren E, Arregui ME (eds) *Ultrasound for the surgeon*. New York: Lippincott-Raven, 1997: 120–135

Ryan J, Rich N, Morgans B, Dale R, Cooper G. (eds). *Ballistic trauma, clinical relevance in peace and war*. London: Arnold, 1997

Scalea TM, Rodriguez A, Chiu WC, Brenneman FD, Fallon WF Jr, Kato K, McKenney MG, Nerlich ML, Ochsner MG Jr, Yoshii H. Focused assessment with sonograpy for trauma (FAST): results from an International Consensus Conference. *Journal of Trauma* 1999; 46: 444–472

Schonfield A, Ziv E, Stein L, et al. Seat belts in pregnancy and the obstetrician. *Obstetrical and Gynecological Survey* 1987; 42: 275–282

Sclafani SJ, Shaftan GW, Scalea TM. Non operative salvage of computed tomography diagnosed splenic injuries: utilisation of angiography for triage and embolisation for hemostasis. *Journal of Trauma* 1995; 39: 818–827

Sherck JP, Oakes DD. Intestinal injuries missed by computed tomography. *Journal of Trauma* 1990; 30: 1–7

Smith JS Jr, Wengrovitz MA, Delong BS. Prospective validation of criteria, including age, for safe non surgical management of ruptures of the spleen. *Journal of Trauma* 1992; 33: 363–368

West JG, Trunkey DD, Lim RC. Systems of trauma care: a study of two counties. *Archives of Surgery* 1979; 114: 455

Wherry DC, Punzalan CMK. Imaging in abdominal trauma. *Trauma* 2000; 2: 283–290

Zantut LF, Ivatury RR, Smith S, et al. Diagnostic and therapeutic laparoscopy for penetrating abdominal trauma: a multicentre experience. *Journal of Trauma* 1997; 42: 825–831

Chapter **28**

Maxillofacial trauma

David R. J. Parkins

INTRODUCTION

The maxillofacial area may be defined as extending from the upper margins of the orbits to the lower border of the mandible. This is a vital region to all of us; not only is the face intimately involved with eating, drinking, taste and speech, we also use this area to express the emotions of anger, joy, surprise, horror and sexual arousal. Our face is what we present to the rest of the world as our identity. As a result of its prominent position, the face is also on the receiving end of a significant amount of traumatic injury. Such trauma not only has implications regarding physical treatment of the injury inflicted, but also may cause prolonged psychological morbidity to the patient.

CLINICAL ANATOMY

The anatomy of the face is complex and consists of an underlying facial skeleton (Figure 28.1) with attached musculature, soft tissues, and skin. There are also several specialised areas, including the eyes, nose and the mouth, in addition to the salivary glands and the lacrimal apparatus, providing a variety of special senses including smell, vision, taste, speech, eating, breathing and facial expression.

Facial bones

The main bones of the facial skeleton and their principal functions are shown in Box 28.1.

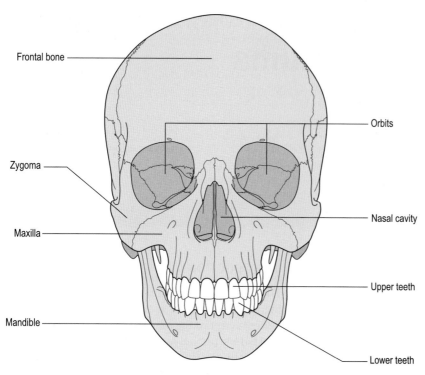

Figure 28.1 Anterior view of the facial skeleton.

Frontal bone

Orbits

Zygoma

Nasal cavity

Maxilla

Upper teeth

Mandible

Lower teeth

Box 28.1 Main bones of the facial skeleton and their functions

Maxilla	Bearing the upper teeth
Zygoma (malar)	Providing the prominences of the cheekbones
Nasal Vomer Ethmoid }	Providing and supporting the nasal complex
Palatine	Posterior part of the hard palate
Mandible	Bearing the lower teeth

The facial muscles are attached to the facial skeleton and are supplied by the seventh (facial) cranial nerve with the exception of the muscles of mastication (chewing), which receive their innervation from the motor branch of the fifth (trigeminal) nerve. These latter muscles are associated with chewing in that they move the mandible and thus the lower teeth in relation to the maxillae bearing the upper teeth. The muscles supplied by the seventh cranial nerve are termed the 'muscles of facial expression'. This nerve travels through the facial canal behind the ear and passes through the parotid salivary gland on the side of the face. It is, therefore, very susceptible to injury, either due to damage within the canal, often as a result of fracture of the temporal bone, or from facial lacerations, which may cut the nerve as it crosses the side of the face. Injury to this nerve can result in permanent facial paralysis.

The nose is a specialised structure consisting of two external nares (nostrils), which give way to the nasopharynx via the nasal airway. The nose is associated primarily with smelling by the first cranial (olfactory) nerve, although this function has a major role in providing taste sensation also. Owing to its prominence in the middle of the face, the nose is at risk from traumatic injury.

The mouth is the first part of the gastro-intestinal tract and is primarily associated with the preparation of food for swallowing. This is achieved by means of the teeth and the tongue. Saliva is added to the food, and this acts not only as a lubricant but also adds enzymes to food to begin the process of digestion. The mouth is also involved with breathing and with speaking.

MAXILLOFACIAL TRAUMA

Aetiology

As has already been mentioned, interpersonal violence is the commonest cause of facial injury (Telfer et al., 1991), although motor vehicle collisions (MVC) still account for a significant number and are a major cause of facial fractures. Alcohol is a significant factor in the majority of facial injuries in both the assault and MVC groups. Most victims are young, in their late teens to early 20s and male.

In addition to fights and MVCs, maxillofacial injuries may also result from:

- sport, particularly of the contact variety (e.g. rugby, boxing)
- industrial injuries
- falls, especially in the elderly and those with epilepsy.

Injury to the facial bones is rare in children. The facial skeleton forms from fibrous tissue and the bones of children are particularly soft and pliable. When fractures are seen in children, this suggests significantly high levels of energy dissipation and the possibility of non-accidental injury must always be considered.

In current UK practice, the vast majority of facial injuries are blunt, with penetrating trauma and significant tissue loss, as seen in the so-called 'military-type injury', very rare indeed.

Basic management principles in facial injury

Injuries to the facial area may be isolated, but many patients have other injuries; these may be more serious and more of a threat to life. Associated injuries may, therefore, take priority over facial wounds. Nevertheless, given the close anatomical relationship of the facial tissues to the airway and also as a result of the copious blood supply to the facial tissues, maxillofacial trauma may well be life threatening.

> Facial injuries may be life threatening either because of airway obstruction or blood loss

The initial management of the patient who has sustained maxillofacial trauma is no different from the management of any other patient,

---

Box 28.2	The mnemonic 'AMPLE'
A	Allergies
M	Medication (including prescription, over-the-counter and recreational drugs)
P	Previous medical history
L	Last time of eating/drinking
E	Events surrounding the incident i.e. 'What happened?'

following the fundamental principles of primary survey, resuscitation and then secondary survey.

History

It is important to try to obtain a full history, either from the patient or from friends, relatives or emergency medical service personnel. The mnemonic 'AMPLE' is useful for ensuring adequate history taking (Box 28.2).

The primary survey of patients with maxillofacial injuries follows the standard ABCDE pattern as promulgated in 'Advanced trauma life support' (ATLS®; American College of Surgeons, 1997) courses:

- airway with cervical spine control
- breathing
- circulation with haemorrhage control
- disability
- exposure/environment.

Airway obstruction

Airway obstruction is often a feature of facial trauma. This may be due to swelling of the oral tissues, loosening or detachment of the teeth which may then be inhaled, or a result of the tongue falling back in the airway. The tongue is attached via the genial tubercle to the inner surface of the mandible in the midline. In bilateral fractures of the body of the mandible, this tongue attachment is lost and the so-called flail mandible results. The tongue is thus free-floating and, if the patient is supine, the airway is at risk. If immediate airway control is not available, these patients are best nursed either in the recovery position or else prone, where gravity will pull the tongue forward, and also allow secretions and blood to run out of the airway. Consideration must be given to possible injuries of the cervical spine before repositioning the patient.

When viewed from the side, the facial skeleton appears to be attached to the base of the skull at an angle of 45° (Figure 28.2). This means that, when direct force is applied to the front of the face, the entire facial skeleton can detach from the base of the skull, and tend to slide downwards and backwards (Figure 28.3).

This has the effect of occluding the airway, and relief of this requires urgent disimpaction and reduction of the facial skeleton to its previous position. This may require placing the fingers behind the palate and pulling the entire face forwards and upwards to restore the patency of the airway. This task may need the attention of the on-call maxillofacial team. If it proves impossible to reduce the dislocation, then a surgical airway may be required.

Early airway management with endotracheal intubation is indicated in patients whose airway is at risk following facial injury. Owing to the swelling, bleeding and associated disruption of

the anatomy seen with facial injuries, expert anaesthetic involvement is required at an early stage. As a result of the difficulties in airway management that these patients present, emergency departments (EDs) should discuss with

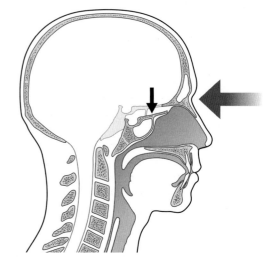

Figure 28.3 Basal skull fracture with potential airway obstruction.

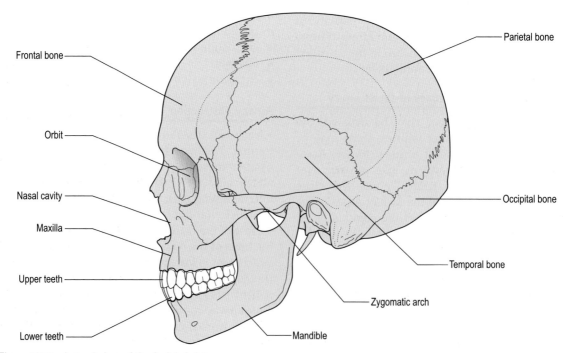

Figure 28.2 Lateral view of the facial skeleton.

their anaesthetic departments what equipment should be available for difficult intubation cases. Such items as right-handed and McCoy laryngoscope blades, intubating laryngeal mask airways (ILMA®), retrograde intubation sets and fibreoptic laryngoscopes should all be considered for provision in the emergency department. An anaesthetic machine for gaseous induction of anaesthesia may also be necessary.

Haemorrhage

The facial structures have a particularly profuse blood supply. This can be advantageous in that wounds heal rapidly without serious risk of infection. The negative aspect of this is that injury to the face can result in severe and potentially life-threatening bleeding. Haemorrhage of facial injuries is managed as for any injury with blood loss, control of bleeding, large-bore intravenous access and fluid replacement.

Controlling bleeding may be very difficult in some complex facial fractures and early involvement of the maxillofacial team to reduce the fractures is indicated. Direct pressure on the tissues may control soft tissue bleeding and, in the case of severe blood loss from the cheeks and lips, bimanual pressure can be applied from both within the mouth and externally. When the bleeding is intraoral, the patient should be encouraged to spit out blood rather than swallow, since this can precipitate vomiting. The use of intranasal packs may be life saving in some instances of nasoethmoidal fracture with profuse haemorrhage (Dyer and Greaves, 1995).

FRACTURES OF THE FACIAL SKELETON

Fractures of the facial skeleton are usually the result of direct trauma and the forces involved are often severe, so cervical spine and skull injury should always be suspected. Facial fractures in themselves are not generally life threatening unless they compromise the airway or cause severe blood loss. Most fractures of the facial skeleton can safely be left until the patient is stabilised as part of a head-to-toe examination in the secondary survey. Indeed, definitive management of most facial fractures can be delayed for

several days until the multisystem trauma patient is more stable.

Types of facial fracture

Fractures of the facial skeleton can be classified as follows:

- middle third of the facial skeleton (Le Fort I, Le Fort II, Le Fort III)
- nasal complex
- zygomatic
- mandibular (lower third of the facial skeleton)
- dentoalveolar.

Middle third fractures

Le Fort I, II and III fractures were first classified by René Le Fort in 1901. Le Fort was a surgeon in Paris who produced facial injuries in cadavers by dropping weights from varying heights. The facial fractures thereby induced were examined by dissection of the subjects. He found that, although all facial fractures cause gross comminution of the facial skeleton, with some several hundred fragments of bone caused by one blow, all fractures broadly fell into three categories (Figure 28.4): low-level (Le Fort I); mid-level (Le Fort II) and high-level (Le Fort III).

Management of middle third fractures

Initial management of these patients follows the basic principles of the primary survey with ongoing resuscitation. Attention to airway, cervical spine, breathing, circulation, disability and exposure takes first priority.

> Patients who have sustained fractures to the middle third of the face are at risk of having sustained cervical spine and head injury

Patients who have sustained middle third fractures are at risk of having sustained cervical spine and head injury, and these should be sought if suspected. There is usually generalised swelling of the face, often with elongation of the face itself. When viewed from the side, there is frequently a 'dished-in' appearance to the face. The patient frequently complains of being unable to close the teeth together normally. This often indicates

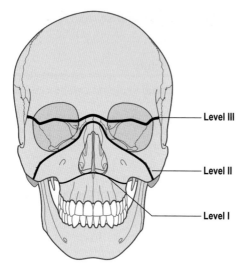

Figure 28.4 Le Fort classification of fractures of the middle third of the facial skeleton.

downward and backward displacement of the facial skeleton and is a result of the patient closing together on to the back (molar) teeth, leaving the anterior teeth wide apart. This is known as 'anterior open bite'. Patients with middle third fractures may show loss of a clear fluid from the nostrils. This may be a cerebrospinal fluid leak from the brain. This indicates fracture of the cribriform plate of the base of the skull within the anterior cranial fossa. There is a risk of infection and antibiotic cover is indicated in these patients; penicillin is usually the agent of choice, with erythromycin being given in penicillin-sensitive individuals.

Diagnosis of the exact type of Le Fort fracture sustained can be difficult; indeed, some patients may have different types of fracture on opposite sides or may even have several fracture levels on one side. In truth, the exact level is immaterial in the initial management of these patients. Common features on examination are altered sensation over the frontal and infraorbital areas, a so-called 'cracked-cup' sound on percussing the upper incisors and the entire facial skeleton may be mobile. This last sign is elicited by grasping the upper anterior teeth with the fingers of one hand and attempting to move the face in and out. The fingers of the other hand may be placed over the frontonasal area to detect mobility of the middle

third of the face. Examination inside the mouth may reveal splitting of the palate in the midline, and there is also usually bruising and swelling of the buccal sulcus, between the cheeks and the teeth-bearing bony ridge.

Definitive diagnosis can be deferred in severe trauma patients until initial resuscitation and management is complete. First investigations will include plain radiography with 'facial views' (i.e. occipitomental 15° and 30°). Owing to the complex anatomy, and the fact that most of these fractures are severely comminuted, interpretation of the radiographs can be difficult. Most centres now advocate the use of computed tomography (CT) or magnetic resonance imaging (MRI) for definitive investigation and pre-operative planning in these cases.

Patients who have sustained middle third fractures frequently have intraoral bleeding. They should be encouraged to spit out this blood rather than swallow, since this can precipitate vomiting. Such patients should be offered oral hygiene procedures, since dried blood and saliva in the mouth can be particularly uncomfortable and distressing.

Nasal fractures

The nose is one of the most prominent parts of the face and is, therefore, particularly susceptible to traumatic injury. The nasal bones are especially thin and fragile, and so comminuted fractures of these bones are common. Broadly speaking, trauma to the nose can come from one of three directions: the left, the right or the front. Blows from the side usually result in fracture with deviation of the nasal prominence away from the side of the attack; indeed, it is often possible to surmise on which fist has been used to deliver the blow! If a right-hand-dominant assailant hits their victim with a 'right cross', that is coming from the victim's left, then this will tend to push the entire nose over to the right. Usually, left- or right-sided displacement is a simple injury to treat.

With frontal blows, the nasal bones tend to collapse into the face, and particularly into the nasoethmoidal complex. These injuries can be severely disfiguring and may well be technically very difficult to treat successfully. Typically the patient presents with 'dishing-in' of the nasal complex with broadening and flattening of the nose; compromise of the nasal airway is common.

In assessing the patient with suspected nasal fracture, it is important to take a full history of the alleged mechanism of injury. Diagnosis is essentially a clinical entity, with radiology not being indicated in the initial management. It is vital when first seeing the patient with nasal fractures to exclude septal haematoma. This appears as a red swelling on the nasal septum; it can present either unilaterally or bilaterally. If present, this represents a surgical emergency. Incision and drainage of the blood contained therein is essential, otherwise septal perforation may occur.

If no septal haematoma is detected, the patient may safely be discharged providing no other injuries need managing. Before definitively treating the fracture, it is important to allow the swelling to subside. Patients may, therefore, be discharged from the emergency department with analgesia and general advice; they must particularly be told not to blow their nose, since this may cause surgical emphysema and infection to develop. An outpatient appointment for 5 days time should be made with either the maxillofacial or ear, nose and throat (ENT) team, according to local guidelines. Head injury warning advice may also be appropriate. Written advice sheets regarding nasal fractures can be also helpful.

Zygomatic fractures

Zygomatic fracture is the commonest bony injury to the facial skeleton in UK practice. This bone provides the lateral and inferolateral aspects of the orbit, so such injuries are very frequently associated with eye injury. In one survey, 90% of all zygomatic fractures showed concomitant eye damage of varying degrees (Al-Qurainy et al., 1991). The muscle attachments of the eye are often deranged, causing problems with eye movement and resultant double vision. Eye examination and assessment is, therefore, mandatory when examining patients with zygomatic complex injury. Al-Qurainy et al. have devised the Canniesburn scoring system for detecting patients at high risk of eye injury with associated zygomatic trauma. This is shown in Table 28.1.

Table 28.1 Canniesburn ocular trauma score

Clinical findings after trauma	Score
Visual acuity	
6/6 or better	0
6/9–6/12	4
6/18–6/24	8
6/36 or less	12
No light perception	16
Zygomatic fracture	
Comminuted	3
Blow-out	3
Other	0
Eye movement disorder (e.g. diplopia or post-traumatic squint)	
Present	3
Absent	0
Retrograde or post-traumatic amnesia	
Present	5
Absent	0

Add 1 if final score is 11, and: patient is female; age is 30–39; if cause is road traffic accident.
If final score is: 0–4, no referral necessary; 5–11, consider routine ophthalmic referral; 12+, consider emergency ophthalmic referral.

Zygomatic fractures may be classified according to the anatomical involvement and the degree of displacement of the zygoma itself. This system is of little help in managing these injuries in the emergency department and, since these fractures in themselves are not life threatening, their management can be deferred to the secondary survey phase. Diagnosis of these fractures is a combination of clinical examination and radiology.

The patient will almost invariably have a history of direct trauma to the cheekbone with or without other traumatic injuries. The other injuries may well take precedence over the zygomatic trauma. There is characteristically swelling and bruising over the cheek, and this often extends into the orbit. There may be associated altered sensation over the infraorbital area; if this is suspected, sensation on the contralateral side must be assessed and the two sides compared for sensory function. There may be excess watering of the eye, suggesting damage to the lacrimal apparatus and full assessment of the eye itself is, of course, necessary (see earlier). Palpation of the zygoma must include the zygomatic arch and the entire orbital rim. Any stepping or loss of bony continuity is suggestive of bony injury. When viewed from above the top of the head, depression of the arch may be seen, although in the early postinjury phase, soft tissue swelling may mask this sign. Arch fractures are often associated with inability to open the mouth fully or problems with moving the lower jaw from side to side.

In suspected zygomatic fracture, facial radiographs are indicated, the standard views being occipitomental (OM) taken at 15° and 30°. For arch fractures, the submentovertex, or *'jug-handle'* view is indicated. The OM views can be difficult to interpret, but it is essential to try and visualise the orbital margins for integrity of bony continuity, and also to assess the maxillary sinuses on each side. Clouding or reduction of the apparent size of this air space is pathognomonic of zygomatic fracture, whilst a so-called 'tear-drop' sign hanging from the floor of the orbit is indicative of a blow-out fracture of the floor of the orbit. In this injury, the orbital contents, including parts of the inferior rectus muscle, herniate from the orbit through the orbital floor into the sinus. Classically, these patients are unable to look upwards with the affected eye. Plain radiographs are frequently insufficient for operative planning and the maxillofacial specialist team may well request either CT or MRI imaging at some stage prior to surgical repair.

Initial management of these patients involves initial management of life-threatening injuries followed by secondary survey to find and assess other injuries. Appropriate referral to maxillofacial or plastic teams will be according to locally agreed guidelines and availability of these specialists. If possible, these patients are best nursed in a head-up position to aid drainage and to reduce swelling. Nose blowing must be strongly discouraged, even if the patient is not requiring hospital admission, since surgical emphysema and infection may result. Since these are almost inevitable open fractures, prophylactic antibiotics should be given according to the locally agreed protocol. Regular assessment of the eyes for pupil reactions, visual acuity and movement is essential to detect potential problems, particularly with bleeding into the orbit. This condition, termed retrobulbar haemorrhage, is a potential threat to sight and requires emergency decompression of the orbit to save the patient's sight.

> Retrobulbar haemorrhage is a potential threat to sight and requires emergency decompression of the orbit to save the patient's sight

Retrobulbar haemorrhage is suggested by: a hard tense eyeball with a dilating pupil, reducing range of eye movements, increasing pain behind the eye, decreasing visual acuity, pale optic disc and proptosis. If this condition is suspected, an immediate ophthalmic opinion must be sought. Emergency management of a retrobulbar bleed is both medical and surgical.

Medical management consists of:

- acetazolamide 500 mg intravenously;
- hydrocortisone 100 mg intravenously;
- mannitol 20% 200 ml intravenously.

Surgical management consists of emergency decompression of the orbit. This may be undertaken by the maxillofacial team caring for the patient, or may be deferred to an ophthalmic surgeon or a plastic surgeon

Mandibular injuries

Given its prominent and isolated position at the lower part of the face, it is not surprising that fractures of this bone are common. Interpersonal violence and motor vehicle collisions are the commonest causes, with sporting injuries also accounting for a significant number of injuries. The site of fracture depends upon the mechanism of injury; these sites, in descending order of their frequency of occurrence, are:

- condyle – 36%
- body – 21%
- angle – 20%
- symphysis – 14%
- coronoid process – 3%
- ramus – 3%.

The patient typically presents with a history of direct trauma, and often complains of pain at the site or sites of fracture, malocclusion of the teeth, facial swelling and the inability to open the mouth normally. In the dentate patient and where the fracture passes through a tooth-bearing part of the mandible, there is often intraoral bleeding, emphasising the fact that such fractures are classified as open. Examination of the patient may reveal facial deformity with associated pain, trismus and paraesthesia of the mental nerve, crepitus, malocclusion, sublingual haematoma and intraoral bleeding.

As always the first priority is with airway, breathing and circulation. The airway may be particularly compromised in mandibular fractures in the so-called 'flail mandible' (see earlier). If such patients are nursed supine, the tongue may fall back in the pharynx causing obstruction of the airway. As a result of these fractures, the patient is unable to maintain tongue protrusion and may, therefore, asphyxiate. Placing the patient on the prone or the recovery position may be life saving, although care must be taken in suspected cervical spine injury.

> Patients with maxillofacial injuries may be nursed in the prone or recovery position; extreme care must be taken in suspected cervical spine injury

Alternatives are airway adjuncts, if tolerated by the patient, or traction on the tongue with a large suture placed through the body of the tongue musculature, a so-called 'tongue suture'. Alternatively, if the patient is conscious but cannot maintain his or her own airway, rapid sequence induction (RSI) of anaesthesia with endotracheal intubation must be considered. Given the fact that these patients have not been starved and that they have considerably deranged anatomy as a result of their injuries, RSI should be left to an experienced anaesthetist. If the airway cannot be maintained by any of these more conventional methods, then consideration should be given to performance of a surgical airway technique.

Radiological investigations are essential in the diagnosis of mandibular fractures. As a minimum, the patient with a suspected fracture of the lower jaw should have an orthopantomogram (OPG) performed. In addition a postero-anterior view of the mandible may be helpful. If OPG is not available, bilateral lateral oblique views of each side of the mandible helps to visualise the angle and body. Specialised temporomandibular joint (TMJ) views with the mouth open and closed may be considered necessary in suspected TMJ fractures.

Definitive management of mandibular fractures has changed considerably in the last two decades. The standard treatment in the 1970s and into the 1980s was reduction of the fracture with intermaxillary fixation (IMF; jaw wiring) for a prolonged period. In areas without access to specialist treatment, this method will still have its role, given that it is possible to apply this therapy with local anaesthesia only. There are several drawbacks with this technique. If the patient vomits, the airway may be at risk and aspiration of vomit is a real risk. Wire cutters used to accompany such patients on each trip around the hospital in case this occurred! The other main problem connected with IMF was malnutrition; inevitably, the patient must stick to a liquid diet for the 6 weeks of fixation and weight loss was inevitable, indeed, jaw wiring was in vogue in the past as a treatment for obesity. The fact that it is no longer used now for this is testament to its lack of success in providing sustained weight loss. In addition to these difficulties, wiring the jaws together by a variety of methods can cause arthritis of the TMJ and also causes problems with dental hygiene, thereby possibly resulting in dental decay and gum disease.

Nowadays management of mandibular fractures is generally by open reduction of the fracture; with the patient under general anaesthetic fixation of the fractures is maintained by microplating techniques. Many mandibular fractures with little or no displacement are frequently amenable to being managed conservatively with soft diet, physiotherapy and analgesia. Whatever the injury, involvement of the on-call maxillofacial team at an early stage is mandatory.

Soft tissue injuries of the face

As a result of the abundant blood supply to the facial tissues, injuries to this area may result in quite profound blood loss either externally or internally. This munificent supply means that any disruption to the facial tissues heals quickly and usually without significant sequelae. These wounds are particularly resistant to infection. Management of soft tissue wounds of the face is frequently left to the on-call maxillofacial team but such a facility may not always be available and, in some circumstances, repair may have to be undertaken by ED staff. These wounds can be some of the most difficult but also the most rewarding to treat. The basic principles are the same as for any other soft tissue repair but there are certain specific considerations to bear in mind.

Patient preparation is vital to success, with adequate lighting, anaesthesia and cooperation being essential. Instruments should be capable of handling fine suture material, either 5-0 or 6-0 without causing cutting of the material or slipping through the jaws of the needle holders. The provision of fine suture packs for use only on facial injuries should be considered. Wound closure in layers is essential in facial wound repair to prevent subsidence of the repair; a fine absorbable suture (e.g. 5-0 Vicryl®) should be used.

DENTOALVEOLAR AND DENTAL INJURIES

These injuries primarily involve the teeth as well as the supporting tissues, that is the alveolar bone of the mandible and maxilla, and the associated soft tissues, the gums (gingivae) and the adjacent oral mucosa.

The teeth themselves may be fractured, subluxated (dislocated) or luxated (avulsed). Fractures of the teeth may be classified as follows (Figures 28.5 and 28.6):

1. enamel only
2. enamel and dentine without pulpal exposure
3. enamel and dentine with pulpal exposure
4. fracture of the root of the tooth, below the level of the alveolar ridge.

Teeth that have been fractured but which are still retained in the socket will need to be seen by a dentist as a matter of urgency. The enamel fractures are not too painful and need treatment primarily for aesthetic reasons. Those fractures involving dentine will require dressing with a sedative coating (usually calcium hydroxide paste) and may also need removal of the pulp and root filling at some stage (endodontic therapy).

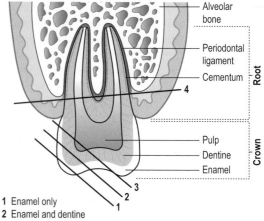

1 Enamel only
2 Enamel and dentine
3 Enamel, dentine and pulp
4 Fracture below level of alveolar ridge (root fracture)

Figure 28.5 Anatomy of incisor tooth and fracture classification.

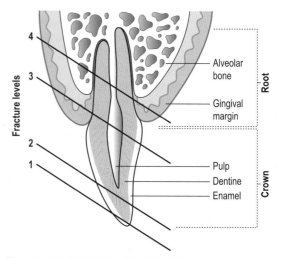

Figure 28.6 Sagittal section of tooth.

Fractures where the dental pulp is exposed require endodontic therapy both for pain control, and also to prevent dental infection and abscess formation. Antibiotic cover may be indicated for this category of patient. In cases where there is a root fracture, there will usually be some degree of subluxation of the tooth and also associated fracture of the alveolar bone. Again antibiotic cover is indicated, and these patients should be referred to the on-call maxillofacial team or a dental surgeon for definitive care.

Dental fractures are usually caused by direct or indirect trauma, and the cause varies with age and sex. In younger children, fractures of the deciduous dentition are rare and usually indicate significant violence. The possibility of non-accidental injury must always be considered. In older children, dental fractures become more prevalent in boys, usually as a result of contact sports. It is commonly the incisors that are involved and particularly the upper incisors, especially if these teeth are more prominent. All children involved in any contact sport should be encouraged to wear custom-fitted dental guards; these are particularly efficient at reducing dental fractures and, in high school football in the USA, they are mandatory for all players. In young adults, interpersonal violence is the principal cause of dentoalveolar injury, with sport and falls accounting for a large percentage of the remainder. Epileptic patients are also at significant risk from dental trauma, sustained during the course of seizures.

Finally, iatrogenic trauma may either present to the emergency department or, indeed, may even be caused within the department by over-enthusiastic insertion of airway adjuncts, commonly oropharyngeal airways or injudicious manipulation with a laryngoscope. Patients who have already sustained trauma to the teeth are particularly at risk from having dental injuries further exacerbated by this means. In patients with reduced level of consciousness, any very loose or avulsed teeth should be removed to avoid potential inhalation during their continuing management in the emergency department.

Where a tooth has been lost from its socket, there is a matter of urgency in replacing it. The earlier this is done, the higher the success rate for reimplantation. If a patient or carer telephones for advice on this subject, they should be advised to attend for care as considered appropriate. If the patient is fully alert and has full comprehension of the situation, the caller should be told to place the tooth in the patient's buccal sulcus (i.e. between the lower teeth and the lip or cheek). There is good evidence that this is the most appropriate and most physiological place to keep the tooth in transfer, with the highest reimplantation success rate. Ideally, the caller should be given instructions on direct reimplantation, if this is deemed convenient, and particularly if there is a

long period before treatment will become available. Of course, this option may not be appropriate in many cases. If it is not possible for whatever reason for the tooth to be transported in the buccal sulcus, then the following are appropriate alternatives:

- gently wrap in Clingfilm
- place in milk within a clean receptacle
- place in saline within a clean receptacle or wrap in saline-soaked gauze
- place in water within a clean receptacle.

On arrival at the A&E department, the patient should be generally assessed for injuries and the luxated tooth should be inspected. Reimplantation is really only applicable to anterior teeth and, if there is any fracture of the tooth, then specialist advice should be urgently sought. If reimplantation is considered to be the correct treatment, then the tooth should be gently irrigated in normal saline, attempting to remove any debris or blood clot, but with minimal disturbance to the adherent soft tissue, the periodontal ligament. Integrity of this is essential to the success of the procedure. Next the socket should be examined and any clot gently removed; infiltration of local anaesthetic may help with this procedure, and will certainly make the reimplantation easier. To effect reimplantation, the crown of the tooth is gently inserted into the socket and inserted into what appears to be an acceptable position. It is vital to ensure that:

1. the tooth is correctly orientated (i.e. not 'back to front'
2. if there are two or more teeth for reimplantation, each is inserted into its appropriate socket.

After reimplantation, it is necessary to splint the tooth *in situ*. This is ideally done by a dentist with adhesive cement but, in an emergency, a splint can be fashioned from a piece of aluminium foil; a milk bottle top, if available, is the ideal size for this. It is folded in half, and applied to both anterior and posterior aspects of the tooth, moulded around all of the teeth, and cemented in place with a 'runny' mix of dental cement. Dental referral is necessary for definitive care and the reimplanted tooth will almost invariably require endodontic treatment. Once again, antibiotic cover and tetanus prophylaxis are essential.

Alveolar fractures usually result in subluxation of the adjacent teeth. In these injuries, careful assessment of the vitality of the teeth is necessary as well as appraisal of the fracture by intraoral radiography. Vitality testing can be carried out by placing a small pledget of cotton wool soaked in ethyl chloride on to the tooth. A tooth is said to be 'vital' (i.e. have intact nerve function), if the cold sensation can be felt.

The main priority is to relocate the tooth or the displaced alveolar bone into its anatomical position. As a temporary measure, local anaesthetic infiltration of the adjacent oral mucosa may allow digital reduction of the fractured alveolar plate until definitive treatment can be accessed. This will allow the subluxated tooth or teeth to be reapproximated into a more anatomical position.

Early specialist referral is indicated. The aforementioned technique of splinting reimplanted teeth may also be used in subluxated teeth after reduction, to ensure stability of the tooth and adjacent bone.

CONCLUSION

Maxillofacial injuries are a common consequence of trauma, especially among the young and as a consequence of motor vehicle crashes. All are potentially life threatening owing to the risk of airway obstruction and significant blood loss, and must be afforded a high clinical priority. Concomitant head injury or cervical spine injury must always be considered, and must be assumed until proven otherwise. Caution must also be exercised when positioning these patients to prevent exacerbation of coexisting injuries.

References

Al-Qurainy IA, Dutton GN, Ilankovan V, et al. Mid facial fractures and the eye: the development of a system for detecting patients at risk. *British Journal of Oral and Maxillofacial Surgery* 1991; 29: 363–367

American College of Surgeons. *Advanced trauma life support student course manual*. Chicago: American College of Surgeons, 1997

Dyer D, Greaves I. New methods for controlling major maxillofacial bleeding. *Journal of the British Association for Immediate Care* 1995; 18

Telfer MR, Jones GM, Shepherd JP. Trends in the aetiology of maxillo-facial fractures in the United Kingdom (1977–87). *British Journal of Oral and Maxillofacial Surgery* 1991; 29: 250–255

Further reading

Hawkesford J, Banks JG. *Maxillofacial and dental injuries*. Oxford: Oxford University Press, 1994

Hutchison I, Lawlor M, Skinner D. Maxillofacial injuries. In: Driscoll P, Skinner D, Earlam R (eds) *ABC of major*

trauma, 3rd edn. London: BMJ Publishing Group, 2000: 42–47

Mitchell DA, Mitchell L. *Oxford handbook of clinical dentistry*, 2nd edn. Oxford: Oxford University Press, 1995

Chapter 29

Ocular trauma

Janet Marsden

CHAPTER CONTENTS

INTRODUCTION

Assessment of ocular trauma is straightforward and a good deal less complicated than generally considered. This chapter aims to provide clear and systematic information to enable clinicians to care for patients with ocular trauma confidently. Basic information relating to the equipment needed for effective assessment of patients with eye and adnexal injuries will be addressed, followed by the assessment itself and its three critical elements, namely, history, visual acuity and examination. Ocular trauma is then divided into sections that address injury to the eye (the globe), injury to the lids and injury to the orbit. Globe trauma is subdivided into surface trauma, blunt trauma, penetrating trauma and burns.

THE BASIS OF EYE ASSESSMENT

Minimal equipment is required for an adequate assessment of the eye. Local anaesthetic eye drops, fluorescein eye drops (which show damaged areas of epithelium by fluorescing in cobalt blue light) and a bright light source (preferably a pen torch with a cobalt blue filter or an ophthalmoscope with a blue filter) are required. A magnifying loupe and slit-lamp are advantageous; having the skills to use them effectively should be the standard to which emergency department (ED) staff aspire. Cotton-tipped applicators or cotton buds are essential for use whilst everting the lid and removing foreign bodies. These should be moistened before the globe is touched, as moist epithelium will stick to a dry cotton tip which is likely to result in loss of cells and more severe injury than that with which the patient attended. Equipment for the accurate assessment of visual acuity must be available.

As with all body structures, a working knowledge of the anatomy and physiology of the eye is essential to make accurate judgements about the extent and importance of injury (Figure 29.1). The eyes and surrounding structures are areas where many non-specialist clinicians feel disadvantaged. These are, therefore, areas where particular attention should be paid regarding triage training and the training of those trauma nurses involved in nurse practitioner roles who undertake the evaluation, treatment and referral of patients with ocular trauma.

ASSESSMENT OF OCULAR TRAUMA

Assessment of trauma essentially comprises three different steps: eliciting an accurate history, examination of the structures involved and, in the case of ocular trauma, assessing visual acuity.

History

The history of the incident(s) that led to presentation may often lead to a working diagnosis before the actual examination takes place. The patient's history is critical in predicting what type of damage may have been sustained to the eye and surrounding structures. For example,

grinding or drilling is likely to lead to a metallic corneal foreign body and no ocular penetration. Use of a hammer and chisel, however, which results in high-speed metal particles being directed towards the eye, may result in an intra-ocular foreign body. A good history is rarely given spontaneously and children, in particular, may give a misleading or unreliable history, especially if they have been doing something they should not. Good questioning techniques are, therefore, essential.

Questioning should elicit the following: a detailed description of the mechanism of injury; symptoms both at the time of injury and at time of presentation; concurrent injuries; first-aid treatment administered (e.g. removal of foreign bodies, area involved, irrigation performed, agents used, duration of irrigation); medical and ophthalmic history; and allergies.

Visual acuity

The patient's best-corrected visual acuity should be ascertained before any other intervention takes place. Exceptions to this are where the patient has a chemical injury and where irrigation should be commenced, or where there is acute pain, when local anaesthetic may be instilled to enable the visual acuity to be recorded accurately. Only after the visual acuity is completed and a brief examination of the eye has been carried out can an accurate and informed triage decision be made.

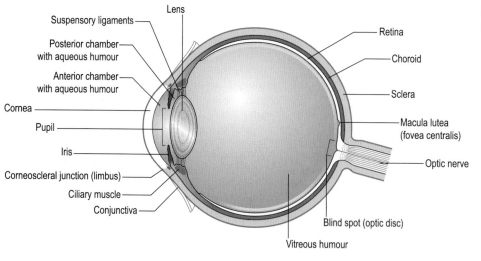

Figure 29.1 Cross-section of the eye.

An informed triage decision can only be made after the visual acuity has been assessed and a brief examination of the eye has been carried out

The patient's affected or poorest eye should be tested first and the other occluded with a card, an occluder or the palm of the patient's hand. (Some patients do not perform this test accurately and look through their fingers.) If the patient wears glasses for distance, these should be worn. Reading glasses should be removed, as it is the best-corrected distance vision that is being assessed. The patient should be asked to read from the top of the Snellen chart downwards making an attempt at all possible letters (Figure 29.2).

Visual acuity should be recorded as the distance at which the eye is being tested (usually 6 metres), over, the last line read by the patient. The number for this line is indicated on the Snellen chart just above or just below the letters.

If part of a line only is read, this is reflected in using a + or − sign; for example, if the patient reads the 6/9 line plus one letter of the line below, the visual acuity is recorded as 6/9 + 1. If all of that line is read other than one letter, 6/9 − 1 would be recorded. If the patient's vision appears poor (less than 6/9), a pinhole (a small hole in a card or a commercial pinhole) can be held in front of the eye to remove the effects of any refractive error. The visual acuity should be recorded with and without pinholes; the use of spectacles or contact lenses should also be included.

If the patient is unable to read the top letter on the Snellen chart, the distance between the chart and the patient should be reduced until the patient can see the top letter, i.e. 5/60, 4/60, etc. to 1/60. If the patient cannot see the top letter at 1 metre, it should be ascertained whether he or she can *count* the assessor's *fingers* (CF – on a couple of occasions to remove any guesswork), see the assessors *hand movements* (HM), or just *perceive light* (PL) at 1 metre. Lack of light perception is recorded as *no perception of light* (NPL). Normal visual acuity is 6/6 or greater, but normal visual acuity for the patient may be less than this for a variety of reasons.

Problems with accurate visual acuity assessment may occur if the patient does not have English as a first language or is not able to read. Strategies to overcome this may include the following.

- The use of a recognition chart so that letters or shapes may be matched using an interpreter or family member to translate for the patient;
- Children are often very cooperative if picture tests, such as the Kay picture test, are used. The procedure is made into a game, and carers used to occlude the child's eye in order to calm and reassure him or her.

EXAMINATION OF THE EYE

Pointers about diagnosis may come from the history but reliance on this may lead to false confidence about the patient's problems, and less obvious signs and symptoms may be missed. Eye examination, therefore, must always be systematic. The classical examination technique starts at the 'outside', the eye position and surrounding structures, and then works 'in' to consider the globe itself.

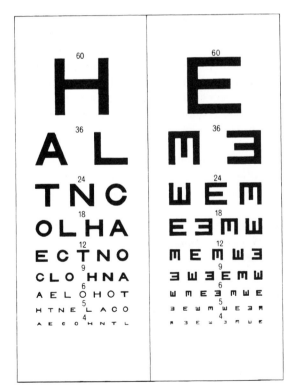

Figure 29.2   Snellen chart.

During a systematic eye examination, the clinician should consider the eyes, the eyelids, the conjunctiva, cornea, anterior chamber and iris.

The eyes

The position of the eyes should be checked to determine whether they are in the normal position for the patient and whether they are at the same level on each side of the nose. Evidence of sunken eyes (enophthalmos) or proptosed eyes (exophthalmos) should be ascertained. Movement should be assessed to determine its normality, any complaints of pain or double vision and, if so, in which gaze positions they occur.

The eyelids

The position of the eyelids should be checked, looking for entropion (lids turning inwards) or ectropion (lids turning outwards). The integrity of the eyelids should be checked, looking for lacerations; if lacerations are present, their depth and possible damage to underlying structures should be assessed. Whether the lash lines are intact, lashes ingrowing, crusting or infestation should also be determined. Swelling either to the whole lids or parts of them, or swelling pointing on to the lid margin on one or both lids should be assessed. Correct functioning when the lids close, whether the globes are exposed and whether the eyes can be opened to the same extent as each other should be ascertained.

Conjunctiva

The integrity of the conjunctiva is important. The presence of lacerations, inflammation (whether localised or generalised) and the structure should be assessed, looking at smoothness; the presence of follicles, papillae, conjunctival cysts or pterygia, pingueculae should be noted. Similarly, subconjunctival haemorrhage and chemosis, and whether it extends posteriorly are also notable, as these may be suggestive of orbital haemorrhage after severe trauma. The type, amount and frequency of any discharge must be determined in addition to examination of the fornices, both lower and subtarsal areas, looking for the presence of concretions or foreign bodies.

Corneas

The integrity of the corneas is notable and, in particular, the presence of lacerations, abrasions or ulcers. Clarity of vision and any haze or opacity must be determined, and the features of the iris visualised. Any foreign bodies must be assessed and their depth noted.

Anterior chambers

The depth of the anterior chamber (i.e. the distance between the curved cornea and the iris) is generally equal in both eyes; any deviation from this should be noted. Red blood cells or other abnormal contents should be assessed. Inflammation is difficult to see without the use of a slit-lamp.

Irises

The colour of the iris may be dull, if there is inflammation in the anterior chamber. Changes in its integrity may also occur in both blunt and penetrating trauma. Positioning is important, as a deviated pupil may be indicative of perforation. The size and shape of the pupil should be noted; whether one is smaller or larger than the fellow eye, or is round or oval are significant. Reaction to light should be assessed to determine whether there is a direct response (constriction with bright light), consensual response (constriction when bright light is shone into the other eye) or a near response (constriction when the patient focuses on a near object).

Findings should always be compared with the fellow eye. What appears to be an abnormality may be bilateral and normal for the patient.

> Findings should always be compared with the fellow eye. What appears to be an abnormality may be bilateral and normal for the patient

INJURY TO THE EYE

Surface trauma

While surface trauma is generally minor, the pain associated with it is often severe, especially when the cornea is abraded. Instillation of local anaesthetic drops (oxybuprocaine 0.4%, amethocaine 1% or proxymetacaine 0.5%) may be necessary in order to facilitate adequate examination. Local anaesthetic drops should only be used in the emergency department and should never be prescribed or dispensed as they retard epithelial healing.

Subtarsal foreign bodies

Patients often present with a foreign body sensation and a history of something falling or blowing into the eye. The lid should be everted and any foreign material wiped off with a moistened cotton tip. The eye should then be stained with fluorescein and examined for any corneal or conjunctival epithelial loss, which is often linear, superficial and quite characteristic of this type of injury. If epithelial loss is minimal, a 'stat' instillation of antibiotic ointment is usually sufficient. If larger abrasions are present, they should be treated as corneal abrasions.

Traumatic subconjunctival haemorrhage

This is a common but trivial component of some surface injuries. Fluorescein should be used to rule out conjunctival abrasions or lacerations. This is a self-limiting condition that does not require treatment. Traumatic subconjunctival haemorrhages, which extend backwards so that the posterior borders are not visible, may be indicative of significant orbital trauma and will need further investigation if the history and other findings are suggestive. Subconjunctival haemorrhages generally resolve within 2–3 weeks. The patient needs reassurance of this and the fact that the spread of blood under the conjunctiva may appear worse before it begins to resolve.

Conjunctival abrasions and foreign bodies

Foreign bodies rarely penetrate the conjunctiva and are usually easy to wipe off using a moistened cotton bud after instillation of local anaesthetic. Any abrasion should be treated with a broad-spectrum antibiotic ointment such as chloramphenicol. (Although a drop of the same drug is quite adequate, the use of ointment can give the patient some pain relief, as a greasy layer is formed between the abraded tissue and the lid that moves

over it. This is an important consideration in the treatment of corneal abrasion.) Padding is unnecessary and the eye is generally gritty rather than particularly painful.

> Any abrasion should be treated with a broad-spectrum antibiotic ointment

Corneal abrasions

Corneal abrasions are common, as the corneal epithelium is fragile. Pain levels may be high and the patient will experience tearing and reduced vision. Accurate assessment of the abrasions is necessary to rule out any deeper lacerations; if there is any suspicion of this, referral to an ophthalmic unit should follow. Scarring will result from corneal laceration, whereas superficial corneal injury usually resolves without visual disturbance. Topical anaesthetics may be needed in order to examine the eye effectively. The extent of the abrasion should be documented after the instillation of fluorescein.

Corneal abrasions are painful and out of all proportion to the size of the injury. Treatment is concerned with minimising pain and aiding healing. Spasm in the ciliary muscle is often a component of corneal abrasion pain and may result in a very slightly sluggish pupil. Dilating the pupil with, for example, cyclopentolate 1% as a stat dose can relieve this. Once the corneal epithelium is breached, infective organisms can enter the globe itself quite easily and intraocular infection is extremely difficult to treat. Any breach in the corneal epithelium, therefore, necessitates the use of prophylactic topical antibiotics. Chloramphenicol is again often used, as it is available in ointment form, which gives a greater degree of patient comfort than drops and tends to stay in the eye longer.

Eye padding is used for patient comfort, as there is little evidence that padded abrasions heal faster. Padding the eye after instillation of a dilating drop and antibiotic gives the patient the experience of the eye pad and the comfort levels it produces. Many patients find that an eye pad makes the eye much more comfortable and, if this is the case, the pad should remain in situ for 24 hours before being removed and antibiotic treatment commenced. If the patient is less comfortable with the pad, they may remove it and commence antibiotic treatment immediately. After removal of the pad, chloramphenicol ointment should be instilled four times daily for 5–7 days. Corneal abrasions generally heal within 48–72 hours. Abrasions which appear slow to heal or involve loose epithelium should be referred to an ophthalmologist.

In the case of human, animal or vegetable material scratches, the cornea may be at particular risk of infection, slow healing or recurrent abrasion. It is important that the patient is aware of this and uses the antibiotic ointment at night, for a period of 3–4 weeks, even after the eye feels completely better to prevent this occurring. Follow-up visits are not usually necessary unless the abrasion is particularly large or the clinician has concerns about the patient.

If padding is required, the following method should be used. One pad should be halved and placed over the closed eyelids after instilling the necessary medication. This fills the socket and helps to keep the eye closed underneath the pad. The second pad should be placed flat over the first and secured with tape. The eye should never be padded merely because local anaesthetic has been used. Anaesthetic drops last for only around 20–30 minutes and the risk of the patient sustaining any further injury because of an anaesthetised eye is remote.

Patients who are driving home should not have eye pads applied. This is likely to invalidate their insurance and is also extremely dangerous both for themselves and for other road users. Patients are much more likely to comply with advice and treatment if they are enabled to drive home and advised how to apply their eye pad when they arrive. A drop of local anaesthetic before leaving the department will enable a pain-free journey.

If both eyes are affected, the worst may be padded and pads given for use at home for the other eye, if necessary. Padding both eyes should be avoided by the patient and should never be carried out in the department. This is intensely disorientating, limits movement and sensory input, and the benefits do not compensate for the limitations and problems they may cause.

Corneal foreign bodies

Superficial foreign bodies are often easily removed with a moistened cotton bud after instillation of local anaesthetic.

Removal of impacted corneal foreign bodies with a needle is a procedure that must be carried out with extreme care. The edge of a 21-gauge needle, mounted on a cotton-tipped swab or syringe to aid mobility should be held tangentially to the cornea, with the hand resting on the patient's cheek or nose and the foreign body gently lifted or scraped off the cornea. Although the cornea is robust, it is only around 1 mm thick and, therefore, penetration with a very sharp needle is always a possibility. If a foreign body is 'dug' out too enthusiastically, the deeper layers of the cornea will be damaged and a corneal scar will result. Scarring can cause visual problems if it involves the visual axis, but many patients who present with foreign bodies have obvious old corneal injuries from previous particles and have unaffected vision. Insufficient local anaesthetic or insufficient time for it to work, fear or previous experience may make it difficult for the patient to keep their head or eye still, further complicating the process.

If the department possesses a slit-lamp, it should be utilised for the removal of corneal foreign bodies so that both a high degree of magnification and support for the patient's head are possible. Unless highly skilled and confident, clinicians may feel most comfortable removing only peripheral foreign bodies and referring central ones. If in any doubt, the patient should be referred to an ophthalmic unit.

Treatment of the foreign body site is similar to that for a corneal abrasion, although since little epithelium is lost, the degree of pain will not usually necessitate padding. Opportunities should be taken for health education about the use of eye protection. X-ray examination is rarely indicated. If there is a definite history of a high-speed foreign body hitting the eye (e.g. hammer and chisel) and no foreign body can be found, this may be worthy of consideration.

Superglue injuries

Superglues of various sorts may be instilled into the eye, as their containers often resemble eye-drop containers. Patients present with a considerable degree of pain and with their eyelids stuck together. Superglue does not penetrate the eye and, as the eye is permanently wetted by the tear film, the glue does not tend to stick to the tissues of the eye but hardens and forms a plaque inside the lids which abrades the cornea as the eye and lids move. The glue is often not adhered firmly to the lids, as they are also moist, but holds the lids firmly together by gluing the eyelashes together. Topical anaesthetic applied to the lids and allowed to drain between them to act on the cornea will relieve pain, and allow examination and treatment. The eyelashes may need to be cut very close to the lid margin and then the remaining glue picked off the lashes in order to allow the lids to be opened. This process needs extreme care and a very fine pair of scissors, as laceration of the lid margin must be avoided. Once the lids are opened (and this may be a lengthy procedure necessitating repeated topical anaesthetic and much patience), the plaque of glue may be removed from the eye. Care must be taken to remove all particles of the hard glue and any resulting abrasions may be treated as corneal abrasions. Children may be much less cooperative than adults and may need a general anaesthetic for this procedure. Referral to an ophthalmic unit should be considered. Lids stuck together with superglue will take a considerable time to open on their own and practitioners should not be tempted to 'let nature take its course'. These abrasions are likely to be extremely painful, as the glue plaque will abrade as long as it is in the eye, and the loss of corneal epithelium will provide an entry point to the eye for pathogens.

Blunt trauma

The globe itself is fairly rigid in an adult. A blow to the globe will cause it to compress, and will stretch and distort tissues. Any or all of the intraocular structures may be damaged in this process. A variable degree of visual reduction usually results. A simple 'black eye' may cover a severely damaged globe. It is important that visual acuity is assessed accurately and that the eye under the bruised lids is assessed. If the lids cannot be opened enough for a formal assessment

of visual acuity, the patient should be encouraged to open them and a subjective assessment recorded. If the patient says that their vision is reduced in any way, further investigation is necessary and the patient should be referred to an ophthalmologist.

Intraocular structures and how they may be damaged by blunt trauma

- The iris may bleed leading to blood in the anterior chamber, which may settle into a layer seen in the bottom of the anterior chamber, or which may diffuse, seen as a reddish haze (i.e. hyphaema); this may result in raised intraocular pressure. The iris may be separated from the ciliary body, leading to the appearance of a 'hole' in the iris at its periphery (i.e. iridodialysis).
- The sphincter muscle may be damaged leading to a dilated pupil (i.e. traumatic mydriasis). It may become inflamed owing to the insult, and may exude white blood cells and protein into the anterior chamber (traumatic iritis), which will result in reduced vision, and an aching pain in and around the eye.
- The drainage angle may be stretched, which may eventually lead to aqueous drainage problems and glaucoma.
- The lens may be partially or complete dislocated owing to rupture of the ligaments (zonules) holding it in place. Blunt trauma may also result in a cataract, either initially or eventually.
- Distorting forces may lead to ruptures in the choroid, which underlies the retina and provides part of its nutrition. If the damaged choroid lies under the most sensitive retinal area, the macula, gross permanent reduction of central vision may result.
- A retinal tear or detachment may give rise to symptoms of flashes of light and new floaters, curtains covering vision, or spider webs or hairs in vision.
- Retinal oedema and haemorrhages (commotio retinae), which result in a reduction in vision that may or may not be permanent.
- Haemorrhage may also occur in the vitreous humour thereby reducing vision. The optic nerve may be contused or even avulsed.

- At its most extreme, blunt trauma may cause the globe to distort sufficiently for it to rupture. A squash ball or even a finger in the eye may cause this devastating injury. A posterior rupture of the globe may be difficult to recognise and, therefore, it is essential that patients with any reduction in vision are referred to an ophthalmologist. Patients with signs of ocular damage, such as those above, should be referred urgently.

Penetrating trauma

Penetrating injuries and intraocular foreign bodies may cause damage to the globe by the following means.
- Disruption of tissues that occurs at the time of the injury.
- Long-term damage owing to the formation of scar tissue. Retinal scars will contract and cause retinal detachment while corneal scars will distort or disrupt vision.
- The introduction of foreign material to which the eye reacts. Organic material may introduce infection or produce inflammation. Metallic foreign bodies degrade and deposit pigment in the tissues of the eye leading to loss of function.
- Pathways for infection are allowed to enter the globe.

Large penetrating eye injuries are obvious, but small perforations may be easily missed, as the eye may look completely intact. The wound may have self-sealed, or iris tissue may have moved to block the hole, resulting in an iris prolapse. The upper lid may obscure the wound; examination must always include all aspects of the anterior part of the globe, asking the patient to look in each different direction so that all segments may be examined. As the patient looks down, the upper lid should be retracted so that the upper portion of the globe may be seen. All penetrations of the lid should lead to a high index of suspicion about the state of the globe.

Corneal perforations always leave a full-thickness scar even if they are very small. Overlying subconjunctival haemorrhages may mask scleral perforations. A small hole in the iris may mark the passage of a foreign body. Patients with penetrating trauma should be referred urgently to an ophthalmologist.

> Patients with penetrating trauma should be referred urgently to an ophthalmologist

In the interim, care of these patients should include the following.

- Considering the administration of analgesics and antiemetics, as vomiting may lead to expulsion of the contents of a perforated globe.
- Protecting wounds with retained foreign objects using rigid shields, such as cartella shields or gallipots. No perforating objects should be removed from the eye.
- Covering the eye with a single pad in cases of penetrating injury where no foreign objects are present (no pressure is applied to the eye), and using cartella shields or gallipots.
- Patients should be transported lying flat in order to reduce intraocular pressure and, therefore, reduce the risk of further injury or loss of ocular contents.

Ocular burns

Ocular burns may be divided by their cause: chemical, thermal or radiation (of which only ultraviolet will be considered here). Chemical eye injuries are the only category of ocular trauma that should be triaged as priority one without any consideration of life threat. They are immediately sight threatening.

> Chemical eye injuries are immediately sight threatening

Chemical burns

Alkalis, acids or solvents may cause chemical burns. Substances such as petrol, perfume and alcohol may cause solvent injuries and, although initially painful, are essentially self-limiting. Tiny areas of fluorescein stain may be seen on the cornea and these may be treated as corneal abrasions with dilating drops and antibiotic ointment to prevent any secondary bacterial infection.

Many household and industrial chemicals are alkaline. The most usual forms are sodium or potassium hydroxide (used as cleaning agents), calcium hydroxide (a major component of plaster, mortar, cement and concrete) and ammonia (in fertiliser or as a liquid). Alkalis rapidly penetrate tissue combining with cell membrane lipids in the cornea and resulting in tissue disruption. Alkali soon appears in the anterior chamber and may cause damage to the iris, ciliary body and lens. Damage to vascular channels leads to ischaemia.

Acids are less penetrating and most damage is done during and soon after initial exposure. Acids damage tissues forming barriers against deeper penetration and localising damage to the point of contact. Car battery acid (sulphuric acid) burns are common, and some complex organic and inorganic compounds are acidic. Acetic acid is normally a very weak acid but in its glacial form, used in industry, may cause severe injury. Hydrofluoric acid, used in the etching of glass and stone, may cause progressive damage similar to alkaline substances.

Solvent burns, although very painful, usually cause only transient irritation and damage.

Thermal and/or contusion injuries may cause concurrent injuries owing to the temperature or pressure at which the chemicals hit the eye.

Irrigation The initial treatment of ocular chemical injuries involves copious irrigation to dilute the chemical and remove particulate matter. Irrigation should commence immediately, using whatever source is available. Generally, the irrigating fluid of choice is normal saline (0.9%) via a giving set to provide a directable and controllable jet. Sterile water may, however, be used and, in areas where neither of these fluids is immediately available, tap water is an adequate substitute. Indicator paper may be used to ascertain the pH of the chemical, but this should not delay irrigation and neutralising solutions are not used. Adequate topical anaesthesia is needed to allow the patient to cooperate and this may need to be repeated throughout the procedure. Contact lenses should be removed and all aspects of the globe irrigated thoroughly with the patient looking in all aspects of gaze. All particles should be removed; the lids must be everted so that particles may be removed from under them. The irrigation time and volume of fluid used depends on the nature and physical state of the chemical, its amount in the eye and the patient's condition. Wagoner (1997) suggests that it is impossible to overirrigate a chemically injured eye and, therefore, irrigation should continue for between 15 and 30 minutes. Adequate irrigation requires lengthier time periods where particulate rather than liquid chemicals are present.

Indicator paper, while useful to check pH, is not a substitute for thorough irrigation. The pH of the tear film should take place 5 minutes after irrigation is finished to ensure that it is tear film and not irrigation fluid that is tested (Wagoner, 1997). If the pH is still abnormal, delay in irrigation may lead to further tissue damage. Following irrigation, the patient's visual acuity should be assessed and the eye examined.

All but the most trivial chemical injuries should be referred to an ophthalmologist. Ophthalmic management usually includes a combination of:

- a mydriatic agent to dilate the pupil, thus reducing ciliary spasm and pain, and stopping the iris from adhering to the lens just behind it
- topical antibiotics and steroids to prevent infection and reduce inflammation
- topical or systemic potassium ascorbate or ascorbic acid to aid tissue healing
- admission to hospital where irrigation may, in the most severe cases, be combined with therapy over a number of days.

Thermal burns

The very fast lid reflex, closing to prevent harm to the globe, usually ensures that thermal burns are confined to the lids. Treatment is similar to that of thermal burns elsewhere on the body. Superficial burns to the eyes or lids, such as those caused by tobacco ash, may be treated as abrasions. More severe burns may necessitate major reconstruction of the eyes and surrounding structures. Thermal burns involving the lids should be referred to an ophthalmic unit owing to the possibility of adhesions forming between areas of lid tissue, resulting in impaired motility.

Radiation burns

Radiation burns are likely to be caused by ultra-violet light in the form of sun lamps or from welding equipment. Symptoms range from mild discomfort to severe pain, photophobia and lacrimation, and are often delayed by 6–10 hours. This is due to the cornea absorbing the ultraviolet radiation, and those cells most affected slowly dying and then being removed from the cornea by the lid, leaving erosions on the cornea. Local anaesthetic drops may be used to facilitate examination and treatment similar to that for a corneal abrasion. Opportunities may be taken for health education advice about adequate eye protection.

Eyelid injury

Intact eyelids are vital to protect the globes from injury and to keep them moist. A number of structures are within or underlie the tissues of the lid. The lacrimal drainage system comprises an upper and lower punctum (tiny holes at the nasal end of each lid), which lead to canaliculi or tear channels that drain eventually into the lacrimal sacs. The lacrimal glands, which secrete part of the tear film, are mostly located in the orbits but a portion extends into the upper eyelids. A number of muscles, the tarsal plates, and the medial and lateral ligaments form part of the structure and function of the lids. Thus, when repair of lid injuries are considered, all these structures must be taken into account. Accurate apposition of all structures is vital, if the eyes are not to be exposed by notches in the lid margins or by entropion caused by damaged ligaments. Damage to drainage apparatus may lead to chronic watery eyes with all their consequences for the patient.

The eyelids have a very good blood supply and primary repair of the lids is successful up to 48 hours after injury (Cheng et al., 1997). Patients with eyelid lacerations should, therefore, be referred to ophthalmologists for repair of all but the most superficial wounds.

Orbital injury

The force involved in producing a 'black eye' may also damage the orbit. The orbit is weakened where the infraorbital nerve runs in the infra-orbital canal, and its medial wall and floor are also fragile. Orbital rim fractures usual result in paraesthesia of the area supplied by the infraorbital nerve and the cheek. No treatment is generally undertaken unless the fracture is associated with an orbital floor fracture.

An orbital floor fracture is often referred to as a blow-out fracture, and occurs when a force hits the bones of the orbit directly and displaces the globe and orbital tissue backwards putting extra force on the orbital floor. Patients often present complaining of double vision (diplopia), loss of sensation in the cheek, or may have blown their nose and found that their lids immediately swell as air is forced from the sinus into the lid tissues resulting in subcutaneous emphysema.

Diplopia is caused by orbital fat or muscle tissue becoming trapped in the orbital fracture and restricting eye movement. The eye may look sunken compared with the other eye (enophthalmos). Patients may have normal vision in the primary position (both eyes looking ahead) with diplopia only present if the patient looks to the side, up or down. It is important that all aspects of gaze are considered when assessing the extent of double vision (straight up, up and left, up and right, straight ahead, left, right, straight down, down and left, down and right). In general, ophthalmologists refer all patients with double vision to an eye unit in order that this may be measured accurately, and trapped tissue and muscles considered along with repair of the fracture.

Raised pressure within the orbit may occur as a result of haemorrhage owing to blunt trauma. This compromises eye movements and may cause permanent loss of vision owing to compression of the optic nerve. Any proptosis of the globe following trauma should be monitored and an urgent referral to an ophthalmologist should follow. Visual acuity must be assessed frequently and, if the patient complains of any reduction of visual acuity, an immediate ophthalmic opinion should be sought, as orbital decompression may be required. This may be undertaken as a lateral canthotomy, performed under local anaesthetic, to reduce pressure in the orbit.

CONCLUSION

Adequate assessment of ocular trauma comprises three main stages: eliciting an accurate history, examination of the structures involved and, in the case of ocular trauma, assessing visual acuity. This involves skill in the use of appropriate techniques, and a structured and systematic approach to ensure the assessment of all structures and to avoid potentially preventable complications, which may have devastating consequences for the patient.

References

Cheng H, Burdon MA, Buckley SA, Moorman C. *Emergency ophthalmology*. London: BMJ Publishing Group, 1997

Wagoner MD. Chemical injuries of the eye: current concepts in pathophysiology and therapy. *Survey of Ophthalmology* 1997; 41: 275–313

Further reading

Cheng H, Burdon MA, Buckley SA, Moorman C. *Emergency ophthalmology*. London: BMJ Publishing Group, 1997

Eagling EM, Roper-Hall MJ, *Eye injuries: an illustrated guide.* Sevenoaks: Butterworth and Co., 1986

Kanski JJ. *Synopsis of ophthalmology*. London: Wright, 1990

Marsden J. Ophthalmic trauma in accident and emergency. *Accident and Emergency Nursing* 1996; 4: 54–58

Marsden J. Care of patients with minor eye trauma. *Emergency Nurse* 1998; 6(7): 10–13

Marsden J. Systematic eye examination in A&E. *Emergency Nurse* 1998; 6(6): 16–19

Marsden J. The use of eye drops and ointments in A&E. *Emergency Nurse* 1998; 6(8): 17–22

Marsden J. Ocular burns in A&E. *Emergency Nurse* 1999; 6(10): 20–24

Perry JP Tullo AB (eds). *Care of the ophthalmic patient*, 2nd edn. London: Chapman and Hall, 1995

Snell RS, Lemp MA. *Clinical anatomy of the eye*. Oxford: Blackwell Scientific Publications, 1989

Tannen M, Marsden J. Chemical burns of the eye. *Nursing Standard* 1991; 30(6): 24–26

Wagoner MD. Chemical injuries of the eye: current concepts in pathophysiology and therapy. *Survey of Ophthalmology* 1997; 41: 275–313

Chapter **30**

Paediatric trauma

Ian Maconochie

INTRODUCTION

Trauma is the leading cause of death in children over the age of 1 year, with almost one-half of all trauma deaths occurring immediately or within a few minutes of the incident. Survivors may die within a few hours from potentially preventable problems associated with the airway, breathing or circulation, or may die weeks or months later from complications such as multiorgan failure, pulmonary embolism, fat embolism or sepsis.

By adopting the same structured approach to managing these children as that used in adults, problems associated with hypoxia and hypovolaemia, the leading causes of trauma deaths, may be rapidly identified and treated, and potentially adverse sequelae minimised. As with adults, life-threatening disorders discovered in the primary survey must be dealt with in the order in which they are discovered before moving on to the next component of assessment.

The aim of this chapter is to enable trauma and emergency care nurses to manage children who have suffered trauma, to know when to ask for help and to follow a logical, sequential approach. Inherent in this is the need to remember that trauma can affect children differently, not only physically and physiologically, but also psychologically. Although minor injuries constitute a large proportion of paediatric attendances and presentations to emergency departments and minor injuries units, this chapter will focus mainly on those who have suffered more moderate or severe injuries, as indicated by their mechanism of injury.

EPIDEMIOLOGY

Children comprise between 20% and 35% of all patients attending emergency departments each year. In the UK, it is also estimated that, in any one year, around 3.5 million children visit emergency departments as a result of injury; this translates into around one-fifth of all children (A&E Services for Children, 1999). The potential impact on the care delivered to children and to society is, therefore, significant, and should not be underestimated.

Common mechanisms of injury in children and their associated patterns are shown in Table 30.1.

Paediatric trauma due to road traffic crashes, whether as car occupant, pedestrian or cyclist, is the leading mechanism of injury-related death in all age groups. Drowning, near-drowning and immersion injuries follow closely behind, and form the second leading cause, with deaths due to house fires and associated burns or smoke inhalation also accounting for a significant number. Falls are common but rarely cause major injury unless the length of the fall is greater than the child's height. As they represent a small physical target for the dissipation of mechanical forces, children involved in road traffic crashes or other serious trauma commonly suffer multisystem injury; in these circumstances, all systems should be considered to be at risk.

Injury prevention programmes have been shown to be most effective where they focus on injuries that are frequent and severe, and for which proven prevention strategies exist that are available and accessible.

A STRUCTURED APPROACH TO MANAGING THE INJURED CHILD

Major trauma affects children and adults in different ways – physically, physiologically and psychologically. Despite this, and the fact that traumatised children have a number of unique problems, the need for a structured approach to their management is not invalidated (Box 30.1). By following the simple sequence of airway with cervical spine control (Ac), breathing (B) and circulation (C), followed by assessment of disability (i.e. neurological status) detecting the

Table 30.1 Common mechanisms and associated patterns of paediatric injury. (Reproduced from *Pediatric education for pre-hospital providers*, 2000: 134)

Mechanism of injury	Associated patterns of injury
Road traffic crash (child is passenger)	*Unrestrained* Multiple trauma, head and neck injuries, scalp and facial lacerations *Air bag* Head and neck; facial and eye injuries *Restrained* Chest and abdominal injuries, cervical and lower spine injuries
Road traffic crash (child is pedestrian)	*Low speed* Lower extremity fractures *High speed* Chest and abdominal injuries, head and neck injuries, lower extremity fractures
Fall from a height	*Low* Upper extremity fractures *Medium* Head and neck injuries, upper and lower extremity fractures *High* Chest and abdominal injuries, head and neck injuries, upper and lower extremity fractures
Fall from a bicycle	*Without helmet* Head and neck injuries, scalp and facial lacerations, upper extremity fractures *With helmet* Upper extremity fractures *Hitting handlebar* Internal abdominal injuries

Box 30.1   The structured approach

- Primary survey
- Resuscitation
- Secondary survey
- Emergency treatment
- Definitive care

presence of concomitant injuries and determination of blood glucose level, life-threatening problems will be identified and treated in order of priority.

The primary survey and resuscitation are performed simultaneously

The trauma team

Dealing with a seriously injured child requires a uniform approach by the different members of the trauma team. A calm, ordered approach provides comfort to the members of the team caring for the traumatised patient and allows for optimal management to take place. One person, the most senior and appropriately trained present, should lead the team and give clear commands with roles having been allocated to other team members. Where there are sufficient members of the team, one person can be delegated to manage the airway in conjunction with another whose role is to assist with maintaining in-line cervical stabilisation. Others may be tasked with dealing with assessment of breathing and circulation. Clear reporting of the clinical findings are made aloud in sequence to the team leader, who continues to remain in command throughout.

Airway and cervical spine

The airway

In infants, the head is disproportionately large in relation to the rest of the body, hence the need to ensure optimal airway positioning with the infant's head in the neutral position. Care should be taken to avoid pushing on the soft tissue structures underneath the jaw line, as this can cause airway obstruction. Older children should

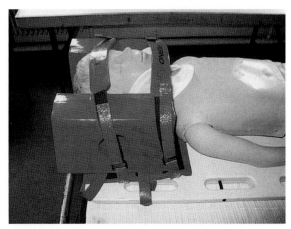

Figure 30.1   Application of cervical spine collar with blocks.

be managed in the 'sniffing the morning air' or head tilt–chin lift position. Attention *must* be paid to the cervical spine; hence a combination of jaw thrust with in-line cervical stabilisation is mandatory in the seriously injured child.

The importance of communication must be reinforced, and the need to ensure that children are spoken to and given explanations regarding all actions and interventions to be performed, even if they appear obtunded.

The cervical spine

The cervical spine must be kept stable until any possibility of injury to the spine has been ruled out (Figure 30.1). This involves assessment of the child's peripheral and central neurological status, and the use of cervical x-rays. The lateral shoot through of the cervical spine can reveal bony injury to the cervical spine; however, the absence of any x-ray injury does not exclude the possibility of damage to the spinal cord. This phenomenon, known as SCIWORA (spinal cord injury without radiological abnormality) is due to the ligaments encasing the vertebral bodies being very strong, so much so that, when the wedge-shaped structures of the developing vertebral bodies move forward, the posterior part of the vertebral bodies damage the spinal cord. The vertebral bodies at the full forward position of their travel from the impulse of the trauma, are then brought back into their normal alignment by the strength of the intervertebral ligaments.

The absence of x-ray abnormalities on cervical spine films does not exclude the presence of cervical spine injuries

All children who have been involved in serious trauma should have had cervical collars fitted by the attending ambulance crew at the scene and their cervical spines immobilised. If this has not happened, one of the trauma team members should immediately assume responsibility for this, placing their hands on either side of the child's head, being careful not to obstruct or occlude the ears. The position of the hands should maintain the neck in line with the rest of the spine. The airway should be assessed and maintained at the same time and, if there are sufficient members of the trauma team, the correct size of cervical collar measured, selected and applied by another. Cervical collars that are too small may cause flexion of the head and potentially worsen spinal cord damage; collars which are too large will not give any protection, and may indeed give the carer a false sense of security and false reassurance that cervical spine stabilisation has been achieved. Cervical collars should be applied by gently and carefully slipping them around the neck whilst in-line stabilization is being maintained, and then securing them into place. This procedure is followed by tape being placed across the forehead on to the non-mobile section of the trolley the patient is lying on, taking care to avoid covering the child's eyebrows; the other is applied at the lower part of the patient's chin.

An alternative method of securing the cervical spine is the placement of two soft blocks, one on either side of the child's head, with holes cut in the sides so that the child can hear. This is particularly important, as the child may be in pain, confused and probably disorientated, and in the presence of strangers. These soft blocks have two straps that should be positioned in a similar fashion to that for the tapes outlined above (see Figure 30.1).

It is only when these three separate points of attachment to the head are secured that manual in-line stabilisation can be released. The hands used in stabilising the head should be carefully and slowly withdrawn in order to avoid any tilting or movement of the head on the cervical spine. The cervical spine can only be cleared if the cervical spine x-rays and neurological examination are normal. Children who are ventilated, paralysed and sedated by drugs cannot have their cervical spines cleared; as their neurological examination is incomplete, the cervical spine must be protected until such time as the neurological examination can be performed. Failure to consider cervical spine damage in trauma victims can mean long-term disability or may even lead to death.

Airway assessment and management
Where children are making noises, the airway is open. Ongoing assessment and review of the airway to ensure its continued patency throughout the resuscitation is of paramount importance. The relevant trauma team member must *look, listen* and *feel* for air being inspired and expired by the patient.

High-flow oxygen should be given to all traumatised children at a rate of 15 litres/minute. Unlike adults, children do not develop chronic obstructive pulmonary disease (COPD). Accordingly, whereas when 100% oxygen is administered to certain adults, such as those with COPD, a decreased respiratory rate and loss of hypoxic drive may result owing to their physiological dependence on blood oxygen levels. This situation does not arise in children, as their ventilatory controlling mechanism relates to blood carbon dioxide levels; 100% oxygen should, therefore, be given. In the awake and spontaneously breathing child, an oxygen mask with reservoir bag should be used (Figure 30.2).

All children who have suffered trauma should be given high-flow oxygen

As the child inspires, the side vents in the mask close, thereby avoiding entrainment of room air into the mask; the valve covering the reservoir opens, so the higher concentration of oxygen from the reservoir is inspired by the child. When the child exhales, the reservoir valve is closed and the side vents opened so that exhaled carbon dioxide does not enter the reservoir bag but instead goes into the surrounding room air.

The person providing in-line stabilisation of the neck may also perform a jaw-thrust manoeuvre. Suction of the oropharynx may be required, as

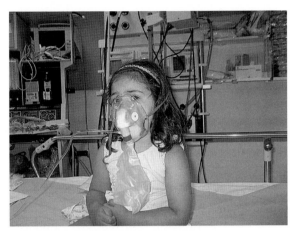

Figure 30.2   Oxygen mask and reservoir bag in a spontaneously breathing child.

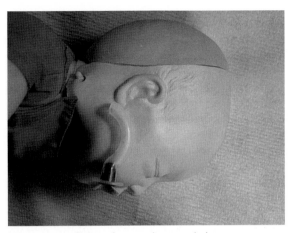

Figure 30.3   Sizing of an oropharyngeal airway.

blood, secretions or foreign bodies can prove a threat to the airway. Adjuncts, such as oropharyngeal airways, must be used with caution as they can induce the gag reflex, which can result in the aspiration of gastric contents. Nasopharyngeal airways should be avoided if there is the possibility of mid-facial frontal head injuries, as the cribriform plate may have been damaged. Under these circumstances, nasopharyngeal airways could be inserted directly into brain tissue.

The internal diameter of nasopharyngeal airways can be determined by comparing the size of one of the child's little fingers with that of the matching diameter of the nasopharyngeal airway. The correct length is given by the distance from the tip of the child's nose to the tragus of the ear on the same side. Conventionally, the right nostril is used for insertion; the nasopharyngeal airway is lubricated using a non-irritant substance such as K-Y jelly and inserted along the bottom of the floor of the nostril. A gentle twisting motion can be used. If the area around the nostril appears to blanch, this indicates that the chosen nasopharyngeal airway is too large and pressure necrosis could occur, if it is used.

As previously mentioned, nasopharyngeal airways should not be used where basal skull fractures are possible. Nor should they be used in the presence of coagulopathy, as their use may result in damage to the adenoids; in the presence of bleeding disorders, the adenoids can become a significant source of haemorrhage.

Oropharyngeal airways are also used as adjuncts to manual airway opening techniques; however, as with nasopharyngeal airways, their presence alone does not signify that the airway is secured. Aspiration of gastric contents into the lungs is possible, with potentially serious consequences for the child. Oropharyngeal airways tend to be used in children who have a lowered level of consciousness, as the gag reflex is unlikely to be evoked; nasopharyngeal airways may be used in situations when the level of consciousness is likely to improve. When used, oropharyngeal airways must be sized appropriately; correct sizing may be achieved by placing it on the cheek, one end starting at the angle of the jaw and the other where the incisors are, or would be in a toothless infant (Figure 30.3).

Using oropharyngeal airways that are too large can obstruct the airway, whereas those that are too small can push the tongue backwards, also leading to potential airway obstruction. The technique for insertion is straightforward, albeit different from adults, with the airway inserted directly over the tongue, thereby following the curve of the airway. The use of tongue depressors or laryngoscope blades may be of assistance. The paediatric insertion technique differs from that of adults, as considerable damage may be caused to the child's mouth by running the pharyngeal end of the airway along the hard palate. The presence of an oropharyngeal airway should lead to consideration of the need to secure a definitive airway by endotracheal intubation.

> The presence of an oropharyngeal airway should lead to consideration of the need to secure a definitive airway by endotracheal intubation

Suction of debris in the oral cavity and removing secretions and blood can help maintain airway patency. Yankeur suction catheters are the most commonly used and are available in a range of sizes. Most have an end hole with tonsillar holes so that, if the tongue or other soft tissues adhere to the end of the catheter, the side holes can still drain fluid. In those used in adults, there is often a hole in the middle part of the catheter, which may be occluded by the user; this permits a degree of control over the pressure generated at its distal end. The smaller paediatric suction catheters do not have this feature, hence there may be considerable sucking forces that can cause tissue damage. Where this type of catheter is used in children, a small hole cut in the connecting tube from the wall-mounted pressure regulator to the paediatric Yankeur suction catheter can allow the operator more control over the suction pressure and so lessen the risk of soft tissue damage.

Bag mask ventilation is the next step in providing further ventilation in the child with respiratory failure and an inadequate respiratory effort; the ensuing step is definitive management and endotracheal intubation.

Definitive airway management – endotracheal intubation

Experienced help may be required to place an endotracheal tube; indeed, many trauma nurses are proficient in performing this intervention. As with oropharyngeal and nasopharyngeal airways, the need to select appropriately sized devices is key. A useful formula to use, which relates the age in years to the internal diameter of the endotracheal tube is:

$$\text{Internal diameter of the endotracheal tube (mm)} = \left\{ \frac{\text{Age (years)}}{4} \right\} + 4$$

For example, a 3-year-old child would require an endotracheal tube sized 4.75 mm (i.e. 3/4 + 4). As endotracheal tubes are only available in whole and half sizes, the required tube sizes would be 4.5 mm and 5 mm internal diameter.

Once the endotracheal tube is in situ, its location must be checked by auscultation of the apices and bases of the lungs. Good air entry should be heard in these sites when the patient is ventilated using a bag-mask device. No air entry should be heard when listening to the stomach. A complication commonly found is that of the endotracheal tube being inserted too far into the airway so that it comes to lie in the right main bronchus. As the angle of the right main bronchus is steeper than the left, foreign bodies tend to lodge preferentially within it.

Capnometers may be attached to the endotracheal tubes to measure end-tidal carbon dioxide levels. Carbon dioxide is only produced by the lungs; therefore, on the expiratory phase of ventilation, carbon dioxide should register in the exhaled gas. If the tube is displaced or misplaced, such as being in the oesophagus, then no carbon dioxide will be detected. Loss of the airway when endotracheal tubes are in place may occur when they become blocked by secretions, thus preventing gas exchange. Suction catheters can prove invaluable in overcoming blockages due to secretions and blood. Where it is certain that loss of the airway is not due to *displacement* or misplacement of the tube (this may be evidenced by direct visualisation of the tube beyond the vocal cords and end-tidal carbon dioxide registering on the capnometer), that ventilation is not improved with suctioning of the endotracheal tube (i.e. there is no *obstruction*), that there is no *pneumothorax* present, and that the *equipment* is working, then the tube must be removed and replaced. This sequence of checks – DOPE – can be extremely helpful in investigating the loss of the airway and effective ventilation (Box 30.2).

> **Box 30.2 Investigating breathing problems in intubated patients – (DOPE)**
>
> D   Is there displacement or misplacement of the endotracheal tube?
> O   Is there any obstruction of the endotracheal tube?
> P   Is a pneumothorax present?
> E   Is all equipment functioning?

Breathing

Once the airway has been secured and the cervical spine controlled, breathing should be assessed. This assessment includes observing the rate and effort of breathing, detecting the presence of intercostal and sternal recession with or without the use of accessory muscles, and relating these to the child's overall condition (Box 30.3). For example, the rate may be abnormally fast for the child's age, as in compensated shock, or abnormally slow, as in decompensated shock. Grunting is important to detect, as this signifies respiratory difficulty; it helps the child to maintain the volume of air within his lungs.

Upper airway obstruction may be indicated by stridor, whereas lower airway obstruction may be heard as wheeziness on auscultation of the chest. Efficacy of breathing is determined by listening for air entry in the lungs and observing patterns of chest expansion. The knock-on effect of inadequate ventilation is to cause tachycardia (as seen in compensated shock) initially followed by bradycardia (decompensated shock) as the body's physiological mechanisms begin to fail. At this stage, children tend to become more agitated owing to cerebral hypoxia, and increasingly 'shut down' and acidotic as a consequence of tissue hypoxia. Where the child's respiratory effort is insufficient or ineffective, bag mask ventilation should be maintained with high-flow oxygen at a rate of 15 litres/minute. Early intervention to secure a definitive airway should be considered at this stage, if not already established.

The airway should be secured definitively in the following circumstances:

- flail chest
- pulmonary contusion
- ventilatory requirements due to inadequate ventilation
- thermal burns to the airway, as tracheal obstruction due to tissue oedema may occur very rapidly.

Clinical signs of thermal injury include singed eyebrows, the loss of nasal or facial hair, sooty carbonaceous deposits on the tongue, nose or face, and red or inflamed oral mucous membranes; in severe cases, burns may be seen on the face and within the buccal cavity. Patients who present with hoarseness are at risk of losing their airway owing to oedema of the larynx and upper part of the trachea.

> Patients who present with hoarseness following thermal injuries or burns are at risk of losing their airway

Certain life-threatening conditions may be noted within the breathing component of the primary survey and must be treated immediately. These include: open pneumothorax, tension pneumothorax, haemothorax and flail chest.

Open pneumothorax

Open pneumothoraces are visible on inspection of the chest wall and, where greater than two-thirds of the internal diameter of the trachea is involved, will preferentially allow air to enter into the thoracic cavity. These should be covered with occlusive dressings, and taped down on three sides to prevent further air entry on inspiration, removing the potential for converting an already serious situation into an even more serious one – a tension pneumothorax (Figure 30.4).

Tension pneumothorax

The diagnosis of tension pneumothorax can be made from diminished chest wall movements

---

> **Box 30.3   Assessment of the adequacy of breathing**
>
> **The work of breathing**
> - Recession
> - Respiratory rate
> - Inspiratory or expiratory noises
> - Use of accessory muscles
> - Flaring of the alae nasi
>
> **Effectiveness of breathing**
> - Breath sounds
> - Chest expansion
> - Abdominal excursion
>
> **Effects of inadequate respiration**
> - Heart rate
> - Skin colour
> - Neurological status

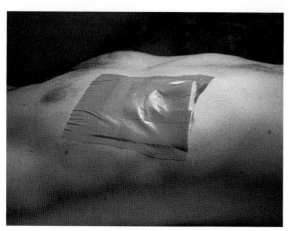

Figure 30.4 Application of a three-sided occlusive dressing in an open pneumothorax.

on the affected side, increased resonance of the affected side on percussion of the chest wall, and decreased air entry on the same side. A tension pneumothorax poses an immediate life threat as air accumulates within the chest wall cavity, thereby limiting normal lung expansion on inspiration; the pressure within the chest cavity increases greatly and compresses venous structures, such as the inferior vena cava, thus impeding venous return. If allowed to develop, the pressure generated within the chest cavity can result in a shift of the solid structures of the chest cavity (*mediastinal shift*), causing the trachea to deviate away from the affected side. Tracheal deviation is a late and pre-terminal sign.

> Tracheal deviation is a late and pre-terminal sign of a tension pneumothorax

The immediate management of a tension pneumothorax is to perform a needle thoracocentesis. Here, a cannula is inserted into the child's second intercostal space in the mid-clavicular line on the side of the tension pneumothorax. A hiss may sometimes be heard as the air, under pressure, rushes out of the cannula, relieving the tension within the chest cavity. The insertion of a formal chest drain will be required; this is relatively urgent but should not impede the primary assessment of the child. Chest drains are inserted into the fifth intercostal space between the mid-axillary line and the anterior axillary line on the affected side. Local anaesthesia is infiltrated down to the layers of the pleura and a small lateral incision made above the sixth rib. Once the skin has been breached, blunt dissection with forceps is carried out until the pleural layer is reached. When the pleural layer is broken, a finger sweep is made to remove or free tissue plugs or fat tags, and the chest drain inserted into the pleural cavity. The drain must then be connected to an underwater seal, or Heimlich valve equivalent, and secured so that it cannot be displaced.

Haemothorax

The presence of a haemothorax represents considerable blood loss into the chest wall cavity. Given the potential blood loss, two wide-bore cannulae must be inserted into the venous circulation prior to insertion of a chest drain, which is the definitive management of this condition. Chest drains are required urgently after this to prevent the tamponading effect of the haemothorax.

Flail chest

Where two or more ribs have been broken in two or more places so that they are free floating and are not connected to the rib–vertebral connections posteriorly, a flail chest is said to exist. This is an extremely painful condition owing to irritation of the pleural lining caused by fracture segments rubbing against it. This pain limits the effort of breathing, and decreased ventilation and decreased chest wall movements ensue. On examination, the ribs may be felt to be free floating and crepitus may be felt as the rib segments move against each other. The fractured ribs will exhibit paradoxical breathing (i.e. the rib cage moves up and out on inspiration); however, the flail segment will be drawn inwards due to the negative pressure generated by the intrathoracic pressure, which normally draws air into the lungs. The converse is true on expiration.

Treatment of a flail chest is early recourse to elective ventilation, the provision of adequate pain-relief, for example, by intercostal nerve block, and appropriate analgesia.

Burns may also pose a threat to life when they extend around the thoracic cage. Full-thickness circumferential burns may cause diminished chest wall movement, as normal expansion is not possible owing to a cuirass of burnt tissue. This leads to inadequate ventilation and resultant hypoxia and hypercarbia. Surgical assistance may be needed to perform escharotomies, so that the chest wall can move with expiration and inspiration.

Where any deterioration in the patient's condition occurs, the airway should be examined and reassessed immediately, followed by a similar assessment of the breathing and circulation.

Cyanosis is a late pre-terminal sign

Circulation

Assessment of the circulation comprises the rapid determination of the heart rate, capillary refill time, skin colour and peripheral temperature, respiratory rate and mental status. These parameters enable an estimation of blood loss to be made. The systolic blood pressure is maintained until late in hypovolaemic shock, hence hypotension is an ominous sign. It is a poor marker of peripheral perfusion.

Hypotension is a pre-terminal sign

Two large-bore intravenous cannulae should be inserted for peripheral access. Up to three attempts may be made to secure vascular access; if unsuccessful after these attempts, intraosseus access should be performed. Central venous access takes more time and should ideally be performed by a practitioner skilled in performing this technique on a regular basis. Following cannulation, blood samples should be taken for full blood count, urea and electrolytes, blood glucose level and an urgent cross-match. Rapid access to type O-negative blood should be available within the emergency department to manage severe blood loss. Type-specific cross-match can take up to 30 minutes and a full cross-match 1 hour, dependent upon local circumstances and arrangements.

Fluid administration

Fluid therapy should be commenced by administering crystalloid or colloid solutions in aliquots of 20 ml/kg. In such emergency situations, familiarity with formulae for calculating the child's weight may be useful. One such formula that may be used in pre-pubertal children is:

Weight of child (kg) = [Age (years) + 4] × 2

Given as a bolus, either as an intravenous or intraosseous push, the child is reassessed after the first aliquot to determine their response to the fluid bolus in relation to their physiological parameters. Where there is little or no effect, a repeat bolus of 20 ml/kg of crystalloid or colloid should be given. If further fluid is indicated after this, blood is required and may be given either as whole blood (20 ml/kg) or as packed cells (10 ml/kg). These signs vary with the age of the child.

With the loss of up to 25% of the circulating blood volume, the body's physiological response is tachycardia, mild tachypnoea and mild agitation. The skin may also feel cool; however, the systolic blood pressure will be maintained at its age-appropriate value. With a loss of between 25% and 40%, the tachycardia becomes more marked, the pulse volume diminished and the blood pressure may start to decrease, with the peripheries feeling cold and appearing mottled. Capillary refill time will typically be longer than 3 seconds. Marked tachypnoea may be evident, with recession and considerable respiratory effort. The child may appear lethargic and may become obtunded. With losses of more than 40%, children are in grave danger of losing their lives as their compensatory processes fail. The heart rate may drop, along with the systolic blood pressure and pulse volume, which is termed *decompensated shock*. The child's skin typically feels cold with a greatly prolonged capillary refill time. Respirations may be agonal and the child only reactive to pain.

Assessment of blood loss is summarised in Table 30.2.

Up to 40% of the circulating volume may be lost before a measurable drop in blood pressure occurs

Disability

A brief neurological assessment of the child's neurological status can be determined by the following:

1. Noting pupillary reactivity and size, looking to ensure that they are equal. An increasingly

Table 30.2   Assessment of blood loss. (Reproduced from European Paediatric Life Support, 1997)

Sign	< 25%	25–40%	> 40%
Heart rate	Tachycardia +	Tachycardia ++	Tachycardia/bradycardia
Systolic blood pressure	Normal	Normal or falling	Falling
Pulse volume	Normal/reduced	Reduced +	Reduced ++
Capillary refill time (normal < 2 seconds)	Normal/increased	Increased +	Increased ++
Skin	Cool, pale	Cold, mottled	Cold, pale
Respiratory rate	Tachypnoea +	Tachypnoea++	Sighing respiration
Mental state	Mild agitation	Lethargic/uncooperative	Reacts only to pain

dilating pupil on the side of a head injury may indicate an ipsilateral collection of blood within the skull, which needs urgent neurosurgical specialist referral.

2. Determining the conscious level of the child according to the AVPU scale, where A signifies an alert child, V one who responds to voice, P one who responds to painful stimuli and U an unresponsive child.

3. Noting the child's posture; a decerebrate posture may be demonstrated clinically by the arms being held out in extension, whereas decorticate posturing may be demonstrated by flexion of the upper limbs. In both these conditions, the lower limbs are extended.

Exposure

The whole of the child's body, both front and back, needs to be inspected, palpated and, where appropriate, auscultated to ensure that all injuries have been identified. For children whose cervical spines have not been cleared, a controlled log roll will be required. Responsibility for coordinating all actions, manoeuvres and communications lies with the trauma team member maintaining in-line cervical stabilisation. Ensuring that the child is kept warm after completion of the head-to-toe examination should not be overlooked.

INVESTIGATIONS AND MONITORING

X-rays of the chest and pelvis can be taken at this time, if the child is clinically stable. The lateral shoot-through to obtain a cervical spine view can also be taken, whilst bearing in mind the caveat that, to rule out cervical spine injury, a full neurological investigation is mandatory.

> A full neurological investigation is mandatory to rule out cervical spine injury

Radiography of the cervical spine with a lateral view demonstrating all seven cervical vertebrae, chest and pelvic x-rays are mandatory in all children who have suffered multiple injuries, and should be obtained as soon as possible. In many instances, it may be preferable for these to be taken in the resuscitation room, with the child only being moved once stabilised. Ideally, the chest film should be taken before the pelvic x-rays, with the cervical spine cleared after this; cervical spine immobilisation must be maintained throughout. X-rays to confirm or exclude other associated injuries may be taken after this time, ideally in the x-ray department once the patient is stabilised. The need for computed tomography scans or other more sophisticated images may be confirmed after this time.

Monitoring of physiological vital signs, heart rate and rhythm and neurological observations, as well as blood glucose measurements, capillary refill, oxygen saturation, arterial blood gases and other pathology tests may also be taken after this time. These can provide valuable information in relation to haemodynamic and respiratory status, and provide a useful baseline upon which to gauge future progress. Monitoring of fluid input and output provide useful indicators of circulatory status and adequacy; detailed records of hourly urine volumes and all fluids administered or ingested may help to provide a more accurate picture. Catheterisation in boys is contraindicated where there are signs of urethral trauma, such as blood at the urethral meatus or a scrotal haematoma. The ideal output is 1 ml/kg per hour of urine in children and 2 ml/kg per hour in infants. Insertion of nasogastric tubes may be useful as they decompress the stomach, thereby minimising pain and distress; where mid-face fractures or signs of basal skull fractures are evident, the gastric tube should be passed orally rather than nasally.

SECONDARY SURVEY

After the primary survey has been completed and the patient resuscitated and stabilised, the secondary survey may then be performed. This is a much more detailed examination of the body to look for *any injury* that the child might have sustained.

The head, face and neck

This examination commences at the top of the head, examining for any boggy swellings, lacerations or bleeding from the scalp. Considerable blood loss can occur from scalp lacerations and direct pressure on the sources of bleeding is required. Any open fractures, full-thickness lacerations or depressed areas of skull are all causes for concern, as injury to the brain and the risk of intracranial bleeding is high. The ears must be examined to determine whether blood is present behind the tympanic membrane, or present in or around the ear. Blood around the ear particularly posterior to the pinna – Battle's sign – is indicative of a basal skull fracture and can be a late sign, appearing hours after the trauma to the head.

Similarly, the nose must be inspected to detect any rhinorrhoea or septal haematoma, which may require referral to ear, nose and throat specialists. The scalp, the forehead, facial bones, nose, teeth and the oral cavity must be examined. Evidence of any bruising, swelling, wounds, deformity, bleeding and dental injuries should be noted. The jaw must also be carefully palpated to ensure that it has not been broken. Where the middle third of the bony skeleton of the face is mobile, the airway is at risk of obstruction from the soft palate; vigilance is, therefore, essential in the non-intubated child.

To examine the neck, the child's head must be held still and the collar removed to enable full visual inspection and palpation. Manual in-line immobilisation of the cervical spine must be maintained throughout. The back of the neck and head can only be properly inspected during the log roll. Any swellings, bruising, wounds or deformities should be noted, palpating for surgical emphysema, bony tenderness or steps between the vertebrae. The collar should be carefully replaced upon completion of this phase of the secondary survey.

The chest

Inspection of the anterior chest wall should begin with establishing the position of the trachea, in particular, determining whether it is centrally placed or has deviated from its normal midline position. The neck veins should not be distended, such as may be seen in cardiac tamponade. Movements of the anterior chest wall should be observed and studied to ensure their equal and symmetrical movement. Where pneumothoraces and haemothoraces are present, the affected side will have reduced excursion. The chest note will be increased on percussion on the side with a tension pneumothorax, as previously mentioned, whereas the note will be dull with a haemothorax. Auscultation of the chest wall in tension pneumothorax and haemothorax will reveal decreased breath sounds.

In children, the presence of rib fractures means that considerable force has been applied to the chest wall, as the ribs are generally very pliable. Rib fractures may require early intervention for respiratory support, as there may be underlying pulmonary contusion. Other potentially severe but not immediately life-threatening conditions that must be identified and excluded include great vessel, bronchial or oesophageal injury, diaphragmatic injury and myocardial contusion.

The abdomen and pelvis

The abdomen should be carefully examined by inspection, palpation, percussion and auscultation. Insertion of a gastric tube will deflate the stomach and may facilitate the examination, making it more comfortable for the child and the clinician. Any bruising, grazes, swellings, masses, tenderness, guarding and rigidity should be noted, including rebound tenderness. The perineum should also be inspected; however, rectal and vaginal examinations should only be carried out by the surgical teams with responsibility for the child's care, if absolutely necessary. Where signs of perineal injury are evident, such as scrotal bruising, swelling or laceration, or blood is present at the urethral meatus, a high index of suspicion for trauma to the urinary tract should be maintained and specialist intervention sought.

Emergency surgery is indicated when the shocked child has an acutely tender abdomen. Referred pain, for example, to the shoulder, is an important symptom. In other cases, the need for repeated examinations may be required. Having completed the abdominal examination, the pelvis should be examined, noting any crepitus and bony instability on palpation.

The limbs

Each limb should be inspected and palpated looking for signs of bone and joint injury, such as tenderness, crepitus or hypermobility. Peripheral pulses and neurological function distal to the injury sites should also be assessed, especially where fractures and dislocations are involved. Compartment syndrome, which is characterised by swelling and tenderness of the compartment, numbness affecting the compartmental nerve and pain on stretching the compartmental muscles, must be excluded. If found to be present, urgent specialist referral is warranted. Photographs should be taken of all open fractures after any gross contaminants have been removed. The wounds should then be covered with antiseptic dressings, appropriate broad-spectrum antibiotics commenced and tetanus immunisation status addressed and acted upon where relevant. Where fractures are present, bones should be realigned into their anatomical position and then splinted to relieve pain, bleeding and shock.

Pain relief should never be withheld from the injured patient. Signs of abdominal injury are not masked or diminished by the judicious use of intravenous opiates.

The use of charts

There is great variation in the weight of children, however, there is a helpful linear relationship of weight to length before the onset of the growth spurt in early adolescence. Emergency department workers may have recourse to using the Oakley chart or Broselow tape, which provide information on the doses of emergency drugs as well as the size of adjuncts used in resuscitation.

CHILD PROTECTION/CHILD PROTECTION ISSUES

Children can present with numerous abuse-related presentations ranging from neglect and emotional abuse to physical and sexual abuse; any one child may experience a combination of any of these forms. Abuse may occur in all social strata; there may also be a past history of abuse in the perpetrators.

The diagnosis has important consequences for the child and his family as well as the perpetrator of the abuse, hence the importance of attention to detail, and the need to ensure a caring and considered approach throughout all interactions with children and their attendants. A thorough history and detailed examination are required, and careful documentation is essential. The roles of nursing and medical staff are manifold: to ensure that any injuries suffered by the child are treated; to ensure that social services are informed and are able to address the welfare needs of the child; and to take part in the multidisciplinary and multiagency processes by which the optimal management of the child and his or her situation can be determined.

Attending clinicians must not appear to be judgmental but must present themselves sympathetically to the child. Clinicians should not ask any leading questions and must not express shock or disbelief, but should react in a kind, understanding and sympathetic manner, particularly if the child is showing signs of distress. Frequent attendance at the local emergency or multiple presentations at different emergency departments are seen in cases of abuse.

NEGLECT

Neglect may present as the child being unkempt, or displaying inappropriate behaviour. He or she may have been deprived of decent clothing or food, adequate supervision, shelter, medical care and/or education. Play may be an unfamiliar idea to the child and the perturbing picture of *'frozen watchfulness'* recorded; here, the child looks on at normal playing activities without apparent facial expressions of emotion.

Emotional neglect alludes to the absence of any affection and care for the child. This may also be associated with unusual and sometimes unruly behaviour, and he or she may take part in high risk-taking activities. Self-esteem and body image may be poor. The child may have undergone repeated rejection, have been ignored, not spoken to or have been isolated from other family members.

Sexual abuse may present due to medical illnesses, such as vaginal discharge, or may arise from questioning abnormal behaviour in the child. This may be reported by teachers or other carers, and may include sexually explicit behaviour or inappropriate language.

Physical abuse shows signs, as there may be evidence of beatings or injuries. There are often injuries that are highly suspicious (see Box 30.4). Physical abuse can be life threatening; every paediatric intensive care unit (PICU) will see between three and four children per annum who have suffered severe injuries. In enquiries relating to children who have died from abuse, many of the cases could have been picked up at an earlier stage in their maltreatment; hence it is important to have a high index of suspicion when the history is odd, the examination of the child reveals elements of concern, or the clinical findings do not match with the history as given.

The *shaken baby syndrome* is a well-recognised form of physical abuse, which occurs in infants, particularly under the age of 6 months. In this circumstance, the child is held by the upper part of the trunk and shaken robustly. This can cause small tears within the brain and is associated with significant morbidity and mortality.

Factitious illness is a much less common condition, which occurs when the child is brought to the attention of medical services owing to a fabricated illness, or has an ailment which is caused by the carer. This is typically more often due to the mother of the child rather than the father. Presentations include fevers that settle when the

---

Box 30.4   Child abuse or non–accidental injury

Neglect
- Failure to thrive
- Unkempt appearance with poor dentition and marks on the body
- Repeat attendance to medical services, often with poorly explained injuries
- Not immunised and little contact with health visitor services
- Concern about behaviour expressed at nursery or school

Emotional abuse
- Odd behaviour:
- Inattentiveness
- Frozen watchfulness
- Lack of socialisation
- Rocking of the body
- Fearfulness
- Passivity or aggression

Physical abuse
Classic lesions such as:
- Slap marks, e.g. hand-shaped marks
- Bruises
- Pinch marks
- Linear marks from beatings with straps, rulers or solid bars
- Cigarette burns
- Torn frenulum – oral, genital

Lesions in certain distributions such as the axillae, the perineal region, on the buttocks and on the lower back are less common sites of accidental injury in toddlers; further detail must be obtained regarding how they occurred

---

child is on the ward, increased weight gain of an otherwise failing to thrive child whilst an in-patient, or even more bizarre presentations such as odd-coloured urine, apnoeic episodes or periods of fitting, which are not apparent following admission.

In all forms of abuse, there may have been repeat attendances to medical services. Some of the presentations may include injuries or events that are incompatible with the history given as the explanation. The child may have been brought in at odd times, for example, late at night, or have had a delay in presentation. Effective liaison between colleagues working in the community such as health visitors, school nurses and community paediatricians, as well as general practitioners and other related agencies, such as social services and the child protection branch of the police service, must be maintained.

Obtaining a history

Obtaining a detailed clinical history is an essential part of all clinical assessments and examinations. This is particularly the case with the vulnerable in society, including children who are often unable to speak for themselves and who rely on others to serve as their advocate.

With regard to children and the possibility of non-accidental injury, a number of areas give rise to concern. These include a story inconsistent with the developmental age of the child; for example, a story may be relayed of a baby rolling off his or her bed even though he or she had been placed in the middle of it. This would immediately register concern, as 2-week-old babies cannot make themselves roll over. In some instances, the story given relating to the events in question changes each time it is recounted and there may be inconsistencies in the details given. Similarly, serious injuries that are attributed to siblings or relative minors may cause alarm bells to ring. The identification of signs of non-accidental injury when the child presents with another complaint, which is often relatively minor, may also signify the need for closer observation. For example, a child may present with an upper respiratory tract infection but also has a 3-day burn to his or her leg that is incidentally found by nursing staff. Other examples of histories that cause concern include delays in seeking medical help, injuries of varying ages, particularly when the explanations are dubious or inconsistent, and the attendance of children with injuries for which the carers can give no attributable account for their severity or inappropriate mechanisms of action.

Examination

The weight and height (or length in an infant) must be measured and documented in all children; this may include any previous data from hand-held parent records.

Marks

Linear marks may be present on the child's back and limbs owing to injuries inflicted using belts or sticks. Cigarette burns characteristically provide central discrete burns that have clearly demarcated borders with central third-degree burns. There may also be multiple bruises of different ages; although it may be difficult to date these lesions precisely, there may be a range of colour from fresh marks to those with a yellow–orange discolouration. The outline of fingers can sometimes be seen following episodes where children have been slapped; the individual fingers causing the lesion can sometimes be discerned. Bruising to the ear over the cartilaginous element is indicative of a considerable force having been applied. Perioral pinch marks are seen in babies who have had their feeding bottles forced into their mouths. Bite marks may also be visible; notably the size of the bite and of the lesion can provide useful forensic information.

There are four frenula that may be disrupted in abuse. These are the upper and lower alveolar frenula, the lingual frenulum, and the penile frenulum. The *upper alveolar and lower alveolar frenula*, arising from the upper and lower gums, respectively, insert into the buccal side of the lips. Where blows are delivered to the closed mouth, these may be torn. The *lingual frenulum* originates from the floor of the mouth and inserts into the tongue; blunt objects pushed forcefully into the buccal cavity may break this. The *penile frenulum* is attached to the dorsal surface of the penis inserting into the base of the foreskin. This may tear if forced backward.

The most common sites for pre-school children to have bruises due to accidental knocks include the lower legs and the forehead, as these are relatively large structures. Marks on the back and buttocks from normal play are uncommon. Recording of clear and thorough details outlining all marks seen should be undertaken as soon as possible after the examination and contemporaneously, if possible; this includes measuring the size of any lesions with a tape measure, and giving their distances from fixed bony points. Drawings of the lesions should be made, official charts made and each lesion numbered and individually described in clear, succinct, unambiguous words.

Where photographs are taken, a centimetre-marked ruler should be placed beside each photographed lesion. Digital cameras should be avoided on the whole, as their images can be manipulated; ordinary photographs on 35 mm film should be used. Disposable cameras may also be used with the complete reel used for each patient, and sent off to the photography department with an accompanying referral letter. This should be clearly documented in the child's notes.

If there is any suggestion that the child has been sexually abused, examinations should not be commenced and expert help sought immediately. The designated nurse or designated doctor for child protection should be contacted with the safety, security and well-being of the child uppermost in the minds of his or her health care workers. A calm atmosphere must prevail.

Social services can be contacted to see if the child is on the 'at-risk register'. Should the child not be registered, this fact should not detract from making the diagnosis or seeking the assistance of team members. Where concerns are present, these must be expressed to senior medical staff as well as to social services.

All health care workers have a duty to inform the designated or named nurse/doctor within their Trust about concerns they may have regarding potential suspected abuse in children. This includes cases of domestic violence between adults giving rise to injuries sustained by one or the other; this is a high-risk group. It is well recognised that there is a higher incidence of abuse within families where the parents have themselves been victims of abuse.

A high index of suspicion is required when caring for all vulnerable patients and children in particular. As the majority of Trusts have child protection guidelines relating to their local Area Child Protection Committee (ACPC), all health care workers should familiarise themselves with these, with local procedures and with the details of those to be contacted in the event of emergencies arising.

EFFECTIVE INJURY PREVENTION

Education, alteration of environmental hazards and the implementation of safety legislation are the three cornerstones of injury prevention. Terms such as primary, secondary and tertiary prevention schemes are used when considering how the effects of accidents may be diminished.

Primary prevention relates to the prevention of an unintentional injury (e.g. use safe playground material), secondary prevention to reducing the effects of the accident (e.g. promoting bicycle helmet use) and tertiary prevention to diminishing the morbidity/mortality by the effectiveness of the emergency services. Courses such as the European Paediatric Life Support course and Pre-hospital Paediatric Trauma courses are examples of tertiary prevention, and are directed towards teaching professionals how to deliver effective management of injured children, so improving their outcome after the traumatic event.

Voluntary organisations, such as those listed below, have a role to play in injury prevention:

- The Royal Society for the Prevention of Accidents (www.rospa.co.uk)
- Children Accident Prevention Trust (www.capt.org.uk)
- TraumaCare (www.traumacare.org.uk).

The first two organisations are concerned with primary and secondary prevention. TraumaCare is directed towards tertiary prevention by encouraging a multidisciplinary approach, from the pre-hospital setting to rehabilitation. Their websites detail their activities and are good sources of further information.

The government has directed considerable resources towards injury prevention: The saving Lives: Our Healthier Nation (OHN) White paper (www.ohn.gov.uk) was published in 1999; this set a target of reducing 'death rates by at least one fifth and to reduce the rate of serious injury by at least one tenth by 2010', saving an estimated 12 000 lives. Subsequently, there have been many initiatives, such as 'Safe Routes to School', 'Healthy Citizens Program' and 'Think! Road Safety'.

The cost of unintentional injury to the National Health Service is estimated to be about £12 billion per annum, and the average cost of dealing with a childhood injury is £1300, with over 10 000 patients being permanently affected every year. This burden on the health care services and society as a whole means that injury should continue to be high on the list of priorities for government action.

SUMMARY

When trauma occurs to children as a result of accidental injury or child abuse, the use of a structured approach will ensure that life-threatening problems are identified and dealt with rapidly. Adherence to the well-established ABCD care pathways will minimise the risk to the child and will contribute to a swift resolution.

Consideration of the use of parents and carers to comfort their children in the treatment process will help the medical and nursing staff fulfil their duties in a calm and structured way.

It is the duty of all clinicians to ensure that the possibility of child abuse should be kept at the forefront when considering the cause of unusual injuries or presentations in children. Prevention is always better than cure, and emergency department staff have a duty to ensure that appropriate advice is offered when relevant.

Reference

A&E Services for Children, 1999

Further reading

Advanced Life Support Group. *Pre-hospital paediatric life support*. London: BMJ Publishing Group, 1999

American Academy of Pediatrics. *Pediatric education for pre-hospital professionals*. Elk Grove Village, IL: American Academy of Pediatrics, 2000

Candy D, Davies G, Ross E. *Clinical paediatrics and child health*. London: WB Saunders, 2003

Capehorn DMW, Swain AH, Goldsworthy LL. *Handbook of paediatric accident and emergency medicine – a symptom-based guide*. London: WB Saunders, London, 1998

Davies FCW. *Minor trauma in children – a pocket guide*. London: Arnold, 2003

European Paediatric Life Support Group. *Advanced paediatric life support*. London: 2004

Gill D, O'Brien N. *Paediatric clinical examination*. Edinburgh: Churchill Livingstone, 1998

Gill D, O'Brien N. *Paediatric clinical examination made easy*. Edinburgh: Churchill Livingstone, 2003

Goldbloom RB. *Paediatric clinical skills*. Edinburgh: Churchill Livingstone, 1997

Greaves I, Porter K. *Pre-hospital medicine: the principles and practice of immediate care*. London: Edward Arnold, 1999

Harden A, Weston R, Oakley A. A review of the effectiveness and appropriateness of peer-led promotion and interventions for young people. London: Evaluation of Health Promotion and Social Interventions, 1999: 1–180

Lissauer T, Glayden G. *Illustrated textbook of paediatrics*. Edinburgh: Churchill Livingstone, 2003

Meadow R. *ABC of child abuse*. London: BMJ Publishers, London, 1993

Mott A, Rolfe K, James R, Evans R, Kemp A, Dunstan F, Kemp K, Sibert J. Safety of surfaces and equipment for children in playgrounds. *Lancet* 1997; 14: 316–320

Polin RA. *Paediatric secrets*. Edinburgh: Churchill Livingstone, 1997

Sibert J. *Accidents and emergencies in childhood*. London: Royal College of Physicians, 1992

Chapter **31**

Care of the patient with major burns

Lesley Jenkins

'We had this house fire and there were children…. I thought where do you start with these kids… they were so badly burnt, one of them was unrecognisable but alive.' (Jenkins, 1999: 62)

INTRODUCTION

It is difficult to imagine the disruption caused to a person and their loved ones as a result of a thermal injury to the skin. Sometimes visually overwhelming, caring for the burn victim can be a daunting experience and the smell of burnt flesh can linger long after the experience.

Many people rely on the skills of the nursing staff in the trauma room, yet as the quote above illustrates, at times one may wonder where to start. The place to start, as with any trauma patient, is with the trauma management principles laid down by the Advanced Trauma Life Support Course (ATLS®; American College of Surgeons, 1997). This provides a structure within which the burn patient can be initially assessed and managed. This chapter will be developed using these guidelines to underpin the specific focus on burn trauma. The aim is to provide information that will help develop the nurses' understanding of burn trauma, and establish a systematic approach to assessment and care of the patient with severe burns.

TRAUMA ROOM PREPARATION

Preparation includes the measures taken to facilitate the resuscitation of any trauma patient.

The burn-injured patient is particularly susceptible to hypothermia as a result of poor thermoregulatory control and specific preparation to prevent this includes pre-warming the trauma room. The patient's trolley should be covered in a clean or sterile sheet with plastic undersheeting to reduce the risk of wound contamination.

HISTORY

One of the major pitfalls in burn trauma is failure to suspect or recognise coexisting injuries and conditions. The appearance of the burn can distract even the most experienced eye, with the focus placed on the burn alone.

Establishing and documenting a clear history of the mechanism of injury is paramount. Pre-hospital personnel are witnesses to the scene and can provide information that may indicate a potential for other injuries and problems. Important information available from the pre-hospital team is summarised in Table 31.1, and the history relevant to the actual thermal injury in Table 31.2.

To emphasise the importance of clear history taking and how coexisting injuries and problems may be suspected, the following case studies are outlined.

Case study 31.1

A 25-year-old man presents to the emergency (ED) department with severe burns to his lower torso following a house fire. Paramedics note that the patient jumped out of the second-floor bedroom window to escape the fire, landing on concrete. Associated injuries included a pelvic injury and fracture to the right mid-shaft femur.

Case study 31.2

A 22-year-old man with full-thickness burns to his face and upper torso is brought to the emergency department unconscious and

Table 31.1 Important information about the history of injury

Mechanism of injury	Considerations
Road traffic accident	Speed
	Unrestrained occupant
	Damage to vehicle
	Ejection
	Fatality at scene
Fall from a height	Height of fall > 20 feet/6 metres
Electrocution	Voltage
House fire	House severely damaged
	Escape attempted
	Conscious level at scene
	Burning materials produce toxic gases
Explosion/blast	Type of explosion – gas/chemical
	Distance thrown
Scalds	Hot water
	Oil
	Steam
Self-inflicted injury	Drug toxicity
	Psychiatric problems
Collapse	Epilepsy
	Alcoholism
	Hypoglycaemia
	Cardiac event
Assault	Concealed injuries

Table 31.2 History specific to the thermal injury

History	Significance
Time of injury	Fluid replacement calculated from time of burn injury
Burning agent – temperature and duration of exposure	Helps determine depth of burn
What clothing worn	Synthetic fabrics ignite and burn rapidly at high temperatures
First-aid measures	Helps determine depth of burn
Burned in enclosed space, e.g. building or car	Potential inhalation injury
Conscious level at scene	Indicates possible severity of inhalation injury
Identity of chemical	Potential systemic complications
Voltage of electrical injury	High voltage can cause associated injuries
Inappropriate history	Consider non accidental injury in children
	Consider criminal injury

tolerating an oral airway. Paramedics say the patient was involved in a gas explosion at work and was thrown against metal railings. The patient required theatre for the emergency management of a ruptured spleen and bowel perforation.

Case study 31.3

A 24-year-old lady presented to the emergency department with 45% full-thickness burns after dousing herself in petrol. Paramedics found empty packets of paracetamol and aspirin at the scene. Patient management included treatment for paracetamol and salicylate poisoning.

Establishing a clear history of the mechanism of injury can help establish the presence of co-existing injuries and problems

PATIENT ASSESSMENT

Assessment begins with a rapid primary survey. ATLS® (American College of Surgeons, 1997) describes the primary survey as a sequential process where life-threatening conditions are identified and treatment priorities established. Priorities for the burn patient are the same as for those of any trauma victim and it is vital that the burn does not detract from these priorities of assessment.

Primary survey

Specific considerations include the following.

Airway maintenance with cervical spine protection
Rapid assessment to determine upper airway patency should be made with the provision of high-concentration oxygen (ideally warmed humidified oxygen) via a non-rebreathing mask with a reservoir bag. Airway management is performed with simultaneous protection of the cervical spine, if the mechanism of injury is suggestive of a possible cervical spine injury.

Effective assessment of the airway of a burn victim requires knowledge of the effects of heat and smoke on the airways. These are discussed later.

Breathing and ventilation
- Smoke inhalation injury may impair ventilation.
- Circumferential full thickness burns to the chest may impair the efficiency of ventilation.
- In children, full-thickness thermal injury to the anterior and lateral chest wall, and upper abdomen may impair ventilation.

Circulation with haemorrhage control
Prompt *vascular access* and initiation of fluid therapy should be established by inserting two large-bore cannulae (14 gauge) preferably through unburnt skin. Burnt skin does not deter the placement of a cannula, if the vein is accessible (American College of Surgeons, 1997). It may be difficult to secure vascular access in extensive thermal injuries and a venous cut-down may have to be used. During the resuscitation of children up to 6 years of age, intraosseous infusions can be used when there is collapse of the circulation and peripheral access has failed.

Routine blood samples should be taken for:

- full blood count
- urea and electrolytes
- serum glucose
- type and cross-match
- pregnancy testing in women of childbearing age.

In addition, carboxyhaemoglobin levels should be taken. No significant difference has been found between carboxyhaemoglobin concentrations taken from either venous or arterial samples (Touger et al., 1995).

Other considerations include:

- haemorrhage from other injuries should be considered in addition to fluid lost from the thermal injury
- extensive burns to the limbs may cause difficulties in palpation of pulses and measuring of blood pressure
- skin pallor and capillary refill may be difficult to evaluate
- altered conscious level may be indicative of blood volume loss as well as airway compromise, smoke inhalation and head injury

- impaired perfusion to limbs and the need for escharotomy/fasciotomy should be identified.

Assessment to determine the size of the burn and calculate the fluid needs from the thermal injury are time consuming, and can be safely deferred until resuscitation priorities have been identified and treatment established.

Disability (neurological evaluation)

A brief neurological assessment should be made to determine the level of consciousness and pupillary response. The causes of a decreased conscious level may include:

- hypoxia
- hypovolemia
- head injury
- coexisting medical problem.

Exposure with environmental control

- Fully undress to assess for further injuries.
- Poor thermoregulatory control can quickly lead to hypothermia.
- Keep patient covered to maintain warmth.
- Remove inappropriately placed wet soaks to prevent hypothermia.
- Remove jewellery.

After completion of the primary survey and the institution of resuscitative measures, the secondary survey is completed so that the patient can be fully evaluated. This comprises a top to toe examination of the patient, including a log roll, if it has not already been done. The focus now shifts to a more in-depth assessment of the burn and determination of the fluid needs from the thermal injury. Pain control is also addressed and managed.

PAIN CONTROL

Thermal trauma can result in the most severe form of acute pain experienced. The severity of pain may vary depending on the extent of thermal injury, together with the individual's own unique response. It is essential to address pain control early.

> All burns are painful

Analgesia should not be given via the intramuscular route because it is likely to remain in the muscle and thus will be poorly absorbed during the resuscitative phase of care. An intravenous opiate such as morphine is advocated, given in small incremental doses, to achieve the desired effect.

Many health care workers are taught that full-thickness burns are not painful as nerve damage is severe; however, it should be remembered that at the edges of all full-thickness burns are areas of burn that are less severe, and these areas are painful.

AIRWAY MANAGEMENT AND INHALATION INJURY

Inhalation injury encompasses various insults to the respiratory system that can injure different parts of the respiratory tract in different ways. Furthermore, the inhalation of toxic fumes can have a severe systemic toxic effect. The patient may have one or more of these types of injury, which can be classified according to the anatomical site of injury.

Upper airway injury

The airway above the larynx is particularly susceptible to the effects of heat. Inhaling hot gases, usually in a confined space, causes a direct thermal injury to the upper airway. Generally, this injury can be compared to the changes that take place in a cutaneous thermal injury; however, the mucosa of the airway swells more than the skin. Within minutes, swelling may be visible on inspection of the airway and this may progress to airway obstruction as a result of pharyngeal and laryngeal oedema. Furthermore, external burns to the face and neck can lead to immense oedema necessitating early definitive airway intervention.

Lower airway injury

A common misconception is that smoke inhalation causes a true thermal injury to the lower respiratory tract. Direct thermal injury to the airway below the larynx is rare, principally owing to the protective element of cooling by the naso-pharynx (Papini and Wood, 1999), and the reflex opening and closing of the glottis, which protects it from the effects of hot dry air (Harvey, 1997). The exception is inhalation of steam, which has the potential to liberate sufficient heat to cause a direct thermal injury beyond the carina (Pruitt et al., 1975).

Airway injury below the larynx is caused by the effects of inhalation of the byproducts of incomplete combustion and causes a chemical injury to the lung. Smoke contains irritants, mainly carbon, which are deposited in the respiratory tract. Depending on what products are burning, toxic chemicals are also produced. These compounds dissolve in water contained in respiratory mucus, producing acids and alkalis, which damage the mucosa, leading to inflammation, cell death, sloughing and obstruction. Papini & Wood (1999) identify three stages of lung injury:

- respiratory compromise and bronchospasm up to 12 hours postinjury
- pulmonary oedema, 6–12 hours postinjury
- bronchopneumonia up to 60 hours postinjury.

Effects of toxic fumes

Carbon monoxide and cyanide are two important chemical compounds produced by fire that have a systemic toxic effect.

Carbon monoxide

Carbon monoxide (CO) is an odourless and colourless gas sometimes referred to as the *silent killer*, which is responsible for a large number of deaths at the scene of a fire. Owing to its greater affinity for combining with haemoglobin than oxygen (200–250 times greater), it diffuses rapidly into the bloodstream. The binding of carbon monoxide to haemoglobin forms carboxyhaemoglobin (COHb) and, once formed, reduces the oxygen carrying capacity of the blood, resulting in tissue hypoxia.

There are other mechanisms whereby carbon monoxide exerts its toxicity in addition to the reduction in the oxygen-carrying capacity of the blood. Those that cause a direct cellular toxicity are (Bird, 1999; Turner et al., 1999):

- poisoning of intracellular oxygen-carrying haem proteins

Table 31.3   Expected symptoms related to levels of carboxyhaemoglobin

Carboxyhaemoglobin	Expected symptoms
0–15%	No signs – levels typically found in cigarette smokers
15–30%	Headache, nausea, irritability,
30–40%	Dizziness, vomiting, visual disturbance, disorientation
40–60%	Tachycardia, tachypnoea, ataxia, hallucinations, convulsions, coma
> 60%	Coma, cardiopulmonary arrest, death

- cytochromes – cellular respiration is reduced;
- myoglobin – skeletal and myocardial function is reduced
- distortion of the red blood cell membrane.

The effects of acute carbon monoxide poisoning depend on a number of factors, such as the concentration levels at the scene and the duration of exposure in the burning environment. Symptoms can relate to levels (Table 31.3).

Diagnosis of carbon monoxide poisoning is based on a history of exposure, with blood samples taken to confirm the presence and degree of carboxyhaemoglobin. Blood levels in the ED do not give an accurate picture of the severity of exposure. Carboxyhaemoglobin levels begin to fall as soon as a patient is removed from the toxic environment. It has a variable half-life of 4 hours breathing room air or 90 minutes when breathing high-concentration oxygen (Turner et al., 1999). By the time samples are taken, levels may fail to represent the initial exposure level. Clarke et al. (1981) found that carboxyhaemoglobin levels broadly correlated to the degree of smoke inhalation and reported that severe inhalation injury can be expected with peak levels of 30–35%.

A patient may have one, or a combination of injuries to the airways – upper airway, lower airway and systemic toxic effects. An important message is that establishing a clear history of the pre-hospital events, together with a record of the patient's initial presenting symptoms can help determine the possible severity of respiratory injury. **The main value in detecting a raised carboxyhaemoglobin level is demonstrating that**

an inhalation injury has occurred and is, therefore, an important marker to help indicate the potential severity of upper and lower airway injury. Ultimately, management of carbon monoxide poisoning focuses on administering high-concentration oxygen via a mask with a reservoir bag, as early as possible.

Cyanide

Cyanide is a cellular poison and is rapidly absorbed through the skin and respiratory tract. Cyanide fumes are emitted as a product of burning plastics and can cause loss of consciousness, convulsions and death. There is no rapid test for establishing blood cyanide levels in current practice; however, patients who are likely to have high cyanide levels are those with high carboxy-haemoglobin levels (Clarke et al., 1981). Although there are specific antidote treatments for cyanide poisoning, they can be toxic in themselves.

> Early management of carbon monoxide and cyanide gas inhalation focuses on provision of high-concentration oxygen and adequate ventilation

RECOGNITION AND MANAGEMENT OF AIRWAY PROBLEMS

Acute airway problems

Initial management is determined by the degree of airway compromise and respiratory distress. Airway compromise may be due to a number of factors (Box 31.1).

Upper airway injury and external burns to the face and neck can quickly lead to obstruction owing to pharyngeal and laryngeal oedema. Patients presenting with thermal injury above the larynx must always be intubated (Hilton & Hepp 2001). Endotracheal tubes should not be pre-cut, as progressive facial oedema may potentially displace the tube in the trachea. Ideally, the burn patient should be nursed semirecumbent to reduce swelling but this may be contraindicated, if measures are being taken to manage a potential cervical spine injury. A surgical airway is avoided owing to risks associated with infection. However, the technique may be life saving when other means of maintaining an airway have failed.

Delayed airway problems

Compromise to the airway and breathing may not always be immediately obvious. Signs of airway obstruction and respiratory difficulty may be subtle and insidious, developing over a period of time. Assessment includes the following.

- A high index of suspicion of inhalation injury based on the injury history:
  - entrapment of patient in a confined burning environment (e.g. car, building);
  - patient unconscious/altered conscious level, when rescued from scene;
  - fatalities at scene, if history of confinement in a burning environment;
  - explosion of gas or chemicals.
- The presence of clinical warning signs (Table 31.4). The patient may not initially present with all of these signs and inhalation injury can occur in the absence of a cutaneous injury. Obstruction may evolve gradually, so frequent reassessment is vital.

Decisions to secure the patient's airway definitively may be based on:

- altered conscious level
- increasing signs of obstruction
- respiratory distress
- associated injuries
- prolonged transfer to burns unit.

Early discussion with a senior burn anaesthetist is important for advice on appropriate airway management.

> Signs of airway obstruction may not be obvious immediately

The following case history illustrates the management of a patient with an acute airway problem.

Case study 31.4

A 16-year-old male driver of a car is brought to the ED following a high-speed collision into a brick wall. The car ignited shortly after impact and the patient was dragged from vehicle by a passing motorist.

Box 31.1   Possible causes of airway compromise

General
- Glasgow Coma Scale ≤ 8
- Head injury
- Maxillofacial trauma
- Alcohol intoxication
- Drug toxicity

Specific
- Airway burns
- Circumferential neck and chest burns
- Smoke inhalation
- High carbon monoxide levels
- Effects of a blast injury

Table 31.4   Clinical signs of inhalation injury

Site of burn	Clinical signs
Facial burns	Carbonaceous sputum
Perioral burns/ mucosa inflamed	Soot in nostrils
Neck burns	Singeing of nasal hairs and eyebrows
Excessive coughing	Stridor
Voice change	Difficulty in breathing
Hoarseness	Altered level of consciousness

On arrival, the patient smells strongly of alcohol and is shouting loudly. He has superficial facial burns and soot in his nostrils. Inspection of the patient's airway reveals swelling and soot deposits. There is also a large full-thickness burn to his abdomen and thighs.

High-concentration oxygen is given via a mask with reservoir bag and his SaO$_2$ is 96%. COHb level approximately 1 hour postinjury is 9%. During assessment in A&E, the patient's airway becomes noisy and his behaviour more agitated. He is then intubated and ventilated.

The patient has a direct thermal injury to his upper airway as a result of inhaling hot gases in a confined space. This rapidly caused airway obstruction due to progressive pharyngeal and laryngeal oedema, and necessitated early endotracheal intubation.

Pulse oximetry

Pulse oximetry is a useful adjunct to measure and monitor patients' oxygen saturation levels. However, false high readings may be given in carbon monoxide poisoning because carboxy-haemoglobin absorbs light similarly to oxyhaemo-globin (Buckley et al., 1994).

Escharotomy

In circumferential full-thickness burns, the skin loses its elastic qualities and is unable to expand, as progressive oedema forms beneath the eschar. This results in a tourniquet effect, which can lead to circulatory compromise in limbs and decreased chest wall compliance when the burn is around the chest. In children, because breathing is mainly diaphragmatic, ventilation may be impaired when there is full thickness injury to the anterior and lateral aspects of the chest wall and upper abdomen [Australia and New Zealand Burn Association (ANZBA), 1996].

To release the effects of circumferential pressure, an escharotomy is required. This is a surgical incision made through the entire thickness of the eschar down to subcutaneous fat. This procedure is not usually required within the first 6 hours postburn (American College of Surgeons, 1997). However, if there is an urgent need to improve the efficiency of ventilation, this procedure may be indicated in the emergency department after consultation with the burns team.

BURN ASSESSMENT

Assessment of the burn includes determination of its size and depth. In order to map the area of the burn and assess its size, the practitioner needs to be able to differentiate between different depths of injury.

Estimation of the depth of burn

The depth of injury may be variable and its differentiation can be difficult. Essentially assessment is subjective, and accuracy depends on the skill and experience of the practitioner. Also the appearance of the burn can alter from the time of initial assessment to arrival at the burns centre.

Depth of injury is classified according to the depth of tissue damage, and is dependent on the temperature of the burning agent and duration of exposure. Burns may be classified according to the causative burning agent:

- thermal:
  - scalds
  - flame
  - contact
- electrical
- chemical
- radiation.

Terms used are *superficial, partial thickness, deep partial thickness* (also referred to as deep dermal) and *full thickness*. It is important that a partial-thickness injury is distinguished from a full-thickness injury, as the outcome of the area of burned skin is dependent upon the level of tissue destruction. Figure 31.1 illustrates the structure of the skin and its relationship to the depth of injury.

In superficial burns that involve only the epidermis, healing usually takes place within 3–6 days. Partial thickness burns can be further subdivided into superficial partial thickness and deep partial thickness. Superficial partial thickness burns involve the epidermis and part of the dermis and usually heal within 7–10 days. However, deep partial thickness (deep dermal) burns involve the entire epidermis, but extend much deeper into the dermis and take much longer to heal (3–4 weeks). They are associated with scarring and functional impairment, and usually require excision and skin grafting. Bacterial infection can convert a partial thickness injury into a full-thickness injury.

In full-thickness burns, all layers of the skin are destroyed and the tissue destruction may extend to fat, muscle and bone. These burns require excision and skin grafting. Knowledge of typical wound characteristics at different depths of injury

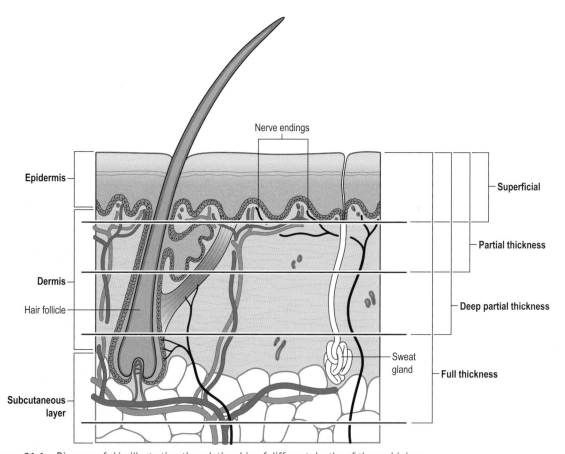

Figure 31.1   Diagram of skin illustrating the relationship of different depths of thermal injury.

Table 31.5   Burn depth characteristics

Depth	Characteristics
Superficial	Red Painful Brisk capillary return
Partial thickness	Red or pink Wet surface ± blisters Very painful Brisk capillary return
Deep partial thickness/ deep dermal	Dark pink or a mottled red Wet ± blisters ± pain Sluggish or absent capillary return
Full thickness	Appearance varies: – White, waxy – Charred brown – Dry, leatherlike – Thrombosed vessels – Painless – No capillary return

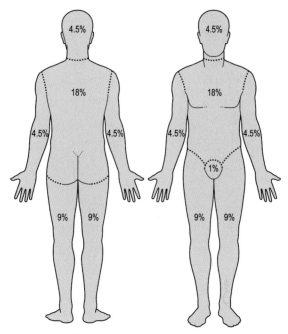

Figure 31.2   Estimation of surface area using the 'rule of nines'.

is fundamental in the assessment of burn depth. These are summarised in Table 31.5.

Other factors to consider are the age of the patient, the burning agent and the location of the burn on the body. The skin of an infant is thin, gradually increasing in thickness with age until, in the elderly, the skin becomes thinner once again. Therefore, infants and the elderly are burned more easily and deeper than adults, with a burning agent of the same temperature. Typically, flame can cause deep burns, and high-voltage electrical injury is likely to result in full-thickness burns that may extend to deeper structures. Contact burns from hot fluids are more unpredictable and it may take several days to determine their depth accurately.

Estimation of the size of burn

Assessment includes an estimation of total body surface area (TBSA) burnt and the depth of injury. Appropriate fluid resuscitation is dependent on the accuracy of assessment of TBSA; however, this can vary depending on the skill of the referring team. Laing et al. (1991) found that assessment in the ED was often inaccurate, leading to suboptimal treatment and referral. However, attendance of patients with major burns to the ED can

be infrequent, so there is little opportunity to develop expertise. Familiarity with one method of assessment should be obtained.

Assessment methods

One of the most familiar methods for estimating body surface area is the 'rule of nines' (Figure 31.2). The body surface is divided into areas of 9% or multiples of 9%, leaving 1% for the genitalia/perineum. It is easy to remember and useful to obtain a quick estimation. Although relatively accurate in adults, it is inaccurate in small children. This is due to different body surface proportions. Children have proportionally larger heads than adults and smaller lower extremities. Although the method can be modified (Figure 31.3) to take account of this, more accurate estimations can be achieved by using an age-dependent diagram such as the Lund and Browder chart (Figure 31.4). Both methods rely on an accurate representation of the burn on the chart. Areas of simple erythema are considered unburnt tissue and must be excluded. In extensive burns, it may be easier to estimate the unburnt area and subtract this from the total.

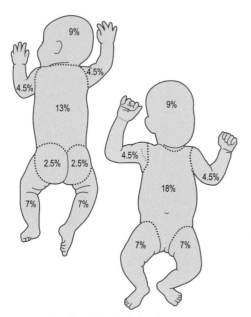

Figure 31.3 Paediatric 'rule of nines'.

Another useful method, especially for calculating small awkward areas, is using the palmar surface area of the injured patient's hand. This area, excluding the fingers, is identified as representing approximately 1% of the patient's body surface area (American College of Surgeons, 1997). It is worth noting that there seems to be some discrepancy as to what constitutes the area described as the hand and the size this represents. Rossiter et al. (1996) found that, in general, the UK describes the palm including the fingers as representing 1%. The Lund and Browder chart identifies the palm including the fingers as 1.5%. Apparently there is a gender difference. The area of the palm alone represents 0.5% in males and 0.4% in females. The area of the palm, including the fingers, was found to represent 0.8% in males and 0.7% in females (Rossiter et al., 1996). It was found that, if the size of the burn is estimated with the hand alone, the percentage of TBSA could be overestimated.

FLUID RESUSCITATION

Children with burns over 10% TBSA, and adults with burns greater than 15% TBSA, require fluid resuscitation and admission. Burn trauma results in an intravascular hypovolemia, sometimes referred to as 'burns shock'. Immediately following a thermal injury, mediators are produced that have a significant effect on increasing cell permeability. Increased permeability disrupts the normal exchange of blood plasma into the extracellular space at the site of injury, resulting in rapid fluid loss. In burns greater than 20%, there is generalised systemic oedema, resulting from widespread increased vascular permeability (ANZBA, 1996). There is also a visible fluid loss occurring from exudate, blisters and oedema, and an evaporative loss at the burn surface. Fluid loss occurs rapidly in the first 8–12 hours following injury and, by 18–36 hours postinjury, cell permeability returns towards normal, therefore, the overall duration of fluid resuscitation is variable.

Estimation of fluid requirements

The aim of fluid resuscitation following a burn injury is to maintain organ perfusion. Several burn resuscitation formulas exist and all merely provide an estimate of the fluid requirements following a burn injury. Calculations for fluid requirements are based from the time of injury, and not the time the patient arrives at hospital or when fluid therapy is commenced. The most important principle to remember is that the amount of fluid given is based on the patient's physiological response and is adjusted accordingly.

A crystalloid resuscitation formula is advocated by the ATLS® (American College of Surgeons, 1997). A total of 2–4 ml of Hartmann's solution per kilogram body weight per percentage burn is given in the first 24 hours. One-half is given over the first 8 hours postburn and the remaining half over the next 16 hours postburn. The formula takes account of the gradual reduction of fluid loss from oedema by decreasing the estimation of fluid requirements over the period of time. In the following groups of patients, fluid needs are likely to be greater and the higher range of the formula (4 ml/kg body weight per %TBSA) is used:

- inhalation injury
- associated trauma
- high-voltage electrical injury
- extensive depth and surface area burnt
- patients intoxicated with alcohol

CHART FOR ESTIMATING SEVERITY OF BURN WOUND

Name.. Ward......................... Number.......................... Date..........................

Age.......................... Admission weight...........................

Lund and Browder charts

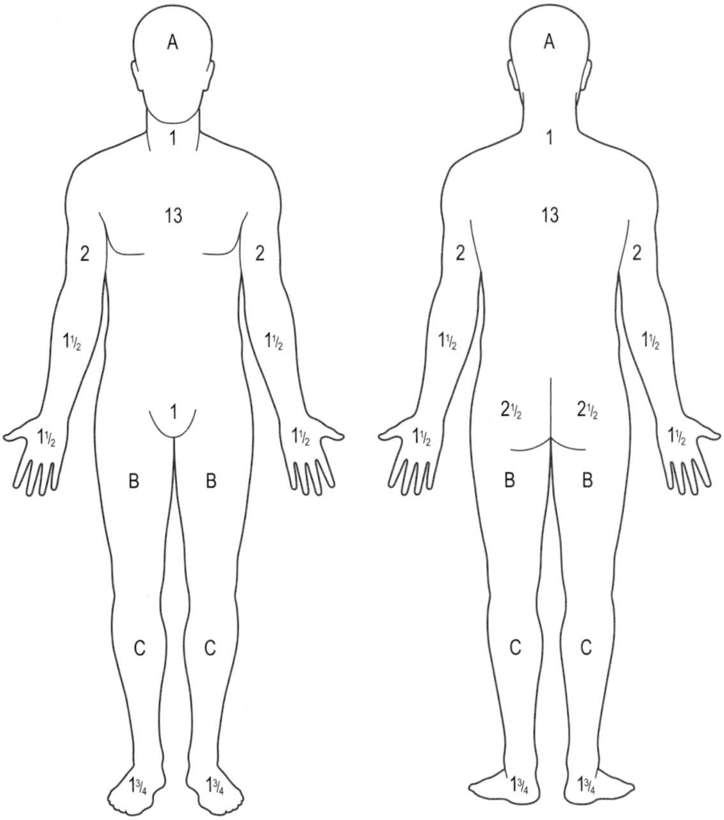

IGNORE SIMPLE ERYTHEMA

Partial thickness loss (PTL)

Full thickness loss (FTL)

	%	
Region	**PTL**	**FTL**
Head		
Neck		
Ant. trunk		
Post. trunk		
Right arm		
Left arm		
Buttocks		
Genitalia		
Right leg		
Left leg		
Total burn		

Relative percentage of body surface area affected by growth

Area	Age 0	1	5	10	15	Adult
A=1½ of head	9½	8½	6½	5½	4½	3½
B=1½ of one thigh	2¾	3¼	4	4½	4½	4¾
C=1½ of one leg	2½	2½	2¾	3	3¼	3½

Figure 31.4   Lund and Browder chart for more accurate estimation of the surface area burnt. (Reproduced with permission from Smith & Nephew.)

- delayed resuscitation
- children.

In children less than 30 kg, additional maintenance fluids are given to compensate for increased fluid needs compared with adults. There are a number of reasons for this: a higher body surface area to weight ratio; higher blood volume per kilogram of body weight – 80 ml/kg (adult 60–70 ml/kg); kidneys less able to reabsorb water from the urine to maintain blood volume. Therefore, formulae based on body weight tend to underestimate fluid requirements in children.

The maintenance fluid used is 4% dextrose/ 0.18% saline solution at a rate of:

4 ml/kg per hour up to 10 kg body weight
plus 2 ml/kg per hour from 10–20 kg
plus 1 ml/kg hour from 20–30 kg.

A dextrose-containing solution is used because children have lower stores of glycogen and are more susceptible to hypoglycaemia.

The following case histories illustrate the implementation of fluid resuscitation.

Case study 31.5

A 27-year-old man sustained 30% partial- and full-thickness burns, with evidence of a severe smoke inhalation injury, following a house fire. The patient's weight is estimated at 75 kg.

FORMULA
4 ml/kg per % TBSA.

FLUID
Warmed Hartmann's solution.

CALCULATION

4 ml × 75 kg × 30% TBSA = 9000 ml

to be given intravenously over 24 hours following the time of injury.

ADMINISTRATION
4500 ml to be administered over the first 8 hours and the remaining 4500 ml over the next 16 hours. The injury occurred 2 hours ago, therefore, the first half of the fluid needs to be administered over 6 hours.

Case study 31.6

A 27 kg child presents to the ED with 40% severe full-thickness burns following a road traffic accident. The patient also has a fracture to the right mid-shaft femur.

FORMULA
4 ml/kg per % TBSA.

FLUID
Warmed Hartmann's solution.

CALCULATION

4 ml × 27 kg × 40% TBSA = 4320 ml in 24 hours

(2160 ml over the first 8 hours, then 2160 ml over the next 16 hours).

MAINTENANCE FLUID CALCULATION
4% dextrose/0.18% saline solution:

4 ml/kg × 10 kg = 40 ml
2 ml/kg × 10 kg = 20 ml
1 ml/kg × 7 kg = 7 ml

Maintenance fluids = 67 ml/hour administered simultaneously with estimated burn fluid requirements.

Evaluation of adequacy of fluid resuscitation

Monitoring the adequacy of fluid resuscitation is vital. Consequently, insertion of a urinary catheter is necessary to evaluate the patient's response. Fluid is administered to maintain an average urine output of 0.5 ml/kg per hour (30–50 ml) in adults and 1 ml/kg per hour in children less than 30 kg. A urometer is essential to measure urine output accurately. If the urine output is inadequate, this indicates poor tissue perfusion and extra fluid is required. Conversely large urine output is indicative of excessive fluid resuscitation.

Following severe burns, particularly electrocution injury and burns affecting muscle, haemochromogens – myoglobin from muscle cells (rhabdomyolysis) and haemoglobin from red blood cells (haemolysis) – are released into the circulation. They are then excreted by the kidneys but in high concentration can form deposits in the renal tubules leading to acute tubular necrosis.

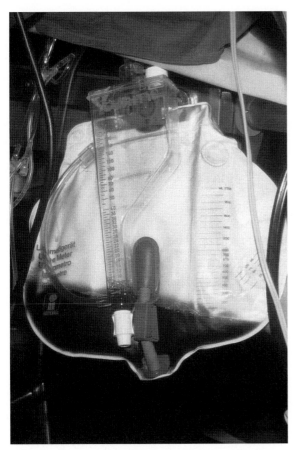

Figure 31.5 The presence of haemochromogens in the urine of a patient who sustained a high-voltage electrical injury.

The presence of haemochromogens in urine (myoglobinuria or haemoglobinuria) colours it dark red (Figure 31.5). When present, the urine output should be increased to 1–2 ml/kg per hour until the urine is clear (ANZBA, 1996).

Wound management

Attention can be paid to the burn wound when treatment priorities have been established. Complicated dressings are time wasting and unnecessary, so the initial goals of wound management are to stop the burning process, to alleviate pain, to prevent infection and establish tetanus prophylaxis.

First-aid measures include removal of clothing, which can retain heat and continue burning. Synthetic fibres rapidly ignite and burn at high temperatures. These garments can melt and adhere to skin making them difficult to remove. If the garment is firmly adhered, the non-adherent cloth can be trimmed, leaving the adherent piece in place. To prevent constriction to oedematous limbs, jewellery must be removed.

In an attempt to limit tissue destruction, first-aid measures include rapidly cooling the area with cold running water for about 20 minutes. It is recommended that the temperature of the water should be 15°C, and ice or iced water should not be used, as this may deepen the injury. In major burns, the main problem is preventing hypothermia, which is a significant risk, especially in children. In this situation, application of cold water should be discontinued, as this can rapidly cause hypothermia.

During the resuscitative phase of care, the burn can quickly be covered in a temporary dressing, such as 'Clingfilm' or a clean sheet. This helps alleviate pain from air currents passing over the surface of exposed nerve endings and reduces risks of wound contamination. It also reduces evaporative losses from the wound. When applying Clingfilm, care should be taken to avoid compromising circulation. To reduce the risks of infection, an aseptic technique should be followed when dealing with the wound and any invasive procedures. The tetanus immunisation status of the patient should be established and, if there is uncertainty, tetanus prophylaxis may be required.

SPECIAL BURN CONSIDERATIONS

Electrical injury

Electrical injury can be deceiving. An innocuous-looking cutaneous injury may be the mere tip of the iceberg in terms of the magnitude of concealed problems. Electrical current enters the body at its point of contact, although, at extremely high voltage, the current may arc through air and direct contact is not required. It then travels along the path of least resistance, usually blood vessels and nerves, exiting through the earth contact. Tissue is damaged as a result of the generation of heat. The amount of heat produced depends on the voltage, electrical resistance of tissues and duration of exposure. Consequently, high-voltage injuries

(> 1000 volts) are most damaging because of the extent of heat generated. Low-voltage (< 1000 volts) injuries usually result in a local thermal injury.

Massive underlying tissue destruction can occur as the current flows freely through deep tissues. Fractures and dislocations may result secondary to tetanic muscular contractions, and other associated injuries may occur as a result of the casualty falling or being thrown. Rhabdomyolysis is a further complication, resulting in myoglobin release, which can cause acute renal failure.

Fluid resuscitation in electrical injuries

Fluid requirements in the patient who has sustained a high-voltage electrical injury are likely to be greater. If haemochromogens are detected in the urine, fluid resuscitation is increased to achieve a urine output of at least 100 ml/hour in order to eliminate the pigments from the kidneys.

Dysrhythmias

Cardiac dysrhythmias may initially be seen or delayed for up to 24 hours. These include sinus tachycardia, sinus bradycardia, right bundle branch block and focal ectopic dysrhythmias. ST elevation and QT prolongation are other non-specific changes (Sutcliffe, 1998) associated with severe burns. A 12-lead electrocardiogram should be obtained and cardiac monitoring undertaken.

Compartment syndrome

High-voltage electrical injury to an extremity often leads to compartment syndrome. This is secondary to tissue oedema in the muscle compartment and may necessitate fasciotomy. The increase in pressure results in severe pain and increasing neurological deficit. Loss of a palpable distal pulse is usually a late sign. Assessment includes a high index of suspicion for the potential complication, together with recognition of clinical signs.

Chemical injury

Chemical burns are caused by tissue reaction to a variety of substances, usually acid or alkali. The main problem results from substances continuing to burn long after the initial contact. The extent of tissue destruction depends on the chemical substance, its quantity and concentration, the length of exposure, its mechanism of action and first aid administered. The aim of treatment is early removal of the chemical, usually by irrigation with copious amounts of water, sometimes for many hours. In addition to direct cutaneous damage, some agents can be absorbed, resulting in systemic toxicity. Specialist advice about the chemical agent and its treatment can be sought from the local poisons information unit, although few have specific antidotes.

Burns to special areas

The anatomical location of the burn influences healing. Of particular concern are burns to the head, face, neck, hands, feet and genitalia. Facial burns can create problems with airway management as a result of tissue oedema. The pinna of the ear is difficult to heal, as the structure is cartilaginous and has a poor blood supply. It is difficult to prevent infection in burns to the perineum and prevention of wound contamination necessitates early catheterisation. Thermal injuries over joint surfaces are predisposed to the development of contractures and may lead to mobility problems. Although the size of thermal injury may be small, referral and admission to a burns unit may be necessary.

CRITERIA FOR REFERRAL TO A BURNS CENTRE

The British Burn Association identify the following criteria for referral of patients to a burns centre:

- burns > 5% TBSA in children
- burns > 10% TBSA in adults
- full-thickness or deep partial-thickness burns > 5%
- burns with inhalation injury
- chemical burns
- electrical burns
- burns involving special sites – hands, feet, face, joints, perineum, genitalia
- circumferential burn injuries
- burns in patients at the extremes of age

- burns in patients with pre-existing medical conditions
- burns with associated trauma.

The thermally injured patient with associated trauma may have other, more urgent priorities to deal with before stabilisation can be achieved and transfer to a burn centre arranged.

Role of the burns unit

The teams providing care for the burn victim and their family face unique challenges. Apart from complex changes to the body, disturbing psychological and emotional problems may compound the patient's recovery. Centralisation of burn care enables specialist support from a range of multi-disciplinary team members, who are equipped to deal with the challenges faced by both patients and their families.

Transfer

Transfer to a definitive unit is a potentially dangerous time in the management of any trauma patient. The overriding aim is to ensure a safe transfer. Communication between the ED and the burns unit should be coordinated by the referring and receiving teams. Before leaving, the following should be considered.

Airway and breathing care during transfer

The patient's airway should be secure and high-concentration oxygen continued via a mask with reservoir. There may be a need for endotracheal intubation before leaving the ED, especially when there is a prolonged transfer time. Any concerns about airway management should have been discussed with the burns team beforehand.

Circulatory care during transfer

Intravenous access should be established and well secured. Patients requiring fluid resuscitation need placement of a urinary catheter and output measured with a urometer.

Pain control during transfer

Reassess the effectiveness of pain relief before leaving and ensure that adequate supplies of medication are taken for the duration of the journey.

Burn wound and tetanus

Clingfilm or clean dry sheets are suitable temporary wound coverings to enable safe transfer of the patient. Tetanus prophylaxis should be administered in the ED, if required.

Communication

Appropriate documentation should be completed. Telephoning the burns unit with an estimated time of arrival can be helpful when the patient leaves the ED. This enables appropriate team members to be prepared, especially if the patient is intubated and ventilated.

CONCLUSION

Extraordinary challenges can be faced by the multidisciplinary team caring for the patient who has sustained a major burn. The thermal injury might constitute only part of the patient's overall injuries and problems. Rapid assessment and management can be dealt with according to principles of the ATLS® (American College of Surgeons, 1997).

References and further reading

American College of Surgeons. *Advanced trauma life support, student course manual*, 6th edn. Chicago: American College of Surgeons, 1997

Australia and New Zealand Burn Association (ANZBA). *Emergency management of severe burns course manual*. Kelvin Grove, Queensland: ANZBA, 1996.

Bird D. Inhalation injuries. *Emergency Nurse* 1999; 7(7): 19–23

Bosworth C. *Burns trauma*. London: Baillière Tindall, 1997

Buckley RG, Aks SE, Eschom JL, et al. The pulse oximetry gap in carbon monoxide intoxication. *Annals of Emergency Medicine* 1994; 24: 252–255

Carrougher GJ. *Burn care and therapy*. St Louis: Mosby, 1998

Clarke CJ, Campbell D, Reid WH. Blood carboxyhaemoglobin and cyanide levels in fire survivors. *Lancet* 1981; 1: 1332–1335

Harvey GA. Care of the burns patient with inhalation injury. In: Bosworth C (ed.) *Burns trauma*. London: Baillière Tindall, 1997: 76

Hilton PJ, Hepp M. The immediate care of the burned patient. *British Journal of Anaesthesia*. CEPD Reviews. Vol. 1. Number 4, 2001.

Jenkins L. *A&E nurses' perceptions of the effect of trauma training in clinical practice*. Unpublished MSc thesis. Swansea: University of Wales, 1999

Laing HE, Morgan BDG, Sanders R. Assessment of burn injury in the Accident and Emergency department: a review of 100 referrals to a regional burns unit. *Annals of the Royal College of Surgeons of England* 1991; 73: 329–331

Muir IFK, Barclay TL, Settle JAD. *Burns and their treatment*, 3rd edn, Butterworths, London, 1987

Papini RPG, Wood, FM. Current concepts in the management of burns with inhalation injury. *Care of the Critically Ill* 1999; 15: 61–66

Pruitt BA Jr, Erickson DR, Morris A. Progressive pulmonary insufficiency and other pulmonary complications of thermal injury. *Journal of Trauma* 1975; 15: 369–379

Rossiter ND, Chapman P, Haywood IA. How big is a hand? *Burns* 1996; 22: 230–231

Sutcliffe AJ. Electrical injuries and the critical care physician. *Care of the Critically Ill* 1998; 14: 102–105

Touger M, Gallager EJ, Tyrell J. Relationship between venous and arterial carboxyhaemoglobin levels in patients with suspected carbon monoxide poisoning. *Annals of Emergency Medicine* 1995; 25: 481–483

Trofino RB. Nursing care of the burn injured patient. Philadelphia: FA Davies, 1991

Turner M, Hamilton-Farrell MR, Clark RJ. Carbon monoxide poisoning: an update. *Accident and Emergency Medicine* 1999; 16: 92–95

Chapter 32

Blast and gunshot injuries

Teresa Griffiths and Karl Trimble

INTRODUCTION

Injuries caused by ballistics and blast are increasing in incidence and are no longer restricted to the military (Cooper et al., 1983). The constant evolution of weapons and their widespread availability has resulted in civilian populations being ever more vulnerable to trauma previously restricted to areas of war and conflict (Leibovici et al., 1996).

Since the Crimean War, nurses have held a pivotal role in the management of penetrating trauma in conflict situations. However, the increase in civilian firearms-related crime and terrorist incidents dictates that all nurses involved in trauma management require a working knowledge of the management of ballistic and blast-related injuries.

Ballistic injury results from the interaction with the body of a missile, bullet or fragment. Blast injury is caused by the exposure of the body to the kinetic energy of an explosion that radiates from the blast source or fragments mobilised by the explosion.

In general terms, the management of these injuries is not dissimilar to that of other high-energy trauma casualties. However, the following chapter aims to identify and discuss specific injury mechanisms that will allow accurate and stepwise management of the ballistic or blast injured patient, and identify potential pitfalls that may be avoided by appreciating the complex nature and biomechanics of these injuries.

EXPLOSIVE BLAST

An explosion results when a material (the explosive) is rapidly converted into an expansile mass of heat and gas accompanied by a varying amount of mobilised fragments. Explosions are termed high or low explosive capacity. Conventional or low explosives rely on heat of combustion to initiate and propagate the explosive reaction. This process of combustion is slow when compared to high explosives, which propagate the reaction electrically or chemically, thus causing an instantaneous detonation and explosion.

The expanding mass of gas and energy creates a pressure wave that alters surrounding atmospheric pressure (Figure 32.1). Following the explosion, atmospheric pressure instantly rises to a maximum value known as peak overpressure (Ppeak). The surrounding pressure then falls towards ambient but, before it stabilises, there is a negative phase that is important to appreciate when considering blast injury.

Following an explosion, the gas, heat and mobilised fragments radiate out from the blast source as an expanding mass of energy known as the blast wave. The blast wave comprises the shock wave, blast wind and the thermal front (Figure 32.2).

> The blast wave comprises the shock wave, blast wind and thermal front

The shock wave, which is the leading edge of the blast wave, travels at speeds greater than sound in air and releases energy when incident upon the body or surroundings. Energy release is maximal at interfaces of substances with different acoustic impedance (similar to density), for example, air and solid. Trailing the shock wave is the blast wind, which is composed of the products of detonation, and mobilised fragments and debris. These fragments include, for instance, the casing around the explosive or debris from the surrounding environment.

The thermal front is formed by the heat energy of the explosion. Figure 32.2 demonstrates the components of the blast wave in diagram form, which, as can be seen by Figure 32.3, are identical in real life. Trees can be seen in the foreground to give an idea of scale and the shock wave, highlighted by atmospheric conditions, and the fireball containing the blast wind and thermal front can be identified.

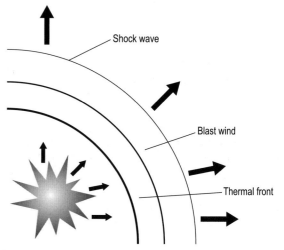

Figure 32.2 Diagram showing the blast wave.

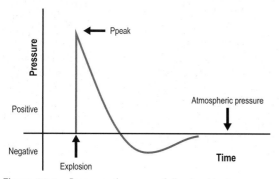

Figure 32.1 Pressure–time curve following blast.

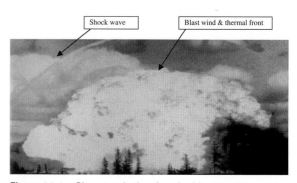

Figure 32.3 Photograph showing the blast wave.

BLAST INJURY

The interaction of the blast wave with the body causes blast injuries that are classified as primary, secondary or tertiary. Primary blast injury results from the shock wave. Secondary blast injury results from fragmentation and debris mobilised by the blast (blast wind) and tertiary blast injury results from the effects of the surroundings on the body.

Primary blast injury

As explained above, the interaction of the shock wave with the body causes injury by the release of energy at interfaces of different acoustic impedance (Cooper et al., 1991). This is most pronounced at interfaces, such as air and solid, or air and fluid, and thus air-containing viscera are most vulnerable to injury (i.e. the lungs and the gut). Primary pulmonary blast injury or blast lung is caused by the rapid expansion and contraction of the alveoli that induces alveolar rupture, haemorrhage and oedema. This is often instantly fatal but, if the patient survives, they are severely respiratory distressed and can present many hours later with an acute respiratory distress syndrome (ARDS)-like picture. Primary thoracic blast injury has been shown to induce a reflex triad of apnoea, bradycardia and hypotension that is not present after isolated primary abdominal blast injury (Guy et al., 1998). Primary gastro-intestinal blast injuries result from the rapid expansion and often rupture of abdominal viscera, with hollow viscera perforations being commonplace.

> Primary blast injury results from the shock wave. Secondary blast injury results from fragmentation and debris mobilised by the blast (blast wind). Tertiary blast injury results from the effects of the surroundings on the body

Secondary blast injury

Fragmentation and penetrating injuries are the commonest forms of secondary blast injury. The fragments are produced primarily from the structures surrounding the explosive or debris from the environment. The injuries either involve the limbs, if severe enough, causing traumatic amputations, or involve the thorax and abdomen, causing penetrating chest and abdominal injuries. Fragmentation injuries can be classified as ballistic injuries (Figures 32.4 and 32.5) and can be treated as such. However, they may be complicated by associated primary or tertiary blast injuries.

Tertiary blast injury

The interaction of the body with the surroundings and the surroundings with the body are termed

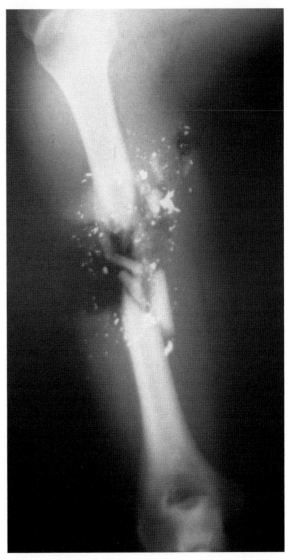

Figure 32.4 Open fracture of humerus caused by gunshot showing multifragmentation owing to high-energy transfer.

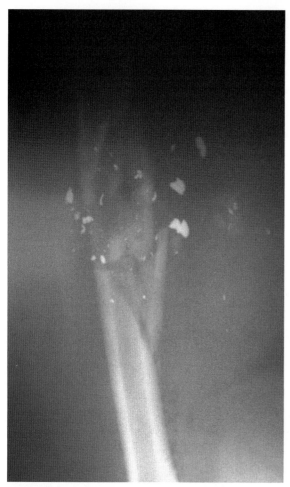

Figure 32.5 Open fracture of femur caused by gunshot showing multifragmentation owing to high-energy transfer.

tertiary blast injury. The blast wave can induce high bodily displacements and casualties can be thrown considerable distances, often on to surrounding objects. Head injuries and traumatic amputations are common.

ASSESSMENT, CLINICAL EXAMINATION AND TREATMENT

Priorities at the scene

With the expanding role of nurses in pre-hospital medicine, it is important to reinforce specific aspects of care regarding blast and ballistic injury pertinent to this environment. Immediate care involves the resuscitation and stabilisation of the seriously injured patient, and recognition and prevention of complications specific to blast.

The environment at a blast scene is austere, unpredictable and fraught with chaos and confusion. In such a situation, it is important that organisation and leadership is established as soon as possible, thus ensuring the safety of all personnel on scene and the effective delivery of medical assistance to the injured. A structured approach using the priorities listed in Box 32.1 can assist in the management of the critical incident.

Personnel required to work at the critical incident scene must ensure safety at all times for themselves, the scene and their patients following the 1-2-3-safety rule (Box 32.2). Personal protective equipment must be worn prior to entering the scene or access may be denied. The designated medical incident officer and ambulance incident officer are responsible for ensuring the personal protection of medical personnel at the scene. The safety of all personnel within the inner cordon is the responsibility of the police/fire service.

Medical personnel should only approach the scene once it has been declared safe by the security services present and authority to move forward from the outer cordon has been given. Cordons are used by the emergency services for a variety of reasons (Box 32.3) predominantly to restrict access to the site, ensuring only those personnel required

Box 32.3   Aims of a cordon

- To prevent personnel straying into danger
- To prevent evidence being disturbed or destroyed
- To provide security

to be on scene enter the inner cordon. The distance of the cordon is dictated by the police and tends to be guided by the size of the device.

Personnel not required within the inner cordon should stay well back, outside the outer cordon, away from glass doors and windows and out of line of sight of the device. This is not the time for sightseeing. If you can see the device, you are too close! Secondary devices are common after the initial explosion. Radio silence should therefore be maintained at all times to avoid the triggering of secondary radio-controlled devices.

Secondary devices are common after the initial explosion

Of all the management and support priorities listed above, triage is the key element to the successful medical management at the scene of any explosion. The main objective of a terrorist bomb is to create fear and panic in the targeted group, causing multiple casualties by the indiscriminate nature of the device.

In a study of 200 bombings over a 25-year period, Frykberg and Tepas (1988) found the overall mortality rate to be 25%, the majority of which occurred at, or immediately following, the time of detonation, with the majority of survivors requiring medical intervention. A total of 30% of survivors required hospital admission. It is also worth remembering that many of the survivors at the scene will be without physical injury, but will be in a state of great confusion and disorientation.

With this in mind, it is critical that those casualties who sustain injury are rapidly identified and sorted into priorities for treatment. This is achieved by using the *triage sieve*, as it easily identifies those in greatest medical need. The *triage sort* allows a more detailed inspection of the casualty based on anatomical and physiological parameters, but should only be attempted once

adequate medical resources are in place. Triage is a dynamic process that requires repetition throughout the evacuation chain, and as the condition of casualties deteriorates or improves.

Priorities at the hospital

Organisational

As with all multiply injured patients, resuscitation of the blast victim is dependent on good preparation (the environment, personnel and equipment). This commences in the resuscitation room. Responsibility for checking that the room is fully stocked and that all equipment is in good working order and ready for use is the responsibility of the nurse at the beginning of each shift and following each resuscitation event.

Owing to the large numbers of personnel attending a trauma call, it has been identified that trauma resuscitation is most efficient if undertaken by a 'formal team' using a predetermined system, personnel and roles. This allows the team to provide fast, effective care where team members complete pre-allocated tasks competently and simultaneously. This is known as 'horizontal organisation' and has been shown to improve team efficiency (Driscoll and Vincent, 1992).

It is essential that all team members have a clear understanding of their own pre-allocated role and those of their colleagues. *Aide-memoires* or posters displaying the specific tasks of each individual inside the resuscitation room may benefit team members from straying outside the boundaries of their allocated roles. All written documentation must be clear, accurate and comprehensive.

Prior to the patient's arrival, all members of the trauma team should be pre-assembled in the resuscitation room, ensuring that personal protective clothing is worn (gloves, plastic apron, lead apron and glasses). Extra care is required when undressing the blast patient as glass, shrapnel and other sharp debris is frequently found in the patients' clothing, hair and skin.

Clinical

Casualties attended to in the resuscitation room following blast exposure present with a spectrum of injuries owing to the multifactorial biomechanical effects of blast as described earlier. However, advanced trauma life support (ATLS®; American College of Surgeons, 1997) treatment principles remain the same with attention to the:

- Airway with cervical spine management
- Breathing and ventilation
- Circulation with haemorrhage control.

As with all high-energy trauma, six potentially life-threatening conditions may be identified in the primary survey. These can be remembered using the mnemonic ATOMFC (Box 32.4).

BLAST AND BALLISTIC INJURIES

Fragmentation

Penetrating limb and torso injury can produce life-threatening haemorrhage that should be identified and controlled according to ATLS protocols. It is important to appreciate that vascular injury requires urgent surgical intervention with proximal control of the bleeding vessel, in the resuscitation room, if necessary.

Pulmonary blast injury

Historically, the majority of casualties who sustain a pulmonary injury die at the scene, as they have a multitude of injuries, including non-survivable penetrating injuries owing to their close proximity to the blast. Pulmonary injury typically occurs in up to 5% of blast survivors and must be considered in all blast casualties. However, with the change in weapon design, shock wave formation is becoming more prominent and fragmentation a less prominent feature. As a result, an increase in the incidence of survivors presenting with pulmonary injury may be seen (Cernak et al., 1999). It is important to appreciate that an apparently stable casualty may have suffered a moderate to severe lung injury and may deteriorate at any stage. Respiratory failure occurs owing to alveolar disruption causing alveolar haemorrhage, pulmonary oedema and sometimes pneumothorax, which may prevent efficient gaseous exchange. In severe respiratory distress, urgent ventilatory support may be indicated with the provision of supplemental oxygen. It must be remembered that thoracic blast injury induces the reflex physiological triadic response of apnoea, hypotension and bradycardia. These clinical findings may be confusing when assessing a casualty with multiple injuries and must be borne in mind when making decisions on treatment.

> Thoracic blast injury induces the reflex physiological triadic response of apnoea, hypotension and bradycardia

Gastrointestinal injury

The interaction of the blast wave with the fluid–air interfaces in the gut induces bowel contusion, disruption and perforation. The shearing forces that occur at the junction of the hypermobile and fixed points (i.e. the hepatic and splenic flexures) can also cause torsion. Penetrating abdominal trauma from mobilised debris can cause life-threatening intra-abdominal haemorrhage, and must be identified and dealt with rapidly, usually requiring laparotomy. Not all contusions identified at laparotomy require excision. Small bowel contusions of less than 15 mm and large bowel contusions of less than 20 mm may be treated conservatively (Cripps and Cooper, 1997).

Burns

Burn injury is common following blast exposure, and may be cutaneous or inhalational. Airway management is essential early on, as oedema can make later management difficult. Fluid resuscitation is important, and burns resuscitation charts and protocols should be used.

Crush injury

Tertiary blast injuries referred to earlier involve the interaction between the body and the

---

Box 32.4 Conditions identified in the primary survey

A	Airway obstruction
T	Tension pneumothorax
O	Open pneumothorax
M	Massive haemorrhage
F	Flail chest
C	Cardiac tamponade

surroundings. Crush injuries are common owing to the high bodily displacements that can occur following blast wind exposure, leading to impaction of the body onto the surroundings and injury from falling masonry and debris. Apart from the direct injury, secondary injuries from limb ischaemia and open fractures may result, including fat embolus syndrome and renal failure secondary to myoglobinaemia.

Psychological effects

The psychological strain on the casualties, their families, emergency service personnel and the general population watching events on television may be considerable, and is often delayed in presentation. Historically, this effect has been utilised by weapons designers who rely on it to unnerve the opposition in warfare. This is especially true of antipersonnel mine injuries, which although sometimes fatal, usually produce devastating survivable injuries that place a huge logistical and psychological burden on the opposing force (Trimble and Clasper, 2001).

Summary – blast injuries

An explosion causes an instantaneous increase in surrounding atmospheric pressure that leads to the formation of the blast wave. The leading edge is called the shock wave, trailed by the blast wind and the thermal front. The shock wave releases energy at interfaces of different acoustic impedance, affecting air-containing viscera, such as the lung and gut. The blast wind causes fragmentation injury and whole body displacement, and the thermal front causes burn injury. The clinical management is similar to that of all high-energy trauma, remembering that thoracic-blast injury can cause reflex physiological changes that may be confusing to the assessor. These include hypotension, bradycardia and apnoea, which can be present in the absence of any obvious injuries.

GUNSHOT WOUNDS

Ballistics is the study of missile-induced injury and also includes fragmentation injury caused by blast (secondary blast injury). A wounding missile

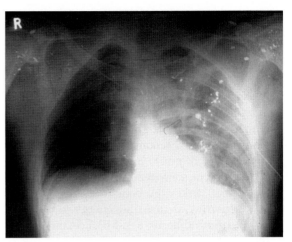

Figure 32.6   X-ray of chest showing fragmentation injury.

is defined as one that has the capacity to be projected and includes bullets, flechettes or fragments that may be pre-formed or shrapnel (Figure 32.6). Pre-formed fragments are those that are intentionally placed adjacent to the explosive device, often within the ammunition casing, to act as secondary missiles thus causing fragmentation injury (e.g. a nail bomb).

> A wounding missile is defined as one that has the capacity to be projected and includes bullets, flechettes or fragments that may be pre-formed, or shrapnel

Missile effects

Missiles induce injury by the transfer of energy when incident with the body. As the missile traverses body tissues, it transfers energy to the surrounding structures directly or indirectly by producing a cavity and leaving a wound track. Direct effects involve the direct interaction with a structure producing a permanent wound track with *temporary cavitation*. Indirect missile effects cause temporary cavitation and induce injury through energy transfer by the passage of a shock wave.

Kinetic energy

In ballistics, it is the energy transfer rather than the absolute velocity of the missile that is of importance. The available missile energy is equal to $1/2\,mv^2$, where m is equal to the mass of the fragment and v is equal to the velocity, and the energy transfer is the difference between the entrance and exit kinetic energy. Thus, the slower a missile travels on exiting the body, the more energy has been transferred. For instance, a small fragment travelling at high velocity may enter and exit a limb without making contact with the bone. Although it will induce injury, the effects are far less than that of a fragment travelling at half the velocity that strikes the bone and does not exit, thus transferring all available energy to the bone and the surrounding tissues. Missiles are defined as high energy if they have a kinetic energy of greater than 1000 J, medium energy if they have energy of approximately 500 J and low energy at 250 J.

Weapon type

The type of weapon used is an important factor when considering wound severity. Different weapons are able to produce different muzzle energies (i.e. the maximum missile energy available when exiting the gun muzzle) (Table 32.1), which affect the wound characteristics.

As well as mass, velocity and muzzle energy, flight of a missile is also important with regard to energy transfer in the tissues. As a missile travels, it may alter orientation without altering direction of flight (i.e. it may *tumble*, *yaw* and *spin*). This may also occur in the tissues themselves, increasing the surface area presented, and thus the transfer of energy and the cavitation. The direction of the missile track within the body is variable and is related to the flight characteristics of the missile, the density of the medium in which it is travelling, the structures it encounters and the tissue planes (Figures 32.7 and 32.8). It must be remembered that: (1) the presence of an entrance wound does not imply an exit wound; (2) the exit wound may be far distant to and in a different body area to the entrance wound; and (3) more than one body cavity may be involved with a single missile track. The higher the energy transfer, the greater the size of temporary cavity produced. As the cavity is produced, the pressure within it is subatmospheric, and air and debris are drawn in. The cavity is only a temporary structure and when it collapses down, a contaminated permanent wound track remains.

Despite knowing the weapon type and thus the muzzle energy available, it is vital that, above all, you *treat the wound and not the weapon*.

> The presence of an entrance wound does not imply an exit wound
> The exit wound may be far distant to and in a different body area to the entrance wound
> More than one body cavity may be involved with a single missile track

Wound factors

Energy transferred can be estimated using Coupland's wound factors tool (Box 32.5). Wounds can be graded 1–3; low- to high-energy transfer.

Wounds are graded as follows:

Grade 1: E + X < 10 C0 F0/F1
Grade 2: E + X < 10 C1 F2
Grade 3: E + X >10 C1 F2.

Table 32.1	Weapon type and muzzle energy		
Weapon type	Missile mass (g)	Velocity (m/s)	Muzzle energy (J)
AK47	8	700	1960
NATO .556 mm	4	920	1693
.44 magnum	15.6	440	1540
.22 S&W	5.5	210	121

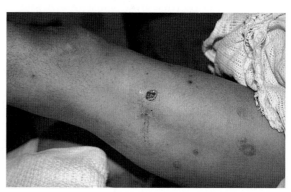

Figure 32.7 Entry wound into thigh caused by bullet (small wound).

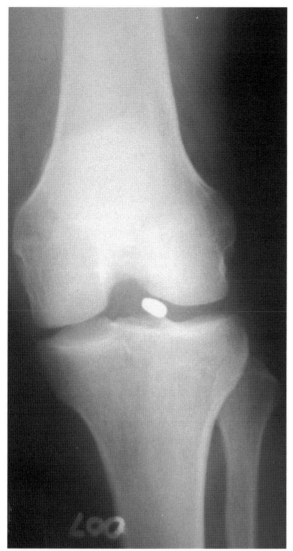

Figure 32.8 Intra-articular involvement of bullet owing to variable wound track. This image relates to that shown in Figure 32.7.

This image relates to that shown in Figure 32.7.

Clinical considerations

The overall clinical strategy is the same as for all high-energy trauma, although Box 32.6 provides a useful guide to history, examination and management of a gunshot wound. Attention should be focused on maintaining an airway, assisting ventilation, controlling haemorrhage and keeping the patient warm. This will hopefully avoid the triad of acidosis, hypothermia and coagulopathy. There is much debate as to the

---

Box 32.5   Coupland's wound factors

E		Entry wound (cm)
X		Exit wound (cm)
C	0	No cavity
	1	Cavity
F	0	No fracture
	1	Simple fracture
	2	Complex fracture
V	0	No vital structure
	1	Vital structure
M	0	No metallic fragment on x-ray
	1	Single fragment
	2	Many fragments

Box 32.6   Useful history, examination and management guidelines

History
- Time of injury
- Situation
- Weapon type
- Range
- ? tetanus status
- ? antibiotics given

Examination
- ATLS (ABC)
- Entry wound size
- Exit wound size
- Cavitation
- Fracture
- Contamination
- Photograph wound

Management
- Resuscitation
- Clean and lavage
- Cover with sterile dressings
- Tetanus and antibiotic cover
- Transfer to operating unit

---

amount of fluid that should be infused during both the pre-hospital and pre-operative phases of resuscitation. Although ATLS guidelines currently advise two litres of Ringer's lactate solution, concern exists about clot-disruption from vessels that have already undergone haemostasis, by raising the mean arterial pressure, disrupting clotted vessels and diluting sparse clotting factors

(Bickell et al., 1994). Advice should be sought at a local level as to the fluid resuscitation policy.

If operative intervention will be undertaken in less than 6 hours, a betadine dressing is of benefit. After 6 hours betadine-soaked dressings can act as a culture medium for bacterial growth and dry dressings should be used. Although some wounds can be treated conservatively, the majority require exploration especially if: (1) they are high energy; (2) there is contamination; (3) a cavity is present; (4) a fracture has been sustained; or (5) transfer to the treating centre has been significantly delayed (Figure 32.9).

In a sterile environment, wounds should be thoroughly debrided and lavaged, removing all unviable tissue, including skin, muscle and bone. Muscle viability may be assessed using the 'four Cs' rule: colour, contractility, consistency and capillary bleeding. Wounds should not be closed primarily and may require several subsequent debridements before delayed closure is allowed. *The solution to pollution is dilution!*

> Wounds require exploration, especially if they are high energy, there is contamination, a cavity is present, a fracture has been sustained, or if transfer to the treating centre has been significantly delayed

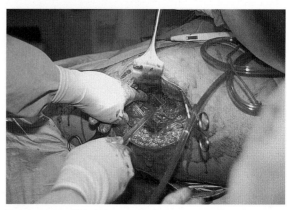

Figure 32.9 Debridement of wound track and cavity.

Summary – ballistic injuries

The management of a casualty with a gunshot wound is similar to that of all high-energy trauma. The available energy for transfer is equal to $1/2\,mv^2$, where m is equal to the mass of the fragment and v is equal to the velocity. It is useful to know the weapon type but remember to 'treat the wound not the weapon'. Important wound factors include entrance and exit wound size, cavity size, amount of contamination and the presence or absence of a fracture. The majority of wounds will require exploration. 'The solution to pollution is dilution'.

References

American College of Surgeons. *Advanced trauma life support, instructor course manual*, 6th edn. Chicago: American College of Surgeons, 1997

Bickell WH, Wall MJ, Pepe PE. Immediate versus delayed fluid resuscitation for hypotensive patients with penetrating torso injury. *New England Journal of Medicine* 1994; 331: 1105–1109

Cernak I, Savic J, Ignjatovic D, Jevtic M. Blast injury from explosive munitions. *Journal of Trauma* 1999; 47: 96–103

Cooper GJ, Maynard RL, Cross NL, Hill JF. Casualties from terrorist bombing. *Journal of Trauma-Injury Infection and Critical Care* 1983; 23: 955–967

Cooper GJ, Townend DJ, Cater SR, Pearce BP. The role of stress waves in thoracic visceral injury from blast loading: modification of stress transmission by foams and high-density materials. *Journal of Biomechanics* 1991; 24: 273–285

Coupland RM, Korver A. Injuries from anti-personnel mines: the experience of the International Committee of the Red Cross. *British Medical Journal* 1991; 303: 1509–1512

Cripps N, Cooper GJ. Risk of late perforation in intestinal contusions caused by explosive blast. *British Journal of Surgery* 1997; 84: 1298–1303

Driscoll P, Vincent C. Organizing an efficient trauma team. *Injury* 1992; 23: 107

Frykberg ER, Tepas JJ. Terrorist bombings: lessons learned from Belfast to Beirut. *Annals of Surgery* 1988; 208: 569–576

Guy RJ, Kirkman E, Watkins PE, Cooper GJ. Physiologic responses to primary blast. *Journal of Trauma* 1998; 45: 983–987

Leibovici D, Gofrit ON, Stein M, Shapira SC, Noga Y, Heruti RJ, Shemer J. Blast injuries: bus versus open-air bombings; a comprehensive study of injuries in survivors of open-air versus combined-space explosions. *Journal of Trauma* 1996; 41: 1030–1035

Trimble K, Clasper J. Anti-personnel mine injury: mechanism and medical management. *Journal of the Royal Army Medical Corps* 2001; 147: 73–79

Chapter **33**

Sports injuries

Peter L. Gregory

INTRODUCTION

Health professionals may attend sports events in their professional capacity, often requested by organisers or team management or, in some instances, they are paid to attend. More often, they are spectators when their assistance is requested. In either situation, the same standard of care is expected (i.e. the standard provided by a reasonable health professional). Nurses are, therefore, expected to provide the standard of care that most other reasonable nurses would provide.

The priorities of treatment when managing injured athletes at sports events is the same as with other facets of medicine and health care: to save life, to do no harm and to prevent further harm. Fundamental to this is the need to prepare facilities, equipment and to be skilled in anticipation of any problems that may arise. In particular, it is essential that all health care professionals managing sports events know and understand the need for a safe approach to life-threatening situations and are familiar with a structured approach to clinical assessment. In all trauma patients, protection of the cervical spine and management of concussion are vital; this is especially true of the athlete who has sustained a traumatic injury. Achieving haemostasis in the event of open wounds with consideration given to hygiene and the prevention of secondary infection are also of importance, not only in the acute phase but also in the follow-up and rehabilitative phases.

In all situations, the aim, as far as possible, is to enable athletes to return to play with no or little residual weakness or disability; the assessment of musculoskeletal injury is, therefore, vital. The following chapter aims to outline and discuss a structured regime for the management of some of the most common sports injury presentations within such a context.

> Priorities of treatment are to save life, to do no harm and to prevent further harm

PREPARATION FOR THE EVENT

Well-planned preparation is the key to doing things well, and to achieving success. Top sportsmen themselves illustrate this through their attention to detail in every aspect of their sporting events. Their preparation involves psychological preparation, equipment design and purchase, travel logistics, nutrition and hydration planning, sleep, health and the obvious traditional physical training. It is recommended that health professionals become as meticulous in their preparation to be 'pitch-side'.

Anticipation

Knowledge of the sport and, in particular, knowledge of injury patterns associated with that sport can provide information regarding the types of situation that may be encountered. This information may come from a range of sources including epidemiological sports medicine studies. It may also be obtained from those with a history of being involved with the sport, particularly in relation to the types and patterns of injuries that they have come across. Other health professionals with experience of the sport may also provide valuable sources of information.

In general, lower limb injuries are more common than upper limb injuries. Interestingly, this applies to those sports that at first consideration may seem to put more stress on the upper body, such as tennis or cricket. However, most sports depend on the firm base provided by the legs and involve running, often explosively. In these situations, the lower limb muscles and tendons tend to be torn, resulting in strains and, when ligaments are damaged by injuries that involve twisting forces, sprains. Contact sports, such as rugby and football, have a high incidence of bruises and lacerations, as well as sprains and strains that are also common in strenuous non-contact sports, such as squash, tennis, baseball and cricket. The greater the forces transferred to the body in these strenuous impact sports, the greater the incidence of fractured bones. In boxing events, boxers aim to knock out their opponents; indeed, concussion is a significant risk. As a consequence, a doctor must now be in attendance during boxing bouts. Information on the injury risk classifications of sport can be found in the American Academy of Pediatrics Committee on Sports Medicine (1988) and Table 33.1. Included in this are the risk of physical contact with other players, the possible impact with other solid objects and an outline of how strenuous the sports are.

When preparing for any sporting event, it is essential to anticipate and prepare for the most common injuries. The ability to be flexible and to adapt to unexpected catastrophes is also crucial; for example, the tennis patient stabbed by a spectator or the golfer hit on the head by a stray shot or a ricochet. Spectators might also be taken ill and may require clinical intervention. At large sporting events with large numbers of spectators, regulations require that a doctor with responsibility for the crowd is available to attend;

Table 33.1 Injury risk classification of sport	
Risk classification	**Sports activities (examples)**
I – Contact/collision	Soccer, rugby, hockey
II – Limited contact/impact	Basketball, squash, skiing
III – Non-contact/strenuous	Running, swimming
IV – Non-contact/moderately strenuous	Badminton, table tennis
V – Non-contact/non-strenuous	Golf

however, the majority of sporting events are not large enough for this. Spectators are of various ages and states of health; medical emergencies, such as myocardial infarctions or hypoglycaemic attacks, therefore, are as likely as injuries from serious trauma. Preparations should take account of such eventualities.

Skills

The skills required of clinicians at sporting events, including nurses, are varied extending from wound assessment and management techniques and the management of soft tissue injuries, to basic and advanced resuscitation and the control of haemorrhage. Those attending and providing 'cover' must also be able to immobilise the cervical spine safely in situations where the mechanism and type of injury suggest a potentially unstable cervical spine fracture. Education and training in relation to such skills may be obtained from a variety of sources, including the MSc in Sports and Exercise Medicine at the University of Nottingham, and the National Sports Medicine Institute (NSMI).

Facilities

Facilities for medical care vary enormously and health professionals should investigate them well in advance of the event. Information relating to the facilities may be gained by contacting the clubs or venue directly, or by personal review and inspection of the site. At motor racing tracks, such as Silverstone, 'mini-hospitals' with teams of doctors, paramedics and sometimes nurses with facilities for x-ray and more complex imaging have been established. Operating theatres are also available on site, so that no time is lost in managing the critically ill or unstable patient. However, the establishment of such a system is a rarity; indeed, sometimes there are no facilities. Health care professionals may find themselves in the rain beside a pitch with no shelter. Sometimes no running water is available. Consideration must be given to the location of the nearest hospital and plans for transfer of any seriously injured patients. In the event that a large number of patients are expected, effective liaison with the wider multidisciplinary team and associated agencies,

including emergency departments and the ambulance service is vital. Some sports clubs have medical rooms, but these may be dirty and the lighting may be poor. Arriving early to clean them and provide some additional lighting may improve the working environment. At some venues, it may be necessary to bring portable trolleys or couches in the event of it being necessary to examine and treat patients lying down.

> Effective liaison with the wider multidisciplinary team, including external agencies, is essential

Equipment

Responsibility for ensuring the provision and availability of adequate equipment falls to health care professionals. They are also responsible for ensuring that they are familiar with and skilled in the use of all equipment. The following list provides a resumé of typical equipment that may comprise part of the requirements at any sporting event: defibrillator, electrocardiogram monitor, oxygen therapy, a range of oropharyngeal and nasopharyngeal airways, advanced airway devices (including laryngoscope and endotracheal tubes), bag-valve-mask devices, intravenous cannulae, a variety of fluids for intravenous administration, emergency medicines, spinal board, gloves, torch or penlight, stethoscope, scissors, range of dressings (including swabs, bandages and tape), splints, wound management devices and products (including sutures and suture packs), sphygmomanometer, ice box, towels, blankets, and effective communication devices (including mobile telephones or hand-held radios).

The cost of and payment for such equipment may be raised as an issue. If they are necessary, it is proposed that the sports organisations should finance them. Health care professionals may provide their own personal equipment and may charge accordingly. In the event that the sports organisations are not prepared to pay for equipment that is considered necessary, it is suggested that health care professionals withdraw their services and advise that the sports events are cancelled on the basis that the organisers are risking the health of participants and putting health care professionals in an indefensible position.

> Health care professionals must ensure that all essential equipment is available prior to the event

PRIORITIES OF CARE

The priorities of care of someone injured at a sports event are common to the management of any patient and are based on fundamental principles that the public has a right to expect: that the health professional will 'do no harm' and will act 'to prevent further harm'.

Do no harm

Harm occurring intentionally is a criminal offence, but harm may be caused unwittingly. For example, rugby patients may be removed from a pitch to examine them following a brief concussion, and may become paralysed because the risk of a cervical spine injury failed to be recognised. Removing a motorcyclist's helmet may have similarly disastrous effects, particularly if there is an unstable cervical spine fracture. Helmets are now widely used in a variety of sports, including American football, hockey and cricket. If there is doubt regarding the technique for helmet removal or the potential for cervical spinal injury, the helmet should be left in situ until it can be removed with careful immobilisation of the neck. Patients could also potentially become infected with the hepatitis B virus owing to the use of non-sterile suturing equipment. Vigilance is required to prevent situations such as these arising. Health care professionals must ensure that they follow their guiding principle (i.e. to 'first do no harm' – translated from the Latin motto *premum non nocere*).

Prevent further harm

Having first ensured that they are causing no harm, health care professionals must ensure that they act to prevent further harm. It is natural to focus on the injured sportsmen or sportswomen; however, the safety of health care professionals and those around them, such as spectators, officials and other competitors, must also be

considered. If injured, they will be unable to help anyone, and if others are injured, the added difficulty of dealing with several patients at the same time will ensue.

To yourself

Imagine the situation where a jockey is thrown at a fence and appears to be seriously injured. You are the health care professional and he needs your help. You administer treatment to him when the horses come around again. Unaware that you are just over the fence, the horses jump and land on you, causing you to sustain worse injuries than the patient.

In this type of situation, where help is required, it is essential that officials stop the race or divert the horses from this area before the injured jockey is attended. Similar risks are associated with attending drivers at motor sports events. It is vitally important that carers do not put themselves at risk.

To others (spectators, other competitors, officials)

Some sports injuries result in severe bleeding. It is well known that blood can transmit infection, such as human immunodeficiency virus (HIV) and hepatitis B or C. Other players are also likely to have sustained open wounds. The risk of contact between the blood and other players should be limited by removing the injured player from the pitch or other relevant arena to attend the injuries. Sterile wound pads should be available and accessible to compress such wounds. Gloves must also be worn for protection. Alcohol-based solutions, or even neat alcohol, may also be available for cleansing purposes; this should be used on areas where blood has run before the game is allowed to continue.

To injured sportsmen and sportswomen

Having assessed the situation and deemed it safe, attention should then be turned to the patient. Preventing further harm may be as dramatic as attempting to save their life. Patients may be unconscious, may have stopped breathing or there may be catastrophic bleeding. The risk of the 'second impact syndrome', which may be devastating, must be considered; for example, prior to authorising a patient's return to play after a head injury. Knowing the limitations of one's practice or the limitation of the circumstance, and being prepared to arrange safe transfer to hospital are also key considerations, especially given the impossibility of closely observing patients and attending to other possible patients, if the game proceeds.

Sometimes other people cause the harm. This should be prevented as far as possible by taking firm control of the situation. For example, fellow team mates of the rugby players with a head injury may drag them off the pitch, thinking that they are helping, or maybe just wanting to get on with the game. Referees will try to maintain control of the game and may continue to exert their control over the situation regarding the injured patient. This should not be allowed. Other potential hazards come in the form of keen amateurs who have undertaken first-aid courses and who are keen to practice. It must be remembered that you are the professional and retain professional responsibility for actions and interventions. Assertiveness and confidence in making decisions are, therefore, crucial.

UNCONSCIOUS ATHLETES

One of the most serious situations that may be encountered involves that of a patient who goes down and stays down. The referee quickly calls for your help. As you approach, the patient is still down and is not moving. The assessment has already begun, and questions asked relating to events leading to the incident and mechanism of injury, including any history of loss of consciousness asked. In such situations, the 'AVPU' mnemonic may be used as an *aide-memoire* to rapidly assess conscious level (Box 33.1).

AVPU

In the alert patient, a medical history may be obtained as inspection is commenced. In such patients, it must be remembered that a period of loss of consciousness may have ensued prior to this. Injury to the cervical spine must always be assumed, particularly where the extent of head trauma has been sufficient to cause loss of consciousness. *Such patients must not be moved.*

Box 33.1 AVPU scoring system	
A	Alert
V	Responds to Verbal command
P	Responds to Painful stimuli
U	Unresponsive

Instead, they should be encouraged to remain still and not to move until they have been assessed; this may involve gentle restraint. Where patients are responsive but not alert, they may be concussed. As before, they should not be moved and their cervical spine must be protected (see Fig. 33.3). Where patients are unresponsive both to verbal commands and to painful stimuli, they are unconscious. In the most serious cases, breathing may be absent and a cardiac output may not be detectable. Such situations could deteriorate in the failure of rapid action and intervention. The severity of the situation must be communicated to those in the highest relevant authority and help summoned. Liaison with the ambulance service is essential, as transfer to hospital is almost certain.

Assume injury to the cervical spine in patients who have sustained head trauma or trauma above the clavicles

ABC OF BASIC LIFE SUPPORT

Airway – with cervical spine control

Whilst delegating the task of summoning help, attention must be focused on the airway. The airway must be clear to allow breathing and may require positioning of the patient to facilitate resuscitation. If such positioning involves rolling the patient from the supine or side-lying position, this could exacerbate an unstable cervical spine fracture and cause neurological damage. This will be irrelevant, however, if the patient is not resuscitated. The tongue cannot block the airway when prone; it is reasonable, therefore, to try to assess the patient's breathing while in this position. If satisfactory breathing has been confirmed, there is no need to move the patient at this stage. Where there are doubts about breathing, the patient should be placed in the supine position. Help will usually be available and the patient should be moved using a controlled log-roll technique. The risks should be explained, clear instructions given and overall control of the manoeuvre maintained by the senior health care professional, ensuring that the head and body are in alignment at all times.

Once the patient is supine, a jaw thrust should be performed to ensure that a patent airway is established and maintained. The jaw thrust is a safer manoeuvre than a chin lift to perform in this situation where a cervical spine injury may have occurred. In this way, the 'A' of airway in the ABC of basic life support (BLS) sequence is addressed. The use of an oropharyngeal airway may be considered at this stage to help secure the airway, although this will not be tolerated in athletes who are not deeply unconscious, nor will this adequately secure the airway when used alone.

Breathing

Breathing should now be assessed using the look, listen and feel approach for a minimum of 10 seconds. Hearing may prove to be very difficult, particularly if there is a large crowd; other senses of feeling and vision should also be relied on. If breathing cannot be detected, two rescue breaths should be given, and the chest observed for its rise and fall confirming their effectiveness.

Circulation

Assessment of circulation by palpation over the carotid artery for a minimum of 10 seconds should be undertaken. If no cardiac output is detected, cardiac compressions must be commenced and an attempt at resuscitation performed following the European Resuscitation Council basic life support algorithm. The advanced life support algorithm should also be followed and instituted as early as possible. The most useful way to support breathing is by using inspired oxygen; this should be delivered at its maximum concentration and flow rate.

Glasgow Coma Scale

The unconscious patient may have maintained effective breathing and an acceptable cardiac output from the start, or these may have been restored following successful resuscitative interventions. Yet, the patient may be unconscious still. More detailed assessment of conscious level may be required using a tool that will enable ongoing observation and measurement so that any deterioration may be quickly identified and acted upon. The Glasgow Coma Scale is one tool that performs this function that is used and understood by hospital teams (Teasdale and Jennett, 1974). A potential disadvantage, however, is that some find difficulty in recalling all components when required to do so. To avoid this, it may be useful to carry a laminated *aide-memoire* outlining this information in emergency equipment kits. Of particular importance is ensuring that trends are identified and recorded to enable a longitudinal record to be compiled.

The Glasgow Coma Scale comprises three elements: eye opening, best verbal response and best motor response, each having a designated minimum and maximum score. The maximum score that may be achieved is 15 with the minimum being three. Anyone having a score of less than eight will be deemed to be comatose (Box 33.2).

It should be remembered that unconscious patients vomit and are at risk of aspirating gastric contents. The prone position, which is the ideal position for resuscitation, can prove to be catastrophic should they vomit when in this position. Vomitus may be aspirated and may compromise the airway, possibly causing a pneumonitis. As before, the aim of management is to prevent further harm by protecting the airway or placing the patient in the recovery position.

Secondary survey

With the patient's life saved, other problems should now be identified and managed as appropriate. Some problems will be obvious, such as lacerations with severe haemorrhage, while others may be occult. All must be sought or they may be missed and the patient's condition may deteriorate. The search must be systematic and thorough, if further harm is to be prevented. The secondary survey outlined in the 'Advanced trauma life support' (ATLS®; American College

Box 33.2   Glasgow coma scale

Eye opening

Spontaneous	4
To speech	3
To pain	2
None	1

Best verbal response

Orientated	5
Confused	4
Inappropriate words	3
Incomprehensible sounds	2
None	1

Best motor response

Obeying commands	6
Localises to pain	5
Normal flexion	4
Abnormal flexion	3
Extension	2
None	1

Box 33.3   Components to be assessed during the secondary survey

- Neurological system – Glasgow Coma Score, neurological function
- Neck
- Head – face, eyes, ears, nose
- Thorax, abdomen, pelvis
- Upper limbs
- Lower limbs
- Back

of Surgeons, 1997) methodology is a useful system to follow. This incorporates assessment of neurological function, the neck and head, thorax, abdomen, pelvis, upper and lower limbs and back (Box 33.3).

Strong scissors will be required to facilitate the rapid removal of clothing and a thorough examination. Evidence of bleeding, deformity, pain or loss of function should be sought. Any bleeding should be controlled and any deformity managed. Deformity, which may be bony in nature owing to fracture or joint separation, or owing to haematoma or oedema, may be strongly indicative of underlying damage. Problems should be prioritised and dealt with accordingly, paying particular attention to conscious level, respiration and circulation. Function may then be assessed.

THE BLEEDING ATHLETE

Bleeding should be dealt with quickly and efficiently to prevent patients losing dangerous amounts of blood. Steps should be taken to protect oneself and other patients from acquiring possible blood-borne infections. Gloves should be worn at all times. Sterile wound pads should be used to compress bleeding points, the first step in

controlling haemorrhage. Patients should be removed from the field of play as soon as their condition allows; indeed, the rules of some sports such as rugby demand this and have the 'blood bin' as a characteristic feature. The risk of contamination of other patients may be minimised by pouring alcohol on blood spilled on the pitch or field of play. Adequate wound toilet should minimise the risk of infection. The rare, but potentially fatal, illness of tetanus that may occur in some wounds, particularly those involving soil, must be considered and prophylactic treatment instituted.

The objective of management in the bleeding athlete is to stem the bleeding as rapidly as possible (Fig. 33.1). Sustained compression alone can achieve haemostasis within a few minutes in many injuries, while elevation will stop most venous bleeds. Many superficial wounds require treatment with adhesive paper strips such as 'steristrips' or 'band-aids', while deeper wound may require suturing. Temporary closure with two or three sutures approximating the wound edges and the application of a robust dressing often provides a rapid, but temporary solution. Patients can then return to the contest. Afterwards, the wound should be reviewed and, if necessary, managed with more carefully positioned sutures. Tissue adhesive products, such as Histoacryl, may be helpful in achieving rapid wound closure and are particularly useful on the scalp, where it is difficult to suture without shaving an extensive area. Although relatively expensive, they may be economical when compared with the cost of sterilising suture packs. The structures underlying wounds should also be

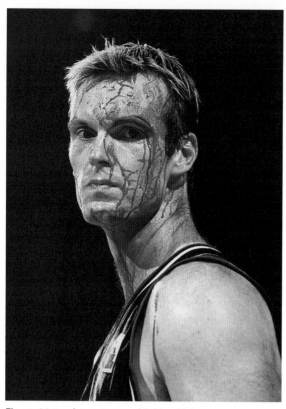

Figure 33.1   A sportsman with blood injury.

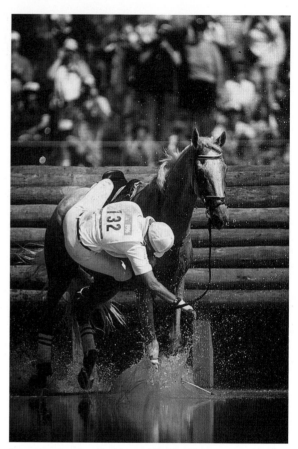

Figure 33.2   A typical horseriding accident.

considered. Superficial tendons may be damaged, hence the need to test their function by assessing movements as appropriate. Nerves may similarly be affected, hence the importance of checking for numbness, especially distal to the injury. Where fractures underlie wounds, compound fractures are said to exist and bones may become infected. The presence of osteomyelitis can delay or prevent healing of fractures; wounds must, therefore, be debrided in hospital and antibiotic therapy administered.

Heavy bleeding may occur without any obvious external sign. This bleeding may be so severe that shock may rapidly follow. Fractures of long bones are key examples. Femoral fractures require splinting and urgent transfer to hospital for definitive treatment. Pelvic fractures may occur in equestrian sports when jockeys are thrown (Fig. 33.2). In such situations, blankets wrapped tightly around the pelvis may go some way to controlling bleeding, whilst transfer is arranged.

Tachycardia is one of the first clinical signs of shock to become manifest, followed by diminished capillary refill. Establishing intravenous access and administering intravenous fluids are important early interventions as long as they do not delay the patient reaching hospital. The administration of excessive fluid may increase blood pressure and restart bleeding; generally speaking, it is best to administer sufficient fluid to maintain a radial pulse, which is estimated to equate with a systolic blood pressure of approximately 90 mmHg.

MUSCULOSKELETAL INJURY

Mechanism of injury

Soft tissue injuries are the most common type of injury encountered by those covering sports events. Unusually for health professionals, there may be an opportunity to witness the moment of injury; this should be watched avidly. Nevertheless, the incident will not always be witnessed and it may, therefore, be necessary to obtain the history from the injured patient, as occurs in other situations. As much information as possible should be gathered regarding the mechanism of injury, as this can often provide guidance on the likely diagnosis. Other patients, officials and spectators should also be questioned about the mechanism of action to complete the picture.

Mechanisms of injury fall into four main types: impact, twisting, strain or spontaneous. Impact injuries tend to occur in contact sports, such as boxing or soccer. Here, the tissues may be crushed and damaged. Bleeding results in the formation of haematomas and severe impacts may fracture bones. Twisting injuries may occur in many sports, most of which involve turning at a fast pace. Sometimes both these elements are involved, for example, a patient tackled while trying to side-step. Twisting injuries result in sprains, which are essentially injuries of joints. Ligaments are the main structures injured in sprains. Many injuries occur when athletes are physically straining to move powerfully. Tendons or muscles may be ruptured, resulting in injuries that are aptly called 'strains'. Occasionally, athletes who develop pain state that they were doing nothing to bring on an injury at the time in question. These 'spontaneous' problems provide greater diagnostic problems but require equally careful assessment. It should be remembered that athletes suffer the range of problems also seen in the general population; for example, calf pain could be suggestive of a deep vein thrombosis, chest pain could indicate a possible myocardial infarction and abdominal pain may suggest appendicitis.

> Soft tissue injuries are the most common type of injury encountered at sports events

Examination

The key principles underpinning structured examination include inspection, palpation, assessment of range of movement and assessment of function (Box 33.4).

Box 33.4   Examination principles

- Inspection – deformity, swelling
- Palpation – tenderness
- Active range of movement
- Passive range of movement
- Resisted contractions
- Function (sporting)

Assessment of injured patients on the field needs to be speedy and adequate. Examination should begin while taking the history. Clinical *inspection* should be commenced while obtaining information on the nature of the complaint (e.g. what hurts or what activities are prevented or restricted). Deformities should be looked for, such as abnormal alignment of the limbs, which may indicate the presence of fracture or joint dislocation. Swelling may be due to haematoma or oedema, and is most commonly seen an hour or two after the injury rather than immediately after the event. The affected part should be *palpated* for areas of tenderness. Knowledge of surface anatomy will help to interpret this tenderness and relate it to damage of particular structures.

Checking first active and then passive movements tests musculoskeletal function. This involves engaging the patient's cooperation, and asking them to demonstrate a full *range of movement* of the affected joints, with consideration given to the joint above and below the site of injury. Any restriction in the range of active movement and pain experienced during movement should be noted. Complete muscle rupture may lead to a restriction in movement brought about by that muscle, but with less pain experienced than that which occurs when the muscle is partially torn. The range of motion may be less affected in a partial tear. Passive movement should not be restricted, as the examiner is taking over the action of the damaged muscle. Patients may restrict passive movement, particularly if movements are very painful; these must be performed slowly in order to gain the patient's trust. A flap of damaged cartilage, or meniscus, may lodge in the knee joint, restricting both passive and active ranges of movement.

Isometric contractions enable muscle *function* to be tested. Examiners use their own strength to resist maximal contraction encouraged of the patient. Should there be weakness relative to the examiner, patients should be positioned so as to assess whether the contraction is strong enough to overcome gravity. This forms part of the muscle strength grading system. A muscle or tendon rupture will cause significant weakness, whereas motor nerve damage will weaken or paralyse muscles.

> Always assess the joint above and joint below the site of injury

Return to play

Competitors will want to know whether they can continue in the event. When the clinical examination outlined above is satisfactory, function should be assessed in an increasingly challenging way until confident that the patient is safe to return to play. This part of the assessment should be speedy and should be undertaken confidently to satisfy patients, sports colleagues and coaches. A well-rehearsed and structured approach relevant to the sport in question may facilitate this.

Lower limb injury - graded tests of function
After lower limb injuries have been sustained, simple, active, non-weight-bearing movements should first be used progressing to resisted, weight-bearing activity and then simulated sporting activity relevant to the event (Box 33.5). Such assessments may often be carried out on the touchline so as to avoid delaying play. Pressure may sometimes be exerted by referees who are eager for patients to be taken off or left to

> **Box 33.5   Lower limb injury – graded tests of function**
>
> 1. Stand
> 2. Walk
> 3. Run
> 4. Sports specific – jump, cut, sprint

> **Box 33.6   Upper limb injury – graded tests of function**
>
> 1. Full active range of movement
> 2. Sports specific – catching, throwing, tackling

continue. Similar pressure may also be exerted, for example, on the touchline, by coaches who want the patient to be declared fit or who want early warning to make substitutions. It is important, nevertheless, to ensure that patients can perform all activities required of them on the field, before agreeing to their return to play.

Upper limb injury – graded tests of function
Testing upper limb function may involve throwing a ball to the patient or asking them to fetch one they have thrown (Box 33.6). It may also be necessary to simulate an opponent to enable patients to try out tackles. Some sports involve bearing weight on the upper limbs. This applies particularly to some gymnastic exercises; however, the resistance of the water provides similar effects in swimming and diving. Athletes should be encouraged to try out simple skills before returning to full activity. If they are unable to cope with these, they are unlikely to contribute to their team's performance. Nor are they likely to do themselves justice; indeed, they may aggravate their injuries by returning to play. In such circumstances, they should be advised not to resume activities and their coaches informed that their further involvement could not be approved. Some coaches will disagree strongly believing that they know better and may try to override this decision. Health care professionals should be prepared to argue this stance and maintain their standpoint. Documentation of interventions and advice given should be completed as soon as is feasible. This may provide useful testimony and protection at a later date if patients are subsequently reinjured and health care professionals challenged for allowing them to return play.

> Document all findings and decisions taken

Fractures or joint separation may be suspected. Fractures may need to be immobilised with splints until transfer and effective analgesia given; ideally, patients should remain nil by mouth in the event that surgical fixation is required. Certain dislocation may be reduced on site, if the skills to perform this are available; however, these are usually best treated in hospital where preliminary x-rays can be performed. Fractures are frequently associated with dislocations and these can be demonstrated radiographically before reduction. This protects against possible accusations that the fractures occurred as a consequence of the manipulation.

ACUTE MANAGEMENT OF SOFT TISSUE INJURIES

The mnemonic 'PRICE' is a useful *aide-memoire* when dealing with acute soft tissue injuries and represents the sequence of events followed in management of the acute phase: protection, rest, ice, compression and elevation (Box 33.7).

Protection reiterates the important principle of preventing further harm. Using immobilisation devices and stretchers to remove patients from the field when they have sustained lower limb injuries is a good example. Where stretchers are not available, it may be possible to assist patients in avoiding weight bearing by acting as a 'human crutch'. Collar and cuff devices or slings may similarly protect the shoulder or clavicle from undue movement, while strapping or ankle braces may offer support to sprained ankles.

Rest may involve cessation of activity or may involve resting a particular injured structure. Cricketers who have injured the shoulder of their throwing arms may continue play if they avoid throwing with this arm, or they may arrange for the captain to set them in close catching positions where throwing is less important. Like protection, the aim of rest is to prevent further harm that may occur by repeated use of an injured structure.

The application of crushed *ice* for 15–20 minutes serves to decrease the temperature of tissues beneath the ice (Fig. 33.3). Such tissues respond to cooling by vasoconstriction, which reduces haematoma formation and the tendency to swell. This cryotherapy also has significant analgesic effects. The infliction of 'ice burns' to the skin is possible if the ice is applied directly and for longer than the recommended periods. Supervision is necessary to prevent this happening.

Commercial cooling systems are available that circulate cooled fluids in cuffs around injured body parts. These concomitantly apply *compression*, which aims to prevent the build-up of fluid and, therefore, swelling around injured parts. This swelling can restrict movement,

Box 33.7   Acute management of soft tissue injuries – PRICE
P   Protection
R   Rest
I   Ice
C   Compression
E   Elevation

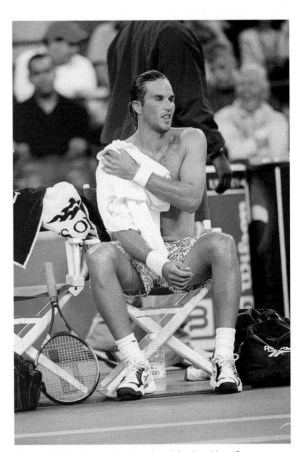

Figure 33.3   A tennis player ices his shoulder after an injury.

possibly leading to muscle atrophy and joint stiffness within a few days. Compression of injured limbs with tubular elastic bandages of variable size to suit the injured part is indicated; bandages must not, however, be so tight that the circulation is compromised. Colour and temperature of the limb distal to the bandage should be assessed at regular intervals.

Elevation of injured parts can also reduce blood flow and help disperse fluid. Legs may be raised above the body when patients are supine, and arms elevated in slings.

The Association of Chartered Physiotherapists has investigated the use of these 'PRICE' guidelines for the management of acute soft tissue injuries and has obtained sufficient evidence to support their ongoing use. Little benefit is likely to be gained by prolonging this treatment or management plan beyond 72 hours of the injury or its exacerbation.

COMMON PROBLEMS AT SPORTS EVENTS

Anterior cruciate ligament rupture

The knee is the most commonly injured joint in sport. Soccer and rugby are especially high-risk sports for knee injuries, about 40% of which involve the ligaments. Of these knee ligament injuries, approximately 60% affect the anterior cruciate ligament (ACL) (Miyasaka et al., 1991). The cruciate ligaments – anterior and posterior – link the femur to the tibia at the knee, forming a strong 'cross' that gives stability to the knee at various angles of flexion. The ACL is taut when the knee is extended, and a primary restraint of anterior displacement of the tibia on the femur. It is also a secondary restraint of varus, valgus and rotation when the knee is in full extension. The primary restraints of varus and valgus are the lateral collateral ligaments and the medial ligament complex, respectively. Thus, in more extensive injuries that have initially damaged collateral ligaments, the ACL may also be ruptured.

Typically, ACL injuries occur whilst twisting when bearing weight through the knee. Athletes may decelerate rapidly whilst the tibia is rotating externally relative to the femur at the moment of injury. The ACL is even more likely to tear if there is an additional valgus force. This commonly occurs when soccer patients change directions whilst being tackled. Miyasaka et al. (1991) found that 13% of knee ligament injuries involve both ACLs and medial collateral ligaments. The medial collateral ligament is bound to the medial meniscus, which may be damaged concurrently. The combination of an ACL rupture, sprain of the medial collateral ligament and tear of the medial meniscus is known as the 'unhappy' triad of O'Donahugh.

Bollen and Scott (1996) reviewed 119 anterior cruciate ligament injuries and found that 90% had presented with four features: history of an injury sustained twisting whilst bearing weight through the affected knee; hearing a 'snap' or feeling a 'pop'; swelling of the knee occurring within 4 hours of the injury; and, later, the complaint of recurrent giving way of the knee on changing direction (Box 33.8). Thus, the pitch-side medical attendant may well witness the mechanism of injury and be told of the 'pop' heard by the patient at the moment of injury. Observation over the ensuing hours may confirm the rapid onset of swelling, which is due to bleeding in the joint. Bloodstained synovial fluid may be aspirated. Where swelling accumulates more slowly (i.e. more than 4 hours later), it is more likely that the injury involved the meniscus only and not the ligament.

When anterior cruciate ligament injuries are suspected, the leg should be immobilised in a long leg brace and the patient referred urgently to a sports physician or orthopaedic surgeon specialising in knee problems. Other clinicians have a tendency to miss this diagnosis (Bollen et al., 1996). Patients should be encouraged to see an

---

Box 33.8 Key features of anterior cruciate ligament injuries

- History of injury sustained when twisting whilst bearing weight through the affected knee
- Hearing a 'snap' or feeling a 'pop'
- Swelling of the knee within 4 hours of the injury
- Recurrent giving way of the knee on changing direction

orthopaedic surgeon specialising in knee injuries soon after sustaining any severe knee injury. Instability typically follows ACL injury. Many patients cannot return to sport, as their knee lets them down. During such moments of instability, damage to the menisci are likely. Reconstruction of the ACL can be achieved with patellar tendon graft or semitendinous tendon graft.

Unless there are other associated knee injuries, early surgery is reported to give poor results when compared with delayed surgery, with a higher re-rupture and fibrosis rate. Athletes should initially undergo extensive rehabilitation programmes under the expert guidance of skilled physiotherapists. Using these alone, 62% of patients functioned satisfactorily and did not require surgery (Daniel et al., 1994). However, those involved in sports demanding great stability of the knee are less likely to cope without reconstruction. These include sports such as soccer, basketball and high level skiing.

Meniscal tears

The meniscal cartilages of the knee deepen the socket for the rounded femoral condyles and hence contribute to the stability of the knee. They also serve to absorb forces in the knee. Two meniscal cartilages can be found in each knee, one medial and the other lateral. Both are 'C' shaped and sometimes referred to as semilunar cartilages. Statistics show that the medial meniscus is damaged five times more often than the lateral meniscus. The mechanism is often twisting of the knee and, not uncommonly, impact with another person at time of injury. Meniscal injuries most commonly occur in contact collision sports, such as soccer and rugby. The menisci may degenerate in older patients and are then vulnerable to injury during less extreme activities. Meniscal injuries typically cause sudden pain, sometimes locking or blocking of the knee movement, and usually swelling several hours later. Persistent locking may be due to the torn part of the meniscus becoming lodged in the joint. This is most likely with a partial circumferential tear, which allows a rim to lift up, referred to as a 'bucket handle tear'. Should the knee remain locked, patients should be transferred to hospital for release under anaes-

thesia. Arthroscopic debridement of the damaged portion of the meniscus usually resolves symptoms of meniscal tears.

Inversion sprain of ankle

When most ankle sprains occur, the toes are pointing down with the feet rotated inwards. These are inversion injuries. When the forces involved take the restraining structures beyond their normal length, tearing occurs. In 70% of inversion ankle sprains, there is damage to the anterior talofibular ligament fibres only. In 20%, the calcaneofibular ligament is also damaged. Severity of the injury varies from tearing of a few fibres giving rise to pain, minimal swelling and no deterioration in function, to complete rupture of one or more ligaments with associated fractures, cartilage damage and tendon rupture. The latter gives rise to severe pain with swelling, bruising and inability to bear weight on the affected leg. In these situations, sportsmen and sportswomen have to cease activities and attend emergency departments (EDs) for assessment and further management. Guidance followed by those working in emergency departments, produced by Stiell et al. (1992), helps to determine which patients presenting with ankle sprains require radiographs to look for associated fractures. These are known as the *Ottawa rules* (Box 33.9).

Box 33.9   Ottawa rules

Request ankle x-ray series
- Pain near the malleolus and inability to bear weight at the time of injury
- Pain near the malleolus and inability to bear weight at the time of examination
- Point tenderness over the bone at the posterior tip of either malleolus

Request foot x-ray series
- Pain at the mid-foot and inability to bear weight, both at the time of injury
- Pain at the mid-foot and inability to bear weight, both at the time of examination
- Bony tenderness at the navicular or at the base of the fifth metatarsal

The anterior talofibular ligament resists anterior movement of the ankle relative to the end of the leg. Its rupture gives rise to persistent instability symptoms, such as the ankle giving way when walking over uneven ground, and recurrent pain and swelling. Patients are also susceptible to further ankle sprains. A gentle range of dorsiflexion and plantarflexion exercises may be started after 2 or 3 days, and further rehabilitation supervised by physiotherapists. A full return of strength around the ankle with attention to regaining proprioception that has inevitably been lost in this type of injury is important for reducing the risk of reinjury. Regardless of the grade of ankle sprain, the injured part should be cooled with ice and compressed using an appropriate bandage. Injured joints should be protected from further damage by advising athletes to stop training or competing, and to use braces or crutches if available.

Acromioclavicular joint injury

Impact with the point of the shoulder causes injury to the acromioclavicular joint. This occurs in falls or where patients sustain blows to the shoulder region, for example, in ice hockey, rugby, martial arts or equestrian events. Patients feel pain in the superior aspect of the shoulder near to the joint, which is tender. Injuries vary in severity and may be classed as first, second or third degree. Injuries with minimal deformity and no evidence of increased anteroposterior movement of the acromioclavicular joint are referred to as 'first degree'. These are associated with swelling and bruising around the joint owing to microscopic tears in the ligaments. First-degree acromioclavicular sprains may be treated conservatively with activities encouraged within the limits of the patient's pain. Second-degree sprains involve tearing of the joint capsules and result in instability of the acromioclavicular joints. Increased anteroposterior movement of the joint suggests this injury, although movement is restricted when the strong coracoclavicular ligaments are intact. This prevents the inferior displacement of the acromion, indicated by a step in the shoulder contour, in those with third-degree injuries. Those with second-degree sprains of the acromio-clavicular joint should avoid further blows to the shoulder until the original injuries have healed, as this can convert them to third-degree injuries. Removal from play is, therefore, indicated until tenderness has resolved. Slings may provide comfort. Third-degree sprains need to be assessed for surgical treatment.

Glenohumeral dislocation

Acute traumatic dislocations of the shoulder are common in rugby, gymnastics and wrestling. The most common mechanism of action is a large force exerted on the abducted, externally rotated shoulder, which drives the humeral head anteriorly. This occurs when rugby players attempt to tackle opponents to one side. This is known as *anterior dislocation*, with patients invariably presenting in pain and often supporting the injured side under the elbow with the opposite hand. It is not unusual for patients to realise what has happened and for them to tell you that the 'shoulder has come out'. Any rotation of the shoulder will be painful. Removal of clothing is required to facilitate a complete examination, which will reveal loss of deltoid contour.

Longitudinal traction for several minutes until the shoulder muscles have relaxed is often all that is required to allow the humeral head to slip back into the glenoid fossa. Several techniques are available to reduce the dislocated shoulder; these should be used in hospital after appropriate x-rays have excluded fractures. The axillary nerve, which lies close to the glenohumeral joint, may be damaged when the shoulder is dislocated. This results in numbness over the outer aspect of the upper arm. Sensation should be assessed and any loss (e.g. from pinprick stimuli) documented.

Should prompt attention at hospital prove impossible, shoulder reduction should be attempted. Firm traction should be applied to the arm in a slightly abducted position, and the body restrained at the axilla. The foot of the therapist should then be placed in the patient's axilla or, if there is a gate nearby, the patient's arm placed over this. Another technique involves the patient lying prone and hanging their arm over the edge of the table on which they are lying. After a few minutes, the therapist should feel a slight 'give' as the muscle spasm is overcome, and the arm then brought into slight adduction. If reduction is not achieved at this stage, the arm can be internally rotated a little; this is usually effective. Postreduction sensory deficit is again checked and findings documented prior to taking the patient to hospital for x-rays.

The capsule of the glenohumeral joint will be torn in the primary glenohumeral dislocation or it may become detached with the labrum from the glenoid margin. The labrum is a rim of cartilage which deepens the socket provided by the glenoid for the humeral head. If these injuries do not heal, the shoulder is liable to dislocate again. Redislocation rates are very high, especially in the young, with rates of 80–90% quoted in those aged less than 20 years. Immobilising the shoulder in a sling for 6 weeks, and undergoing intensive rehabilitation may reduce the risk of dislocation. This involves carrying out isometric contractions in the sling for 3 weeks, followed by strengthening out of the sling. Patients should avoid the combination of external rotation and abduction for 8 weeks.

Fractured clavicle

The clavicle is the most commonly fractured bone. Falling on the outstretched hand or falling on to the point of the shoulder may cause fractures. The bone tends to fracture at the junction of the middle and outer third. Satisfactory treatment for most clavicular fractures involves a sling with healing likely within 8 weeks. Children tend to heal more quickly. Should broken ends of the clavicle pierce the skin, surgery may become necessary.

Head injury

Severe head injuries may lead to unconsciousness. Management of these situations has already been dealt with earlier in relation to the unconscious patient. Occasionally, athletes may suffer short periods of unconsciousness after sustaining a bang on the head (Fig. 33.4). Some may appear confused and questioning may reveal memory loss. However slight the psychological deficit, structural brain damage associated with concussive injury will have occurred and must be taken seriously. The duration of memory loss is indicative of the degree of diffuse brain damage sustained. This may be referred to as *retrograde*

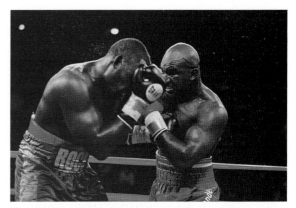

Figure 33.4   Boxers take heavy punishment during a bout.

or *post-traumatic amnesia*, where the memory loss relates to events preceding and following the incident, respectively. Health professionals ought to question athletes frequently to assess memory function. Initial questions are best thought out before the event, as it may be difficult to think of suitable ones when they are required.

Head injuries may cause contusions or lacerations of the cerebral cortex and shearing lesions of the brainstem. Skull fractures over the temporal bone may tear the middle meningeal vessels leading to extradural haematomas. These and other intracranial haematomas compress the brain, resulting in potentially life-threatening situations if not controlled. Diffuse brain swelling may also be life threatening, causing athletes to deteriorate and die after talking, and is thought to arise particularly in young people owing to a disturbance in autonomic regulation of the cerebral circulation.

Speculation abounds that a 'second impact syndrome' may occur in which a second and often minor head injury occurs before patients recover completely from the first, leading to possible death within a few hours. Some cases may satisfactorily fit this description; however, McCrory (2001) argues that these may be manifestations of diffuse brain swelling as described earlier. Should patients continue to play when not fully recovered from their head injury, diminished concentration and impaired judgement may make them susceptible to further injury. Attending sports clinicians should not condone this behaviour, and should instead remove concussed patients from play until confident that they have made a full recovery. This may be difficult to assess, as normal neurological examinations are not sensitive. Other examination techniques, such as the digital substitution test, have been proposed, which require recording baseline performance in the pre-participation phase and comparing this with the postinjury situation. Some sports such as rugby have rulings that patients who have been concussed during an event should not play again for a given period (e.g. 3 weeks) after apparent full recovery. Although evidence to support this is minimal, it would nevertheless seem to be a sensible and cautious approach on the part of sports governing bodies.

> The attending clinician is responsible for ensuring that a full recovery has been made prior to allowing players to return to play

The value of protective headwear cannot be overstated. All those involved in sport have a responsibility to ensure that appropriate protection is available and used properly by those training or competing in sport. The England and Wales Cricket Boards now insist that all batsmen under the age of 18 years wear helmets unless signed legal disclaimers are presented to umpires prior to events. Young wicketkeepers must also wear helmets when standing up to the stumps. The Board of Control for Boxing now insists that suitably trained doctors and paramedics (and perhaps nurses in the future) are in attendance for all professional boxing bouts, and that neurosurgical facilities and teams are prepared. This is aimed at avoiding delays in treatment that may have led to the devastating effects for Michael Watson in 1989.

Cervical spine injury

Horse riding is the sporting activity associated with the highest risk of cervical spine injury. Diving, gymnastics, rugby and American football also have a high incidence of similar injury. Spinal cord injury may also have occurred with tetraplegia; a possible disastrous outcome. Cervical spinal injury must be considered in all athletes who are rendered unconscious as a result of trauma. Even those who are conscious may have sustained serious neck injuries. As many as one in six patients who have suffered a fracture of the second cervical vertebra will not complain of pain at the time of injury. Three-quarters will not complain of symptoms attributable to the nervous system or signs of abnormal neurology on examination. Thus, it is dangerous to assume that a cervical spine injury can be excluded without hospital assessment and appropriate radiological investigation.

> Cervical spine injury must be considered in all traumatic events, and must be assumed to have occurred in all injuries above the clavicle
> One in every six patients who have suffered a fracture of the second cervical vertebra will not complain of pain at the time injury

The role of first aid must, therefore, be to ensure that movements of the neck are minimised until trained paramedics can immobilise patients securely and arrange safe transfer to hospital. The event may need to be stopped. Conscious patients should be warned to keep still, with their heads firmly restrained using manual methods. Hard cervical collars may also be applied if appropriate sizes are available. Transfer to hospital should be carried out using a long board, scoop stretcher or vacuum mattress (Fig. 33.5).

The mechanism of injury is often hyperflexion of the neck, such as that which occurs in the collapsing rugby scrum or the dive into shallow water. Torg (1979) recognised that American football players used their heads like battering

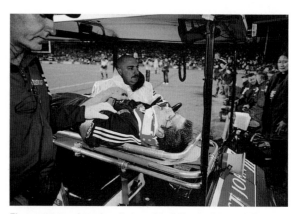

Figure 33.5   A rugby player with full spinal immobilisation.

rams in tackles. This activity, known as 'spearing', causes axial loading in the cervical spine and accounts for 52% of cases of tetraplegia occurring in that sport. In rugby, the dangerous practice of the high tackle may lead to hyperextension injury. Sports authorities have attempted to reduce these injuries by well-informed rule changes; indeed, collapsing the scrum and high tackles are now offences in the sport of rugby. Those particularly involved in rugby are the front row forwards, and players now have to be specially trained to play in these positions. Both knowledge and the use of appropriate techniques and neck strengthening exercises are important for these 'props' and 'hookers'. Neither can be replaced by anyone other than those also trained in these positions, even if this means that the game or event has to be abandoned.

Injured players may lie with their arms parallel to the trunk, and elbows flexed at right angles with forearms across the chest. This presentation is characteristic of a spinal cord lesion at the level of C6/C7, where the flexors are unopposed by the paralysed extensors of the arm. If the lesion occurs at the level of C5/C6, the arms may be abducted by the deltoid. Lesions above this level lead to the arms flailing in no specific pattern as all muscles supplied by the brachial plexus are paralysed. Where lesions are sustained at the level of C3/C4, patients cannot breathe unassisted as the diaphragm is paralysed. In tetraplegic patients, the outlook is poor, especially if this is obvious immediately after the event. Safe transfer to hospital must be arranged as quickly as possible as treatment with dexamethasone may help to reduce the neurological deficit.

Epistaxis/nasal fracture

Epistaxis or a nosebleed is not uncommon in sporting settings, even in the absence of trauma to the nose. Sport is often played in hot dry environments. The increased airflow over the nasal mucosa as athletes breathe has a tendency to make it dry and, therefore, more susceptible to cracking. Superficial blood vessels just inside the vestibule on the medial aspect of the nose, an area known as Little's area, are vulnerable. Damage to this area results in epistaxis. Another aetiological

factor associated with sport that may affect the incidence of epistaxes is the rise in blood pressure that can accompany intense activity, such as weight lifting.

Most epistaxes stop with firm pressure applied over the bleeding point. Squeezing the nostrils together is, therefore, usually effective, if maintained constantly for approximately 10 minutes. Cooling the nose towards the bridge with crushed ice whilst this pressure is maintained may also be helpful owing to local vasoconstriction. Where clots are present, these should be removed prior to commencing compression. The bleeding point may be obvious on inspection inside the nostrils, aided by a strong light. Where a great deal of blood has collected in the nose, this can spill backwards into the back of the throat, especially if the patient lies back. It is, therefore, preferable to ensure that patients remain sitting up, unless they are clinically shocked. If bleeding persists in spite of these first-aid measures, the nose will either need packing or the bleeding site cauterised.

Nasal fractures, the most common facial fractures, should be suspected in all cases of bleeding after trauma. They are associated with fractures of the maxilla and frontal bones, both of which should be considered as possibilities when assessing sportsmen and women thought to have sustained nasal fractures. Hallmarks of nasal fractures are deformity, which can be from deviation of the nasal septum or soft tissue swelling, pain and epistaxis. Deviation of the nasal septum may cause the nostril to occlude, either partially or fully. This may be tested by gently occluding each nostril with a finger whilst the patient closes the mouth and attempts to breathe through the nose. Lack of airflow through that nostril indicates occlusion. Firm side-to-side pressure at the bridge of the nose will often cause crepitus when the nose is fractured. Bruising is often soon apparent and blood may track from the nose causing a periorbital haematoma.

Management of the suspected nasal fracture primarily involves controlling epistaxis as discussed above. The application of crushed ice may also provide some pain relief and patients may benefit from analgesia. Reduction of fractures may be carried out on scene by experienced clinicians, although there is no disadvantage in delaying reduction for up 2 weeks when soft tissue swelling has usually subsided, thereby allowing the cosmetic result to be assessed more easily. Septal haematoma formation is a potential complication of nasal fractures. This may present as a bluish swelling of the septum on inspection with a good light source, and may account for any nasal occlusion noted. It is important that septal haematomas are drained. The perichondrium separates from the cartilage under pressure of accumulating blood and this can lead to septal necrosis and subsequent collapse of the cartilage. This reveals itself as the so-called 'saddle deformity'. Early after injury, the accumulating blood is still in fluid form; needle aspiration is, therefore, generally effective. Later, incision and removal of clotting blood is required for drainage. Where clear fluid is found draining from the nose after trauma, the possibility of a cribriform plate fracture must be considered. This is a serious injury that requires hospital management. Infection may ascend into the brain and must, therefore, be prevented.

Auricular haematoma

The external ear is vulnerable to trauma in sport. This is particularly so in rugby, where the ears are subject to serious friction during scrummaging. Punches frequently land on the ears in boxing and wrestlers are often seen to hold on to or drag their opponents' ears. Initially, there may be pain and swelling of the ears, which may be the start of a perichondral haematoma. In situations similar to that of septal haematomas of the nose, failure to drain these haematomas may lead to necrosis of the cartilage of the pinna. The resulting deformity, known as a 'cauliflower ear', requires aspiration with a sterile needle and syringe if managed within 24 hours. Formal incision and drainage will be necessary later when the blood has congealed. A pressure dressing and ice should be used to reduce the chance of the haematoma accumulating again.

Muscle strain

Muscle damage may occur as a consequence of extrinsic or intrinsic injuries. Extrinsic injuries include those sustained in crushing tackles in rugby union, causing sudden compression of the quadriceps muscle, vastus lateralis, against the underlying femur. This may give rise to muscle contusion, the resultant haematoma being either intermuscular or intramuscular. Blood tracks in the connective tissue surrounding the muscle bundles in intermuscular haematomas, arising from damage to blood vessels in the muscle sheaths or surrounding fascia.

In intramuscular haematomas, muscle fibres are damaged; bleeding, therefore, occurs within the fascial sheaths that surround the muscle bundles. Pressure increases inside the fascial sheath owing to the accumulation of blood and provides internal compression of the bleeding vessels. Bleeding in this situation tends, therefore, to be self-limiting. Intramuscular haematomas tend be locally tender with marked reduction in power of the muscle and pain on stretching. The bruising or swelling of intermuscular haematomas tends to track away from the site of injury under the influence of gravity. Muscle function is generally less severely affected than with intramuscular haematomas and recovery is usually quicker.

When the elastic and physiological properties of muscle are exceeded, intrinsic injury to the muscle may result. These are referred to as *strains* and commonly occur in sport. Experiments by Garrett (1986) showed that muscles tear when stretched to approximately 25% of their resting length. The majority of tears occur near to the muscle tendon junction, which is presumed to be the weakest point in the musculotendinous unit. In adolescents, another weak point is the attachment site of a tendon to the bone. Avulsion of this bony attachment is typical in this age group. Those muscles that pass over two joints are more vulnerable to strains than those passing over one joint. Hence, in the lower limb, the thigh muscles (i.e. the rectus femoris), the hamstring group and the gastrocnemius of the calf are most commonly strained. Injury often occurs during eccentric contractions where the muscles are being pulled and, therefore, lengthened, but are simultaneously contracting to decelerate the movement. These are sometimes referred to as *distraction strains*. The forces through muscles that are involved in explosive actions, such as sprinting, are great;

muscle strains often occur, therefore, in soccer or athletics.

The severity of strains varies considerably. In some, there may be discomfort during movement, but no discernible weakness or loss of range of movement. Tenderness is localised to the area of the injury. Athletes may initially be unable to compete; however, healing and recovery is rapid. These are *first-degree strains* in which there is no appreciable tear of muscles. In *second-degree strains*, muscle fibres are torn but some fibres remain intact, such that the continuity of the muscle persists. Pain is usually more severe than in first-degree strains and attempts to contract the muscle are painful and often ineffective. Athletes can rarely continue playing in the presence of such injuries. Tenderness and swelling are common, and bruising may be apparent the next day. Complete rupture of muscles is rare. These *third-degree strains* may initially be very painful, but become less painful than second-degree strains. Weakness is more marked, although recruitment of agonist muscles may allow some strength to persist. The divided ends of the muscle tend to retract from the site of rupture. Defects are often visible and are usually palpable in the muscle. They are tender and, in time, may become filled with fluid and blood lost from the damaged muscle.

Athletes typically suffer sudden sharp pain during explosive actions, particularly at the beginning of a game or training session after an inadequate warm up. Warm up is thought to improve blood flow through the muscles and improve their flexibility, making them less susceptible to injury. Strong muscles are able to withstand higher forces without damage, therefore, those who have prepared adequately ('getting fit to play' rather than 'playing to get fit') are less likely to be injured. However, the antagonist muscles generate the stretching force on a muscle; thus, achieving muscle balance is also important in the prevention of muscle strains.

Initial management of muscle strains should include protection, rest, ice, compression and elevation (PRICE). Protection from further injury may require removing the player from the game or event. In second- or third-degree strains, splints or strapping may be applied to restrict range of movement. Cooling with crushed ice and compression may help to reduce bleeding and oedema. Massage, heat and vigorous stretching during the first 72 hours may cause further bleeding and are, therefore, not advised. Significant defects palpable in the muscle and significantly diminished muscle strength indicate second- or third-degree tears. The torn ends of the muscle can be sutured; however, the muscle soon retracts away from the defect and this may prevent the ends coming together. Early surgical referral is, therefore, indicated.

Whether athletes undergo surgery or not, all require a rigorous graded rehabilitation programme. This should aim to restore strength and flexibility of the muscle. Before returning to sport, functional assessment should be made and any deficiencies addressed. Isometric contractions do not involve a length change in the muscle and are less likely to cause further damage; these should, therefore, be introduced early in the programme. Contractions achieving movement through the painless range should then be encouraged, but initially without resistance. Concentric, muscle-shortening contractions are potentially less damaging than eccentric contractions and should next be attempted using progressively increasing loads. When athletes cope well with high loads, eccentric strengthening exercises should be commenced. Here external forces tend to stretch the muscle and are resisted by athletes. Progression through the programme is determined by pain. Athletes should return to a lower level in the programme in the event that new exercises cause pain. The final stages involve functional work. Once more, less demanding activity comes first; walking will, therefore, come before jogging, before sprinting, before jumping or before cutting and weaving.

> All athletes who have suffered muscle strain require a rigorous graded rehabilitation programme before returning to sport

Contusion injuries causing deep intramuscular haematomas near the underling bones have a propensity to the complication of *myositis ossificans*. In this condition of disturbed healing, new bone is laid down within the muscle. Pain persists in the injured muscle and the range of motion is restricted. Diagnosis is confirmed by characteristic appearances on plain radiographs. The problem may recur after surgical excision, which should not be undertaken for at least 2 years, when the ossification process is generally complete. As management of this condition is far from satisfactory, prevention is the key. Recurrent impacts on areas of intramuscular haematoma may cause further injury and interfere with the normal healing process. Even strenuous activity may cause further insult; sport should, therefore, be stopped whilst intramuscular haematomas settle. A full painless range of motion and return of strength should be checked and confirmed before advising a return to sport.

Achilles tendon rupture/calf strain

Patients complaining that they heard a noise similar to a 'crack like a gunshot' at the same instant when a sudden pain began in the back of their leg have probably ruptured their Achilles tendon. In their confusion, they will often believe that opponents have kicked or hit them on the calf, but in reality no opponent was close to them. The tendon undergoes a degenerative process in some people and the tendon may 'give' under a sudden increase in load, such as pushing off to sprint. Typically, this happens early in a game of squash, badminton, tennis or cricket before a player, who has played little recent sport, has warmed up. The explosive contraction of the calf muscles required for jumping may also lead to this injury. The rupture tends to occur some 2–5 cm above the calcaneum; a gap may be felt in the tendon at this point. Injured patients will find it difficult to walk following the injury and, in particular, will have difficulty plantar-flexing. This may be demonstrated by asking them to perform a heel raise when standing or to push the toes down when lying down. Swelling soon develops and later bruising. Achilles tendon tears may be partial or complete. Surgery to suture together the tendon ends may be offered to those who have suffered total rupture, though immobilisation in a plaster of Paris cast may allow satisfactory healing. Special boots are now available, which allow the degree of dorsiflexion

to be increased incrementally during the healing process. Many athletes with this injury take 12 months to return to their sport.

A sudden pain higher in the calf during strenuous activity is probably due to rupture of the gastrocnemius muscle. This injury is not as devastating to the athlete as the Achilles rupture and many will return to sport in 8 weeks. The 'soleus' muscle can also be ruptured, resulting in tenderness deep in the calf. Bruising tends to occur after 24 hours or more, becoming visible on the inner side of the leg. Both calf muscles bring about plantarflexion. Damage weakens this movement; therefore, resisting the contraction of these muscles will be painful. Initial management should be along the lines of the PRICE guidelines referred to earlier. Athletes should then work through a programme of stretching and strengthening the affected muscle before progressing through gradually more demanding functional exercises. When these exercises are managed without pain, the player may return to sporting activity.

Collapse in the endurance event

Athletes of various ages and with a variety of medical conditions take part in endurance events such as the London Marathon (Fig. 33.6). Even with sensible pre-race advice and screening of medical information supplied, the collapse of a number of athletes should be anticipated. The differential diagnosis is considerable, making appropriate management difficult for the attending clinician. The effects of heat and dehydration may be contributory factors in some climates. Core temperature should be recorded, although temperatures of 40° C are not unusual in those exercising strenuously in hot climates. Cooling with iced towels and fans may help to reduce excessive temperatures more quickly. Hypotonic oral fluids should be given; if this is not possible, intravenous access should be established and fluids given in this way.

Some competitors might describe chest pain preceding their collapse. Myocardial infarction or angina may be the cause. Rapid transfer to hospital is required for electrocardiographic diagnosis and thrombolysis in the event that a

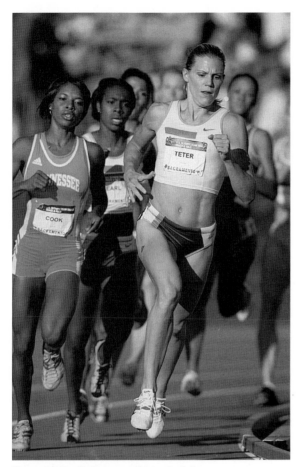

Figure 33.6   Endurance athletes in full cry.

no history of trauma, cardiac arrhythmias and, in particular, ventricular fibrillation should be considered and appropriate action instituted. Insulin-dependent diabetic patients may become hypoglycaemic during prolonged activity. Medical alert bracelets may prompt this diagnosis, although many patients do not wear these. Measurement of capillary blood glucose levels on anyone who collapses in an endurance event is vital. Hypoglycaemia may successfully be treated with buccal glucose solution or gel, or the administration of glucagon by intramuscular injection. Persistent hypogylcaemia may require intravenous injections of concentrated glucose solutions.

SUMMARY

The priorities of treatment when managing injured athletes at sports events are the same as with other facets of medicine and health care: to save life, to do no harm and to prevent further harm. It is essential that clinicians attending events in their professional capacity are familiar not only with the sport and its associated injury patterns, but also with the environment, equipment and systems for communicating with the statutory emergency services. Prior planning and preparation are vital. Maintaining a high index of suspicion with regard to the mechanism of injury, and following a structured approach to assessment and treatment will ensure that appropriate medical care is provided. Modes of transport to facilitate rapid transportation to hospital must also be agreed at an early stage to optimise chances of survival and recovery.

myocardial infarction has been confirmed. If clinicians are available, aspirin, nitrates and morphine for analgesia may be administered. Where competitors are unconscious and there is

References

American Academy of Pediatrics Committee on Sports Medicine. Recommendations for participation in competitive sports. *Pediatrics* 1988; 81: 737–739

American College of Surgeons. *Advanced trauma life support, student course manual*, 6th edn. Chicago: American College of Surgeons, 1997

Bollen SR, Scott BW. Anterior cruciate ligament rupture: a quiet epidemic? *Injury* 1996; 27: 407–409

Daniel DM, Stone ML, Dobson BE, Fithian DC, Rosman DJ, Kaufman KR. Fate of the ACL-injured patient. A prospective outcome study. *American Journal of Sports Medicine* 1994; 22: 632–644

Garrett WE. Basic science of musculo-tendinous injuries. In: Nicholas J, Hershman EG (eds) *The lower extremity and spine in sports medicine*. Mosby: St Louis, 1986

Miyasaka KC, Daniel DM, Stone ML, Hirschman P. The incidence of knee ligament injuries in the general population. *American Journal of Knee Surgery* 1991; 4: 3–7

McCrory P. Does second impact syndrome exist? *Clinical Journal of Sports Medine* 2001; 11: 144–149

Stiell IG, Greenberg GH, McKnight RD, Nair RC, McDowell I, Worthington JR. A study to develop clinical decision rules for the use of radiography in acute ankle injuries. *Annals of Emergency Medicine* 1992; 21: 384–390

Teasdale G, Jennett B. Assessment of coma and impaired consciousness *Lancet* 1974; ii: 81–84

Torg JS, Truex R, Quedenfeld TC. The national football head and neck injury registry. Report and conclusions. *JAMA* 1979; 241: 1477

Further reading

Cantu RC. Head injuries in sport. *British Journal of Sports Medicine* 1996; 30: 289–296

Cantu RC. Second-impact syndrome. *Clinical Sports Medicine* 1998; 1: 37–44

National Collegiate Athletic Association (NCAA) Committee on Competitive Safeguards and Medical Aspects of Sports. Concussion and second-impact syndrome. In: *NCAA sports medicine handbook*. Overland Park, KS: NCAA, 1994

Peterson L, Renstrom P. *Sports injuries – their prevention and treatment*. London: Martin Dunitz; 1992

Stiell IG, McKnight RD, Greenberg GH, et al. Implementation of the Ottawa Ankle Rules. *JAMA* 1994; 271: 827–832

Williams JGP. *A colour atlas of injury in sport*. London: Wolfe Medical Publications, 1990

Chapter **34**

Management of traumatic wounds

Fiona Churchill and Linda Stark

INTRODUCTION

A wound is a breach in the external surface of the body. This can be caused by sharp or blunt trauma. The list is not exhaustive as to where a wound can occur and what can cause it, making wound management interesting yet complicated. Some wounds will be straightforward in their assessment, healing with no real complications, whilst others may cause debilitation, disfigurement and death. Wound assessment and management must, therefore, be methodical, following a systematic approach to prevent serious errors in judgement.

The principles of wound management are to produce the optimum healing, and to restore function and mobility to the wounded area as soon as possible. However, life-saving assessment must always come first and follow the principles of airway, breathing and circulation.

THE BASIS OF WOUND ASSESSMENT

Every wound is potentially life threatening, but special care must be taken with such areas as the head, face, neck, chest and abdomen owing to the structures involved.

Wounds to the head carry a risk of brain injury and haemorrhage, and will be discussed later; *facial wounds* will also be discussed later, but all carry a risk of airway obstruction and haemorrhage. *Wounds to the neck* also carry a risk of airway obstruction and haemorrhage, and must be regarded with caution. Alexander and Proctor

(1995) describe wounds on the neck in three zones. Zone one relates to wounds found around the structures at the thoracic outlet, zone two wounds in the area between the clavicle and mandible, and zone three wounds between the angle of the mandible and the base of the skull.

The *chest* contains many of the major organs: the heart, lungs and major blood vessels. If the wound is penetrating, there is a high risk of haemorrhage and subsequent ventilatory compromise. Life-threatening emergencies, such as cardiac tamponade, tension pneumothorax, sucking chest wounds and massive haemothorax, must all be excluded prior to more definitive assessment. The *back* must also always be checked for further injuries.

The *abdomen* contains organs with a rich blood supply and blood vessels, which, if injured, could cause the patient to exsanguinate. A high index of suspicion must, therefore, be maintained when assessing wounds in these areas.

Wounds may appear to be relatively small and harmless (e.g. puncture wounds); however, the mechanism and site of injury must always be considered, as underlying structures may be damaged. A methodical and systematic approach to the assessment of all wounds is, therefore, advocated.

> A methodical, systematic approach to all wound assessments must be followed

A SYSTEMATIC APPROACH TO WOUND ASSESSMENT

A summary of this approach is presented in Box 34.1.

Presenting complaint

The presenting complaint is simply a statement of what the patient is presenting with (e.g. cut to the right hand or laceration to the scalp) and is always a good starting point. Obtaining a detailed history relating to the presenting complaint is also helpful in determining the events leading up to the incident, and may provide valuable information relating to underlying illnesses or disease processes.

> **Box 34.1   A systematic approach to wound assessment**
>
> - Presenting complaint
> - History
> - Past medical history, drug history, allergies, tetanus status
> - Examination (inspection, palpation, movement, sensation and circulation)
> - Investigations
> - Diagnosis
> - Treatment
> - Discharge

History

A good history is vital and will essentially diagnose the problem. The history must be clear to the point where the incident can be visualised. Accurate and detailed documentation of the history is also essential. The patient's age and sex must be documented; this is especially important when caring for those in the vulnerable groups. It is generally accepted that children do not comply as well as adults; therefore, the approach and performance should be adapted to 'win them over'. For legal reasons, children under the age of 16 years should not be treated without first obtaining consent from their legal guardian. Exceptions to this include the emergency situation. The elderly may not be able to comply with wound care for many reasons (e.g. poor nutrition, impaired eyesight, reduced mobility, incontinence or dementia). It is important to obtain a social history to determine whether patients live alone, the type of accommodation they live in and the level of social support required.

The patient's occupation should also be documented, as this has an enormous bearing on wound care. If patients work with food, they should cover the wound with a brightly coloured waterproof dressing (HMSO, 1995), and refrain from certain work, if infection is present. Ultimately, the regulations are at the discretion of the environmental health officer. If the patient has a job that is likely to contaminate the wound (e.g. plumber or mechanic), especially if a wound to the hand has been sustained, the patient should not work. Many workers are reluctant to take time off work owing to financial and employment constraints, which, in turn, may contribute to the incidence of wound infections. If an injury to the hand has been sustained, the patient's dominant hand should also be documented.

The mechanism of injury is vital in history taking. What happened and how, why, when and where the injury occurred must all be established. This will enable the severity of the injury to be determined. Whether the wound was caused by a sharp or blunt object, the size and weight of the object involved, the time elapsed from cleansing and the likelihood of contamination are all key to wound assessment and management. If a knife caused the wound, it is important to establish whether it was serrated or smooth, clean or dirty. If the patient was rendered unconscious, their last recall of events should be determined in addition to obtaining a history from witnesses who may be able to verify the duration of unconsciousness and the patient's account of events.

Issues relating to wound toilet are also important. If the wound has been cleansed, the agent used and duration of cleansing should be identified. If it has not been cleansed, the length of time elapsed since the injury should be considered along with any contaminants involved. This will determine the need for antibiotic therapy and antitetanus prophylaxis.

Past medical history

Past medical history, specifically diabetes, bleeding diatheses and disorders of the immune system, can all affect wound healing. A history of asthma, gastric/duodenal ulcer, epilepsy, eczema, cardiovascular or peripheral vascular disease must also be established, as these will raise concern of any confounding factors that could affect medications that may be given and subsequent patient outcomes.

Drug history

Concurrent drug treatment, especially the use of steroids, anticoagulant therapy and immuno-suppressive therapy, must all be elicited, as these may impact upon wound management and healing.

Allergies

Allergies to antibiotic therapies, tetanus, local anaesthetics, wound dressings and tapes/adhesives must be established and documented.

Tetanus status

The patient's immunisation status must be determined and documented. Heavily contaminated wounds must be treated promptly and effectively to avoid the development of infection and subsequent complications.

WOUND EXAMINATION

Having taken a concise and detailed history, a clear picture of what to expect should be envisaged. Good lighting is essential to optimise wound assessment and examine it thoroughly. Examination of the wound consists of four phases:

1. inspection
2. palpation
3. movement
4. sensation and circulation.

> Wound examination consists of inspection, palpation, movement sensation and circulation

Inspection

Wounds should be described with words, pictures and diagrams. The use of photographs should be used where wounds are complex and where review by a number of clinicians is necessary, thus reducing the increased risk of infection. Concise and accurate description is important for legal reasons and should contain the following:

- type of wound
- appearance of wound
- location of wound
- direction and shape
- size
- depth.

> Description of wounds should include their type, appearance, location, direction, shape, size and depth

Types of wound

There are many different types of wounds. The type of wound must be recognised and documented.

- *Cut or incised wounds* are breaches in the skin caused by a sharp edge (e.g. a knife or glass). The wound edges are well defined and often straight with little surrounding bruising.
- *Lacerations* are breaches in the skin caused by a blunt force. The wound may be irregular with tearing of the tissues. The skin is burst rather than cut and possibly ragged. Milroy and Rutty (1997) describe how the distinction between lacerations and cuts is important because describing a wound incorrectly can make the difference between a non-custodial punishment and a prison sentence when giving evidence.
- *Contused wounds* are breaches in the skin with surrounding bruising.
- *Penetrating or puncture wounds* are wounds with a fine pathway made by a pointed object.
- *Contusions* are areas of bruising due to blunt force, without a break in the skin.
- *Haematomas* are subcutaneous collections of blood giving rise to a fluctuant swelling.
- *Abrasions* are grazes caused by a friction force passing across the skin surface, shearing it away.

Other types of wounds, such as flap wounds, crushing wounds, degloving wounds, bites and high-pressure injection wounds will be discussed later in the chapter.

Appearance of the wound

The appearance of the wound should be described, particularly noting any swelling, bruising, erythema, deformity, bleeding (capillary, venous, arterial), infection, necrotic tissue, tissue viability, grazing, foreign bodies and skin loss. Sometimes what may look like skin loss may in fact be elastic retraction of the skin edges. The state of the surrounding skin should also be noted, especially any maceration, oedema, dryness, blisters or fragility. The extent of necrosis, slough, granulation or epithelialisation of the wound bed is also notable, as well as the degree and nature of any wound exudate (i.e. serous, haemoserous

or purulent). Malodorous wounds are also of significance. Erythema should be measured and marked with an indelible pen; this provides a useful guide to whether it is improving or deteriorating.

Location of wound

A clear description of the anatomical position of the wound is necessary, as is the extent of any motor or sensory impairment.

Direction and shape

The direction and shape of the wound must be documented (e.g. V shaped, transverse, longitudinal, oblique, circumferential, circular, crescent shaped or stellate laceration). In addition to providing valuable information regarding wound management techniques and possible problems associated with wound healing, potential damage to underlying structures may also be considered.

Size

The length and width of wounds should be measured accurately using a tape measure. This must be documented as a key part of the patient's history.

Depth

The base of the wound must be visualised (Figure 34.1). If this cannot be carried out at the examination, it must be carried out during the treatment. This must be clearly documented.

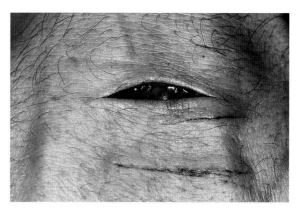

Figure 34.1 Incised wound to the depth of subcutaneous fat.

Damage to underlying structures and exposure of bones and joints carries a risk of chronic infection (MacNicol and Lamb, 1984). Detailed knowledge of anatomy is vital to envisage the structures beneath the wound (i.e. blood vessels, nerves, tendons, bones, vital organs and ligaments). No wound examination is complete without a full examination of the underlying structures and, if necessary, wounds should be gently probed to establish their depth. Wounds should never be closed unless their base has been visualised (Figures 34.2 and 34.3).

> No wound examination is complete without a full examination of the underlying structures

If the wound extends to the level of the tendon, this must be assumed to have been damaged until proven otherwise by an experienced emergency

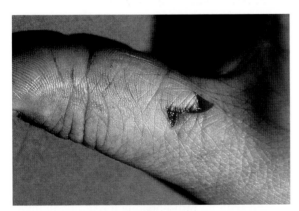

Figure 34.2   Z-shaped incised wound.

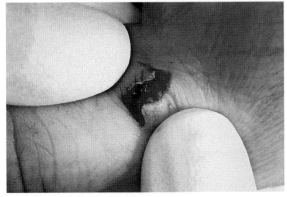

Figure 34.3   The wound shown in Figure 34.2 is opened to reveal its hidden depth.

department (ED) doctor or hand surgeon. Damage to underlying structures may also be revealed by asking the patient to return the injured part to its original position at the time of injury (e.g. a fist punching). This places the structures in the position under the wound at the time of injury. Deep structure injury may be missed if this stage is omitted.

Palpation

Palpation forms the second phase of wound examination. Wounds should be gently palpated feeling for foreign bodies, bony damage, crepitus, abscess, oedema or pain.

Movement

Phase three of wound assessment relates to assessing the degree of movement of the injured part. Three components must be addressed: active movement, where patients move the part themselves; passive movement where the examiner moves the part; and resistive movement where patients move the part against force applied by the examiner.

The area should be checked to determine its range of active movement. Any reduction may indicate damage to underlying structures. The inside of the wound should be observed while assessing the whole range of movement.

The inspection and movement phases of wound assessment and examination are carried out simultaneously. Tendons that are completely divided tend to shrink or be pulled away from the wound by the contraction of muscle and the movement of joints. The degree of function of the affected area should also be visualised and tested.

> The inspection and movement phases of wound assessment and examination are carried out simultaneously

Notes of caution
1. Movement can be carried out by more than one muscle. If one of the muscles is injured, damage may be hidden. This is a common problem in the limbs where tendons moving over distal joints contribute to the movement of every joint they pass over. Familiarity with

appropriate tests that isolate specific tendons and identify specific damage is recommended (e.g. flexion testing of the fingers).

2. If glass is lying in a wound next to a tendon, or there is a partially divided tendon and the tendon is being moved during testing, the injury may be aggravated, converting a partially divided tendon into a completely severed tendon. Resisted testing should be performed to ascertain that the tendon is not injured and the area compared with the opposite side. Patients may have active movement by using a substitute tendon, or a partially divided one, but they should not have full power against resistance. Resisted testing should be carried out carefully owing to the potential for making the injury worse. If there is any suspicion of such an injury, resisted testing should not be performed. Sometimes pain or a fracture will inhibit movement. Clinical judgement and acumen must be exercised at all times. To exclude damage to underlying structures completely, the examiner must be content that active, passive and resistive movements are normal.

MacNicol and Lamb (1984) state that cuts from glass are associated with tendon injury in 50% of paediatric cases.

> To exclude damage to underlying structures completely, the examiner must be content that active, passive and resistive movements are normal

Sensation and circulation

The final phase of wound assessment relates to checking for sensory and circulatory involvement. Ischaemia distal to the wound must be sought and sensation distal to the wound assessed for evidence of nerve damage. The latter can be difficult to gauge in a distressed patient (MacNicol and Lamb, 1984). Response to light touch sensation should be elicited; if altered, this may indicate sensory damage. The tip of a needle may also be used to gauge response gently; similarly, two needles may be used comparing the sensation of one needle to two. The patient's gaze should be diverted to avoid inaccurate findings. With very superficial cuts, it is rare to find evidence of deep nerve damage. A 'numb feeling' may be experienced owing to the injured area being held stiff and dependent along with the local reaction to injury.

Evidence of capillary, venous or arterial bleeding at the wound site should be documented. Circulation distal to the wound should be checked and the capillary refill time found to be less than 2 seconds. The presence of pulses, colour, warmth and sensation should also be assessed. Common sense should be exercised; if *both* hands have a capillary refill time of more than 2 seconds, consideration should be given to whether the patient has just come in from the cold. All evidence should be compiled and a rational clinical decision reached.

Investigations

There are several investigations that may be appropriate in wound assessment. Investigations are used to either confirm or refute suspicion, but they are not absolute; suspicion alone is evidence enough to refer these patients

Soft tissue x-rays should be requested, if there is suspicion of a radio-opaque foreign body in the wound (e.g. glass, crockery, metal, teeth, gravel). Soft tissue x-rays for foreign bodies are essential for all wounds caused by shattered glass. Raby et al. (1999) state that 'all glass is radio opaque'. It is important not to be lured into a false sense of security with the x-ray result; glass can still be in a wound with no radio-opaque foreign body noted on the report.

If there is a risk of an underlying fracture, an x-ray should be requested. Finding a fracture underneath a wound transforms it into a compound fracture, thus requiring prophylactic antibiotics. Similarly, if there is a risk of joint penetration an x-ray should be requested. Two standard views should always be taken; one is not sufficient.

> When requesting x-rays, two standard views should always be taken

If there is evidence of infection, a swab should be taken to assess for culture or a white cell count measured, if there is rampant infection. If blood loss has been severe or the patient is bleeding excessively for no obvious reason, blood may be taken for haematology or clotting profiles.

If there is evidence of significant infection, excessive blood loss or any other pathology that is giving cause for concern (e.g. head injury), regular vital signs must be recorded. Urinalysis and blood glucose measurements may also prove useful in addition to measuring the patient's temperature.

Diagnosis

This should be a brief statement based on the clinical findings (e.g. superficial cut to dorsum of right hand, deep laceration to scalp, or right pre-tibial laceration).

Treatment

An explanation of all tests, investigations and treatment must be given and verbal consent obtained. Explanation of the pros and cons of treatment involves patients in their care. If patients are given an informed choice and have knowledge of what the expected outcome of treatment is, then they may be prepared should the result not turn out as well as expected. Patient compliance will also improve if the patient has been involved in the decision-making process. However, it must be recognised and accepted that some patients are happy to 'allow' practitioners to treat them with minimal involvement in the decision-making process.

Irrigation of the wound is the most important aspect of treatment. Necrotic tissue, foreign bodies, devitalised skin and haematoma must be removed. Tap water and normal saline are ideal for cleaning wounds. Fluids should not be cold but warmed slightly. Miller and Glover (1999) recommend that regular cleansing is not necessary once treatment has commenced, as it removes beneficial exudate and dries the wound.

High-pressure irrigation is the subject of debate. Dearden et al. (2001b) suggest that the pressure range should be from 4 to 15 lb per square inch; this can be approximated by using a 35 ml syringe and a 19-gauge needle. Caution must be exercised with regard to needlestick injuries and splashback. If the pressure is too high, this may traumatise healthy tissue or push dirt further into the wound. However, this form of irrigation can be useful in loosening ingrained foreign bodies that are otherwise impossible to remove (e.g. tiny threads from fabric). Foreign bodies can also be removed with forceps or the point of a needle. If dirt is ingrained, a sterile toothbrush or sponge should be used; local anaesthetic may also be required. If it is not possible to cleanse wounds adequately, these patients should be referred. Povidone–iodine is not recommended for routine wound cleansing owing to its toxicity to fibroblasts and osteoblasts (Cole, 2003).

WOUND CLOSURE

The selected method of wound closure is one that will promote rapid healing, yield the best cosmetic result and prevent infection. Four common types of wound closure are used: adhesive strips, staples, tissue adhesive/'glue' and sutures.

Adhesive strips

These should not be used on the palm of the hand, between the web space, in areas where there is skin loss, on mobile and loose skin over joints or on the lip. Should they become moist or wet, they will become undone. Adhesive strips are not painful to apply and need no local anaesthetic; they are, therefore, less likely to cause tissue ischaemia. Being non-invasive, they are also associated with a lower infection rate and they are usually quick to apply. If applied properly, they are strong and yield a good cosmetic result. They are ideal for dry superficial wounds but are unsuitable for deep, wide, bleeding wounds. They are especially useful in:

- children
- flap lacerations (e.g. pre-tibial lacerations in the elderly)
- finger injuries (beware the tourniquet effect!)
- between sutures
- on the face.

Staples

These are quick and relatively painless to use and do not require the use of local anaesthetic. They are recommended for superficial scalp lacerations but are unsuitable for deep wide wounds, facial wounds, the hands or over joints. The cosmetic result can be disappointing. Should they become wet, staples can be patted dry.

Tissue adhesive/'glue'

Wound/tissue adhesive, or 'glue', is recommended for children, as it is quick to use, is relatively painless and local anaesthetic is not required. It may become moist or wet without losing its function, and cosmetic results are satisfactory. Tissue adhesive may not be used on deep, wide or wet wounds, and is unsuitable for wounds under tension or over joints. It forms a dry scab that normally falls off 7–10 days after application. For application, the wound edges require to be easily opposed.

Sutures

Sutures are the method of choice, if no other method of closure is suitable. Exceptions to this include circumstances where:

- the wounds involve tendons, nerves, muscle, fascia or joint capsules
- there is a crush injury – interstitial pressure causes build-up of fluids resulting in increased pressure
- the skin edges do not easily oppose
- the wound involves puncture injuries with possible damage to underlying tissues and structures (e.g. stab wounds)
- the wound bleeds profusely or requires ligation of blood vessels
- the wound requires debridement of tissues
- the wound requires subcutaneous suturing
- the wound involves sites where undue scarring may result
- the wound is produced by bites from animals or humans
- the wound is older than 6 hours (except on the face) or heavily contaminated. These wounds are better treated by secondary intention or delayed primary suture in 5–6 days owing to the risk of anaerobic infection (gas gangrene or tetanus). All facial wounds should be treated by primary closure regardless of wound age

Table 34.1 Suggested uses of sutures

Body part	Suture size	Removal of suture
Hands	4/0 or 5/0	7 days
Trunk	3/0 or 4/0	10 days
Knees	3/0 or 4/0	14 days
Limbs	3/0	7–10 days
Face	5/0 or 6/0	5 days

owing to the cosmetic effect and the excellent blood supply.

Special care should be taken when suturing wounds involving joints, the face and hands, and wounds associated with bony injury. Suggestions for the use of different sutures are given in Table 34.1.

Prior to suturing, the wound will require to be anaesthetised. This can be carried out using either local anaesthetic or a digital nerve block, and provides an ideal opportunity to re-examine the wound and cleanse it thoroughly. Most wounds heal best if left exposed; however, this is not always possible. Consideration must be given to the location of the wound, the type of wound and the level of patient compliance.

Frequent medications required are analgesia, local anaesthesia, antibiotics, tetanus vaccine and human anti-tetanus immunoglobulin.

DISCHARGE

Discharge advice should cover all aspects of prevention of wound infection and restoration of function of the injured area as quickly as possible. Information must be clear and aimed at the level of the patient's understanding. Patients should be given written information regarding the number of stitches or staples inserted, when they should be removed, how to obtain further dressings if required, how often to take any medication given and when to have further antitetanus vaccinations. Where a head injury has been sustained, patients should be discharged into the care of a sensible adult with written instructions given regarding adverse signs. Patients' injuries should also be related to their occupation/lifestyle, providing a useful opportunity for health promotion.

Analgesia should be offered to patients. Anti-inflammatory medications are not advised as they may interfere with the inflammatory phase of wound healing (Dearden et al., 2001a).

If follow-up or a review is required, this may be undertaken in several ways:

- minor injury clinic/accident and emergency clinic
- general practitioner
- district nurse
- practice nurse
- occupational health service.

If referral is required, specialists may be selected dependent upon the particular area of concern:

- accident and emergency
- orthopaedics
- plastic surgeons
- infectious diseases
- physicians
- surgeons.

SPECIAL CIRCUMSTANCES

Penetrating/puncture wounds

These wounds are caused by long, pointed, relatively narrow implements (e.g. nails, drills, spikes from railings). Puncture wounds to the foot can be highly contaminated by the penetrating object collecting dirt on its journey through the shoe sole. If the object was rusty, a soft tissue x-ray is required. Other foreign matter may also be revealed on x-ray. It can be difficult to estimate the depth of the wound owing to the elasticity of the skin at the time of penetration, even though the entry wound may be very small. These wounds have a high risk of contamination and infection.

Flap wounds

Flap wounds can be problematic if the apex of the flap is more proximal than the base, compromising the blood supply to the flap and resulting in tissue death. Pre-tibial lacerations are the most common of these wounds and are particularly common in elderly females owing to the friability of their skin. Flap lacerations must not be sutured. If there is extensive tissue loss, these patients should be referred to the plastic surgeons;

alternatively adhesive wound closure strips may be applied. The tissues must not be placed under tension. If the wound extends as far as bone, subcutaneous sutures may be necessary. Such patients may require referral.

Crush injuries

History is important, as the wounds themselves may appear to be relatively trivial. Consideration must be given to the forces involved. This type of injury can cause extensive damage to underlying structures (e.g. fractures, tendon injuries, nerve injuries, blood vessel injuries, deep haematomas and muscle compartment syndrome). Degloving injuries may be associated with crush injury. If evidence of this exists, these patients will require immediate referral. X-rays may also be indicated. It may not be possible to oppose these wound edges owing to swelling. If suturing is indicated, these must be loose, using as few sutures as possible. Elevation of the affected area is essential.

Foreign bodies

The history will again indicate whether there is a suspicion that a foreign body is present in the wound. Attention should be paid to the high-speed fragment causing a penetrating foreign body to lodge, which can cause serious damage (e.g. history of chiselling or grinding metal). Injury to the eye requires immediate attention.

Wood will normally only show on x-rays if it is covered in metallic paint. This makes wooden foreign bodies difficult to find and identify. If the patient complains of foreign body sensation, wound healing is delayed or absent, or the wound becomes infected, the presence of a potential foreign body should be considered (e.g.. dirt, hair, metal, glass, grit or teeth). If the wound cannot be adequately cleaned and the foreign body removed, these patients should be referred for further assessment. Ultrasound may serve as a useful adjunct to detecting foreign bodies not seen on x-ray.

Degloving injuries

Any part of the body caught in a rolling mechanism may be degloved (i.e. the skin and subcutaneous tissue may be sheared off their underlying blood supply). The skin should be kept in warm saline soaks and the patient referred immediately. The skin must not be allowed to dry out.

High-pressure injection injury

High-pressure injection guns forcing foreign material, such as wax, paint, grease, oil, solvent and air, into tissues can cause these wounds. The wounds may appear trivial on initial assessment with relatively small wounds observed by the naked eye, but there is always extensive contamination along the tissue planes. Prompt decompression and removal of the foreign material is essential, otherwise chemical inflammation and secondary infection may lead to extensive tissue necrosis, resulting in the possible need for amputation of the affected limb/digit (Wardrope and Smith, 1992; Lamb and Hooper, 1994; Wilson et al., 1997). If the material is visible on x-ray, the finger should be x-rayed.

Scalp wounds

A full neurological assessment should be carried out to exclude head injury, and an assessment of the neck carried out to exclude neck injury. Caution and a high index of suspicion should be displayed where the mechanism of injury has involved an object falling from a height onto the patient's head; this may result in an injury to the cervical spine or a depressed skull fracture.

Blood loss should be estimated and the risk of hypovolaemia evaluated. Attention should be given to those patients who are taking warfarin therapy. These patients may have relatively minor wounds but may have a serious assault to the brain as a result of bleeding caused by the effect of their medication.

The *galea aponeurotica* is a layer of connective tissue that joins the frontalis muscle of the forehead and covers the top of the head below the skin. A large tear in this structure can affect the function of the frontalis muscle, and also makes it easier for infection to spread to the underlying bone of the skull and even into the intracranial space through the deep circulation. If the galea is torn, layered closure using absorbable sutures may be required. Full-thickness scalp lacerations may require closure in layers to avoid a deep haematoma developing.

Facial wounds

A neurological assessment should be carried out to exclude head injury and an assessment of the neck carried out to exclude neck injury. The face bleeds freely owing to its rich blood supply. If there is evidence of muscle injury, these patients need to be referred. Consideration must also be given to damage to the facial skeleton and teeth. The mouth must also be examined for the presence of broken teeth, cuts, lacerations or sublingual haematomas. For cosmetic reasons, debridement should never be carried out; these patients must, instead, be referred.

Deep wounds over the cheek below the zygoma and in front of the ear may penetrate the parotid salivary gland and/or one of the five branches of the facial nerve. Figure 34.4 illustrates the triangular area of danger on the face, if there is a wound present. Important structures are:

- the facial nerve
- the parotid duct
- the lacrimal duct
- the eye.

The *facial nerve* should be tested by asking the patient to:

- wrinkle the forehead and then raise the eyebrows
- close the eyes tightly and test with fingers (i.e. try to open them)
- show teeth, but not a smile
- blow out the cheeks
- purse the mouth and whistle.

The *parotid duct* lies in the middle third of the line joining the external auditory meatus and the angle of the mouth. If there is a deep cut here, injury to the parotid duct should be suspected. The inside of the mouth should be checked; if there is bleeding from the duct orifice (opposite the second upper molar tooth), damage is confirmed.

Where wounds to the *lacrimal duct* and the *eye* have been confirmed, these patients require

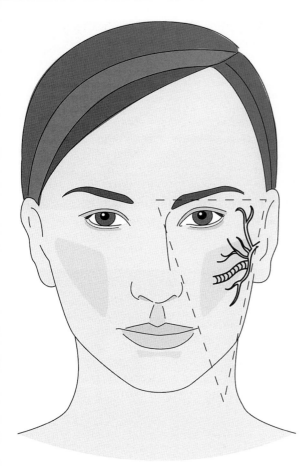

Figure 34.4 Triangular area of danger on the face (outlined with broken lines) if a wound is present.

aspects of the assessment and examination of these patients.

Eyebrows should not be shaved. Where wounds overlie the eyebrows, the supraorbital nerves should be checked by testing sensation over the forehead. These wounds present few problems if damage to underlying structures has been excluded.

Where injuries to the *nose* have been sustained, the patency of the airway must be checked and confirmed. Patients should be asked to breathe through each nostril by blocking the other with a finger. If problems are experienced, these patients should be referred. Septal deviation should be excluded. Septal haematomas, which will be on each side of the septum and look like small cherries, require immediate referral for drainage. If these are missed, patients will end up with necrosis and gross disfigurement. If nasal fractures are suspected, there is normally no need to x-ray unless other fractures of the facial bones are suspected. Depending on the mechanism of injury, the facial skeleton may also need to be checked. Where nasal fractures have been sustained, patients should be followed up in the ear, nose and throat (ENT) clinic 5–10 days after the date of injury. Antibiotics should be considered for all clinical fractures. All lacerations should be referred to the plastic surgery team. All clinical findings should be documented, including a history of epistaxis, where a basal skull fracture should be considered.

Most external *lip* wounds will require suturing. These should be referred to obtain the best cosmetic result. The orbicularis oris muscle may also need to be repaired. The vermillion border should not be sutured unless by very experienced staff. This will avoid an obvious step in the lip margin. Mucosal wounds may be left to heal if they are not deep. The patient's teeth should be checked; any missing teeth must be accounted for (e.g. inhalation or embedded in the wound), and any avulsed teeth placed in a milk medium.

Minor wounds to the *tongue* do not require suturing; deep wounds must be referred.

Wounds to the pinna of the *ear* can be sutured. Where there is cartilage involvement, these patients should be referred, as they may result in perichondritis. If haematomas are present, these

referral. If there are wounds over the inner canthus, the lacrimal duct may be injured. The lacrimal apparatus is more likely to be injured if the wound crosses the lid margin or the eyelid itself. These wounds should not be sutured nor should wounds over the lacrimal gland. These patients should, instead, be referred.

It is important to be familiar with the anatomy of the eye. Caution should be exercised with any injury around the eye. The levator muscle of the upper eyelid can be divided, causing drooping or ptosis of the lid. Caution should also be exercised with penetrating high-velocity foreign bodies (e.g. chiselling). If there is an orbital blow-out fracture, the patient will be unable to look up and down owing to nerve impairment. Checking visual acuity, pupillary equality and reaction to light and range of movement are fundamental patients should be referred to the ENT team for drainage.

Where wounds to the *chin* have been sustained, the mandible, bite, teeth and range of movement should be assessed. Sublingual haematomas must also be excluded.

Hand wounds

Partially divided tendons may retain some of their function, although their actions will probably be weakened. Later, they may divide completely. Complete division of the central tendon of the extensor mechanism of the finger at the proximal interphalangeal joint (PIPJ) may be concealed by the fact that the lateral tendons will continue to work as extensors of the PIPJ, perhaps for days. However, the *boutonniere deformity* will eventually develop and there will be little hope of a good recovery.

The skin on the dorsum of the hand is loose and mobile (Figure 34.5). When a fist is made the skin becomes taught, especially over the knuckles (Figure 34.6).

Scars over joints or skin loss may cause permanent loss of movement. Where there is full-thickness skin loss of more than 1 cm × 1 cm, the patient may need a skin graft or a flap repair, as there is no place in the hand for skin suture under tension (Watson, 1986). Watson recommends the use of 4.0 nylon sutures for repair of hand wounds and removal of only non-viable tissue. Where there is substantial skin loss, the area should be kept moist and the patient referred to the plastic surgeons.

Paronychia

The periungual tissues are swollen and erythematous. There may be evidence of frank pus. If left untreated, the pulp space or flexor tendon could become involved (Wilson et al., 1997). These wounds should be treated with antibiotics. Fluctuant pus can be released using ethyl chloride or a digital nerve block.

BITES

When assessing bites, a systematic approach must be adopted. The use of prophylactic antibiotics for

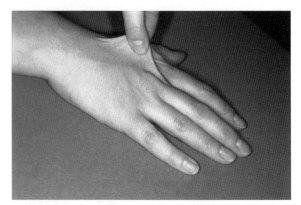

Figure 34.5 Dorsum of the hand showing loose and mobile skin.

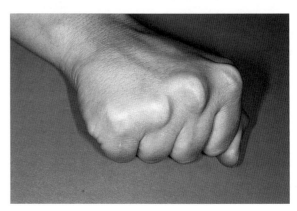

Figure 34.6 Hand formed into a fist showing taut skin, particularly over the knuckles.

animal bites remains controversial. Mellor et al. (1997) stress the need for prophylactic antibiotics, citing their benefit in the case of a patient with life-threatening sepsis after a minor dog bite; others believe that routine prophylactic antibiotics are unnecessary unless the involvement of deep structures is suspected (Wyatt, 1994). Rigorous cleansing of all wounds is essential.

Bites must be left open and not sutured owing to the potential and serious risk of infection. Delayed primary closure can be performed at a later date. Only in special circumstances should bites be sutured (e.g. the face).

Human bites

Human bites are the most serious of all mammalian bites owing to severe complications resulting from infection, commonly staphylococcal and streptococcal. Infectious diseases may also be transmitted, in particular, hepatitis B and, less commonly, human immunodeficiency virus (HIV). Problems may also ensue from clenched fist injuries (i.e. punching a mouth), as these may result in deep cuts to the hand, disrupting fascia, tendons and joints, leading to septic arthritis, osteomyelitis, infection of the tendon sheaths and significant amounts of devitalised tissue. Amputation may be the eventual outcome. Early surgical referral for possible irrigation, debridement and exploration of these wounds is appropriate. Evidence of fractures, teeth, foreign bodies and divided tendons must be actively sought. Other complications including tenosynovitis and cellulitis should also be addressed, and prophylaxis against hepatitis B and HIV considered.

Animal bites

Dog bites are the most common form of bites. When assessing these wounds, several factors must be considered:

- the time the injury occurred and cleansing regime, if any
- the size of dog; large dogs may cause more tissue damage
- the type of dog; certain breeds can cause more damage
- vaccination history of the dog, if known (if the bite occurred in a foreign country, rabies vaccination may be necessary)
- if the dog has a history of biting, this must be addressed
- consideration must be given to the need for x-ray to exclude fractures, joint penetration and foreign bodies.

If the dog is infected with the *rabies virus*, treatment must be started promptly (Canine Crisis Council, 1997). This ruling also applies to apparently minor bites. Tetanus immunisation is required if appropriate.

Cat bites carry a high risk of infection owing to the penetrating nature of their teeth. Their claws can also be grossly contaminated.

Where patients have been bitten by rats, especially sewer rats, systemic infection must be considered.

Insect bites tend to blister and give rise to local erythematous reactions. The erythema in the first instance indicates a localised allergic reaction, usually with itching. This will usually resolve spontaneously or in response to antihistamine therapy or topical steroids. Wilkinson et al. (1993) describe impetigo as a possible complication. New bites are unlikely to show signs of infection; for this reason, it is important to establish the time of injury. After a few days, the bites may be infected and painful. If bites are more than 48 hours old, infection must be considered. Diagnosis is dependent on accurate assessment of the patient (i.e. the presence of pain, erythema, pyrexia, systemic toxicity and lymphangitis).

Wasps are carnivorous (unlike bees) and are able to sting repeatedly. They carry an increased risk of introducing infecting agents when they sting and a greater possibility of infection, as they may feed on rotting flesh. The possibility of anaphylactic reactions and anaphylactic shock must be noted.

Lyme disease as a consequence of tick bites must also be remembered (O'Connell, 1995).

NON-ACCIDENTAL INJURY

Non-accidental injury should be considered when assessing wounds, especially in children. The possibility of domestic violence and deliberate self-harm must also be borne in mind. Such patients may require referral to the mental health team.

WOUND INFECTION

Evidence of infection should be noted. Signs of localised wound infection include localised pain, erythema, warm skin/hot to touch, local oedema/swelling, an increase in exudate, the presence of pus, an offensive odour, wound breakdown, delayed healing and a change in the appearance of granulation tissue.

Redness is a normal feature of wound healing but should not spread beyond the immediate wound edge: Trott (1997) states the distance as 5 mm. Spreading redness (cellulitis) and ascending lymphangitis are also signs of infection.

Systemic symptoms may also be present and include pyrexia, pallor, tiredness, general malaise, lethargy, pyrexia, sweating, nausea, tachycardia and tachypnoea.

Once wound infection has been established, the decision regarding whether to treat the infection locally or systemically will have to be made. Where there is evidence of spread of infection and the patient is systemically unwell, treatment with antibiotic therapy is indicated. Prophylactic antibiotics are commonly prescribed for compound fractures, heavily contaminated wounds, human bites and animal bites. The choice of antibiotic will depend on the causative organism and local policy. Grossly contaminated and infected wounds will require surgical debridement. Infections of the hand require active, aggressive management, including thorough irrigation, local treatment with antibiotics and antitetanus prophylaxis (Gregori and Mackay, 1994).

> Prophylactic antibiotics are commonly prescribed for compound fractures, heavily contaminated wounds, human bites and animal bites

TETANUS

Clostridium tetani is an anaerobic Gram-positive bacillus that lives in the gut of ruminant animals and passes out into the soil in faeces. It forms spores that live in soil and are very resistant. Tetanus bacilli grow anaerobically at the site of wounds and produce toxins that diffuse through motor neurons to the central nervous system, blocking the inhibitory control of motor neurons. This results in tonic spasms of striated muscle, which leads to clonic spasms. Mortality is highest in the very young and the very old, with death occurring from asphyxia or cardiovascular collapse. Elderly women are at the greatest risk of contracting tetanus. The incubation period is between 4 and 21 days. Tetanus can never be eradicated and is not spread from person to person.

Patients with impaired immunity who suffer a tetanus-prone wound may not respond to the vaccine and may, therefore, require antitetanus immunoglobulin. HIV-positive individuals should be immunised against tetanus in the absence of contraindications.

Guidelines on tetanus prophylaxis

1. Tetanus status should be considered for all wounds and burns (Table 34.2).
2. All wounds should receive adequate surgical toilet. Dead tissue and haematomas are ideal culture media for the organism.
3. Immunisation schedule: inducing immunity to the tetanus toxin can prevent tetanus. There are few contraindications to tetanus toxoid. A completed course or booster within the past year is one such contraindication. Pregnancy is not a contraindication.

Tetanus–prone wounds

The following wounds are considered to be prone to tetanus:

- any wound or burn sustained more than 6 hours before surgical treatment
- any wound or burn at any interval after injury that shows one or more of the following

Table 34.2 Tetanus guidelines from immunisation against infectious disease. [Reproduced from Salisbury DM, Begg NT (eds). London: HMSO, 1996]

Immunisation status	Type of wound	
	Clean	Tetanus prone
Last of three-dose course or reinforcing dose within last 10 years	Nil	Nil. (A dose of human tetanus immunoglobulin may be given if the risk of infection is considered high, e.g. contamination with manure)
Last of three-dose course or reinforcing dose more than 10 years previously	A reinforcing dose of adsorbed vaccine	A reinforcing dose of adsorbed vaccine plus a dose of human tetanus immunoglobulin
Not immunised or immunisation status not known with certainty	A full three-dose course of adsorbed vaccine	A full three-dose course of vaccine, plus a dose of tetanus immunoglobulin in a different site

characteristics: a puncture-type wound; a wound contaminated with soil, road dirt or manure; a wound with a significant degree of devitalised or dead tissue; and an infected wound.

In these circumstances, 500 iu of human anti-tetanus immunoglobulin (HATI) should be given if more than 24 hours have elapsed since the injury or there is a risk or evidence of heavy contamination.

There is no need to administer tetanus boosters over the five-dose regime (i.e. the primary course of three in childhood and two further boosters at 10-year intervals). However, Shimoni et al. (1999) advise that tetanus should not be ruled out as a diagnosis in patients who have been immunised fully. 'A number of rare and exceptional cases of tetanus occur despite adequate immunisation' (Vinson, 2000).

Case study 34.1

PRESENTING COMPLAINT
Cut to right hand (Figure 34.7).

HISTORY
A 23-year-old unemployed man punched his fist through a window the previous evening. He says he was under the influence of alcohol at the time. The wound has not been cleaned.

PAST MEDICAL HISTORY
Asthma, claustrophobia.

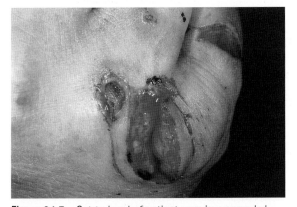

Figure 34.7   Cut to hand of patient seen in a nurse-led minor injury clinic.

MEDICATION
Methadone, ventolin and becotide inhalers.

ALLERGIES
Nil.

TETANUS STATUS
Up to date.

EXAMINATION OF RIGHT HAND
Inspection
Deep gaping wound dorsum of right hand between the metacarpal heads of ring finger and little finger. Wound 3 cm × 2 cm. 0.5 cm circular superficial cut over metacarpal head of ring finger. 2 cm gaping transverse cut over dorsum of proximal phalanx of little finger; partial thickness. No obvious skin loss, clean-looking, no foreign body seen. No obvious signs of infection

Palpation
Tender to touch. No foreign body felt.

Movement
Reduced extension of little finger.

Sensation and circulation
No abnormality detected.

INVESTIGATIONS
X-ray to exclude foreign body and fracture. Result – no foreign body or fracture seen.

DIAGNOSIS
Cuts to dorsum of right hand. ? Penetrating injury to little finger metacarpo-phalangeal joint. ? Extensor tendon damage. High risk of infection as the wound has been open for 14 hours without being cleaned.

PLAN
Cleanse with running water. Apply iodine dressing. Patient to attend accident and emergency department for further assessment by A&E doctor. Notes and x-rays to accompany patient.

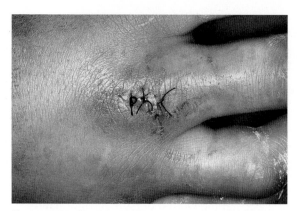

Figure 34.8 Punching injury resulting in a bite over the dorsum of the right metacarpophalangeal joint of the middle finger.

Case study 34.2

CLINICAL PROBLEM

This wound is approximately 14 hours old. The patient was given a prescription for antibiotics by his general practitioner but he did not comply with prescribed treatment. This injury occurred as a consequence of a human bite that was sutured with the obvious complication of infection (Figure 34.8).

There is marked swelling and erythema with pus between the sutures; erythema is seen to track to the proximal metacarpal (lymphangitis).

PLAN

Remove sutures to release pus and assess inside the wound. Look and feel for foreign bodies, teeth, fractures and tendon injury. X-ray for foreign body and fracture. Check for pyrexia and take wound swab.

FINDINGS

Marked reduction in extension and flexion of middle finger, and index and ring fingers. May be due to generalised infection, fracture, swelling, pain and/or tendon damage.

INTERVENTION

This wound will need referral owing to severe infection, possibly involving deep structures. There is a likelihood of a partial or completely severed tendon. Oral and possible intravenous antibiotic therapy is indicated. Surgical intervention is possible. Traumatic injury to the tendon has to be excluded. Consideration should be made to the risk of HIV and hepatitis B transmission. A tetanus booster and human anti-tetanus immunoglobulin are indicated as the wound falls within a 'tetanus-prone' category; last vaccination was more than 10 years ago.

CONCLUSION

Many wounds may appear trivial when compared to other aspects of emergency work. It must be noted, however, that trivial wounds have the potential to disfigure and result in dysfunction, preventing patients from pursuing their hobbies, livelihood and normal activities. The consequences for patients and practitioners can be devastating when wounds are mismanaged. Wound assessment and management should not, therefore, be underestimated.

Once life-threatening conditions have been eliminated, nurses can assess and manage wounds using a methodical systematic approach. This is a logical method that arrives at a clinical decision from which treatment can then safely proceed.

References and further reading

Alexander R, Proctor H. *Advanced trauma life support course for physicians*, 5th edn. Chicago: American College of Surgeons, 1995

Canine Crisis Council. *Humans bitten by dogs*. Leicester: Canine Crisis Council, 1997

Cole E. Wound management in the A&E department. *Nursing Standard* 2003; 17(46): 45–52

Dearden C, Donnell J, Donnelly J, Dunlop M. Traumatic wounds: nursing assessment and management. *Nursing Times Plus* 2001a; 97(24): 52–56

Dearden C, Donnell J, Donnelly J, Dunlop M. Traumatic wounds: cleansing and dressing. *Nursing Times Plus* 2001b; 97(28): 50–52

Gregori A, Mackay G. Prawn bites fisherman. *British Medical Journal* 1994; 309: 1695

HMSO. *The industry guide to good hygiene practice*. London: Chadwick House Group Ltd, 1995

Jones V, Milroy CM, Rutty GN. When and how to use iodine dressings. If a wound is 'neatly incised' it is not a laceration. *British Medical Journal* 1997; 315: 1312

Lamb DW, Hooper G. *Colour guide hand conditions.* Edinburgh: Churchill Livingstone, 1994

MacNicol MF, Lamb DW. *Basic care of the injured hand.* Edinburgh: Churchill Livingstone, 1984

Mellor DJ, Bhandari S, Kerr K, Bodenham AR. Lesson of the week: Man's best friend, life threatening sepsis after minor dog bite. *British Medical Journal* 1997; 314: 129

Miller M, Glover D (eds) *Wound management.* London: Nursing Times Books, 1999

Milroy CM, Rutty GN. *British Medical Journal* 1997; 315: 1312

Jones V, Milton T. When and how to use iodine dressings. *Nursing Times Plus* 2000; 96(45): 2–3

O'Connell S. Lyme disease in the United Kingdom. *British Medical Journal* 1995; 310: 303–308

Raby N, Berman L, De Lacey G. *Accident and emergency radiology.* London: WB Saunders Company, 1995

Salisbury DM, Begg NT. (eds) *Tetanus guidelines from immunisation against infectious disease.* London: HMSO, 1996

Shimoni Z, Dobrousin A, Cohen J. Tetanus in an immunised patient. *British Medical Journal* 1999; 319: 1049

Small V. Management of cuts, abrasions and lacerations. *Nursing Standard* 2000; 15(5): 41–44

Trott AT. *Wounds and lacerations emergency care and closure,* 2nd edn. St Louis: Mosby, 1997

Tsaloumas MD, Potamitis T, Kritzinger EE. Two cases of retention of wooden foreign bodies in orbit of eye. *British Medical Journal* 1998; 316: 1363–1364

Vinson DR. Immunisation does not rule out tetanus. *British Medical Journal* 2000; 320: 383

Wardrope J, Smith JAR. *The management of wounds and burns.* Oxford: Oxford University Press, 1992

Watson N. *Hand injuries and infections.* London: Gower Medical Publishing, 1986

Wilkinson JD, Shaw S, Fenton DA. *Colour guide to dermatology.* Edinburgh: Churchill Livingstone, 1993

Wilson GR, Nee PA, Watson JS. *Emergency management of hand injuries.* Oxford: Oxford University Press, 1997

Wyatt JP. Squirrel bites. *British Medical Journal* 1994; 309: 1694

SECTION **5**

Clinical considerations and their impact on trauma care

SECTION CONTENTS

Chapter **35**

Medical emergencies

Darren Walter and Stefania Walter

INTRODUCTION

Chapter 16 describes a systematic method for the assessment of critically ill trauma patients. It is possible that patients may have suffered a medical insult and that this is the cause of the traumatic injury, or that a medical problem may be a contributing factor in the clinical presentation. This chapter will consider medical emergencies as they relate to the trauma situation and discuss their assessment, investigation and early management.

In keeping with the 'ABC' approach to assessment of the patient, individual conditions will be considered as they might be identified during the primary and secondary surveys.

AIRWAY

If the patient is conscious, they may give a subjective assessment of their airway, for example, complaining that their tongue is swollen or that it is difficult to swallow saliva, suggesting that there may be a problem.

An objective clinical assessment should include direct inspection of the upper airway, looking for evidence of swelling of the tongue or tonsillar fauces, erythema of the pharynx or even pus on the tonsils. The presence of a hoarse voice or inspiratory stridor, or the position in which the patient is holding their head, for example, 'sniffing the morning air', may suggest the cause. Inability to swallow saliva is worrying and suggests the presence of significant pathology in the upper airway. In an unconscious patient, the presence of snoring or gurgling sounds suggest that the airway is not fully patent and that urgent attention, either by airway manoeuvres or through the judicious use of suction, is required.

A summary of medical airway problems is presented in Box 35.1.

Anaphylaxis

Anaphylaxis is a systemic acute allergic reaction that may be rapidly life threatening. For a reaction to occur, there usually has to have been a previous exposure to an antigen followed by a latent period in which sensitisation of the immune system takes place. On repeated exposure to the antigen, a clinical syndrome consisting of oropharyngeal swelling, laryngeal oedema, bronchospasm and cardiovascular collapse, together with effects on almost all other organ systems develops; in some cases in a matter of minutes (Rosen and Barkin, 1998). There is an enormous array of potential triggers from the well-known penicillin sensitivity and bee stings, through foods such as nuts and shellfish to the less well known, such as hydrocortisone and paracetamol.

Box 35.1   Medical airway problems

Obstruction
- Anaphylaxis
- Epiglottitis
- Parapharyngeal infection
  - Quinsy
  - Ludwig's angina
- Foreign body/material

Loss of control
- Depressed level of consciousness
  - Poisoning
  - Alcohol/illicit drugs
  - Fits
  - Intracerebral vascular event
  - Stroke
  - TIA
  - SAH
- Nerve palsy
  - Guillain–Barré syndrome

TIA, transient ischaemic attack; SAH, subarachnoid haemorrhage.

There are two types of reaction: anaphylactic and anaphylactoid. Clinically, they are very similar and the distinction is an immunological one based on the pathophysiology; it has no effect on the management.

Clinical presentation

The first clinical finding is often in the skin, where there is tingling progressing to generalised itching, together with flushing developing into an urticarial rash (red and raised blotches on the skin). If the patient is conscious, they may complain of swelling of the tongue and lips, difficulty swallowing and difficulty with breathing. Their voice may begin to sound hoarse, they may develop inspiratory stridor and the chest will start to wheeze in a manner similar to an asthmatic episode. They will become tachycardic and hypotensive owing to massive vasodilatation and increased capillary permeability, and this may progress to circulatory collapse. Additional symptoms such as gastrointestinal cramping, vomiting and diarrhoea are not uncommon, and are attributed to the development of oedema in the intestinal mucosa.

Treatment and nursing care

On recognising the clinical picture, it is essential to start treatment as soon as possible. There has been considerable controversy about the most effective treatment (Brown, 1998); however, the UK Resuscitation Council has produced guidelines that are widely accepted as the standard of care and are regularly updated (Project Team of the Resuscitation Council, 1999, 2001; Figure 35.1).

The loss of a patent airway is an immediate life-threatening situation and endotracheal intubation may be required to maintain patency. If the patient is able to maintain an open airway, they should be assisted into an upright position. All patients require high-flow oxygen through a tight fitting non-re-breathing facemask with an attached reservoir bag. An injection of intramuscular adrenaline 500 micrograms (causing vasoconstriction and slowing the release of chemical mediators) should be given early followed by an intravenous antihistamine and steroids. Intravenous fluids and even an H_2-blocker such as cimetidine may also be warranted.

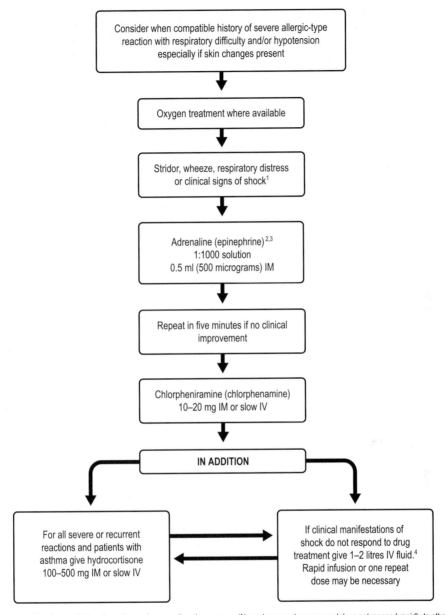

Consider when compatible history of severe allergic-type reaction with respiratory difficulty and/or hypotension especially if skin changes present

Oxygen treatment where available

Stridor, wheeze, respiratory distress or clinical signs of shock[1]

Adrenaline (epinephrine)[2,3] 1:1000 solution 0.5 ml (500 micrograms) IM

Repeat in five minutes if no clinical improvement

Chlorpheniramine (chlorphenamine) 10–20 mg IM or slow IV

IN ADDITION

For all severe or recurrent reactions and patients with asthma give hydrocortisone 100–500 mg IM or slow IV

If clinical manifestations of shock do not respond to drug treatment give 1–2 litres IV fluid.[4] Rapid infusion or one repeat dose may be necessary

[1] An inhaled beta $_2$-agonist such as salbutamol may be used as an adjunctive measure if bronchospasm is severe and does not respond rapidly to other treatment.

[2] If profound shock judged immediately life threatening give CPR/ALS if necessary. Consider slow IV adrenaline (epinephrine) 1:10,000 solution. This is hazardous and is recommended only for an experienced practitioner. Note the different strength of adrenaline (epinephrine) that may be required for IV use.

[3] If adults are treated with Epipen, the 300 micrograms will usually be sufficient. A second dose may be required. Half dose of adrenaline (epinephrine) may be safer for patients on amitriptyline, imipramine or beta blocker.

[4] A crystalloid may be safer than a colloid.

Figure 35.1   UK Resuscitation Council guideline for first-line management of anaphylaxis. ALS, advanced life support; CPR, cardiopulmonary resuscitation; IM, intramuscular; IV, intravenous. [© Resuscitation Council (UK), 2000.]

Once the situation has improved, there is a risk of 'rebound' and a further deterioration up to 6 hours after the initial treatment (Rosen and Barkin, 1998). Observation of the patient is, therefore, required over this period. The patient's airway patency, respiratory and haemodynamic status are the principal parameters to monitor.

Epiglottitis

This is a bacterial infection affecting the base of the tongue and is essentially a cellulitis. It was classically found in young children and caused by *Haemophilus influenzae* type B; however, since the introduction of specific immunization, its incidence has declined. Adults do experience the condition, although it is often less fulminant and is caused by a wider range of pathogens (Fauci et al., 1999).

Clinical presentation

The presentation is very rapid with a systemic pyrexial illness, difficulty in swallowing, progressing to an inability to swallow and drooling saliva. The patient may report a prodromal sore throat and have early dehydration as a consequence of decreased fluid intake. They will appear anxious, usually sitting upright in a tripod position. They are classically described as having stridor and holding their head persistently in a 'sniffing the morning air' position. In this position, the airway remains at its most patent, the danger being the complete obstruction of the airway.

Treatment and nursing care

The patient should be kept calm and positioned comfortably, remembering that agitation can lead to full airway obstruction. Direct inspection of the pharynx is strongly discouraged; if the airway is becoming compromised fibreoptic visualisation and introduction of an endotracheal tube is the ideal intervention (Rosen and Barkin, 1998). Endotracheal tubes one or two sizes smaller than estimated should be readily available as well as equipment for emergency rescue airway interventions (e.g. needle cricothyrotomy).

Specific treatment is based on antibiotics, although the use of humidified oxygen and even nebulised adrenaline may be of benefit.

> In patients with suspected epiglottitis, direct examination of the pharynx should only be undertaken by the anaesthetist

Infective diseases

Other infective problems around the upper airway may cause obstruction. A peritonsillar abscess, colloquially known as a quinsy, can be identified by a swelling on one side of Wallmeyer's ring at the back of the oral cavity, with deviation of the uvula away from the midline. Treatment requires the involvement of ear, nose and throat (ENT) surgeons with possible incision and drainage of the collection, together with intravenous antibiotics. It is usually polymicrobial in origin.

Ludwig's angina is a cellulitis of the floor of the mouth, often attributable to poor dental hygeine, which rapidly spreads to the neck. In the pre-antibiotic era, mortality was high; however, this does respond to early antibiotic therapy and securing of the airway (Rosen and Barkin, 1998).

Loss of control

Depression of the level of consciousness can result in relaxation of the muscle tone around the upper airway, allowing the tongue to fall backwards and occlude the airway. This principle applies whatever the cause. Medical causes involving brain injury or poisoning will be considered during the D or 'disability' stage of the ABCD approach.

BREATHING

Once certain that the airway is patent, an assessment of breathing is possible. Respiratory rate is one of the most overlooked of the basic clinical observations and, together with simple observation of the chest, can give a large amount of information about the adequacy of ventilation.

Features that should be looked for and documented include:

- respiratory rate
- chest excursion, extent and equality between sides
- use of accessory muscles of respiration
- the movement of the diaphragm
- autoPEEP (the pursing of lips during

expiration to create a raised end-expiratory pressure, improving the gas exchange).

Pulse oximetry gives an indication of the adequacy of oxygenation and even the conscious level may reflect respiratory function.

There is a wide range of respiratory medical conditions that can affect the care of a trauma patient and influence their assessment (Box 35.2).

Asthma

Asthma is an inflammatory airway disease in which airflow is limited by constriction of smooth muscle within the airway walls; there is development of mucosal oedema and an increase in exudate in the lumen.

The bronchial tree has increased sensitivity and responsiveness to a wide variety of stimuli resulting in a widespread narrowing of the airways. Fully reversible, it usually occurs in brief episodes in response to exposure to a stimulus or following a respiratory tract infection, and responds readily to self-administered treatment through inhalers and, occasionally, the administration of supplemental oral medication. Asthma has a significant prevalence in the community and is quite likely to be a comorbidity in a trauma patient.

Typically, patients have a smooth muscle relaxant medication in the form of a beta$_2$-agonist (e.g. salbutamol) taken as an inhaler to use during an exacerbation. With more intrusive disease, the patient may also be taking an anti-inflammatory medication, such as inhaled glucocorticoids (e.g.

beclomethasone). Recent developments include the introduction of inflammatory mediator inhibitors and these are being used to supplement the above (e.g. montelukast).

Patients need to continue to receive medication throughout their hospital stay and administration may be complicated if there is any form of respiratory compromise or there is depressed level of consciousness

Clinical presentation

The principal step in the care of the trauma patient with asthma is an assessment of the severity of airflow restriction. Subjectively the patient may report shortness of breath, chest tightness, wheezing, increased coughing and sputum production or a combination of the above.

Physical examination should include assessment of the respiratory rate, the use of accessory muscles of respiration and observation of the ability to speak in sentences or only a few words at a time. Auscultation of the chest for wheezing and crackles gives only part of the picture. The most objective means of assessment of asthma severity is by measurement of peak expiratory flow rate, and comparison of this with the rate that could be predicted for a patient of this height, age and sex.

As a separate entity to ongoing asthma, patients may develop an exacerbation of their disease, possibly triggered by an allergen, an infective episode or even stress. This may potentially be life threatening and requires urgent attention.

The severity of the episode is graded on the basis of peak expiratory flow rate (PEFR) measured with a simple meter prior to commencing treatment. This is compared to the flow rate that could be predicted for a patient of this age and sex without asthma. The presence of a PEFR < 50% of predicted is classed as severe disease (Box 35.3).

Box 35.2   Respiratory diseases in the trauma patient

- Asthma
- Chronic obstructive pulmonary disease (COPD)
  - Type 1
  - Type 2
- Pneumonia
  - Bacterial
  - Viral
  - Atypical
- Pulmonary embolism
- Pulmonary oedema

Box 35.3   Features of acute severe asthma

- Cannot complete sentence in one breath
- Respiratory rate > 25 breaths/minute
- Pulse rate over 110 beats/minute
- PEFR < 50% of predicted or best

> **Box 35.4** Life–threatening features of severe asthma
>
> - PEFR < 33% of predicted or best
> - Silent chest, cyanosis, feeble respiratory effort
> - Bradycardia or hypotension
> - Exhaustion, agitation, confusion, coma

This can equate to a patient who clinically cannot complete a sentence in one breath and has a respiratory rate of > 25 per minute. If the PEFR is < 33% or the oxygen saturation measured with a pulse oximeter is < 92%, then this is classified as life threatening (Box 35.4).

If the disease is of this severity, then there may be so little air being moved through the narrow airways that there is no wheeze and the chest is 'silent'. The patient may be agitated, restless or confused, and rapidly becomes exhausted, leading to respiratory arrest. A quiet, lethargic, grey or even cyanosed patient with a silent chest is in danger of imminent respiratory arrest.

Treatment and nursing care

Patients needs to continue to receive their prophylactic medication throughout their hospital stay. Administration of this and 'when required' bronchodilators may be complicated if there is any form of respiratory compromise, chest pain or depressed level of consciousness

Asthma management in the UK, particularly management of exacerbations, has become more organised in recent years with the production of widely circulated guidelines, regularly updated by the British Thoracic Society (1997a).

For exacerbations, the guidelines give very clear instructions on best management:

- high-flow oxygen
- beta₂-agonist (e.g. salbutamol 5 mg administered through oxygen-driven nebulisers with a flow rate of 6 litres/minute)
- steroids (prednisolone 30–60 mg orally or hydrocortisone 200 mg intravenously).

If life-threatening features are present, then the following should be used in addition:

- anticholinergic (e.g. ipratropium 0.5 mg through the nebuliser)
- intravenous aminophylline (250 mg over 20 minutes, if not already taking oral theophyllines) or intravenous beta₂-agonist (e.g. salbutamol 250 µg over 10 minutes) should be administered.

If respiratory function does not improve, then intubation and mechanical ventilation are required. Initially, patients will require both sedating and paralysing, and airway pressures are likely to be very high. For sedation, opiates such as morphine are contraindicated, since they may cause histamine release from mast cells and exacerbate the situation. Fentanyl is the preferred opiate and ketamine, with its bronchodilator properties, as a sedative is the ideal (Rosen and Barkin, 1998). Once the patient has been intubated, continuous observation of the heart rate and rhythm, blood pressure, oxygen saturation and respiratory pressures should be maintained.

With generally increased airway pressures and accumulation of secretions, there is a real problem with risk of pneumothorax or barotrauma, particularly when ventilated. In the intubated patient, a sudden increase in pressure and oxygenation or change in the haemodynamic state suggest this.

In the intubated patient, regular airway suctioning and the use of warmed and humidified oxygen will help to mobilise the mucus plugs and reduce the tenacity of the secretions.

Chronic obstructive pulmonary disease

Chronic obstructive pulmonary disease (COPD) is the internationally preferred collective term for a number of conditions in which there are three components: emphysema (airway collapse), chronic bronchitis (airway inflammation), and some asthma (reversible airway reaction). It is a chronic and progressive disease largely attributable to the effects of smoking and much of the impaired function is fixed, although bronchodilators can produce some improvement in function (British Thoracic Society, 1997b; Rosen and Barkin, 1998).

In caring for the trauma patient, there will need to be ongoing treatment of the underlying disease, but there is also the potential for an exacerbation and respiratory failure associated with this.

Stable COPD

Assessment of the severity of disease is based on spirometric measurement of respiratory function, specifically the FEV_1 (forced expiratory volume in 1 second), as compared to that predicted for age and sex. Clinically, the patient may simply have limited exercise tolerance but, with progression, there is persistent wheezing and overinflation of the chest. With very severe disease there may be central cyanosis or even the features of hypercapnia.

After removal of the precipitant cause (principally smoking), there is an ascending stairway of therapy, beginning with as required and then regular use of beta$_2$-agonists and anticholinergics, then the addition of inhaled or even oral corticosteroids. Home nebuliser therapy may be required. Oral theophyllines may be included, but have an unpredicatable benefit and the side-effect profile may mean that they cannot be tolerated. Long-term oxygen therapy (LTOT) for 15 hours a day is an almost final option (British Thoracic Society, 1997b).

During management of a traumatic injury, these therapies will need to be continued. If, as a result of the injury, the patient is unable to take their regular medication, then movement up the therapy escalator will probably be required to prevent a deterioration of the COPD.

Exacerbation of COPD

In the community, the commonest cause for deterioration in function is a result of respiratory tract infection. In the traumatically injured, impairment of ventilation may well lead to an infection and initiate the exacerbation. The patient's response to the insult will depend on their physiological response to disordered lung function and rising $PaCO_2$. Some, the 'pink puffers' or those with type 1 respiratory failure, respond by greatly increasing their minute volume at the expense of a significant increase in respiratory rate. Others, the 'blue bloaters' or those with type 2 respiratory failure, increase their minute volume only moderately and tolerate an increase in the $PaCO_2$ and more significant hypoxaemia. The response tends to mirror the patient's lead clinical manifestation of COPD. Those with primarily emphysema who complain of exertional dyspnoea with little cough, often associated with weight loss and thin body build, tend to respond excessively to the hypercapnia. Those for whom bronchitis is the predominant feature with a productive cough, often overweight and possibly cyanosed, fail to respond to the falling pH.

There is considerable debate about why there should be these differences in response (Dick et al., 1997). In effect, there are two separate diseases.

Clinical presentation of exacerbation

The patient will complain of increasing shortness of breath and cough with increased sputum production and purulence, together with a decreased activity tolerance. Changes in appetite and sleep patterns are also common.

On physical examination, the patient may appear to be in some respiratory distress with increased use of accessory muscles. The breath sounds may be very quiet and expiration is prolonged owing to air trapping and respiratory bronchiole collapse. Crackles and wheezes may be heard on auscultation. The patient may be febrile, since infection is the most common cause of an exacerbation.

A reduction in the level of consciousness or episodes of syncope are signs of advanced disease, with increasing hypoxaemia and carbon dioxide retention. These patients may have gasping respirations, tachycardia, a bounding pulse, hypertension and are often sweating. Signs of right ventricular failure owing to pulmonary hypertension may also be present.

Treatment and nursing care

The immediate goal of care for patients with COPD is to ensure an adequate airway and optimise the breathing. The aim of treatment is to achieve a PaO_2 of > 6.6 kPa without a rise in the $PaCO_2$ and a fall in the pH to < 7.26. The underlying cause of the exacerbation will also need treatment. The rate of oxygen administration should be titrated to the arterial blood gas response aiming for adequate oxygenation without a rise in the CO_2 level. This may require the use of a Venturi mask with a fixed oxygen flow rate and administration concentration.

Nebulised bronchodilators are needed on a regular basis. In 'blue bloaters', where 6 litres/minute of oxygen would not be tolerated, the driving gas should be air. If supplemental oxygen is required, but at a lower flow rate, then this can be achieved by concurrent use of nasal prongs. The use of systemic steroids is recommended for exacerbations, either prednisolone 30 mg orally or hydrocortisone 100 mg intravenously for 7–14 days.

Secretions should be assessed for quantity, colour, odour and consistency. Sputum samples should be collected for microbiological assessment with microscopy, culture and sensitivity. Antibiotics are warranted if there is an increase in the sputum volume and it has become purulent.

If, despite maximal therapy as described, there is a continued deterioration, then ventilatory support is required. Over recent years there has been a move towards the introduction of non-invasive respiratory support as an intermediate step, together with infusion of the respiratory stimulant doxapram, to avoid the need for intubation (Sivasothy et al., 1998). The aim is to tide the patient over for 24–36 hours until the underlying cause is controlled.

Pneumonia

Pneumonia is the collective term for a group of infections that affect the lung parenchyma and result in inflammation. It is one of the leading causes of death for the population at large and also for delayed death in the patient suffering a traumatic injury. The reduced chest excursion and suppression of the cough reflex as a consequence of chest injury and pain, the reduced gag reflex and risk of aspiration during a period of reduced level of consciousness, and most certainly the use of endotracheal intubation to support ventilation, all bypass the usual defence mechanisms and may result in the development of pneumonia.

With the establishment of the infective process, the alveoli fill with exudate and pus. Ventilation to these areas decreases and produces a ventilation perfusion mismatch and impaired gas exchange.

Clinical presentation

The patient will tend to have a cough and, depending on severity, may have features of respiratory distress. The presence and type of sputum will depend on the infecting organism. They may also complain of stabbing or pleuritic chest pain associated with inspiration, movement and coughing owing to inflammation of the visceral pleural surface.

On physical examination, the patient will be tachypnoeic, tachycardic, febrile and may have shallow respirations. They should be assessed for the use of accessory muscles, grunting, nasal flaring, sternal and intercostal recession and the presence of cyanosis. Auscultation of the chest may reveal crackles and wheezes over the affected lung area. The presence of consolidation may allow the enhanced transmission of central breath sounds giving 'bronchial breathing' and an increased transmission of vibration and sounds from speech; tactile and vocal fremitus.

A chest X-ray should be obtained to determine the extent and distribution of the infection and the possibility of a pleural effusion.

Treatment and nursing care

The patient's breathing should be carefully monitored for signs of respiratory failure, such as increasing respiratory rate, poorer chest excursion and tremor, suggesting CO_2 retention. Patients should be placed in an upright position to facilitate breathing and supplemental oxygen should be administered as necessary. The efficacy of oxygen therapy should be continually assessed with pulse oximetry and arterial blood gas analysis as required. Patients should be encouraged to cough and expectorate to improve ventilation; administration of analgesia needs to be titrated to allow the patient to be pain-free during coughing without suppressing the respiratory drive.

Close monitoring of the temperature is necessary and antipyretics should be administered as required. Fluid loss from fever, tachypnoea and sweating may necessitate intravenous fluid replacement to maintain adequate hydration. If respiratory failure is imminent, nursing interventions should be aimed towards assisting with non-invasive ventilation or preparing for intubation and mechanical ventilation.

Causation

Community acquired pneumonia is very common. It may present in the classical way with a fever, cough productive of purulent sputum, pleuritic chest pain and signs of pulmonary consolidation to examination, or in a more 'atypical' way with a gradual onset, a dry cough and extrapulmonary symptoms. The cause is often bacterial, although it can be viral (Box 35.5). Fungal infection and *Pneumocystis carinii* (PCP) are also possibilities but should raise questions about the integrity of the immune system. Human immunodeficiency virus (HIV) status should be considered.

While patients should receive antibiotic therapy according to local policy, treatment of this type of infection often involves a penicillin, such as amoxycillin, and/or a macrolide, such as erythromycin.

Mycobacterium tuberculosis had declined in significance in Western Europe with the use of antibiotics and widespread BCG (bacille Calmette–Guérin) vaccination. The development of acquired immunodeficiency syndrome (AIDS) and the increase in international travel has led to a resurgence of its prevalence.

Box 35.5 **Causative organisms in community acquired pneumonia**

Bacterial
- Typical
  - *Streptococcus pneumoniae*
  - *Haemophilus influenzae*
  - *Klebsiella pneumoniae*
- Atypical
  - *Mycoplasma pneumoniae*
  - *Chlamydia pneumoniae*
  - *Legionella pneumophila*

Viral
- Influenza
- Respiratory syncytial virus
- Measles

Fungi
- *Histoplasma capsulatum*
- *Coccidioides immitis*

Parasite
- *Pneumocystis carinii*

It is now generally accepted that there is compromise of the immune system when a patient suffers significant trauma (Cooper et al., 1997). The incidence of nosocomial pulmonary infection can rise to in excess of 25% in those who require mechanical ventilatory support. Diagnosis is complicated by a differential that includes adult respiratory distress syndrome (ARDS) and other coexisting lung injuries, such as pulmonary contusion or atelectasis.

The cause is often polymicrobial. Some cases may be caused by contamination of the ventilator circuit or acquired from the hands of the staff providing care, but most cases arise from bacteria colonising the oropharynx and the stomach. The use of antibiotics and acid suppressants, such as antacids or H_2-blockers, alter the oropharyngeal flora and allow colonisation with *S. aureus* and Gram-negative organisms.

While the antibiotic regimen should follow the local hospital microbiology protocol, the underlying therapy will include cover for both aerobic and non-aerobic organisms and should take account of the widespread antibiotic resistance that Gram-negative organisms can acquire.

Pulmonary embolism

Pulmonary embolism is a major cause of death, with 16% noted in the Framingham study (Goldhaber et al., 1983), and found in a far higher proportion of patients dying after traumatic injury. The introduction of thromboembolic prophylaxis against deep vein thrombosis (DVT) has reduced the incidence but the condition is still far more common than is often realised.

Under normal physiological conditions, there is continual formation of microthrombi within the circulation, which are then rapidly broken down by the fibrinolytic system. Deep vein thrombi form in the veins of the calf, thigh and even pelvis, when they escape the normal breakdown system and begin to aggregate. Traditionally Virchow's triad is required for formation:

- venous stasis
- hypercoagulability
- vessel wall inflammation/damage.

Traumatic injury, with its associated surgical procedures and period of immobilisation, together with the intensive care input using central venous lines, all act as further multiplying risk factors for the generation of intravascular thrombus.

Deep vein thrombus causes local vessel damage but it is the risk of clot movement through the venous system to the right side of the heart, impacting in the pulmonary vascular tree, that causes the serious and life-threatening effects. Diagnosis of the condition is notoriously difficult and the positive predictive value of clinical assessment is < 50% (Rosen and Barkin, 1998).

Clinical presentation
The clinical picture consists of a vague spectrum of symptoms – dyspnoea (84%), pleuritic chest pain (74%) and anxiety (59%) – that could be confused with almost any thoracic or upper abdominal condition. Clinical signs are equally non-specific with tachycardia (92%) and wheeze (58%) being the lead findings. Restlessness, headaches, apprehension, pallor or cyanosis may indicate hypoxia, but none are specific.

Small emboli, even multiple small ones, may be asymptomatic. The presence of a sufficiently large embolus, or a sufficient number of smaller ones, in the lungs raises the vascular resistance and generates pulmonary hypertension. This alters right-sided function and may, if significant enough, impair left-sided ventricular filling and lead to cardiovascular collapse. A pulmonary pseudo-shunt is produced, the increased flow through the unaffected part of the vascular tree results in inadequate time for gas exchange and equilibration, and this will impair oxygenation.

Simple investigations can only provide circumstantial evidence to support the diagnosis. The electrocardiogram (ECG) may show a tachycardia, there may be flattening of the T waves and, more helpfully, there may be signs of right-sided cardiac strain with a right axis deviation and changes to the QRS pattern in the limb leads ($S_1Q_3T_3$). The chest x-ray may show some atelectasis, the hemidiaphragm on the affected side may be raised, and there may be visible changes to the vascular tree pattern with proximal vessel distension and an area where the vessels are less clear (Westermark's sign). The classic wedge-shaped 'sail sign' is rare.

Impaired oxygen saturation detected through oximetry and arterial blood gas sampling may show that there is impairment of gas exchange but are not specific. Echocardiography can provide more substantial evidence with hypokinesis of the right side of the heart and dilatation of the ventricle. There may be deviation of the septum to the left and underfilling of the left ventricle. Objective evidence of a pulmonary embolus can be shown using nuclear medicine ventilation-perfusion scanning but, as was shown by the PIOPED investigators (1990), pulmonary angiography is the gold standard for diagnosis.

With the development of computed tomography (CT) scanning technology, the use of spiral scanning after vascular contrast injection can produce a form of angiogram that is increasingly accepted as a less invasive means of confirming the diagnosis. Unfortunately, it is only able to show emboli to the segmental artery level, potentially missing multiple small clots.

Treatment and nursing care
The goals of nursing care for patients with a suspected pulmonary embolus include relief of the respiratory distress and hypoxia, maintenance of the cardiovascular state and alleviation of pain and anxiety.

Patients should be continually monitored for signs and symptoms of hypoxia. Pulse oximetry and vital signs, together with serial arterial blood gases must be carefully monitored. The threshold for administering supplemental oxygen and analgesia, and initiating investigation is low.

Patients may be too sick for the more invasive tests and a balanced decision about therapy needs to be made. Does the risk from investigation exceed that for initiating treatment on clinical suspicion only?

The core treatment is anticoagulation and, in the first instance, this is done with intravenous unfractionated heparin or increasingly with subcutaneous low-molecular-weight heparin with an activated partial thromboplastin time (APTT) of 1.5–2.5 times the normal range. This impairs the extension of the thrombi and allows the fibrinolytic system to dominate, resulting in a gradual resolution of the thrombus. This will take a considerable time and patients are usually transferred to oral therapy with warfarin or coumarin, with an international normalised ratio (INR) of 3–4 (British Thoracic Society, 1997c).

More aggressive intervention to thrombolyse the clot has been recommended but is not yet mainstream therapy. The risk:benefit profile is not favourable and current British practice is to restrict consideration of its use to those with cardiovascular instability. The other option of surgical thrombectomy is now done very rarely and is restricted to those facilities where cardiothoracic surgery is available and where medical and thrombolytic therapy have not been effective.

Pulmonary oedema

While being identified during the assessment of breathing, pulmonary oedema largely reflects a circulation issue. Its causes are numerous and varied but can be divided into two broad groups: cardiogenic and non-cardiogenic (Box 35.6).

The pathophysiological changes are based on alteration of the Starling forces across the alveolar capillary membrane, either through an increase in the pulmonary hydrostatic capillary pressure (usually cardiogenic) or through change of the capillary membrane permeability (usually non-cardiogenic). In both cases, there is an increase in the 'flow' of fluid from the intravascular space to the interstitial tissue of the lung. The pulmonary lymphatics are initially able to cope but, when their capacity is exceeded, there is fluid accumulation in the interstitial space and flooding of the alveoli. The volume of fluid moving from the circulation to the lungs may exceed 1000 ml, potentially resulting in a paradoxical dehydration!

Box 35.6   Causes of pulmonary oedema

Cardiogenic
- Acute coronary syndromes
- Cardiomyopathy
- Valvular heart disease
- Dysrhythmias

Non-cardiogenic
- Sepsis
- Anaemia
- Inhalation injury
- Aspiration
- Neurogenic

Clinical presentation

Clinically patients will present with shortness of breath, an increased respiratory rate and possibly also orthopnoea (inability to tolerate lying flat) and paroxysmal nocturnal dyspnoea (waking from sleep at night because lying flat). This is because there is an increase in venous return to the heart when lying flat, raising the pre-load.

Hypoxia is evidenced initially by agitation and restlessness, and later by lethargy and an altered level of consciousness. The skin will be cool, sweaty and possibly cyanotic. The pulse is often rapid, weak and thready, the blood pressure may be either high or low. Evidence of increased pre-load on the heart includes a raised jugular venous pulse in the neck, possibly some upper abdominal pain from distension of the liver and increased ankle swelling. Auscultation of the lungs will reveal crackles and wheezing in all areas, but predominantly at the lung bases. Severe pulmonary oedema can cause copious production of frothy white or pink-tinged sputum.

Investigations are based on and will reflect the underlying cause. The chest x-ray has changes that show the severity of the congestion (Box 35.7).

Treatment and nursing care

Treatment will depend to some extent on the underlying pathology. Addressing the cardiac ischaemia or dysrhythmia, or treating the sepsis or anaemia are vital; however, there are a number of interventions that can alter the fluid shifts within the lungs.

Because of the reduction in the air-filled space of the lungs, gas exchange is impaired and the first step is to supplement the inspired oxygen concentration through a non-rebreathing mask with a reservoir at 10–15 litres/minute. If possible, the patient should be nursed in an upright position,

---

Box 35.7   Chest x-ray changes in pulmonary oedema

1. Upper lobe congestion of pulmonary vascular tree
2. Kerley B lines
3. Alveolar haziness across the fields
4. Pleural effusions

and the respiratory rate and effort, colour and level of consciousness continually assessed.

Cardiac monitoring should be in place to detect the presence of cardiac dysrhythmias and all vital signs should be assessed at regular intervals. If the patient is not able to maintain adequate oxygenation or persistently retains CO_2, some facilities will try to assist with non-invasive ventilatory support (CPAP or BiPAP) before proceeding to endotracheal intubation and mechanical ventilation. Preparations for this should be made.

In failure owing to a high output state, such as in sepsis or anaemia, the blood pressure is often maintained or even raised, and the cardiac pre-load can be reduced through dilatation of the pulmonary and systemic large veins using intravenous opiates, such as morphine or diamorphine, and nitrates. The latter can be administered either by the sublingual route or by intravenous infusion, although intravenous infusion allows more accurate titration. Furasemide (furosemide) can also be given, both because of its early vasodilatation effect and because of its more delayed diuretic effect.

In the cardiogenic group, the origin of the oedema is a low output state. Hypotension may be present and there may be little room for opiates and nitrates without reducing the blood pressure to inadequate levels for maintaining coronary and cerebral perfusion. Careful titration is needed. Often these patients are intravascularly dehydrated and they may benefit from a judicious fluid challenge in addition to the furosemide. Inotropes such as epinephrine (adrenaline) and dobutamine may be needed to support myocardial contractility and the blood pressure.

The use of positive pressure ventilation can help drive the alveolar fluid back into the circulation and improve gas exchange. The changes in intrathoracic pressure on commencing intermittent positive pressure ventilation (IPPV) can precipitate cardiovascular collapse. The debate about the use of non-invasive ventilatory support is still ongoing. There is little doubt that it can improve the physiology of cardiogenic pulmonary oedema; however, there are suggestions that its use may be complicated by an increased rate of myocardial infarction (Levitt, 2001).

CIRCULATION

Assessment of the circulation is the third step in the systematic approach to the patient (Figure 35.2). Details of the cardiovascular changes in trauma, and their assessment and implications have been considered in Chapters 12 and 13. Heart disease is very common and will be found as a concurrent problem in the care of the traumatically injured patient, particularly in the older age groups.

From a monitoring perspective, there are a number of objective means of assessment that allow the following of trends. The pulse rate and blood pressure are routinely documented. The urine output is a sensitive indicator of the adequacy of renal perfusion and the state of hydration of the patient. This should ideally be 1–2 ml/hour per kg or more generally > 60 ml/hour. Invasive vascular monitoring of

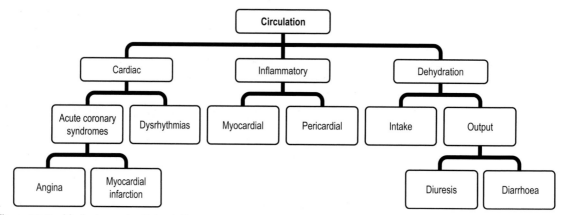

Figure 35.2   Medical aspects of circulation.

both the arterial and venous systems and even the pulmonary tree using a Swan–Ganz catheter may be used.

Specifically, from a cardiac point of view, a monitor continuously following a three-lead trace of cardiac rhythm, supported by a 12-lead ECG on presentation and subsequently with any change in cardiovascular circumstances provides adequate information.

Ischaemic heart disease

Atherosclerosis and consequent narrowing of the coronary blood vessels is an age-related and extremely common condition that can lead to exercise-related or critical ischaemia of the myocardium. The rate of progression is exacerbated by smoking and obesity, and linked to hypertension, hypercholesterolaemia and diabetes mellitus.

Clinical presentation

Cardiac pain can mimic any other thoracic or upper abdominal complaint; suspicion of cardiac origin is important in any chest assessment. Typically, however, the patient will describe tightness across the chest like a tight band, often spreading into the left or both arms, and up into the neck and jaw. There may be associated shortness of breath and nausea, even vomiting. The patient may describe feeling cold and sweating. They are often clammy to the touch.

In its mildest form, with exercise or stress requiring an increase in myocardial activity, there is an increase in the oxygen requirement of the muscle. As a result of the 'furring' or narrowing of the coronary vessels, there is insufficient reserve capacity to meet requirements and an oxygen debt is generated. This creates a cardiac cramping pain known as angina pectoris. Generally, episodes of angina are brought on by exertion, and eased by rest and last from a few seconds to several minutes. If the pain persists longer than 20 minutes, then the problem is more likely to be infarction. The pain may also be eased by the administration of glyceryl trinitrate (GTN) spray or sublingual nitrate, causing coronary vasodilatation.

Many patients who have angina will be on regular medications, such as nitrates or beta blockers, to limit the frequency of symptoms. While being cared for as a trauma victim, these medications should be continued and, if the patient is 'nil-by-mouth' or has an intestinal ileus, then transcutaneous patches and intravenous options may need to be considered.

If there is disruption of an atherosclerotic plaque and fissuring, then a platelet plug will form and narrow the vessel further. This produces a spectrum of critical ischaemia, now referred to as acute coronary syndrome. Unstable angina and myocardial infarction are the two pathologies covered by the term but, in the absence of clear ECG changes suggesting transmural infarction, distinguishing between myocardium that is recoverable and that which will infarct may be difficult and will depend on treatment.

Unstable angina pectoris (UAP)

In unstable angina, there is cardiac-type chest pain with no or minimal exercise. The ECG will not show ST segment elevation to suggest infarction, but part of the myocardium has a critical blood supply and, without intervention, may progress to infarction. Treatment is directed at reducing this risk (Theroux et al., 1998).

Treatment and nursing care

The first principles of treatment are oxygen and analgesia. The administration of high-flow oxygen via a non-rebreathing mask with a reservoir and the relief of pain through titrated intravenous opiates, relieving the physiological stress, may reverse the developing oxygen debt. Intravenous nitrates are used to dilate the coronary vessels and improve the rate of flow; beta blockers are administered to reduce the myocardial work. If these are contraindicated, then calcium-channel blockers can be substituted.

If intravenous nitrates are being used, then they should have a separate intravenous line and should be administered through an infusion pump. A second intravenous line should be available for bolus injections of other drugs or administration of fluids. Continuous observation of the blood pressure is necessary either by a repeated non-invasive automatic blood pressure cuff measurement or an electronically transduced arterial line monitoring system. Continuous cardiac monitoring is also necessary to detect the presence of dysrhythmias.

Since fissuring of a plaque is the likely underlying pathology, anticoagulation and antiplatelet medication are recommended. Aiming for an APTT of 2.0–3.0, intravenous heparin or increasingly subcutaneous low-molecular-weight heparin is used to anticoagulate. Aspirin 75 mg per day alters platelet adhesiveness and is recommended. Clopidogrel is now also suggested (Clopidogrel in Unstable Angina to Prevent Recurrent Events Trial Investigators, 2001).

There has been a considerable amount of research into the use of glycoprotein IIb/IIIa receptor blockers but their place in management is not yet established outside clinical trails.

Myocardial infarction

In myocardial infarction, a coronary vessel has narrowed sufficiently that critical ischaemia progresses to cell death. The clinical presentation is similar in type to that of UAP, although it is often more severe, longer in duration and not relieved by either rest or nitrates.

If a major vessel is involved, then there will be a transmural injury and characteristic ECG changes will be seen in the area of the heart damaged (e.g. inferior, anterior or lateral). If a smaller vessel is occluded and only a subendocardial injury produced, then ECG changes may be minimal; distinguishing the condition from UAP will require the benefit of cardiac muscle injury markers, such as the CK-MB fraction or, more commonly now, a rise in the troponin T level some hours after the presentation.

The criteria for the diagnosis of myocardial infarction and decision to administer thrombolysis are beyond the scope of this text. In simple terms, if there is evidence of significant ST segment elevation on the ECG in two or more consecutive leads of a 12-lead ECG, then, in the absence of contraindications, a thrombolytic agent (e.g. streptokinase or r-TPA) is warranted.

Treatment and nursing care

If an infarction is developing, then the current standard of care is to give a thrombolytic agent to 'dissolve' the clot and reperfuse the injured muscle. Clearly, there is a time factor here to minimise the amount of injury and standards have been set in the UK at government level through the National Service Framework for Coronary Heart Disease (Department of Health, 2000). The target is for assessment and administration of the thrombolytic agent within 60 minutes of calling for help.

In patients who have developed an infarct while in the recovery phase from a significant trauma, a number of the cautions and contraindications to thrombolysis are relevant. The fibrinolysis produced will affect all potential bleeding points and release clots that have already formed. In the presence of significant head injury or after major trauma, especially when there may have been internal bleeding, such as a splenic haematoma, the risk of further bleeding into these areas may outweigh the potential benefit of thrombolysis.

Beyond urgent administration of the fibrinolytic, other measures including high-flow oxygen, intravenous opiate analgesia, beta blockers and aspirin should be provided. Nursing care primarily involves monitoring the actions and side effects of thrombolytics and the other therapies. Hypotension, allergic reactions, reperfusion dysrhythmias, reocclusion and bleeding are all complications. Admission to a high-dependency area with continuous cardiac monitoring is necessary. The risk of further deterioration and development of cardiac dysrhythmias is highest during the first few hours following the myocardial insult.

Dysrhythmias

Many different groups of patients require cardiac monitoring: those with complaints that suggest cardiac dysfunction, haemodynamic instability or respiratory distress; individuals with a poisoning episode; or where there is a depressed level of consciousness. In short, anyone who is acutely ill or whose clinical status can deteriorate or whose treatment may alter the haemodynamic status, should be placed on a cardiac monitor. The trace must be evaluated for heart rate and rhythm at regular intervals along with observation and documentation of all the other vital signs.

There is a wide variety of precipitating causes for cardiac dysrhythmias: as a result of accumulated injury from ischaemic heart disease; as a consequence of an acute coronary syndrome; following trauma to the chest; or even sepsis or electrolyte disturbance. The pattern of electrical conduction through the heart is altered and, while the patient may remain asymptomatic, there may be a profound and life-threatening change in the haemodynamic state.

Cardiac dysrhythmias (or arrhythmias) can be divided into supraventricular or atrial, ventricular, heart blocks and cardiac arrest (Figure 35.3).

In more elderly trauma patients, the most likely cause is development of an acute coronary syndrome on an underlying chronic ischaemic heart disease, the acute management of which has been considered above. Atrial flutter or atrial fibrillation are common here. They reflect disordered electrical conduction within the atria, but this is only transmitted to the ventricles as a tachycardia and/or an irregular rate as a consequence of the conduction delay in the atrio-ventricular (AV) node.

In the presence of haemodynamic compromise, the treatment is electrical cardioversion. If not, then, since the rhythm may be persistent and recurrent, anticoagulation with heparin to prevent the formation of atrial mural thrombus and drug control of the ventricular rate is the treatment of choice (American Heart Association, 2001).

If the area of damaged ischaemic myocardium contains the AV node or part of the His fibres of the interventricular septum, then a heart block may develop. Second-degree block usually indicates the potential for serious problems with bradycardias rather than hypotensive complications directly. Third-degree block may result in a bradycardia of 30–35 beats/minute and will not generate a cardiac output sufficient to maintain adequate coronary and cerebral perfusion. The blood pressure may fall, although the block is often well tolerated.

Treatment of third-degree block is with titrated intravenous atropine and, if this is ineffective, with transvenous cardiac pacing. The aim is to raise the ventricular rate to between 50 and 60 beats/minute and restore the cardiac output without significantly increasing myocardial oxygen demand.

In addition to rhythm disturbance caused by ischaemia, trauma to the chest can produce myocardial injury in any age group (Vogler et al., 2001). The most dangerous of these rhythms is ventricular tachycardia (VT). If consciousness is impaired, then electrical cardioversion is indicated. In the conscious patient, sedation will be required. If the blood pressure is maintained, then the current UK Resuscitation Council guidelines (2001) recommend amiodarone or lignocaine (lidocaine) intravenously over 10 minutes before moving to cardioversion. *Torsades de pointes* is a specific subgroup of VT with a polymorphic and 'rolling' pattern. It is principally found in electrolyte disturbance and correction of this, together with the administration of intravenous magnesium, may terminate the rhythm chemically (Rosen and Barkin, 1998).

Cardiac arrest is said to have occurred when there is loss of cardiac output. Traditionally, there are three rhythms identified with arrest:

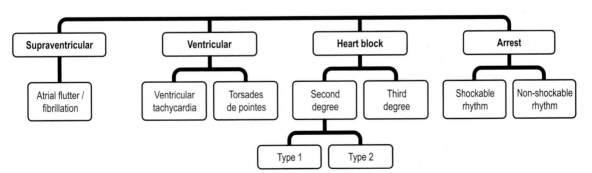

Figure 35.3 Cardiac dysrhythmias.

- ventricular fibrillation/pulseless ventricular tachycardia – loss of coordinated electrical conduction
- asystole – loss of ventricular electrical activity
- pulseless electrical activity – electrical activity consistent with an output is present but there is no detectable cardiac output.

Management of medical emergencies of this type is algorithm driven based on national adaptations of internationally agreed principles. The UK Resuscitation Council (2001) now recommends two different approaches on the basis of 'shockable' and 'non-shockable' electrical rhythms. The reader is referred to the Council for the most recent information (www.resus.org.uk).

Treatment and nursing care

The treatment and nursing care of patients with cardiac dysrhythmias is based on the diagnosis and treatment of the underlying problem as well as following treatment guidelines for cardiac arrest and periarrest arrhythmias from the UK Resuscitation Council (Figures 35.4–35.7).

The immediate goals of nursing care are to ensure an adequate airway, optimise the breathing with sufficient oxygen to relieve hypoxia, and ensure adequate tissue perfusion by maintaining the pulse rate and blood pressure. In addition, steps should be taken to relieve any pain or anxiety.

Cardiac dysrhythmias represent a serious problem for trauma patients and, therefore, their haemodynamic state will dictate the urgency of treatment. Identification of the dysrhythmia in this setting, although necessary, is but a small part of total patient care. A correlation between the history, mechanism of injury, physical findings and subjective assessment must be determined. The patient will require close monitoring and astute observation. Once treatment and interventions have been established, evaluation must take place and continue throughout the crisis period.

Inflammatory conditions

Pericardial inflammation, pericarditis, can mimic ischaemic cardiac pain, although classically it varies with respiration and is described as more sharp and 'pleuritic'. The leading cause is a viral infection, often from the enterovirus group, particularly Coxsackie B, although followed by malignancy and then blunt trauma to the chest. The normal 15–60 ml fluid content of the pericardial space increases and, if developing rapidly, at 200–250 ml reaches the volume capacity. Any further accumulation produces a marked rise in pressure, creating a pericardial tamponade. In a more chronically developing problem, the volume of the space may reach 2 litres.

Clinically, the signs of fluid accumulation are classically described as Beck's triad:

- hypotension
- jugulovenous distension
- muffled heart sounds.

> The signs of fluid accumulation, referred to as Beck's triad include: hypotension, jugular venous distension and muffled heart sounds

There may be ECG changes to support the diagnosis. There is a gradual evolution from diffusely elevated and concave-shaped ST segments through to inverted T waves that may be permanent. It is possible for the ECG to be normal.

Physiologically, the tamponade raises intracardiac pressure and reduces ventricular filling producing a reduction in cardiac output.

Treatment is based on limiting the inflammatory process and uses non-steroidal anti-inflammatory drugs (NSAIDs), such as ibuprofen or indomethacin, and oral steroids, such as prednisolone. If there is evidence of cardiovascular compromise because of the size of the effusion, then drainage through pericardiocentesis is required. This may be ECG guided but is increasingly done under ultrasound control to try to reduce the incidence of complications that may be as high as 15%.

Myocarditis is a less easily recognised and diagnosed condition, and again is often the consequence of a viral infection, the same spectrum of pathogens as for pericardial disease. The patient may present with non-specific signs of infection, such as fever, general malaise and vomiting. Cardiac pain may be present but often there is simply evidence of cardiac failure. The

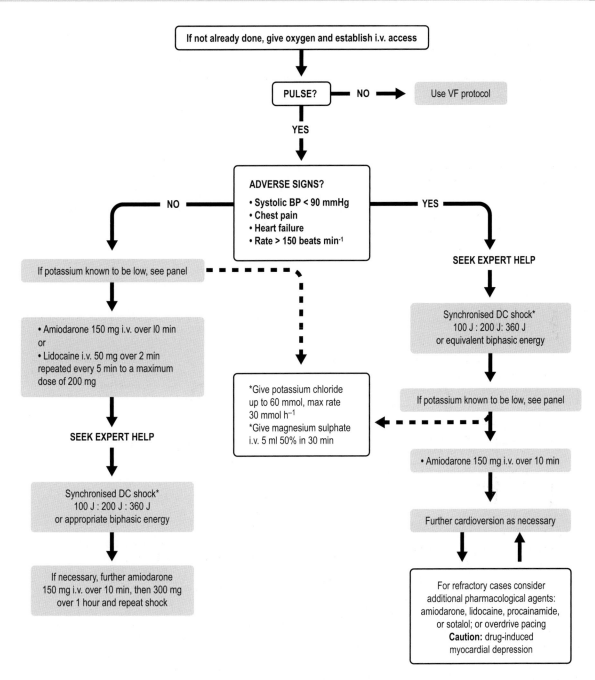

Figure 35.4 Treatment algorithm for broad complex tachycardia. BP, blood pressure; DC, direct current; IV, intravenous; VF, ventricular fibrillation. [© Resuscitation Council (UK), 2000.]

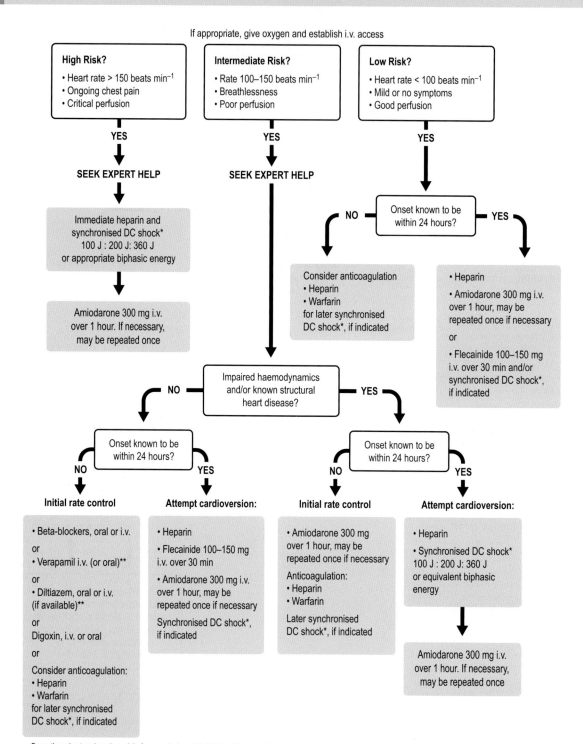

Figure 35.5 Treatment algorithm for atrial fibrillation. DC, direct current; IV, intravenous. [© Resuscitation Council (UK), 2000.]

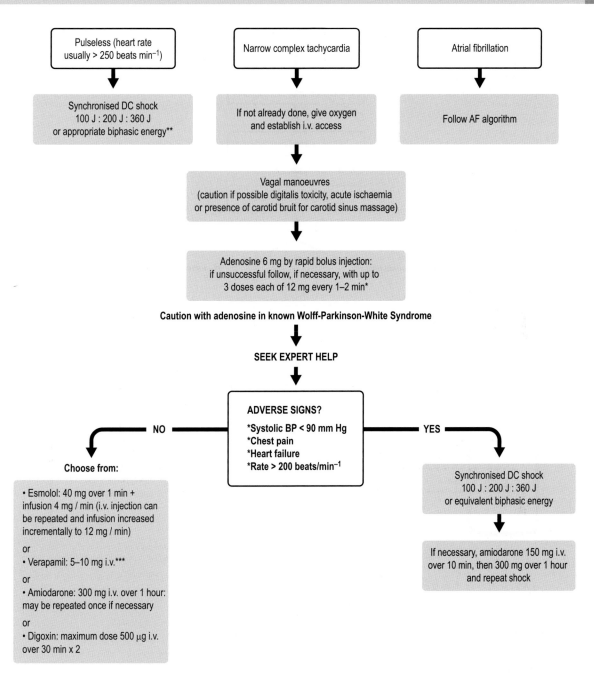

Figure 35.6 Treatment algorithm for narrow complex tachycardia. AF, atrial fibrillation; BP, blood pressure; DC, direct current; IV, intravenous. [© Resuscitation Council (UK), 2000.]

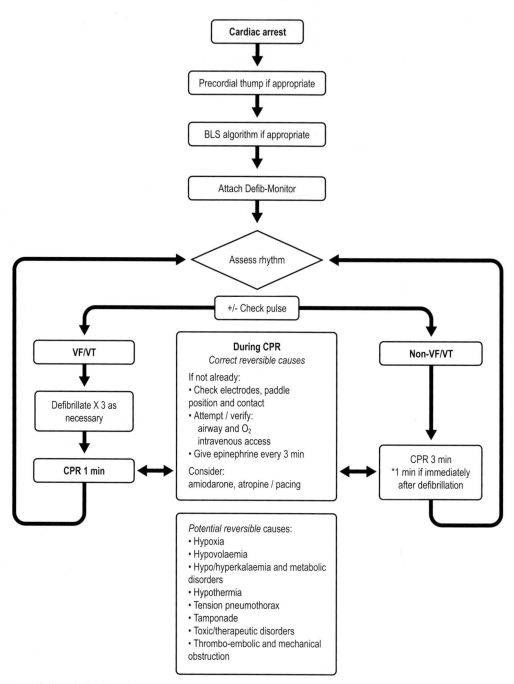

Figure 35.7 Universal algorithm for the management of cardiac arrest in adults. BLS, basic life support; CPR, cardiopulmonary resuscitation; Defib, defibrillator; VF, ventricular fibrillation; VT, ventricular tachycardia. [© Resuscitation Council (UK), 2000.]

inflammatory process within the myocardium increases the risk of dysrhythmias and these can be fatal. Current treatment is based on symptom relief and is supportive only.

Dehydration

While most medical causes of poor cardiovascular status are related to poor pump function, it is important not to forget that there may be hypovolaemia related to lack of intake, excess loss or 'third spacing'.

If fluid intake has been reduced for a prolonged period, for example, an elderly patient who has been immobile on the floor for many hours before being found, then, there may be simple dehydration present, responding rapidly to a careful intravenous fluid challenge.

Excess loss, through diarrhoeal illness, is the commonest cause of death of the young in many developing countries. Together with the electrolyte disturbance following profound diarrhoea, with the potential for severe hypokalaemia, dehydration from this source should be apparent. It is quite possible to be 15% dehydrated before cardiovascular instability presents.

An alternative route of loss is through excess urine production, the commonest being generated in a diabetic with hyperglycaemia, where the glucose acts as an osmotic diuretic. Again the dehydration can be massive.

Third spacing, as may occur with an intestinal ileus or with changes in capillary permeability and leakage of fluid into the interstitial space, as occurs in sepsis, may be less apparent but the patient is still intravascularly 'dry'.

Clinical presentation
The signs and symptoms as well as the different grades of hypovolaemic shock have already been discussed in Chapter 19. The first clinical signs appear in an adult when more than 750 ml has been lost from the intravascular space. There is a gradual development of tachycardia and tachypnoea, then elevation of the diastolic pressure to narrow the pulse pressure before a decrease in the systolic pressure with losses of over 1500 ml. At this point, there may be a deterioration in the mental state. Beyond this, the patient becomes

moribund and ultimately progresses to cardiac arrest of the pulseless electrical activity type through hypovolaemia.

Treatment and nursing care
In all of these cases, direct intravenous fluid replacement is the optimal treatment, with due regard to potential electrolyte disturbance. Judicious administration, gradually titrated to effect, is the ideal but the volume may be quite significant, in some cases of the order 5–6 litres.

As with all the conditions discussed, the goal of nursing care is to observe and maintain the airway, breathing, and circulation. Evaluating the patient's response to fluid resuscitation involves continuous monitoring of tissue perfusion indicators. Improvement in heart rate, blood pressure, skin temperature and moisture, urine output and level of consciousness are objective indicators of the adequacy of volume replacement.

DISABILITY

Once the airway, breathing and circulation have been assessed and attended to, the neurological state can be examined. The trauma neurological examination has been described in Chapters 22 and 25.

The medical examination mirrors this in terms of assessment of the level of consciousness with use of the AVPU scale, supplemented by the Glasgow Coma Score (GCS). The pupil size and reaction to light should be noted, together with any signs of deviation. In the range of medical emergencies, a focal neurological deficit may be more subtle and so careful assessment of the limb position and tone, together with assessment of motor power, sensory function and reflexes is needed. As for the traumatic head injury, the type and rate of change is as important as the actual deficit identified.

If the patient is responsive, a cognitive assessment should be carried out. Is the patient oriented in time, place and person? What is their short- and long-term memory function like? Can they perform the serial sevens (count backwards from 100 in multiples of 7)?

An acute confusional state is a common manifestation of a wide variety of medical conditions;

from hypoxia to inadequate perfusion through hypotension, from sepsis to drug-induced confusion. It does not necessarily indicate cerebral pathology. A thorough physical examination and blood testing for evidence of anaemia, neutrophilia, electrolyte disturbance and glucose level is indicated.

More specific acute neurological problems (Box 35.8) are considered below.

Cerebrovascular event or stroke

Stroke can be best defined as destruction of brain tissue as a result of a vascular event and leading to neurological impairment. The origin in 80% of strokes is due to occlusion of a cerebral vessel by atherosclerotic thrombus or embolism. The remaining 20% are due to haemorrhage and are considered separately. Interruption of the blood supply to brain tissue, which is highly dependent on continual oxygen and glucose supplies, produces rapid loss of function. Over the next 2 hours or so, there are changes in ion flux across the neuronal membranes but the situation is salvageable. Beyond this time, there is irreversible cell injury and the development of local oedema.

In many cases, the origin of the occlusion is described as thrombotic. The pathophysiological process is identical to that producing myocardial infarction. The development of atherosclerosis as a result of age, smoking, obesity, hypertension, hypercholesterolaemia and diabetes produces vessel wall plaques that fissure and result in accu-

mulation of a platelet plug, occluding the vessel. Vasculitis through an autoimmune process, such as giant cell arteritis, may also cause thrombus formation.

A significant number of occlusions result from embolism of platelet clumps from either the carotid vessels (arterioarterial), where the atherosclerotic plaques in the common carotid and its bifurcation have generated platelet plugs, or from the heart. Here the source may be mural thrombus over an area of infarcted myocardium, thrombus within the left atrium in atrial fibrillation or even fragments formed on damaged valves in valvular heart disease.

Clinical presentation
The nature of the focal neurological deficit depends on the location within the brain and there is a clear anatomical/clinical correlation (Table 35.1). The internal carotid arteries divide into anterior and middle cerebral arteries supplying the internal capsule, the frontal lobes and the motor and sensory cortices. The vertebrobasilar arteries supply the brainstem, cerebellum and posterior aspects of the cortex.

Treatment and nursing care
Treatment of a thrombotic or embolic stroke is somewhat controversial at present. Since the pathological process mirrors that in the heart there

---

Box 35.8   Neurological emergencies

Destructive
- Stroke
  - Thrombotic
  - Embolic
- Reversible ischaemic neurological deficit (RIND)
- Transient ischaemic attack (TIA)

Compressive
- Intracranial haemorrhage
- Subarachnoid haemorrhage

Functional
- Seizures
- Epilepsy

Table 35.1   Pattern of stroke syndromes

Artery	Symptoms and signs
Anterior cerebral	Confusion and changes in personality, weakness of opposite lower limb, impaired sensation paralleling weakness
Middle cerebral	Hemiparesis, sensory changes paralleling weakness, loss of half visual field, aphasia
Posterior cerebral	Blindness in half visual field, cortical blindness, lack of visual recognition, altered mental state
Vertebrobasilar	Vertigo and nystagmus, dysphagia, visual field defects, increased muscle tone and ataxia, contralateral pain and temperature sense loss, altered sensation and weakness of the affected side of the face

has been a great deal of interest in the use of thrombolysis. Some very impressive results have been achieved in carefully selected patients in controlled clinical trials where the cause can be determined not to be haemorrhagic by rapid access to CT scanning, and therapy can be administered early. However, there is also a significant increase in deterioration owing to bleeding into the infarcting tissue and extension of the neurological deficit, in some cases sufficient to cause death (Fauci et al., 1999). Currently, thrombolysis should be restricted to clinical trials.

Supportive treatment with supplemental oxygen and intravenous fluids to maintain hydration is indicated. Care must be taken not to overhydrate and increase the risk of generating cerebral oedema. Nursing with the head of the bed slightly elevated may also help to reduce the extent of the oedema. If the patient is hypertensive, then intravenous medication should be used to gradually control it and bring it towards the normal range. Careful monitoring is indicated since the stroke process may still be evolving and there may be further deterioration. There are a number of recognised scaling systems for reporting the severity of a stroke and these can be used to monitor this (Brott et al., 1989).

Approximately 5% of stroke patients will develop seizure activity following the insult and require treatment. The cerebral oedema that develops over the first 48 hours is sufficient to produce a mass effect in approximately 40% of cases. Measures, such as mannitol and furosemide administration, may be indicated to try to limit this (Oppenheimer et al., 1992).

Investigation for an embolic cause requires an ECG and screening for myocardial injury markers. Atrial fibrillation may suggest an atrial thrombus; evidence of a myocardial infarct would suggest a mural thrombus. Duplex scanning of the common carotid vessels may show a significant stenosis. If any of these are present, then anticoagulation, with heparin in the first instance and then warfarin or coumarin in the medium term, are warranted. Significant carotid disease may warrant early endarterectomy (Albers et al., 1999).

The use of antiplatelet medication is an accepted standard of care. Aspirin is the current agent of choice, although the dose is not clearly defined. Other newer agents, such as clopidogrel, have also been shown to be effective at reducing the risk of recurrence (Albers et al., 1999). Other therapies, such as free-radical scavengers, and particularly the calcium-channel blockers, such as nimodipine, are being investigated, but remain experimental (Rosen and Barkin, 1998).

The goals of nursing care involve accurate documentation of the changes in neurological status and interventions to prevent further complications. Careful assessment of the airway and monitoring of the patient's respiratory status are required. Supplemental oxygen should be administered to ensure optimal oxygenation of the brain, and changes to the breathing pattern sought and noted. Measures to prevent complications, such as aspiration, are essential.

Intravenous access should be established and fluids given to maintain the state of hydration. A regular vital sign assessment and continuous cardiac monitoring should take place and a level of consciousness evaluation should be ongoing. Initially, pupil size, responsiveness and equality, together with neurological function of the limbs, should be assessed every 15 minutes to detect any impending deterioration.

> The goals of nursing care involve accurate documentation of the changes in neurological status and interventions to prevent further complications

Ischaemic neurological deficit and transient ischaemic attack

Reversible ischaemic neurological deficit (RIND) and transient ischaemic attack (TIA) form a spectrum of neurological impairment that may present as a stroke but then resolve completely. TIAs are said to clear within 24 hours, although many resolve within 15–20 minutes. RIND may take up to a week to recover (Fauci et al., 1999). The pathological process is thought to mirror that of stroke and might be regarded as the 'less severe' end of a continuous disease spectrum.

In the absence of a clear cardiac embolic cause, routine anticoagulation is not warranted as prophylaxis against further episodes (Liu et al., 2002) and it may even increase the risk of haemorrhage (Algra et al., 2002). The routine use of antiplatelet drugs, such as aspirin and clopidogrel, is the standard of care (Albers et al., 1999).

Intracerebral haemorrhage

Approximately 20% of strokes are caused by a bleed into the brain tissue. Clinically, they may be indistinguishable from a thrombotic or embolic insult, but cause their damage both by local tissue destruction and by pressure on other parts of the brain. They usually occur in the area of the basal ganglia and are linked to hypertensive disease. Alternatively, they may arise from a congenital arteriovenous malformation in any part of the brain. They tend to be found in younger people presenting with a clinical picture of a stroke.

The size of the bleed has a prognostic significance. If the lesion is larger than 5 cm diameter as measured on CT scan, then it is almost universally fatal. While treatment is supportive, as for the other types of stroke, anticoagulation or even thrombolysis are contraindicated.

Subarachnoid haemorrhage

Subarachnoid haemorrhage (SAH) can sometimes follow an extensive intracerebral haemorrhage, but also occurs as a separate clinical entity. Approximately 6% of the population can be identified as having an aneurysmal swelling of one or more of the arteries in the circle of Willis at the base of the brain. When one of these leaks, often only a little, the patient reports a headache and demonstrates signs of meningism (photophobia, neck stiffness). Classically, the headache comes on suddenly ('like I was hit over the head with a spade') and is described as the worst headache that they have ever experienced.

Diagnosis, beyond clinical suspicion, is with CT scanning that shows evidence of bleeding in approximately 90% of cases. If investigation has been initiated, then there is an obligation to follow through with a lumbar puncture to look for xanthochromia (colouring of the cerebrospinal fluid with blood pigment at 6 hours after the onset) to detect those missed by the scan and exclude the condition with any certainty. Full evaluation requires angiography to show the location of the aneurysm.

Table 35.2 Grading system for subarachnoid haemorrhage

Grade	Clinical	Survival
I	Normal MS, no deficit, no meningism	70%
II	Mildly altered MS, focal deficit, severe headache	60%
III	Major alteration in consciousness, mild focal neurological deficit	50%
IV	Stupor, hemiparesis, early decerebrate rigidity	40%
V	Deep coma, decerebrate rigidity, moribund	10%

MS, mental state.

There may often be a 'herald bleed' or small bleed initially and, without neurosurgical intervention, there may be a further extensive and possibly fatal bleed in the following days. Neurosurgical assessment of the severity is based on a well-established grading system (Table 35.2; Alvord et al., 1972).

Management is aimed towards optimising the patient's clinical condition with adequate oxygenation and normalisation of the blood pressure. The use of calcium-channel blockers, specifically nimodipine, is recommended to limit the extent of any arterial vasospasm that may result, increasing the ischaemia to the surrounding brain. A decision is made by the neurosurgeons about evacuation of the haematoma and clipping of the aneurysm based on the clinical condition.

Nursing care related to raised intracranial pressure

The skull is a rigid bone structure containing brain tissue (80% of volume), cerebrospinal fluid (CSF) and blood (20% of volume). The space within the adult cranium is constant and, therefore, any increase in content will result in an increase in the intracranial pressure (ICP). Physiological compensatory mechanisms are present to regulate pressure fluctuations with changes in blood volume within the cerebral circulation. There is a limit to the extent of this adaptation and, beyond this point, there is a rapid increase in pressure.

Specific signs and symptoms of raised intracranial pressure are usually divided into early and late findings (Box 35.9).

Box 35.9   Clinical features of raised intracranial pressure

Early findings
- Decreased LOC
- Pupillary dysfunction
- Limb motor weakness
- Limb sensory deficit
- Cranial nerve palsies (III, IV, VI)
- Headache
- Seizures

Late findings
- Further deterioration in LOC
- Vomiting
- Papilloedema
- Severe headache
- Hemiplegia
- Decorticate or decerebrate limb position
- Changes in vital signs (hypertension, bradycardia, abnormal respiratory pattern), the Cushing reflex
- Impaired brainstem reflexes

LOC, level of consciousness.

The initial management and care of patients suffering an intracranial or subarachnoid bleed mirrors the priorities as with other trauma and critically ill patients: attention to the airway (with due regard to the cervical spine), breathing and circulation. Management principles are aimed at maximising cerebral tissue perfusion (Table 35.3).

Seizures

A seizure or fit is the clinical presentation of an abnormal increase in electrical activity within the brain. It may occur as a result of a stimulus, such as repeated stimulation (e.g. flashing lights), or as a consequence of injury to the brain (e.g. oedema) and necrosis following a stroke or head injury. If seizures occur repeatedly over a period of time and without a clear cause, then the term epilepsy is used.

The full manifestation of the fit will depend on the focus for the increased activity. In the temporal lobes, there may be absence attacks that may self-terminate or progress to generalised convulsions. If the origin is within the motor area of the parietal lobe, then a tonic–clonic seizure may be the first feature.

From a trauma patient perspective, an epileptic will need their regular medication continued during their trauma care. A fall in the anti-convulsant level concentration will predispose the patient to fits and potentially complicate their other care.

While most convulsions will terminate within a matter of 7–8 minutes, this is not always the case. Status epilepticus (SE) is the term used for persistent seizure activity, although there is some variation in its definition. The definition adopted internationally is 'a seizure that persists for a sufficiently long period of time or is repeated frequently enough to produce a fixed or enduring

Table 35.3   Management of raised intracranial pressure (ICP)

Nursing goals	Nursing actions
Maintain adequate oxygenation and ventilation	Ensure an adequate airway Suction secretions, as necessary Administration of supplemental oxygen Pulse oximetry monitoring Maintain PaO_2 and $PaCO_2$ within agreed parameters
Administration of medication	Follow local policy – drugs may include: frusemide and mannitol, barbiturates, anticonvulsants and steroids Sedation and paralysing agents Analgesia for pain relief Inotropes may be required to maintain cerebral perfusion pressure
Prevent further rises in ICP	Positioning to facilitate venous return: head of bed at 30°–45° angle, neutral head alignment, minimal hip flexion Avoid pressures on neck, e.g. tight ET tapes, cervical collar Avoid clustering of activities during nursing care

epileptic condition' (Lowenstein, 1999). In essence, this means that, if two or more seizures occur without full recovery and the duration has lasted for more than 30 minutes, then it is status epilepticus. Consciousness is not regained and, therefore, airway maintenance and respiratory status can be compromised.

Status epilepticus has a mortality rate of 10% (Butler and Lewis, 2001) with complications arising from persistent hypoxia, aspiration, hyperthermia and even rhabdomyolysis. It has a variable response to treatment depending on the underlying origin. That owing to anoxic brain injury or stroke has a longer duration, is more resistant to treatment and has a far worse outcome than that owing to a metabolic photosensitive trigger.

Treatment follows an 'escalating ladder' of therapy (Figure 35.8; Bleck, 1999). Once level four is reached there is a need to secure the airway by endotracheal intubation and mechanical ventilation is needed. Traditionally, in the UK, a thiopentone infusion to produce a barbiturate coma was the preferred therapy but, over the last decade, propofol has been increasingly used. If using these anaesthetic drugs, then EEG monitoring for seizure activity is necessary to ensure that cerebral seizure activity has been suppressed.

Nursing interventions for generalised tonic–clonic status epilepticus are those similar to those discussed under stroke. If intravenous phenytoin is used, then blood pressure and continuous cardiac monitoring are essential, since it can cause hypotension and dysrhythmias during adminis-

tration. Vital signs should be assessed frequently including temperature because of the possibility of hyperthermia.

During seizures there is an increased risk of injury to the patient and to carers. Caution should be taken when handling sharps, bed rails should be padded and the patient must never be left unattended. It should be remembered that fits can be extremely distressing to family members and they too may require support. Once a seizure has terminated, the patient falls into a postictal state that may last from a few minutes to several hours. During this time, they may be drowsy and irritable. There may be a focal neurological weakness, termed Todd's paralysis, or even neurogenic pulmonary oedema.

ENDOCRINE

Endocrine problems are largely a medical issue; however, when adequately treated, patients can lead almost normal lives and can sustain traumatic injury just like the remainder of the population. In this section, issues related to the ongoing care of some of these conditions and how they may be exacerbated by the stress of traumatic injury will be considered. These conditions are:

- diabetes mellitus – hypoglycaemia and ketoacidosis;
- thyroid disorders – thyroid crisis;
- Addison's disease – Addisonian crisis.

Diabetes mellitus

Diabetes is a disease in which control of glucose metabolism has been lost. It is very common, affecting 2% of the British population. There are two main types. In type 1 (insulin-dependent diabetes mellitus; IDDM) there is a loss of β cells within the islets of Langerhans in the pancreas and loss of capacity to produce insulin. In type 2 (non-insulin-dependent diabetes mellitus; NIDDM) there is increased resistance to the effect of insulin at the target cells. Type 1 can only be managed by regular injection of exogenous insulin; type 2 can often be managed by dietary control of carbohydrate ingestion and the use of oral agents to increase the production of insulin or inhibit the production of glucose by the liver.

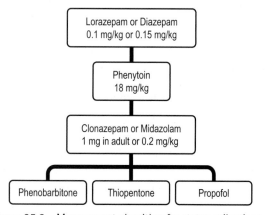

Figure 35.8　Management algorithm for status epilepticus.

In general, the events surrounding a traumatic injury will result in a stress response. This consists of changes driven by both a neurogenic and a hormonal pathway, producing a rapid change followed by a more sustained alteration in metabolism. For a diabetic, the end result is an increase in serum glucose concentration and, in addition, the hypercatabolic state and the poor oral intake in the postinjury phase will disrupt the usual control. Anticipation of potential problems will mean that treatment can be started early. There may need to be an increase in the frequency of glucose monitoring and the introduction of a sliding scale intravenous insulin infusion based on the blood glucose level.

The two main conditions that occur in diabetes, which may be potentially life threatening, are hypoglycaemia and diabetic ketoacidosis.

Hypoglycaemia

Diabetic patients who are insulin dependent (i.e. type 1) are at the greatest risk of developing hypoglycaemia; however, it can occur in those with type 2 and other patients. When the serum glucose falls below the normal range, the patient experiences symptoms that they often recognise. The spectrum varies between patients but is based on a general increase in sympathetic activity.

The early signs and symptoms of hypoglycaemia include weakness and hunger together with sweating, a tremor, palpitations and a tachycardia. Later signs include altered vision, irritability, confusion, slurred speech and amnesia. If left untreated, this will progress to loss of consciousness, fitting and even death.

Treatment and nursing care   A thorough assessment of the patient following the ABC approach is necessary. This should include a full history of events, if possible, the monitoring of all vital signs including temperature, and blood glucose measurements (both reagent strips and formal laboratory tests).

Rapid recognition and treatment are vital to ensure a positive outcome. Treatment is based upon provision of glucose. If the patient is awake and has a gag reflex, oral glucose can be administered. This can be achieved by giving a fast-acting sugar in the form of a drink, such as

Lucozade™ or milk, and then a longer-acting carbohydrate, such as found in biscuits or sandwiches. If the patient is unresponsive, treatment is by rapid administration of an intravenous bolus of 25% or 50% glucose. In the absence of vascular access, then an intramuscular injection of the hormone glucagon (1 mg) will drive the release of glucose from the glycogen stores within the liver.

Once the glucose level has been returned to the normal range, attention to the underlying cause for the hypoglycaemia is needed. Further carbohydrates may be required.

Diabetic ketoacidosis

Diabetic ketoacidosis (DKA) is a biochemical state where insulin, required for the transport of glucose into cells, has been deficient for some time. The cells, unable to use the serum glucose, become hypoglycaemic and generate a 'stress response', producing a serum hyperglycaemia. The cells, still unable to access the glucose, switch their metabolism to use long-chain fatty acids and amino acids for energy. Over several hours, the altered biochemistry produces a dehydrated and acidotic patient with a profound electrolyte disturbance.

Found in type 1 diabetics, DKA is most commonly a result of inadequate insulin administration in response to an underlying infection or physical stress, such as occurs after injury. Inadequate education may mean that insulin is not given if they do not eat or is not increased adequately for the stress response. It can also occur in type 2 diabetes, but residual β-cell insulin production tends to limit this.

In the typical presentation, the clinical picture is one of raised blood sugar, nausea and vomiting, dehydration and feeling generally 'unwell' (Table 35.4). The diagnosis may be more difficult if this is the first presentation of an individual not known to be diabetic, or if other symptoms and injuries serve to mask the ketoacidosis.

Treatment and nursing care   Nursing care should be aimed at the rapid identification and treatment of DKA. It should focus on frequent assessment of the respiratory and haemodynamic status, fluid resuscitation, correction of electrolyte imbalance, careful insulin administration and monitoring of glucose levels.

Table 35.4   Presentation of ketoacidosis

History	Examination
Classic symptoms of hyperglycaemia Increased thirst Increased frequency of urination	**General signs** Ill appearance Dry skin Laboured respirations Dry mucus membranes Decreased skin turgidity
Other symptoms Generalised weakness Malaise/lethargy Nausea/vomiting Abdominal pain Decreased perspiration Fatigue Confusion	**Vital signs** Tachycardia Hypotension Tachypnoea Hypothermia Fever, if infection present Vague abdominal tenderness
Symptoms associated with infections Fever Chills Chest pain Shortness of breath	**Specific signs** Confusion Kussmaul breathing Ketotic breath (not universally present) Coma

Airway support may be required depending on the degree of neurological impairment; a profoundly comatose patient will require intubation and assisted ventilation. High-flow oxygen via a non-rebreathing mask with a reservoir should be administered to reduce tissue hypoxia caused by acidosis. Intravenous access must be obtained with separate lines for the insulin infusion and rehydration fluids. Treatment is aimed at reversing the severe dehydration and, together with the careful administration of intravenous insulin, will gradually reverse the clinical picture that has developed.

Regular pulse and blood pressure measurements, together with hourly observation of the urine output, are required to assess how the patient is responding to rehydration. To this end, a urinary catheter should be inserted at an early stage.

There are also a number of electrolyte disturbances that develop in DKA and they need to be anticipated. The most significant of these is a hypokalaemia and continuous cardiac monitoring should take place to detect dyrrhythmias resulting

from this; a 12-lead ECG may provide further evidence. Potassium supplementation in the rehydration fluid is essential and should be titrated to serum measurement.

Thyroid disorders

Thyroid disease, whether hypothyroidism or hyperthyroidism, is usually a slow and insidious problem. An event causing physical stress, such as traumatic injury, may exacerbate an underlying condition, precipitating its presentation or distorting regular treatment.

Hypothyroidism presents in a non-specific manner with lethargy, weakness and intolerance of cold environments. There are physical changes to the appearance including coarsening of facial and scalp hair and weight gain. There is a decrease in physical activity, even hypothermia, and a loss of mental agility. In the injured patient in an untreated and even undiagnosed state, the slowed metabolism can cause widespread difficulties. There is often depression of respiratory function and even a relative hypoglycaemia. The body response to stress is obtunded. Drug metabolism is impaired, and delayed handling and excretion may lead to toxic consequences.

Management, after confirmation of the diagnosis, is through titrated replacement of thyroxine. This can be given orally, if the patient can tolerate it, although an intravenous formulation is available. Specific assessment of the adequacy of respiratory function and drug level monitoring will be needed.

Hyperthyroidism is a far more dangerous condition. It presents in a wide variety of non-specific ways: tremor, agitation and anxiety, chest pain, shortness of breath and palpitations, even nausea, vomiting and abdominal pain. Medically, it is sought as one of the causes for new-onset dysrhythmias, such as atrial fibrillation. Treatment is targeted at reducing the production of thyroid hormone through the regular use of propylthiouracil. In the longer term, radioactive iodine may be used to eliminate some of the thyroid gland.

Thyroid crisis
Thyroid crisis is rare; approximately 1% of patients with hyperthyroidism will ever experience it

(Kitt et al., 1995). The most common precipitating factors include trauma, infection and metabolic disturbances.

The classic features of a crisis include tachycardia, palpitations, a high fever, anxiety and diarrhoea. Other features include dysrhythmias, dyspnoea, electrolyte disturbance and weight loss. Atrial fibrillation and SVT are the most common rhythm disturbances, together with high-output cardiac failure (Rosen and Barkin, 1998). Serum glucose and calcium levels may be elevated and, depending on the degree of dehydration, other electrolytes may be abnormal.

Treatment and nursing care   Treatment is based on adrenergic blockade, typically using propranolol intravenously, together with specific treatment for the clinical presentation, such as paracetamol for the fever, atrioventricular conduction-slowing drugs, such as digoxin or amiodarone, for dysrhythmias, and diuretics and nitrates for the heart failure (Rosen and Barkin, 1998).

All patients should have cardiac monitoring and a 12-lead ECG is also indicated. Patients in thyroid crisis frequently have fevers up to 41°C; therefore, continuous monitoring of a central core temperature is necessary. Aggressive cooling can be accomplished via cooling blankets, although shivering has to be avoided, since this will further generate heat. Severe dehydration due to sweating, diarrhoea and hyperthermia may occur. Adequate fluid volume and electrolyte replacement is needed. Frequent assessment of the vital signs and urinary output should be performed.

Addison's disease

Addison's disease or adrenocortical insufficiency is a relatively rare condition in which there is a deficiency in the production of corticoid hormone by the adrenal gland. There are a wide variety of causes (Box 35.10).

Under normal circumstances, this is a slowly progressive disease. As adrenal function declines, there is weakness, lethargy, nausea and even vomiting and, eventually, a classic hyperpigmentation of the skin. Management is with oral glucocorticoid supplementation with hydrocortisone in doses of the order 20–30 mg per day. If a patient has been on medium- or long-term oral steroid

---

> **Box 35.10   Causes of adrenal insufficiency**
>
> **Primary**
> - Autoimmune
> - Connective tissue disease
> - Infection
>
> **Secondary**
> - Pituitary infarction
> - Pituitary infection
> - Head trauma
>
> **Functional**

therapy, then the hypothalamic–pituitary–adrenal axis has been suppressed – the functional cause of adrenal dysfunction.

Addisonian crisis

The normal physiological response to stress includes an increase in the endogenous production of glucocorticoids. Patients who are unable to mount an appropriate increase may suffer an Addisonian crisis. Traumatic injury, burns, surgery and even a myocardial infarction can all induce a crisis.

The patient with Addisonian crisis may begin with a wide variety of vague complaints, such as weakness and nausea but, without treatment, will progress to a serious combination of hypotension and hypoglycaemia. There may also be a disturbance of electrolytes with hyponatraemia, hyperkalaemia and hypercalcaemia.

Treatment and nursing care   Treatment requires the replacement of the missing glucocorticoids. This may be either hydrocortisone, the standard therapy or, if cortisol levels are to be measured to confirm the diagnosis, dexamethasone given intraveneously. In addition, steps to correct the electrolytes will be needed. The patients are often volume depleted by up to 20% and require rehydration.

Nursing care should concentrate on administration of steroids, and correction of fluid deficit and hypoglycaemia. Fluid balance needs to be carefully monitored and a urinary catheter should be considered to measure the hourly output accurately. Vomiting can be eased by inserting a nasogastric tube.

Vital signs should be monitored frequently and invasive monitoring may be required. Because of the potential for cardiac disturbances, a 12-lead ECG should be performed and continuous cardiac monitoring maintained.

POISONING AND SUBSTANCE ABUSE

Poisoning covers a very wide spectrum of problems and the intention here is to cover general principles, and consider some of the more common presentations and their management. While not directly relevant to the management of the trauma patient, injury is often sustained while under the influence of drugs, particularly those of recreation.

Poisoning may be the result of a deliberate attempt to self-harm, either a parasuicide or failed suicide attempt (e.g. paracetamol); alternatively, it may be a consequence of the use of drugs for personal pleasure (e.g. cocaine). There may be an ingestion in addition to a fall from height in someone who has attempted suicide, or they may have been experiencing drug-induced delusions or hallucinations and believed that they were 'able to fly'. It may be even be the result of an occupational or accidental exposure to a noxious chemical (e.g. cyanide).

The first concern is for the safety of the carer. Is there any risk of 'off gassing' or absorption through the skin? For example, if patients have sheep dip (organophosphate) on their clothing, then handling them without protective clothing and a respirator may result in staff members becoming significantly poisoned too! Once staff safety has been assured, then the principles of management fall back to the traditional ABC. While assessing these, a search for the causative agent should be made. This may be available from the history, either from the patient or an accompanying person, from the description by the ambulance crew, or even by searching the patient's possessions. A medical prescription, an empty tablet bottle or even the equipment for use of recreational drugs (e.g. needles and syringes, blackened spoon or rolled silver paper) would suggest this. Clearly the patient's consent will be needed if their conscious level is not impaired, but is justified under common law if they are obtunded.

A full set of clinical physiological signs should be taken and documented. Beyond the usual pulse rate, blood pressure and oxygen saturation, a core temperature, formal measurement of the respiratory rate and a 12-lead ECG are necessary.

A search for 'track marks', the tell-tale signs of repeated injection drug use, should be sought. The forearms and antecubital fossae are well known. Less obvious sites, such as the dorsum of the foot, around the ankle and between the toes are used by some, others use their femoral vessels almost exclusively. Another option to consider, particularly if the patient has come from an airport or other point of entry into the country, is the possibility of 'body packing', where large quantities of drugs have been ingested for smuggling purposes and the 'protective' packaging has burst.

With the baseline clinical picture and an idea of the causative agent, information resources on the most up-to-date method of management should be checked. Traditionally, in the UK, this has been through a telephone helpline to the Poisons Information Service, but with the ever-increasing service workload and the development of web-based technology, the use of internet access to Toxbase™ is rapidly becoming the standard. Telephone support is still available for the more difficult situations.

All episodes of poisoning that impair consciousness fall broadly into one of four 'toxic syndromes' (Table 35.5). There are also a variety of cardiotoxic and hepatotoxic agents that present relatively frequently, such as quinine and paracetamol.

The remainder of this section will briefly consider the principles of management of the more common poisonings seen in the UK:

● paracetamol
● aspirin
● tricyclic antidepressants
● benzodiazepines
● narcotics
● amphetamines.

Paracetamol

Paracetamol (acetaminophen in the USA) is an oral analgesic and antipyretic that is a component of a wide variety of proprietary medications

Table 35.5 Toxic syndromes (Kulig, 1992)

Syndrome	Signs	Causes
Sympathomimetic	Tachycardia, hypertension, fever, sweating, increased muscle tone, paranoia, delusions, fits	Amphetamines, ecstasy, LSD, cocaine
Sedative	Bradycardia, hypotension, hypothermia, respiratory depression, coma	Benzodiazepines, narcotics, barbiturates, alcohol
Cholinergic	Confusion, sedation, weakness, salivation, vomiting, cramps, incontinence, fits	Organophosphates, some mushrooms
Anticholinergic	Tachycardia, dry flushed skin, fever, increased muscle tone, retention of urine, fits, dysrhythmias	Neuroleptics, tricyclic antidepressants, antihistamines

available for purchase over-the-counter (OTC). Its ready availability means that it is one of the most frequent substances used in deliberate self-poisoning.

An estimate of time of ingestion is needed to determine treatment. If the tablets were taken within the hour, then there may be some benefit to oral administration of activated charcoal to adsorb and hold some of the paracetamol within the bowel. Peak plasma concentrations are generally reached at 4 hours post-ingestion and a serum paracetamol level is required at this point. With this result, a decision can be made regarding the need for the intravenous administration of N-acetylcysteine (NAC; Parvolex™). This is done using a form of the Rumack–Matthew nomogram (Figure 35.9).

The time since ingestion is plotted against the serum level. If the concentration lies above the toxicity line, then protective therapy is warranted. If it lies below, then NAC is not indicated. The upper line on the nomogram applies to those with no risk factors for increased toxicity, the lower for those who might be anticipated to be sensitive. Treatment consists of a 16-hour infusion of NAC with 5% dextrose. As the nomogram suggests, there may be benefit to administration of supplementary glutathione for up to 24 hours after ingestion.

If NAC is administered sufficiently early, then the degree of hepatic damage can be minimised and liver failure avoided. If significant hepatic damage is going to occur, then between 24 and 48 hours after ingestion, the patient will begin to develop nausea, vomiting and tenderness over the liver. Blood testing will show the liver enzymes

aspartate transaminase (AST) and alanine transaminase (ALT) rising and evidence that clotting is impaired, with a prolonged prothrombin time. At 72 hours, dysfunction will either peak and begin to recover or progress to hepatic failure. If this occurs, then hepatic transplantation will probably be required. At the same time, a proportion of patients also develop proteinuria and haematuria, as renal impairment begins.

Aspirin

Aspirin is also an OTC medication found in many proprietary 'cold' remedies. Assessment of the degree of poisoning may be complicated by 'delayed release' formulations.

In the patient who has ingested a large quantity of aspirin, gastric lavage (to remove any coalesced and solidified aspirin) and repeated activated charcoal administrations are recommended. A serum salicylate (aspirin) level should be taken at a minimum of 6 hours after ingestion and the level matched to a Done (1960) nomogram. If this is above the risk level, then treatment is warranted. If the level is non-toxic but the patient symptomatic, then a repeat level 2 hours later is indicated to detect continued rising salicylate levels through delayed intestinal absorption.

Toxic symptoms begin with stimulation of the respiratory centre and an increase in minute ventilation. The increase is entirely due to deeper breaths rather than respiratory rate. Associated with the respiratory alkalosis may be paraesthesia in the fingers and around the lips. There may be tinnitus and even impaired hearing. With more severe toxicity, vomiting and progressive

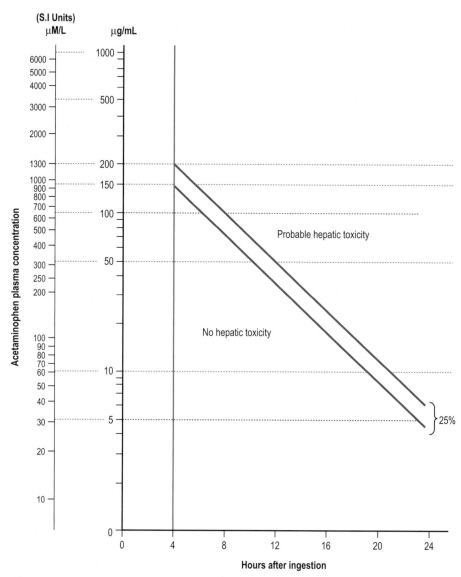

Figure 35.9 Rumack–Matthew nomogram for paracetamol toxicity.

dehydration may occur, together with electrolyte and acid–base disturbance. Hypoglycaemia can be produced. Pulmonary oedema and even cerebral oedema can develop.

Treatment of at-risk aspirin poisoning is based on three approaches (Box 35.11).

Rehydration using crystalloid solutions should be targeted to produce a diuresis of 2–3 ml/kg per hour. Some authorities also encourage alkalin-isation of the urine to enhance salicylate excretion;

this is achieved through the administration of intravenous sodium bicarbonate. The other major electrolyte disturbance is hypokalaemia; potassium supplementation may be required.

Tricyclic antidepressants

Tricyclic antidepressants (TCA) are widely used in the group of patients most prone to deliberate self-harm. Poisoning with this group of agents is

> **Box 35.11   Approaches to the treatment of aspirin poisoning**
>
> ● Prevent further absorption
> ● Correct metabolic disturbance and dehydration
> ● Enhance excretion of salicylate

relatively common in British Emergency Departments.

The signs of toxicity with these agents relate to their anticholinergic effects. Absorption is delayed through reduction of gastric motility and this means that gastric lavage is often of value in the first few hours. Administration of activated charcoal is also warranted.

Patients often have a tachycardia and there may be a degree of hypotension. These are managed expectantly and by intravenous crystalloid fluid administration. Cardiovascular toxicity is relatively high and, through effects on the sodium channels of the myocardium, the QRS complex broadens. This may progress to ventricular tachycardia and other potentially fatal dysrhythmias. Cerebral effects include agitation and delirium with increased muscle tone and hyper-reflexia, and this progresses to significant depression in the level of consciousness. Fits are relatively common, but bear no relation to the level of consciousness. Other anticholinergic effects include the development of an intestinal ileus and urinary retention.

Treatment is entirely supportive. With the obtunded level of consciousness it may be necessary to secure the airway through endotracheal intubation. Acidosis increases the risk of cardiac problems and so adequate ventilation to avoid the development of a respiratory acidosis is advisable. Insertion of a nasogastric tube to administer the activated charcoal and manage the ileus, together with urinary catheterisation may be necessary.

If the QRS complex broadens significantly or a dysrhythmia does develop, then intravenous sodium bicarbonate to alkalinise the serum mildly is the treatment of choice. The standard anti-arrhythmics used in cardiac disease have little effect. Fitting is managed with benzodiazepines and then barbiturates. Use of phenytoin in the presence of the myocardial complications can precipitate further dysrhythmias.

Benzodiazepines

These may be taken during an episode of deliberate self-harm, but they are also used, often in combination, as drugs of recreation. They are purely sedative and amnesic.

The danger with these agents lies beyond simple drowsiness and lethargy with associate amnesia. With deeper sedation, hypothermia and respiratory depression, with potential loss of airway control, can develop.

Poisoning is managed simply by maintaining the airway and ensuring adequate ventilation until liver metabolism eliminates the agent. Flumazenil, as a benzodiazepine antagonist, is available and can be used, but there is a significant risk of inducing convulsions. Few Emergency Departments use it routinely and then only to ensure adequate self-ventilation rather than aiming for complete restoration of level of consciousness.

Narcotics

Diamorphine/heroin and other chemically similar drugs derived from the opium poppy have been drugs of 'recreation' for thousands of years. They are one of the commonest causes of death from self-poisoning.

Opiates as a chemical group are analgesic and depress respiration through a reduction in the respiratory rate. Administration is either through snorting to the nasal mucosa, where absorption is rapid or through intravenous injection. In both cases, the clinical effect has a rapid onset. Excess produces apnoea and depression of the level of consciousness, together with meiosis and nausea. If they survive the profound respiratory depression, a significant proportion develop a pulmonary oedema 12–24 hours after the event.

Management in the acute stage is through maintenance of the airway and assistance of ventilation, aiming for maintenance of adequate oxygenation and a normal pCO_2. An opiate antagonist, naloxone, is available and can be used. When given, the patient will regain consciousness and often becomes combative; they may even develop symptoms of acute withdrawal. The effective half-life of naloxone is 20 minutes when given intravenously and 4 hours when given intramuscularly. If full consciousness is returned, the patients have a tendency to self-discharge from hospital and, once the 'antidote' has cleared, the opiate remains in the circulation unopposed and sedation recurs. Deaths have been reported in relation to this, particularly when opiates with a long half-life, such as methadone, are used.

The tendency in British Emergency Departments currently is to use small aliquots of naloxone intravenously to raise the respiratory rate to an adequate level, but without aiming for a return of consciousness, and then allow the patient to wake gradually as the opiate is eliminated.

Amphetamines

This group of psychoactive drugs includes agents found in some plants (e.g. the herb khat, *Catha edulis*) through to synthetic agents manufactured in illegal drug factories (e.g. Ecstacy).

They are stimulants and fall into the sympathomimetic poisoning group. Acting by promoting release of catecholamines and inhibiting their reuptake, they produce a tachycardia, tachypnoea and fever. Beyond this, they are hallucinogenic, and then produce muscle rigidity, fever and agitation. Inappropriately dilated pupils present a useful clinical sign. Beyond agitation, patients may develop delusions and, in particular, can believe that they have insect infestation beneath the skin. 'Formication', as it is termed, results in intense scratching to the point of self-harm. Rhabdomyolysis can follow the muscle rigidity and ischaemic injury; myocardial infarction and stroke have both been reported, as have dysrhythmias and fits.

Management is based on sedation. Benzodiazepines are the agents of choice to sedate until hepatic metabolism clears the agent. If hypertension is present, then this should be controlled with titratable agents, such as nitroprusside.

Nursing care of the poisoned patient

Nurses should have a high index of suspicion of drug excess in the following situations:

- any patient with altered level of consciousness
- any patient with altered mental status
- cardiac dysrhythmias and pulmonary oedema in young patients

- patients with unexplained metabolic acidosis
- new-onset seizure disorders.

Management of patients with suspected or known poisoning or overdose always begins with attention to the basics of airway, breathing and circulation assessment. Supplemental oxygen should be administered in all cases, except ingestion of the weedkiller paraquat. If patients are unable to maintain a secure airway, or ventilation is inadequate, intubation and mechanical ventilation are indicated. Intravenous access should be established and a nasogastric tube inserted to administer activated charcoal if required.

Frequent monitoring of vital signs, and observation of a cardiac monitor should be performed. Accurate documentation of all findings is important so that changes in the patient's condition can be followed over time.

Alcohol dependency and withdrawal

There is a well-established link between alcohol consumption and an increased risk of being injured. This is a result of a decrease in response or reaction time to stimuli (e.g. poorer driving skills while under the influence of alcohol), and also a change in personality and willingness to take physical risks. Alcohol has been said to contribute to one-third of traumatic deaths (Li et al., 1997).

There is some dispute about the extent to which alcohol augments traumatic injury, related to its cardiodepressive effects, the vasodilatation and possibly even directly toxic effect on injured neurones. It certainly can decrease patient compliance and make assessment of the injured more difficult.

Alcohol withdrawal is a major problem for the ongoing care of the patient who regularly consumes large quantities of alcohol. Chronic alcohol use has a depressant effect on neurological function and its abrupt withdrawal can produce cerebral excitation. In the first instance, this may simply be mild anxiety or even agitation with some minor sympathetic effects, such as a tachycardia or sweating. The initial symptoms of tremor, irritability and insomnia begin 6–12 hours after the last drink. Dehydration occurs during the first 24 hours as a result of vomiting, diarrhoea and sweating. Seizures may be seen in the first 36 hours of abstinence and are tonic–clonic in type.

If left untreated, then *delerium tremens* (or 'the DTs') develops 48–96 hours after the last drink. Autonomic hyperactivity is the hallmark of the DTs with tachycardia, hypertension, sweating, tremor, and visual and tactile hallucinations. Fits are likely.

Treatment and nursing care

These effects of withdrawal can be anticipated and ameliorated. A reducing regime of a benzodiazepine over a week to 10-day period is the current British standard, chlordiazepoxide being the agent usually used. As an adjunct, beta blockers can also be administered to obtund the autonomic effects. Some units prefer to use neuroleptics, such as haloperidol, particularly if there are hallucinations.

Patients in alcohol withdrawal are frequently dehydrated and will benefit from intravenous fluids. Hypoglycaemia is common both in acute intoxication and during withdrawal, therefore, blood glucose levels should be carefully monitored.

Nutrition in chronic alcohol abusers is typically poor and they are at significant risk of Wernicke's encephalopathy. This condition is caused by thiamine deficiency and is potentially life threatening. The syndrome consists of ocular muscle palsies, nystagmus, an ataxic gait and progressive mental impairment. The diagnosis is a clinical one. To prevent this, thiamine should be routinely given in the trauma patient who is at risk of alcohol withdrawal.

> Blood glucose levels should be carefully monitored in patients who have consumed alcohol

Other medical conditions are more likely in patients who are heavy consumers of alcohol, such as gastritis, peptic ulceration, and even cirrhosis of the liver and oesophageal varices. Pancreatitis is also possible. Discussion of these is beyond the scope of this text.

CONCLUSION

In patients who have been injured, consideration needs to be given to the background and history. It is possible that patients may have been driving a motor vehicle and become hypoglycaemic or suffered a fit, resulting in loss of consciousness and a motor vehicle collision. They may have jumped from a building while under the influence of hallucinogenic drugs or as part of a constellation of deliberate self-harm. It is important to keep an open mind when considering the differential diagnosis for signs and symptoms identified in the care of a trauma patient.

While being cared for, deterioration in the clinical condition may not be purely related to injuries that have been identified, suspected or even missed. There may also be a separate medical pathology developing. Whatever the pathogenesis of the problem, the system for management should always follow the standard ABCD approach. Keeping an open mind when developing a differential diagnosis may help to identify intercurrent medical problems.

References

Albers G, Hart RG, Lutsep HL, et al. Supplement to the guidelines for the management of transient ischaemic attacks. *Stroke* 1999; 30: 2502–2511

Algra A, de Schryver EL, van Gijx J, et al. Oral anticoagulants versus antiplatelet therapy for preventing further vascular events after transient ischaemic attack or minor stroke of presumed arterial origin (Cochrane Review). *The Cochrane Library* 2002; 1

Alvord E, Loeser JD, Bailey WL, et al. Subarachnoid haemorrhage due to ruptured aneurysms: a simple method of estimating prognosis. *Archives of Neurology* 1972; 27: 273

American Heart Association. Guidelines for the management of patients with atrial fibrillation: executive summary. *Journal of the American College of Cardiology* 2001; 38: 1231–1265

Bleck T. Management approaches to prolonged seizures and status epilepticus. *Epilepsia* 1999; 40(Suppl 1): S59–S63

British Thoracic Society. Guidelines for the management of asthma. *Thorax* 1997a; 52(Suppl 1): S1–S21

British Thoracic Society. COPD Guidelines. *Thorax* 1997b; 52(Suppl 5): S1–S32

British Thoracic Society. Pulmonary embolism guidelines. *Thorax* 1997c; 25(Suppl 4): S3–S24

Brott G, Adams HP, Olinger CP, et al. Measurement of acute cerebral infarction: a clinical examination scale. *Stroke* 1989; 20: 864

Brown A. Therapeutic controversies in the management of acute anaphylaxis. *Journal of Accident and Emergency Medicine* 1998; 15: 89–95

Butler J, Lewis M. Lorazepam or diazepam for generalised convulsions in adults. Best evidence topic report. *Emergency Medicine Journal* 2001; 18: 116–117

Clopidogrel in Unstable Angina to Prevent Recurrent Events Trial Investigators. Effects of clopidogrel in addition to aspirin in patients with acute coronary syndromes without ST-segment elevation. *New England Journal of Medicine* 2001; 345: 494–502

Cooper G, Graham J. *The scientific foundations of trauma.* Oxford: Butterworth-Heinemann, 1997

Department of Health. *National service framework for coronary heart disease.* London: HMSO, 2000

Dick CR, Liu Z, Sassoon CS, et al. O_2-induced change in ventilation and ventilatory drive in COPD. *American Journal of Respiratory and Critical Care Medicine* 1997; 155: 609–614

Done A. Salicylate intoxication: significance of measurements of salicylate in blood in cases of acute ingestion. *Pediatrics* 1960; 26: 800

Fauci A, Braunwald E, Isselbacher KJ, et al. *Harrison's principles of internal medicine*, 14th edn. New York: McGraw Hill, 1999

Goldhaber S, Savage DD, Garrison RJ, et al. Risk factors for pulmonary embolism: the Framingham study. *American Journal of Medicine* 1983; 74: 1023

Kitt S, Selridge-Thomas J, Proehl JA. *Emergency nursing: a physiologic and clinical perspective*, 2nd edn. Philadelphia: WB Saunders, 1995

Kulig K. Initial management of ingestions of toxic substances. *New England Journal of Medicine* 1992; 326: 1677

Levitt M. A prospective, randomised trial of BiPAP in severe acute congestive cardiac failure. *Journal of Emergency Medicine* 2001; 21: 363–369

Li G, Keyl PM, Smith GS, et al. Alcohol and injury severity: reappraisal of the continuing controversy. *Journal of Trauma* 1997; 42: 562–569

Liu M, Counsell C, Sandercock P. Anticoagulants for preventing recurrence following ischaemic stroke or transient ischaemic attack (Cochrane Review). *The Cochrane Library* 2002; 1

Lowenstein D. Status epilepticus: an overview of the clinical problem. *Epilepsia* 1999; 40(Suppl 1): S3–S7

Oppenheimer S, Hachinski V. Complications of acute stroke. *Lancet* 1992; 339(8795): 721

PIOPED investigators. Value of the ventilation/perfusion scan in acute pulmonary embolism. Results of the prospective investigation of pulmonary embolism diagnosis (PIOPED). *JAMA* 1990; 263(20): 2753–2759

Project Team of the Resuscitation Council (UK). Emergency medical treatment of anaphylactic reactions. *Journal of Accident and Emergency Medicine* 1999; 16: 243–247

Project Team of the Resuscitation Council (UK). Update on the emergency medical treatment of anaphylactic reactions for first responders and for community nurses. *Resuscitation* 2001; 48: 239–241

Resuscitation Council UK. Resuscitation Council guidelines: www.resus.org.uk (2001)

Rosen P, Barkin R. *Emergency medicine. Concepts and clinical practice.* St Louis: Mosby, 1998

Sivasothy P, Smith IE, Shneerson JM. Mask intermittent positive pressure ventilation in chronic hypercapnic respiratory failure due to chronic obstructive pulmonary disease. *European Respiratory Journal* 1998; 11: 34–40

Theroux P, Fuster V. Acute coronary syndromes: unstable angina and non-Q wave myocardial infarction. *Circulation* 1998; 97: 1195–1206

Vogler A, Seaberg DC. Blunt cardiac injury presenting as unsuspected ventricular tachycardia. *Journal of Emergency Medicine* 2001; 19(7)

Chapter **36**

Paediatric emergencies

Rebecca Salter and Ian Maconochie

INTRODUCTION

Responsibility for stabilising and managing seriously ill children fills most health care professionals with fear and trepidation. For many, their lack of experience in caring for time-critical children leads to a lack of confidence in their knowledge and ability; a situation which is perpetuated further unless their exposure to acutely unwell children is considerably increased. The aim of this chapter is to focus on recognising the sick child, providing a structured approach to their clinical assessment and examination, and understanding the need for early intervention and treatment in advance of any sudden clinical deterioration. Common emergency presentations will be reviewed and their immediate management addressed, including the need for rapid transfer and the referral for specialist intervention.

UNDERSTANDING CHILDREN

Children are not small adults, and must be understood, if they are to be properly managed and cared for. Their level of understanding is variable related to their age, progress against developmental milestones, social and family variables, and urgency of clinical condition at the time of presentation. In some instances, the tendency of clinicians, including nurses, is to focus on the mother or other carers rather than the child in an attempt to establish details of the initial complaint rapidly. While this is a vital component of obtaining a clinical history, the child should be central, and this process carried out in conjunction with observation, inspection and communication with the child.

Establishing a good rapport with children and their parents is central to a positive therapeutic relationship. Not only is it essential to listen to parents or carers, and their concerns or anxieties regarding what may be wrong, it is also essential to develop a meaningful and trusting relationship with the child. Understanding typically normal behaviour and activities for children of given age ranges, their general interests and hobbies and type of language used can help to establish this. Interestingly, Gill and O'Brien (2003) have cited a number of attributes that children share with animals including the following: they do not like being stared at; they lie down when sick; repeated food refusal is unusual; they have limited ability to express themselves; they adopt the position of comfort when well; and they have a strong survival instinct. Although unscientific in origin, these characteristics are meritorious.

To care for children appropriately, therefore, one must understand and know how to manage the well infant and child, understand the importance of growth and development, be able to carry out assessments of all age ranges, be able to obtain a good history from parents/carers, and understand the importance of family and social factors in relation to the child's well-being and illness. They should also be able to elicit and interpret findings from the history and physical examination, construct a differential diagnosis and problem list, instigate appropriate investigations and management, and communicate adequately with children and their parents.

Where possible, children should be cared for by specialist clinical teams in an environment tailored to their needs. Having said that, children become unwell and deteriorate in remote, often alien environments, thereby complicating the issue. Whatever the environment, it is essential that those caring for them adopt the same structured approach, applying their knowledge and scientific principles, while at the same time ensuring that psychological and emotional needs are identified, acknowledged and addressed as well as the more obvious physical ones.

ASSESSMENT AND EXAMINATION – A STRUCTURED APPROACH

It is widely understood and accepted that children are not little adults. Of particular significance is the understanding that they can become unwell quickly but can improve equally quickly. Even more importantly, however, is their ability to deteriorate quickly. The need to identify clinical signs and symptoms suggestive of deterioration quickly and to have a low threshold for acting upon findings immediately are paramount, if their chances of survival and a positive outcome are to be optimised. The role of nurses here is vital, with emergency and trauma nurses increasingly taking up the gauntlet of caring for these children. This includes identifying the need for urgent referral and to whom, acting promptly, intervening early rather than waiting until it is too late, and initiating life-saving treatment when required.

> Children can deteriorate suddenly with little or no warning
> Early clinical intervention is vital

Prior to taking the history and carrying out the clinical assessment, however, knowledge of normal anatomy and physiology in relation to differing age groups of children is essential (Table 36.1). As children grow and mature towards adulthood, their physiological capabilities alter alongside their more obvious anatomical developments. Accordingly, their physiological parameters (i.e. their vital signs) change as they progress with normal ranges identified for different age groups. These must be known and understood to enable situations of compromise or distress to be detected and acted upon. For example, a heart

Table 36.1 Normal values for respiratory rate and heart rate for different ages

Age range	Respiratory rate (breaths/minute)	Heart rate (beats/minute)
Birth	35	100–180
28 days–1 year	35–30	100–160
1–5 years	30–20	80–150
5–12 years	20–17	70–110
Adult values	16–12	50–90

rate of 60 beats/minute may be desirable in the fit athletic 16-year-old but would indicate severe cardiovascular compromise in the neonate. Knowledge of the normal age-related value of vital signs and other physiological parameters is, therefore, imperative to perform a meaningful assessment, and to enable variants from normal to be identified.

The terms used to describe children at particular ages are listed in Table 36.2.

Obtaining a history

A comprehensive history forms the largest part of any clinical assessment with examination and the use of diagnostic tests and investigations merely confirming initial impressions and findings. Central to this is the ability to listen, to ask appropriate and pertinent questions and to assimilate these findings, as these can often reveal the diagnosis.

A full paediatric history should make inquiries about the following: pregnancy, delivery, perinatal events, feeding practice, developmental progress, immunisations, infectious diseases, accidents and injuries, hospital admissions and operations, allergies, minor illnesses, medications, school progress and travel. It should also include the role and position of the child within the family, the family unit itself, information relating to the health and welfare of siblings, social and psychological aspects, including the relationship between the child and parents/carer, and other family dynamics. Observing how the child reacts with and separates from his/her parents/carers can also be informative.

Approaching the child

Unless the situation is immediately life threatening, it is important to first obtain a degree of trust and establish some sort of working relationship with the child before touching or examining him/her. The clinician should use all of his/her senses to glean all relevant clinical and related information. Looking at the child, where possible encouraging him/her to look at you, and allowing them to observe you (and you them) as you speak to their parents/carers can facilitate this. Breathing, coughing, stridor and other auditory signs may be assessed at the same time as listening to the child talk, including the nature of his/her cry. Colour and level of activity can be similarly assessed. A brief visual observation of the child can also reveal how well or unwell they are, although physical signs are frequently less florid in the sick child than they are in the sick adult. Worthy of note is remembering that information relayed by mothers or primary carers in particular is usually right until proved otherwise.

Children are best approached in their position of comfort, such as lying flat in infancy, sitting on their mother's knee when toddlers, or on their own two feet when of school age. Lying them down should be avoided unless strictly necessary, as this promotes a feeling of vulnerability and apprehension. Mothers (or other primary carers) should remain close to the child to enhance feelings of safety and security, especially when examinations are concerned.

Assessment

As with all patients, assessment of the seriously ill child should follow the primary survey sequence of airway, breathing, circulation, disability and exposure, with cervical spine control forming part of airway management. Metabolic considerations, particularly in relation to derangement of blood glucose levels are also crucial. For this reason, the primary survey sequence of events has been expanded in children to include 'DEFG' to emphasise its importance – *don't ever forget glucose.*

> A blood sugar measurement should be recorded in all children as part of their baseline assessment

As each of these components is assessed, appropriate treatment should be initiated prior to moving on to the next step. As with adults, the

Table 36.2 Children and their ages	
Newborn, neonate	First month of life
Infant	1 month to 1 year
Toddler	1–3 years
Pre-school child	3–5 years
Schoolchild	5–18 years
Child	0–18 years
Adolescent	Early: 10–14 years
	Late: 15–18 years

order of assessment and treatment must be adhered to throughout, with a return to assessment of the airway, breathing and circulation should any deterioration occur. Following any intervention, satisfaction should be reached that the course of the illness is returning towards the patient's normal physiological status. A systematic ABCDEFG approach will ensure that the seriously ill child has the optimum treatment.

Parents and caregivers need also to be kept informed and receive regular clear explanations about their child's progress.

Airway

In comparison with adults, infants have relatively large heads with comparatively large occiputs; disproportionately so. This tends to lead to flexion of the head on the trunk at the cervical vertebral level when the child is lying supine. The upper airway structures, such as the larynx, are relatively floppy owing to the limited strength of the cartilage at this stage in the child's development. This means that the upper airway can become obstructed owing to pressure on the surrounding soft tissues of the neck bearing on to the laryngeal tissues when flexion occurs.

The optimal airway opening position for the infant (i.e. the child aged up to 1 year) is, therefore, the neutral position. Children over the age of 1 year should have their airway opened by putting the child's head into the head tilt–chin lift or 'sniffing the morning air position' (Figure 36.1). Opening the airway is the top priority in managing the seriously ill or traumatised child. If the child's airway is not open, the child will die.

Where children are talking or making audible sounds, this clearly indicates that their airway is patent and is being maintained. A high index of caution and suspicion should be exercised, however, where they are speaking with a hoarse voice as, when these are associated with findings, such as soot in the nostrils, singed eyebrows, carbonaceous deposits on the tongue, facial burns or involvement in smoke or fume-related incidents, this may herald significant airway problems with an impending threat of obstruction. A similar picture can be found in children in the early stages of anaphylaxis, where the airway

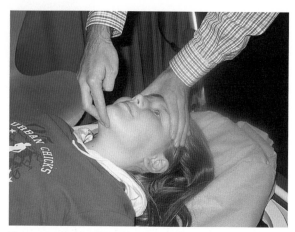

Figure 36.1 Sniffing the morning air position' – head tilt–chin lift.

can rapidly narrow owing to mucosal oedema. A history suggestive of possible involvement with fire or smoke, or suggestive of exposure to allergens with the potential for an acute allergic reaction, signifies the need to seek immediate appropriate help with managing the airway.

> Specialist help should be sought immediately in actual or impending airway obstruction

The epiglottis in the infant is relatively high and anteriorly placed when compared with children over the age of 8 years. In infants it is located at the level of the second cervical vertebral body, whereas in adults it is located at the level of the fourth or fifth vertebral body. Its funnel-like shape is also of significance, particularly when compared with the more mature airway. Blind finger sweeps of the mouth when attempting to remove foreign bodies in the mouth may be considered appropriate in some adult situations; in infants and young children, however, this action may convert a partial obstruction of the upper airway to a total obstruction, as the foreign body can pass from the upper part of the larynx to obstruct the airway completely at the level of the cricoid cartilage.

> Blind finger sweeps must never be carried out in infants or young children

Breathing

Infants and young children

Infants are obligatory nasal breathers; a natural consequence of this is that nasal obstruction from secretions may occur. Secretions due to upper respiratory tract infections may, therefore, cause more discomfort to infants than to adults. A number of conditions, however, can result in respiratory distress and compromise unless recognised and treated promptly. Acute bronchiolitis is one such condition.

Most commonly due to respiratory syncytial virus, acute bronchiolitis causes the production of large quantities of secretions to accumulate within the nasal passages and through the lungs. This leads to 'plugging' of parts of the respiratory tree with adjacent areas of lung becoming hyperinflated. These 'plugged' areas become inadequately ventilated and the hyperventilated areas of the lung poorly perfused. This manifests itself in the child becoming tachypnoeic as part of the body's responding compensatory mechanisms and ensuing signs of respiratory distress

The main muscle of ventilation at this age is the diaphragm. The intercostal muscles are weak and poorly developed when compared with those of adults. Whereas in mature adolescents the ribs act as the bellows of ventilation with the intercostals, this is not the case in infants owing to the cartilaginous nature of the ribs. Abdominal breathing may be seen in a see-sawing motion of the anterior abdominal wall, the force generated possibly causing marked sternal recession to occur. Air hunger results in an increased amount of swallowed air, leading to the stomach becoming distended, thereby limiting downward excursion and function of the diaphragm, the main muscle of ventilation.

Accessory muscles then come into play. These include the sternocleidomastoids; the muscles that control nasal flaring; and, in children, the muscles of the anterior chest wall, namely the pectoralis major and pectoralis minor, and the teres major and teres minor muscles, which form part of the posterior borders of the axilla. These muscles may manifest their accessory role in aiding ventilation by head bobbing, nasal flaring or by fixing the arms on a solid object. Their use indicates moderate to severe respiratory distress. Head bobbing occurs due to the contraction of the sternocleidomastoid muscles, which is attached to the head at the lower part of the mastoid region, and connects to the sternum and to the clavicles. By contracting this muscle and bringing the head backward, the upper portion of the thorax can be elevated and the chest cage dragged upwards, thereby helping with air entry into the chest. It also gives the appearance of tracheal tug.

> Use of accessory muscles of respiration indicates moderate to severe respiratory distress

Nasal flaring is a reliable sign of respiratory distress in infants and is due to the contraction of the levator labii superioris alaeque nasi muscle. This increases the amount of air entering into the upper airways. This is important in infants, who, as previously mentioned, are obligate nasal breathers.

Older children

Older children and adults with respiratory distress tend to hold on to solid objects with their arms. The muscles of the anterior and posterior chest wall, the pectoralis and teres muscles are attached to the upper arm so that, if their upper arm attachments are stable, then by contracting these muscles, the rib cage is drawn out towards the arm, increasing the chest wall diameter and thereby drawing air into the thorax.

Grunting, a physiological mechanism used to prevent the lung deflating completely, is another important indicator of respiratory distress. There is a greater tendency for lung deflation to occur in small children owing to the extremely compliant and relatively lax chest wall comprised of immature ribs and intercostals muscle that have a propensity to collapse inwards. Grunting is a means of closing off the larynx towards the end of expiration, thereby maintaining a positive pressure within the respiratory tree, and preventing these collapsing forces from acting. It requires considerable effort and indicates marked respiratory distress.

> Grunting indicates marked respiratory distress

Every breath humans take is due to a negative pressure within the lung that draws air into the body. The upper part of the airway, such as the larynx, is not within the lung but is subject to these negative indrawing pressures. This does not normally pose a problem; however, where there is mucosal swelling in this area, the effect can be to cause the upper airway to collapse onto itself. When this occurs, it gives rise to the characteristic 'barking-like' noise heard in croup. Stridor is indicative of upper airway narrowing and can be due to other causes other than croup (Box 36.1).

Wheezing represents lower airway narrowing and is heard in illnesses such as acute bronchiolitis and acute asthma. Far more dangerous is when the degree of obstruction to these lower airways leads to loss of the wheezing sound; as no air entry is occurring, the chest is said to be silent. This is a medical emergency as respiratory failure is imminent.

> A silent chest is a medical emergency and signifies imminent respiratory failure

The sustained effort of compensatory tachypnoea, the use of accessory muscles and distension of the stomach, owing to accumulation of air in the air hungry child, leads to exhaustion in the ill child. Following these initial compensatory changes, the child may deteriorate. Evidence of the child decompensating may then be seen, including bradypnoea, the development of clinical signs of central cyanosis, failing respiratory effort and obtundation owing to hypoxia. These are signs of life-threatening respiratory illness and, if untreated, will lead to death.

> Box 36.1   Causes of stridor
>
> - Croup
> - Epiglottitis
> - Inhalation of foreign body
> - Masses, e.g. papillomata, haemangioma
> - External compressive forces, e.g. tumour, thyroid gland enlargement
> - Laryngeal stenosis
> - Vocal cord paralysis

> Bradypnoea, central cyanosis, failing respiratory effort and obtundation signify decompensation

All children who are unwell must be given 100% oxygen via a face mask with reservoir bag; should their respiratory effort be poor or deteriorate, bag mask ventilation may then be required. Senior assistance may be summoned for definitive management of the airway and to aid ventilation. Hypoxia is one of the commonest causes of bradycardia in children.

> Hypoxia is one of the most common causes of bradycardia in children

Circulation

The circulating volume of a child is 80 ml/kg. Fluid loss is a major cause of death with millions of children dying each year worldwide from a range of causes, including diarrhoea and vomiting as well as trauma.

Assessment of the circulation requires observation and measurement of a number of parameters, including the heart rate and rhythm, feeling for peripheral pulses, observing skin colour, feeling skin temperature and determining capillary refill time.

The heart rate can be assessed by palpating the central arteries. In infants, the carotid arteries are often difficult to feel as the neck is very short; in view of this, the preferred pulses are either the brachial artery, located medially to the biceps tendon in the antecubital fossa or the femoral artery, which is halfway between the anterior superior iliac spine and the pubis symphysis. In older children, the carotid artery on either side of the neck can be palpated. The pulse should be counted for at least 10 seconds and the rate considered in terms of normal parameters for the child's age. Tachycardia is an initial response of physiological compensation; bradycardia is a more ominous sign, indicating a loss of normal compensatory mechanisms and the onset of decompensated shock.

> Tachycardia is an initial response of physiological compensation; bradycardia is a more ominous sign, indicating a loss of normal compensatory mechanisms and the onset of decompensated shock

Peripheral pulses are often diminished or absent in marked hypovolaemia; note should be taken of their presence, and whether or not they are easily palpable. With poor peripheral perfusion, there is progressive arteriovenous shunting of blood, so that a gradient of increasing coolness can be felt if the assessor's hand runs from the more central part of the limb outward. A 'line of coldness' that is becoming colder more proximally is a poor prognostic sign. The skin may become mottled and purplish blotches can be seen in very poor peripheral perfusion. Children decrease their perfusion by increasing the amount of arteriovenous shunting. This happens segmentally so that, when one is dealing with a hypothermic child who is gradually being rewarmed, there is noticeable increase in the gradient along his or her limbs; running one's hands along the child's limb, there is a segmental warming increasing from the most proximal parts of the limb as one moves towards the periphery. This is in marked contrast to adults, who are generally speaking cold uniformly over their body surface.

> A 'line of coldness' that is becoming colder more proximally is a poor prognostic sign

Other indicators of peripheral perfusion must also be recorded and, if abnormal, corrected gradually. Capillary refill should be recorded serially to monitor the response to and effectiveness of measures undertaken to improve the child's circulatory status. This measurement is recognised as a better indicator of tissue perfusion than systolic blood pressure.

In infants, two sites show a Gaussian distribution of values for capillary refill: the forehead and the sternum. Where the child has been brought in from a cold environment, the capillary refill may be best measured on an area of covered skin. The technique of measuring capillary refill involves pressing on an area of skin for 5 seconds, releasing the pressure and observing the time taken for the colour of the area that has been compressed to return to the colour of the surrounding tissue. A figure of greater than 2 seconds indicates poor peripheral perfusion. In combination with other circulatory parameters, this simple measure of peripheral perfusion can be measured serially

to monitor the response of interventions performed to improve the child's physiological status.

> A capillary refill time of more than 2 seconds is suggestive of poor peripheral perfusion

Measurement of the systolic blood pressure in children is a poor indicator of peripheral perfusion. This is due to the fact that blood pressure is maintained even though there may be diminishing cardiac output owing to the sensitivity of the arterial system to the merest hint of increased levels of circulating catecholamine, such as adrenaline, which, in the seriously ill child, is elevated as part of the body's normal response mechanisms. However, hypotension is an ominous sign and indicates the failure of normal physiological compensatory mechanisms. Reference must be made to the normal limits of the vital signs relating to the age of the child as decompensated shock reflects the failing of the normal physiological responses.

> Hypotension is an ominous sign and indicates the failure of normal physiological compensatory mechanisms

Where perfusion is poor, intravenous (IV) or intraosseous (IO) access should be established to enable the administration of fluids and drugs. The main sites for intravenous access in infants include the back of the hands, the ventral aspect of the feet as well as the antecubital fossa. The scalp veins tend to be more difficult to cannulate and can interfere, if airway management is required.

The largest appropriate cannula should be chosen and a saline flush prepared along with tape and splints to secure the line when placed. Blood can be obtained to enable estimation of blood glucose levels, urea and electrolytes, full blood count and cross-match in the event of a blood transfusion being required. Other samples, such as toxicology screens, save serum, blood cultures, viral titres and liver function tests may be taken as clinically indicated. Intraosseous access is generally indicated either after two attempts at peripheral cannulation have failed or if the time taken to obtain intravenous access has exceeded 90 seconds. The classic site for intraosseous

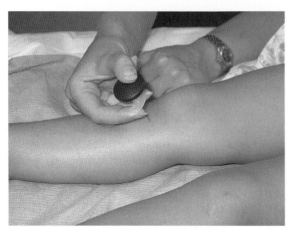

Figure 36.2 Insertion of intraosseous needle.

insertion is two finger breadths beneath the tibial tuberosity and one finger breadth towards the medial surface of the tibia (Figure 36.2). If the child is not obtunded, this area should be anaesthetised using 1% lidocaine, infiltrated down to and including the periosteum. Careful explanation regarding the necessity for this procedure should be given to both the child and caregivers accompanying the child. The technique for insertion of the intraosseous needle is by perpendicular screwing it into the bone. A sudden 'crunch' may be felt, as the cortex of the bone is breached. The needle should remain upright independently, secured into position by the cortex of the bone. Bone marrow can be aspirated and the same samples as indicated for the intravenous route taken. The pathology laboratories should be informed of its origin to avoid confusion. The only difference between the two routes is that samples from the intraosseous route cannot be used for blood gas analysis.

The vein that drains the marrow is much more capacious than the majority of veins seen on the back of the hand or foot. There may be slight swelling of the surrounding soft tissue structures when fluid is given by this route. There are perforating vessels from the bone marrow, which drain into surrounding muscle, and connective tissue and the lymphatic vessels also allow fluid to pass into and out of this space. If there are concerns regarding the possibility of 'tissuing' of the intraosseous needle, fluid should be withdrawn from the cannula and the colour of the withdrawn fluid assessed. This should have a

slightly pinkish hue. Intraosseous needles are associated with a small risk of osteomyelitis. If incorrectly placed, they can also damage the epiphyseal growth plate, leading to asymmetric growth of the leg when compared with the other leg, causing the child to limp in later life.

Fluid can be administered to severely ill or injured children in aliquots of 20 ml/kg over a few minutes. Caution should be exercised in children with raised intracranial pressure; however, hypo-volaemia poses an immediate life-threatening event and takes precedence over such considerations. Fluids must not be withheld in such patients. The effectiveness of fluid administration must be assessed by regular reappraisal of the child's ABC status, including any improvement in circulatory status. If the child's condition has not improved or is worsening, a repeated bolus may be required. Inotropes may also be required to support the failing circulation. Dopamine can be given by the peripheral route but is preferably given centrally; the need for intravenous inotropes often heralds the requirement for invasive arterial blood pressure measurement in order to accurately obtain second to second monitoring of the systolic blood pressure. Such patients may also warrant definitive airway management (i.e. endotracheal intubation and ventilation), as this may reduce some of the work of breathing, enable 100% oxygen to be given and enable close monitoring in the event that pulmonary oedema results as a consequence of increased fluid administration.

Bedside estimation of the child's blood glucose level should be made, as the hepatic reserves are proportionately less than when compared with adults, particularly as the baseline metabolic requirement is higher in children than in older people. Treatment of hypoglycaemia is by a bolus dose of up to 5 ml/kg of 10% dextrose administered intravenously or by the intraosseus route in severely ill children. Blood glucose levels should be subsequently estimated at regular intervals to ensure that the improved level is maintained. *Fifty per cent dextrose is not recommended.*

DISABILITY

Assessment of the conscious level, the child's posture, and the pupillary size and reactivity are basic elements of examination of the child's neurological status. 'AVPU', the mnemonic for establishing the conscious level, depends on the child's response to stimulation (Box 36.2). These letters are used as follows: A indicates an *alert* status, V signifies a response to *voice*, P a response to *pain* and U an *unconscious* state. If the child is alert, this is the equivalent to a Glasgow Coma Score (GCS) of 15. If he or she responds to voice, the GCS may be as low as 9. Responding only to pain is associated with a GCS range of between 8 and 4. If the patient is unconscious, this equates to GCS of 3. Any child who responds only to pain must have an assessment of the patency of the airway and of his or her ability to maintain that airway carried out. This is due to associated loss of the protective reflexes that protect the upper airway should vomiting occur, which is the cause of many deaths.

> Any child who responds only to pain must have an assessment of the patency of the airway and of his or her ability to maintain that airway

Posture

Well children are usually too busy to remain still. In severely ill children, however, abnormal posture can give an indication of their neurological status; for example, in decorticate and decerebrate states the lower limbs are in the extensor position, whereas the upper limbs take on different postures. In decerebrate states, the upper limbs demonstrate predominantly extensor activity, whereas in decorticate states the arms are in a flexed position (Figure 36.3).

Pupils

Pupillary size and reactivity can also provide useful information regarding the child's condi-

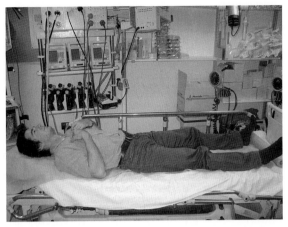

A

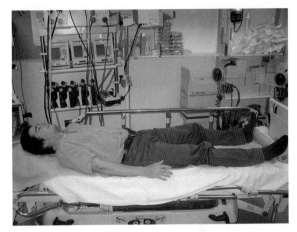

B

Figure 36.3   (A) Decorticate posturing; (B) decerebrate posturing.

tion. For example, the child who has reactivity but pinpoint pupils may have ingested substances such as opiates. Alternatively, the child who has sustained a head injury and who has an ipsilateral dilated pupil warrants *immediate* referral for neurosurgical consultation, as there may be a space-occupying lesion on that side arising from the trauma. The child who has a core temperature below 32°C and who appears to have fixed dilated pupils is not dead, but requires rewarming. This is important as, although the hypothermic child's body displays abnormal physiology, good neurological recovery has been documented in very cold children who have undergone prolonged resuscitation.

The signs of raised intracranial pressure including Cushing's triad, that is, hypertension, bradycardia and Kussmaul breathing (deep sighing breaths), may be seen in almost all intracranial conditions causing cerebral oedema. The management of raised intracranial pressure requires help from senior colleagues, based on ABCDEFG principles. Airway management is important as, if there is raised intracranial pressure, then intubation and ventilation to reduce blood levels of carbon dioxide to the lower end of the normal range is recommended. Ventilation is required to obviate the effect of the Kussmaul breathing pattern observed in this condition. Circulation should also be addressed by considering the child's fluid status; this includes the avoidance of impeding venous drainage from the head (i.e. no necklines should be placed). Mannitol may be required as a temporary measure to decrease the cerebral oedema.

EXPOSURE

It is important that seriously ill children are fully inspected and examined; this includes the front and back of their body as well as from top to bottom. The tone of the anus should also be noted; this is usually only performed once and by an experienced person. This is required in the seriously ill or injured child unless otherwise dictated by the nature of the clinical emergency (e.g. acute abdominal pain). Key information may be gleaned by careful observation of the child's vital signs, the ABC status and any trends noted in charts and careful documentation of findings. It is imperative to repeat these observations at regular intervals, particularly after appropriate interventions have been carried out.

Diagnostic signs, such a non-blanching rash owing to petechiae or purpura, may alert the assessor to the possibility of meningococcal disease. Injuries or burns may be found; the appearance of odd lesions or unexplained marks may raise the possibility of non-accidental injury. Many other conditions may also present themselves as spot diagnoses, such as Kawasaki disease, von Willebrand's disease and Henoch–Schonlein purpura. Kawasaki disease is characterised by the presence of a non-specific macular rash, mucositis, conjunctivitis without pus and large cervical lymph glands, in children who have had a pyrexia for longer than 5 days. Bruising can be a cause of clotting abnormalities, such as von Willebrand's disease, haemophilia, leukaemia or can be also due to less worrying conditions, such as Henoch–Schonlein purpura when the bruises tend to be on the back of the legs and buttocks. Ill children who have a widespread reddened non-specific rash with mucositis and diarrhoea may have toxic shock syndrome, particularly if they have within the past fortnight had a burn or abrasion wherein the toxin-producing bacteria can thrive.

PREPARATION

In all cases of managing seriously ill children, the need for reassessment of the ABCDE is of paramount importance. Should there be a deterioration, then the child *must* be reassessed on this basis from the airway onwards, and effective interventions carried out before proceeding to the next step. To deal with airway, breathing, circulation, disability and exposure, there should be an area dedicated to managing critically ill children. This area must have the specialist equipment for managing the whole age range of the paediatric airway, and equipment for respiratory and circulatory interventions. The team looking after these children must be familiar with this equipment and employ a systematic approach based on ABCDEFG to treating paediatric emergencies.

Aide–memoires

For those who do not specialise in the care of acutely ill children, the ability to remember details of paediatric doses and measurements may prove difficult, if not impossible, not least in the emergency setting. To facilitate safe practice, some units have produced aide-memoires in relation to emergency drug doses and important advanced life support procedures. These may be presented as wall charts, such as the Oakley chart, or come in tape format, such as the Breslow tape. These can be extremely helpful in managing the seriously ill patient and can give confidence to the resuscitating team in establishing the correct dosages. For example, a general formula for calculating the weight of children in relation to their age is: (age in years + 4) × 2 = weight in kilograms. This applies, however, only to children aged over 1 year. For infants, their weight may be estimated from the UK average birth weight at term delivery; at term, this is about 3.5 kg, by 6 months the weight is 6 kg and by 1 year it is 10 kg. These figures are estimates and can vary considerably.

Weight (kg) = [Age (years) + 4] × 2

Similarly, the diameter of the endotracheal (ET) tube in millimeters (mm) = age (in years) divided by 4 and then add 4. Thus, a 6-year-old child may require a 5.5 mm tube, that is, (6/4) + 4 = 1.5 + 4 = 5.5 mm; one size either side of this figure is recommended, so that there should be 5 mm, 5.5 mm and 6 mm size ET tubes to hand should intubation be required. If the condition suggests that there may be narrowing of the airway such as that which occurs in severe croup, then all the endotracheal tubes from size 5.5 should be available. A full-term baby usually requires an ET tube sized 3–3.5 mm, and a baby of 1 year of age a 4–4.5 mm internal-diameter tube.

ET tube = [Age (in years)/4] + 4

There are also formulae to estimate the length of the ET tube at the nose and at the mouth calculated on the basis of age. For the distance from the lips, the ET tube size is given by age (in years) divided by 2 and then 12 cm added; for a nasal tube, the formula is altered to age in years divided by 2 and then 15 cm added.

EMERGENCY PRESENTATIONS

Cardiopulmonary arrest (and respiratory arrest)

The management of cardiopulmonary arrest is based on the fundamental principles of ABCDE.

The initial steps of management are those of instigating basic life support. The child should be approached with caution, with the carers taking care not to become casualties themselves. The 'SAFE' approach, which is shorthand for shout for help, approach with caution, free from danger and

then evaluate, emphasises the importance of this (Box 36.3).

The child should be moved to a place of safety once the scene has been determined to be safe, thereby freeing him or her from further mishap. Where bystanders have been involved, the nature of the problem should be explained to them, and their assistance sought in seeking expert help, asking them to return as soon as possible. This way it will be clear that help has been summoned. Evaluating children simply means gently trying to rouse them. Where there is no response, then basic airway opening techniques should be applied; for infants, the neutral position is adopted, whereas the 'sniffing the morning air' position is required for older children. Where trauma has occurred, a jaw thrust technique should be used to minimise potential movement of the cervical spine (Figure 36.4). If the airway is opened by the chin lift–head lift technique in the presence of spinal cord injury, then the lesion may be exacerbated.

Next, the head should be placed near to the child's mouth and the gaze directed down towards his or her feet, *looking* for rising of the chest wall, *listening* for breath sounds and *feeling*

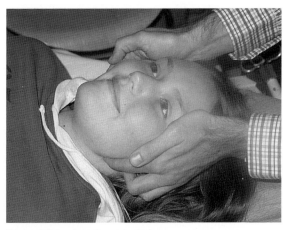

Figure 36.4   Jaw thrust technique.

for breathing against the cheek. This should be continued for 10 seconds. If breathing is not detected, five long slow breaths should be given either by pinching the child's nose and breathing through his or her mouth, or encircling both mouth and nose with the resuscitator's mouth. It is possible to give effective breaths by holding closed the child's mouth and breathing through his or her nose. In all these cases, the duration of each of the five breaths should be about 2–3 seconds, as rapid high-pressure breaths will cause the oesophagus to open with a larger volume going directly into the stomach rather than into the trachea. At least two of these breaths should be effective and cause the chest wall to rise.

The pulse rate should then be sought. In infants, as mentioned earlier, the brachial or femoral pulses are preferred to the carotid, which is the pulse of choice in the older child for measurement of the heart rate. Where the pulse is less than 60 beats/minute, indicating insufficient cardiac output, then cardiopulmonary resuscitation should be commenced. The depth of compressions should be one-third of the anterior posterior diameter of the chest wall. For the infant, drawing an imaginary line between the nipples, and then placing two fingers in mid-sternum one finger breadth down from this line may help to determine the optimal compression site. Two thumbs encircling the chest represent an alternative method of providing compressions. For children aged up to about 8 years, the margin of the rib cage should be tracked up to where it meets the sternum; the heel of one hand should be placed one finger breadth up from this point (i.e. at the xiphisternum). The resuscitator's arm should be directly above this point so that effective compressions can be given.

In children over the age of 8 years (or who appear to be this age by looking at their size), the distance up from the xiphisternum is two finger breadths and the heel of both hands, one on top of the other, should be used to push downwards onto the chest wall to a depth of one-third of the anterior posterior diameter of the chest wall. The ratio of five compressions to one ventilation should be maintained, with 20 of these cycles of 5:1 being delivered every minute. At the end of 1 minute, assistance must be actively sought, if help has not arrived by this stage. In the case of small infants, it may be possible to pick them up and take them to the source of help; older children may have to be left behind in order to obtain the help of emergency services on scene.

Febrile convulsions

Febrile convulsions occur most commonly in young children aged under 2 years, although they may be seen in children aged as old as 5 years of age. They are often benign conditions; at the first presentation of a fit, there must be an attributable focus of infection and other causes excluded by a full history, thorough examination and the use of appropriate investigations to rule out other causes, such as septicaemia, meningitis, acute otitis media, urinary tract infections or other causes of fitting.

The prevalence is higher in boys than girls and a family history may often be present. The mechanism is still unclear; the central temperature is often greater than 38.8°C. The fits occur often during the rise in temperature and do not appear to be related to the duration of the elevated temperature; however, by the time of presentation to medical services, the temperature may have abated or have returned to normal values. Many fits will have stopped prior to arrival to the emergency department. If the child does arrive still fitting, the priorities are the same as those for any seriously ill child, namely airway, breathing, circulation, disability and exposure. Any child who is fitting must have a glucose measurement made; this can often be carried out at the bedside, and any low values corrected by the intravenous (or even intraosseous) administration of 2–4 ml/kg 10% glucose.

The diagnosis of febrile convulsion is a diagnosis of exclusion. Infections, such as urinary tract infection, otitis media, meningitis, septicaemia and other severe infections, need to be excluded by the clinician. Admission to hospital is a frequent occurrence with the first episode, as there is a need to reassure parents and to explain the features of febrile convulsions, including information on recurrences, particularly information relating to the finding that between 95% and 98% of such children do not go on to become epileptic. The most 'dangerous' time for a repeated febrile convulsion is within the first 24 hours of the previous one.

Simple cooling techniques can be used to reduce the temperature; however, cold water bathing is not recommended, as this may increase the probability of a fit due to the central temperature of the body increasing as the peripheral circulation shuts down owing to its exposure to the cold. Parents or the carers of children who have had convulsions may require reassurance about the relatively benign nature of this condition. Education on basic resuscitation techniques, such as positioning the child in the left lateral position and how to ensure that the airway is kept open, may be provided. Such information can be given in the form of information or advice sheets, including what to do in the event of their child suffering another seizure, or in the form of videos or other media.

Meningitis/meningococcal disease

Meningococcal infection is uncommon, affecting about four in 100 000 individuals in the UK each year. However, it is the commonest cause of bacterial meningitis in the UK. *Neisseria meningitidis*, also known as meningococcus, can cause meningitis and/or septicaemia.

- Meningitis is an inflammation of the lining that covers the brain and spinal cord. Infection may be either bacterial or viral in nature.
- Septicaemia is an infection of the blood with bacteria and release of toxins by the bacteria can cause life-threatening illness.

Meningococcal disease is a spectrum of illness, with some individuals having a pure meningitis and some a pure septicaemia, but the majority presenting with some symptoms of both. Meningococcal bacteria are divided into several groups, as listed below.

- Group A: commonest group in the world but mainly confined to hot countries and is rare in UK. Immunisation is available.
- Group B: this is the usual cause of infection in the UK and, as yet, there is no immunisation available against it.
- Group C: this accounted for just under 50%

of cases before 1999, when immunisation was introduced into the standard immunisation schedule in the UK, and it is now rare in the UK.

Meningococcal disease can affect an individual at any age but those under 5 years are particularly at risk. The bacteria are carried harmlessly by one in four people, in their noses and mouth. Close saliva contact is required to pass it on to another, such as by kissing, coughing or sneezing. The bacteria can, on rare occasions, breach the body's natural defences and cause disease. However, what makes some people prone to illness rather than carrier status is as yet unclear.

Children with meningococcal disease may present with many symptoms but the most apparent is that of a petechial, non-blanching rash. This is a red–purple spotty rash that may become confluent and look more like a bruise. These spots or bruises do not disappear under pressure and can most clearly be demonstrated using the tumbler test, whereby a glass is pressed over the spots and, if they do not disappear, then the rash is deemed 'non-blanching' and of serious nature. However, meningococcus can also present with other rashes and may not be present at all. Other symptoms to look for in different age groups are listed below.

Babies may have:

- excessive crying
- a fever
- decreased feeding
- irritability
- drowsiness
- a bulging anterior fontanelle.

Older children and adults may have:

- a fever
- a stiff neck
- a headache
- photophobia – dislike of bright lights
- muscular aches and pains
- confusion and drowsiness
- repeated vomiting.

Treatment

The outcome for meningococcal disease is dependent on swift management and early antibiotic administration. Intensive care is usually required as multiorgan support is often needed.

As soon as meningococcal disease is suspected, high-dose antibiotics should be given, concurrently with assessment of ABC. Pre-hospital antibiotics are as follows:

- Infants < 1 year: benzylpenicillin intramuscular/intravenous (IM/IV) 300 mg.
- Child 1–9 years: benzylpenicillin IM/IV 600 mg.
- Adult/child > 10 years: benzylpenicillin IM/IV 1.2 g.

There has been concern with regard to anaphylaxis but the risk–benefit ratio of giving antibiotics far outweighs these worries.

Initial assessment should include looking for signs of compensated shock, such as:

- tachycardia
- cool peripheries
- increased capillary refill time
- tachypnoea/pulse oximetry < 95%
- confusion/decreased conscious level
- poor urine output < 1 ml/kg per hour
- hypotension.

If present, then IV access and volume resuscitation with 20 ml/kg of colloid should occur and be repeated after further assessment on the way to hospital. In hospital, continued intensive care may be necessary. In the UK, those patients that have meningococcal septicaemia have up to a 50% chance of dying, depending on how quickly treatment is given. Those patients that have meningitis without septicaemia have a 10% chance of dying and, of those that survive, some are left with permanent damage, such as brain injury or deafness.

Contacts Close contacts of a person with meningococcal disease are offered prophylactic antibiotics. Close contact is usually taken to mean a household member or kissing contact within the previous 7 days. Medics, nurses and paramedics who have been in close contact with oral secretions may wish to take prophylaxis, but this is a personal choice and is not universally recommended.

Prophylaxis

- rifampicin (bd for 2 days): < 1year 5 mg/kg, 1–12 years 10 mg/kg, > 12 years 600 mg; or

- ceftriaxone (single IM dose): < 12 years 125 mg, >12 years 250 mg; or
- ciprofloxacin as a single 500 mg dose (adults only).

The local public health department needs to be informed of the need for prophylaxis.

Further information
The Meningitis Research Foundation provides a 24-hour helpline that provides support and information to the general public and health professionals.

- Telephone (24-hour helpline): 0808 8003344 (freephone).
- Website: http://www.meningitis.org/

Poisoning/overdose/ingestion

In the paediatric population, poisoning may be:

- accidental – usually pre-school children
- deliberate – usually teenagers
- fabricated illness – either parents fabricating illness in infants, or older children misusing medication (e.g. insulin-dependent diabetics misusing insulin to control weight gain).

Initial assessment as with any emergency, should be of airway, breathing, and circulation.

- *Airway*: assess for obstruction and, if foreign bodies are apparent, remove carefully. Oral secretions should be suctioned, and the jaw should be held forward and an oropharangeal airway inserted. The patient should be put in the recovery position with head down, ideally to minimise risk of inhaling vomit
- *Breathing*: bag mask ventilation may be required.
- *Circulation*: hypotension is common in poisoning with central nervous system depressants and should be minimised by carrying the patient on a stretcher in the head-down position.

An accurate history of events is vital but it is important to remember that histories from patients may be unreliable, particularly with regard to the amount ingested or inhaled. More than one poison may have been taken, and many poisons can show similar symptoms and signs similar to those of other diseases. Equally, a patient who has been poisoned can be suffering from the effects of another condition (e.g. hypoglycaemia) and head injury may be confused with poisoning, particularly alcohol ingestion.

Presentation may be obvious, as in the case of most accidental poisonings, where a carer comes upon a child ingesting a substance, or may be:

- vomiting, abdominal pain or diarrhoea
- confusion, irritability, slurred speech, ataxia or dizziness
- constricted or dilated pupils
- muscle tremors or convulsions
- respiratory compromise
- circulatory problems (e.g. hypotension, tachycardia or bradycardia)
- pyrexia and sweating
- burns and stains around mouth, or on the skin, if a corrosive or irritant has been ingested
- a history or circumstances consistent with deliberate or accidental poisoning.

Management

The immediate management should start with assessment and stabilisation of ABC and then should be dependent on the site of poisoning as outlined below:

- *Ingestion* – the patient should be kept 'nil by mouth' if drowsy, unconscious or if there is any respiratory compromise. Vomiting should not be induced. If the airway is patent and breathing maintained, then, in the case of ingestion of irritant chemicals, the mouth may be rinsed out with water.
- *Chemicals in the eye* – remove irritant, and irrigate the eye with copious quantities of sterile water or saline for 20 minutes. The pH of the cornea and irrigation fluid should be monitored throughout and irrigation continued until the pH has neutralized. Anaesthetic drops may be necessary to complete full irrigation.
- *Chemical on the skin* – remove contaminated clothing. Irrigate skin with running water or saline for 15 minutes. Continue irrigation until the pH is neutral. Following irrigation, skin lesions should be treated as for burns.

The following signs should be assessed:
- blood glucose, and give glucose, if necessary;
- respiratory rate, blood pressure, heart rate, temperature, oxygen, blood glucose;
- gag reflex;
- GCS;
- pupil size;
- obtain a full history, but this should not delay transfer to the accident and emergency (A&E) department, that is, what substance has been taken, the route of administration, the timing of poisoning, how much was taken, what else was taken, and the previous medical history.

Continuing management

Airway   All patients with GCS < 8, those with an absent gag reflex or are fitting will need airway protection and will need intubation.

Fits   Check patient is safe from injury and check blood glucose. Treat hypoglycaemia and, if fits are continuing, diazepam per rectum or lorazepam IV may be given prior to hospital transfer.

Transfer to the A&E department   All children who have been poisoned should be assessed in the A&E department and referred on appropriately to either the psychiatric unit, or to health visitor liaison or social services in cases of concern, and routinely for accidental poisoning, for education with regard to safe keeping of medicines.

Respiratory emergencies

Croup

Croup, also known as laryngotracheitis, is an inflammation of the larynx, trachea and large airways. It is caused by a viral infection, most commonly parainfluenza, but other viruses may give similar symptoms. Infection with the virus can cause the airways to swell, reducing airflow into and out of the lungs.

Croup commonly affects children between age of 6 months and 6 years. There is a seasonal occurrence with infections being more common in the winter and early spring. The differential diagnosis includes the following:

- Epiglottitis – the child is usually older (4–6 years). There is usually a sudden onset, with a high fever, toxic-looking child, muffled voice and drooling. Fortunately, cases of this are now rare, since the introduction of the Hib vaccine, which acts against *Haemophilus influenzae* group b and is now part of the standard immunisation schedule in the UK.

- Foreign body
- Diphtheria
- Quinsy
- Angio-oedema
- Tracheitis.

The child may present with signs of an upper respiratory tract infection and with a characteristic 'barking' cough. Breathing may be laboured with sternal and intercostal recession. The symptoms are often worse at night and the illness lasts approximately a week.

Assessment of a child with suspected croup should include pulse rate, respiratory rate, oxygen saturation monitoring, and the presence or absence of stridor and sternal recession. The mouth should never be examined, as there is a risk of laryngeal spasm and precipitating a respiratory arrest.

In most cases of croup, treatment is purely supportive with paracetamol for pyrexia, humidified air, such as a steamy bathroom, for comfort of breathing and encouraging the intake of fluids to prevent dehydration. For the more severe cases, nebulised budesonide 2 mg or adrenaline 4 ml of 1:1000 should be given. These may give immediate relief but ongoing treatment with dexamethasone would be required orally on discharge.

Asthma

There are many definitions of asthma, but generally it is taken to mean reversible airway obstruction owing to airway inflammation and bronchial hyper-responsiveness. A clinical definition, which is more useful, is wheeze/cough on two or more occasions over separate occasions over a 3-month period.

Asthma is very common, affecting one in eight children and one in 13 adults in the UK. The cause of asthma is multifactorial, with a partly allergic component with a genetic link to eczema and hayfever, which is known as atopy, and a partly environmental component.

Asthma affects the smaller airways; these become inflamed and swollen and, when irritated, the muscles in the walls of the small airways contract and narrow, and there is an increased production of mucus. This combination leads to narrowing of the airways and causes wheezing and shortness of breath. Attacks are intermittent and often associated with an intercurrent respiratory infection. Whilst asthma is not a trivial illness, with 1400 deaths a year in the UK from asthma, if treated appropriately, attacks can be prevented.

A child may present with cough, wheeze, a tight chest and shortness of breath. Initial assessment should include pulse, respiratory rate, oxygen saturations and an assessment of work of breathing (e.g. intercostals and subcostal recession and tracheal tug). The ability to talk in sentences or to feed in infants are also important indicators of severity of illness.

Once the initial assessment has been made, treatment should follow the British Thoracic Society (BTS) guidelines as shown in Table 36.3. Further guidelines for in-hospital management and for the management of adults can be found at the BTS website.

Anaphylaxis

Anaphylaxis is commonly used to describe hypersensitivity reactions that are mediated by immunoglobulin E (IgE). Anaphylaxis is becoming increasingly common and is associated with an increase in prevalence of allergic disease.

An anaphylactic reaction can occur following exposure to a variety of agents but most commonly are after exposure to:

- insect stings
- drugs
- contrast media
- foodstuffs with peanut and tree nut being common.

Presenting symptoms are likely to include:

- angio-oedema
- urticaria
- dyspnoea
- cardiovascular collapse
- rhinitis

Table 36.3 British Thoracic Society guidelines on the management of acute asthma in children in general practice

Age 2–5 years		Age >5 years	
Assess asthma severity		**Assess asthma severity**	
Moderate exacerbation	Life-threatening asthma	Moderate exacerbation	Life-threatening asthma
• $SpO_2 \geq 92\%$ • Able to talk • Heart rate ≤ 130/minute • Respiratory rate ≤ 50/minute	Severe exacerbation • $SpO_2 < 92\%$ • Too breathless to talk • Heart rate ≥ 130/minute • Respiratory rate ≥ 50/minute • Use of accessory neck muscles	• $SpO_2 < 92\%$ • Silent chest • Poor respiratory effort • Agitation • Altered consciousness • Cyanosis	• $SpO_2 \geq 92\%$ • $PEF \geq 50\%$ best or predicted • Able to talk • Heart rate ≤ 120/minute • Respiratory rate ≤ 30/minute	Severe exacerbation • $SpO_2 < 92\%$ • $PEF \geq 50\%$ best or predicted • Too breathless to talk • Heart rate > 120/minute • Respiratory rate > 30/minute • Use of accessory neck muscles	• $SpO_2 < 92\%$ • $PEF < 33\%$ best or predicted • Silent chest • Poor respiratory effort • Agitation • Altered consciousness • Cyanosis

Age 2–5 years		Age >5 years	
• β_2 agonist 2–4 puffs via spacer ± facemask • Consider soluble prednisolone 20 mg	• Oxygen via face mask • β_2 agonist 10 puffs via spacer ± facemask or nebulised salbutamol 2.5 mg or terbutaline 5 mg • Soluble prednisolone 20 mg	• Oxygen via face mask • Nebulise: – salbutamol 2.5 mg or terbutaline 5 mg + – ipratropium 0.25 mg • Soluble prednisolone 20 mg or IV hydrocortisone 50 mg	• β_2 agonist 2–4 puffs via spacer • Consider soluble prednisolone 30–40 mg	• Oxygen via face mask • β_2 agonist 10 puffs via spacer ± facemask or nebulised salbutamol 2.5–5 mg or terbutaline 5–10 mg • Soluble prednisolone 30–40 mg	• Oxygen via face mask • Nebulise: – salbutamol 5 mg or terbutaline 10 mg + – ipratropium 0.25 mg • Soluble prednisolone 30–40 mg or IV hydrocortisone 100 mg

Age 2–5 years		Age >5 years	
Increase β_2 agonist dose by 2 puffs every 2 minutes up to 10 puffs according to response	Assess response to treatment 15 minutes after β_2 agonist	Repeat β_2 agonist via oxygen-driven nebuliser whilst arranging immediate hospital admission	Increase β_2 agonist dose by 2 puffs every 2 minutes up to 10 puffs according to response	Assess response to treatment 15 minutes after β_2 agonist	Repeat β_2 agonist via oxygen-driven nebuliser whilst arranging immediate hospital admission

Age 2–5 years		Age >5 years	
If poor response, arrange admission	If poor response, repeat β_2 agonist and arrange admission		If poor response, arrange admission	If poor response, repeat β_2 agonist and arrange admission	

Age 2–5 years		Age >5 years	
Good response • Continue up to 10 puffs of nebulised β_2 agonist as needed, not exceeding 4 hourly • If symptoms are not controlled, repeat β_2 agonist and refer to hospital • Continue prednisolone for up to 3 days • Arrange follow-up clinic visit	Poor response • Stay with patient until ambulance arrives • Send written assessment and referral details • Repeat β_2 agonist via oxygen-driven nebuliser in ambulance		Good response • Continue up to 10 puffs of nebulised β_2 agonist as needed, not exceeding 4 hourly • If symptoms are not controlled, repeat β_2 agonist and refer to hospital • Continue prednisolone for up to 3 days • Arrange follow-up clinic visit	Poor response • Stay with patient until ambulance arrives • Send written assessment and referral details • Repeat β_2 agonist via oxygen-driven nebuliser in ambulance	

Age 2–5 years		Age >5 years	
Lower threshold for admission if: • Attack in late afternoon or at night • Recent hospital admission or previous severe attack • Concern over social circumstances or ability to cope at home			Lower threshold for admission if: • Attack in late afternoon or at night • Recent hospital admission or previous severe attack • Concern over social circumstances or ability to cope at home		

NB: If a patient has sign and symptoms across categories, always treat according to their most severe features

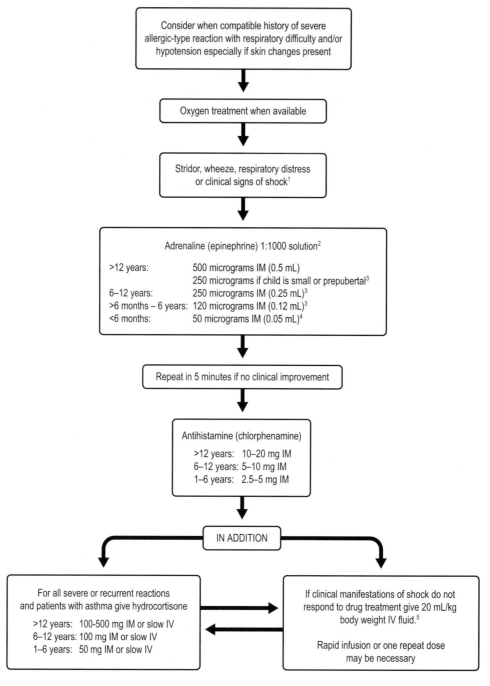

Figure 36.5   The Resuscitation Council (UK) algorithm for treatment of anaphylactic reactions in children by first medical responders.

- conjunctivitis
- abdominal pain
- diarrhoea
- sense of impending doom.

The most important drug in the treatment of anaphylaxis in any circumstance is adrenaline. Adrenaline is an alpha-receptor agonist and works by reversing peripheral dilatation and reducing oedema. It also has beta-receptor activity and this acts to dilate airways, increase the force of contraction of the heart and to reduce mediators of allergic response, such as histamine and leukotrienes. Adrenaline is a very much underused drug in the community and is very safe when given by the intramuscular route, as is recommended in all resuscitation protocols. However, it is a common mistake to give adrenaline via the intravenous route and this may cause myocardial ischaemia. The current recommendations from the Resuscitation Council (UK) for children in the community and for first medical responders, including paramedics, is given in Figure 36.5.

It is important to note that, for some children, anaphylactic reactions may be severe and a recurrent event. In these cases, an Epipen device may have been prescribed for use in such circumstances. These pens provide adrenaline in a predetermined dose, either 300 μg or 150 μg, depending on age and weight. These devices may have already been used by the carer and history of use should be obtained before administering further doses of adrenaline.

Antihistamines are routinely used in the management of anaphylactic reactions to help reverse histamine-mediated vasodilatation. Hydrocortisone is administered to help prevent late sequelae of anaphylaxis and is particularly important in those showing respiratory symptoms. A useful addition to therapy in those with respiratory symptomatology is inhaled or nebulised beta$_2$-agonists, such as salbutamol. Finally, in the case of severe hypotension that does not respond to drug treatment, IV access should be obtained and the administration of crystalloid fluid at a rate of 20 ml/kg should be commenced.

SUMMARY

All emergency and trauma nurses should be able to assess children who have suffered acute illnesses or emergencies, recognise and treat immediate life-threatening problems, stabilise them and manage them until appropriate specialist help arrives or until they are referred on to more appropriate agencies. Following a structured approach will help to ensure this and engender confidence in those entrusted with the care of children.

References and further reading

Advanced Life Support Group. *Advanced paediatric life support*. London: BMJ Publishing Group, 1998

American Academy of Pediatrics. *Pediatric advanced life support*. Dallas: American Heart Association, 1999

American Academy of Pediatrics. *Pediatric education for pre-hospital professionals*. Elk Grove Village, IL: American Academy of Pediatrics, 2000

Candy D, Davies G, Ross E. *Clinical paediatrics and child health*. London: WB Saunders, 2003

Capehorn DMW, Swain AH, Goldsworthy LL. *Handbook of paediatric accident and emergency medicine – a symptom-based guide*. London: WB Saunders, 1998

Gill D, O'Brien N. *Paediatric clinical examination*. Edinburgh: Churchill Livingstone, 1998

Gill D, O'Brien N. *Paediatric clinical examination made easy*. Edinburgh: Churchill Livingstone, 2003

Goldbloom RB. *Paediatric clinical skills*. Edinburgh: Churchill Livingstone, 1997

Greaves I, Porter K. *Pre-hospital medicine: the principles and practice of immediate care*. London: Arnold, 1999

Hull D, Johnston DI. *Essential paediatrics*. Edinburgh: Churchill Livingstone, 1996

Lissauer T, Glayden G. *Illustrated textbook of paediatrics*. Edinburgh: Churchill Livingstone, 2003

Meadow R. *ABC of child abuse*. London: BMJ Publishers, 1993

Polin RA. *Paediatric secrets*. Edinburgh: Churchill Livingstone, 1997

Websites

http://www.brit-thoracic.org.uk/sign/mainframe_download.html

http://www.resus.org.uk/pages/anafig2.pdf

Chapter **37**

Trauma in special circumstances

Tony Simcock and Helen Burdett

INTRODUCTION – THE HOSTILE ENVIRONMENT

Trauma can occur in any variety of situations and places. These can be considered hostile to both the victim and rescuer. A hostile environment may be classified as such if the area is remote from medical help, remote from the hospital where the casualties will be referred to or hazardous with respect to the climatic conditions or environmental hazards, such as a radiation incident.

When assessing an area, the safety for the rescuers and victims should be assessed as a priority, and care taken so no further injuries are sustained by any on the scene.

In the following chapter, unusual situations and circumstances will be looked at to ensure safety for the people involved and also for those at the destination hospital.

DROWNING AND NEAR-DROWNING

Death from drowning causes in excess of 500 deaths in the UK per annum, over 8000 in the USA and an estimated almost 150 000 deaths worldwide. Death from drowning is the second commonest cause of accidental death in children in the USA and the third commonest in the UK, although in 1999 there seems to have been a marked increase in the number of childhood deaths. It may well be that, sadly, the UK figures will move in line with those in the USA. By definition, drowning is 'death by asphyxiation in water'. Near-drowning is defined as initial survival from an immersion incident and it is estimated that near-drowning incidents are 8–9 times more common than actual deaths from drowning. Although there has been a welcome increase in training and activity of life-saving groups through widespread media attention to the importance of resuscitation, this has to be offset by the increase in aquatic activities by the young, middle-aged and elderly population, who have an increased amount of leisure time. Children between the ages of 1 and 4 are particularly at risk, as they have learned to walk but usually not yet learned to swim and have a potentially fatal fascination with water. Young men are three times more likely to die from drowning than young women, although this may reflect the relative numbers of each sex taking part in water sports. The elderly are more at risk from the cardiovascular changes resulting from sudden immersion in cold water, although stroke and myocardial infarction are less common than might be anticipated. Alcohol is undoubtedly a factor in some immersion accidents, such as impulsive midnight bathing and diving into unexpectedly shallow water.

> Drowning is death by asphyxiation in water
>   Near-drowning is initial survival from an immersion incident

Contributing medical conditions

Any pre-existing medical condition that produces unconsciousness or reduced consciousness before the victim enters the water will lead to the airway being unprotected, with water passing through the glottis and displacing air in the lungs. This will lead to a rapid death from the subsequent hypoxia. Unconsciousness can obviously be produced by trauma to the head, causing the patient to enter the water as a result. There are, however, a number of pre-existing medical conditions that need to be considered by those involved in immediate care and initial care at the hospital. Epilepsy is recognised as being a predisposing factor, and certainly people with this condition should always be supervised in water sports and should ensure that their epilepsy is well controlled before engaging in aquatic activities. Similarly, diabetic people should be aware that sudden and un-

expected hypoglycaemia can be rapidly fatal in an aquatic environment. Reference has been made to the increased interest in water sports by the middle-aged and elderly population but, in reality, myocardial infarction and stroke are relatively rare causes of precipitating a drowning incident. Alcohol should be avoided prior to water activities, and a combination of alcohol and drug overdose are a potent combination in precipitating an immersion accident. Drowning is also a recognised form of suicide, although it seems to have a patchy national and international distribution. Those patients with primary muscle disorders must obviously be very careful when close to water; fortunately, this is well recognised and accidents are rare indeed.

> Knowledge of pre-existing medical conditions is essential for accurate patient assessment and management

Pathophysiology

Being plunged into cold water can produce a reflex asystole or ventricular fibrillation, but this is rare. There is an initial involuntary inspiration followed by hyperventilation, and aspiration can occur during this process. Usually the victim will learn to control this respiration, especially if an accomplished swimmer. It has been reported that the hyperventilation can lead to tetany and this would be disabling. If the individual cannot swim, there is a frantic attempt to keep the airway above the water level. This leads to kicking with the legs, outspreading of the arms and extension of the cervical spine. Inspiration takes place only when the water level is below the airway but these efforts will lead to the swallowing of large amounts of what may be very cold water. If the victim is not rescued, however, sooner or later there will be a forced inspiration when under water. This leads to minimal aspiration but severe laryngospasm and, with this, the inability to coordinate inspiration only when the airway is above water. The victim is then in a downward spiral of increasing inspiration under water, increasing aspiration and eventually unconsciousness.

The swimmer will learn to cope with the initial effect of immersion within a second or two, and then will coordinate arm and leg movements with inspiration at appropriate times. Unless the subject is insulated from the environment, there is bound to be cooling if the water is below 30°C. Passage of heat from the body into water is 20–30 times greater than passage of heat from the body to air. Normal mental coordination is maintained until the body reaches a temperature of 35°C, when there is a period of amnesia and a 'switch off' to the danger that the swimmer is in. If rescued at this point, the swimmer may deny that they were in any potential danger whatsoever. Rescue is vital at this point because cooling will continue and a 'dog paddle' type of action has been well documented. The head goes back and rolls from side to side, the feet lie at 45° to the water surface and produce no propulsive action, while the arms produce an ineffectual dog-paddling motion. No forward movement is achieved and unconsciousness ensues. Between 33° and 30°C the victim will become unconscious and, at this point, the airway slips below the water. It may be that the glottic spasm produced by the first inhalation causes cardiac arrest and this is a possible explanation for so called dry drowning. Dry drowning is a post mortem finding of death occurring in the water but minimal aspiration of water in the lungs. This is not completely understood but occurs in less than 10% of drowning deaths.

Exhaustion used to be thought to be a phenomenon associated with shipwreck far from land and only occurring after many hours of swimming in warm water when victims became unable to make the muscular effort required to keep their airway above the water. It is now well documented that an acute exhaustion-like picture can occur in a matter of minutes in very cold water. At 0°C, experienced warm water swimmers may be unable to cope with the initial spasm and involuntary hypoventilation. Even those who cope with this are unlikely to survive long. At 0°C the 50% survival time is 10 minutes. At 5°C, a common winter sea temperature, there are unlikely to be any survivors after 2 hours in the water. The 15°C swimmers can be lost after 2 hours but there can be long-term survivors, particularly those who are familiar with cold water swimming. These times are approximately doubled if the immersion accident occurs with the patient fully clothed.

The final common pathway for death after an immersion accident is a profound right to left pulmonary shunt leading to severe hypoxia, tissue ischaemia and a profound metabolic acidosis. Vomiting is a common terminal event and aspiration with gastric contents is found in 40% of post mortems. Much has been made in the past of the type of water aspirated into the lung. It was thought that aspiration of sea water would lead to osmotic drawing of water from the circulation into the lungs and consequently increasing the degree of pulmonary oedema. Conversely, aspiration of fresh water was thought liable to lead to water passing into the circulation, and causing haemolysis and circulatory overload. In clinical practice, this does not seem to be the case at all. The severity of pulmonary oedema does not seem to be influenced by the type of water and any circulatory change always mimics hypovolaemia. It is the temperature rather than the type of water aspirated that is critical and this will be discussed later.

Rescue and immediate care

The safety of the rescuer or rescuers is paramount. Every year there are several near-drowning incidents that lead to the death of a rescuer. Any rescuer must be a competent swimmer who is aware of the danger of being incapacitated by cold water. Suitable clothing should be worn and wherever feasible wetsuits or drysuits. It is vital that a line attaches any rescuers to a secure place on shore and there is sufficient assistance to be able to retrieve a rescuer, if they get into difficulty. All will be aware of fatalities that have occurred with attempted rescues in ice-covered lakes or stormy sea conditions.

Rescue can be an extremely difficult procedure but, wherever possible, should be achieved with the patient kept in the horizontal position. The use of spinal boards in swimming pools and shallow lakes has definite advantages but requires at least three trained personnel. Bounce and roll techniques can be used to get patients into inflatable dinghies but rescue from deep or stormy water presents its own difficulties. The use of winches and double strops should be used wherever possible to avoid the profound drop in cerebral perfusion pressure that occurs with a vertical lift. After rescue, the victim should always be kept horizontal or in a slight head down position, as this may reduce the risk of postrescue collapse that has been well documented. It is thought this is due to a profound fall in arterial pressure associated with the loss of a 'hydrostatic squeeze' exerted by the water, and venous pooling associated with any head-up position as has occurred during rescue. It has been suggested that initial cardiopulmonary resuscitation should take part in the water before rescue is achieved, wherever possible. Whilst this is ideal, it is unlikely that effective cardiac massage can be performed in the water, but trained personnel should consider airway clearance and expired air resuscitation as soon as is practical. Transport to hospital should be as rapid as possible; any treatment initiated at the rescue site should be continued and the patient should be taken to a well-equipped hospital with intensive care facilities and ability to rewarm.

The importance of immediate care cannot be overemphasised. It is the immediate assessment of the cardiorespiratory state of the patient and the relief of any hypoxia in the shortest possible time that will make the difference between not simply survival but cerebrally normal state. The number of minutes between the airway slipping below the water and the subsequent hypoxia has been referred to as the 'hypoxic gap' and it is the reduction of this to an absolute minimum that is so important. Basic questions to consider after rescue are: (1) is this patient breathing, if so, (2) is this patient breathing adequately?

Once these questions have been asked, treatment will be along the standard guidelines for resuscitation (i.e. airway, breathing and circulation). Once attention has been given to a rapid assessment of these parameters, it should not be forgotten that drowning can be precipitated by events such as head injuries, cervical spine damage and the various medical conditions described previously.

The conscious patient

There will be many immersion incidents where a potential fatality has been avoided by rapid rescue and immediate care. Such patients will usually be

conscious and may not appreciate that they were in potentially grave danger. Anyone who has had to be rescued and treated at the rescue site should be regarded as potentially hypoxic and given high-flow oxygen therapy wherever possible and transported to hospital. The immediate care provider may have to convince not only the patient but, understandably, distraught relatives, that this is an important precaution. Patients who have inhaled water will be very distressed, with wheezing, coughing, retrosternal pain and the production of small amounts of grey–white sputum. They may well be hypothermic and hypotensive and, wherever practical, an intravenous line should be set up. This should not, however, lead to prolonged attempted cannulation of difficult veins or delay the evacuation and transport of the patient to hospital. Where intravenous access is obtained, the infusion of 10 ml/kg of isotonic fluid will help to reverse the circulatory effects of any hypovolaemia and in this volume can do no harm. When available, electrocardiogram (ECG) and blood pressure monitoring should be commenced and pulse oximetry considered. If the extremities are cold and the peripheral circulation shut down, pulse oximetry may result in only a poor signal and misleadingly low values for oxygen saturation (SaO_2). Further treatment is not necessary at the incident site in this group of patients.

The unconscious patient

The unconscious victim of an immersion incident is a medical emergency, as excellent survival rates will be obtained providing the immediate care and hospital management are able to relieve hypoxia and prevent cardiac arrest. When recovered from the water, the unconscious patient will be using mainly diaphragmatic respiration and exhalation may be accompanied by varying amounts of aspirated water. Airway clearance and then assisted ventilation is essential in these patients. Airway clearance with a finger sweep is recommended practice in all but toddlers and infants. Indeed, in small children when there is no reason to think of cervical spine damage, then simple drainage on the left side in the head down position will take only a few seconds and may well be beneficial. Where available, the use of a portable suction unit is invaluable in clearing the upper airways of water and any foreign material or vomitus. Once cleared, the airway must be maintained and it may be necessary to repeat the airway clearance procedure again.

Airway maintenance and the provision of adequate ventilation are vital. If airway clearance and maintenance results in an adequate rate and volume of spontaneous ventilation, then this may suffice until supplementary oxygen is available. This should be given at a high flow of 10–14 litres/minute through a closely fitting facemask. Any question of inadequate ventilation should be treated aggressively at the rescue site and during transfer to hospital. Expired air resuscitation is well known to be compatible with cerebrally normal survival and should be used in the apnoeic or nearly apnoeic patient, if this is all that is initially available. Airway clearance may need to be repeated, if the airway becomes obstructed with water. However, ventilation with 100% oxygen has a high priority here. This may have to be commenced with bag and mask ventilation. However, the airway should be secured as soon as possible by endotracheal intubation, and intermittent positive pressure ventilation with 100% oxygen commenced and continued during transfer to hospital. If endobronchial suction is available, this can be used to clear the upper airways to facilitate ventilation.

The circulatory state will be of peripheral circulatory shutdown with tachycardia, poor pulse pressure and hypotension. Wherever possible, an intravenous cannula should be sited and a volume replacement with 10 ml/kg of crystalloid fluid infused as rapidly as possible. Venous access, however, may not be easy as peripheral veins may well be shut down, and undue time should not be wasted in repeated attempts at venepuncture. For those practised in cannulation, it may be worth remembering that the external jugular vein is frequently prominent when the patient is in the horizontal position. For those with suitable training, venous access can be obtained by cutdown at the ankle, but again this requires expertise, equipment and should not delay transport to hospital. Although the reversal of hypothermia is not a priority at the accident site, it is sensible to prevent further heat loss with some form of blankets or dry clothing; the use of 'space blankets' has now largely been discarded.

The management of cardiac arrest

The diagnosis of cardiac arrest must be made on clinical grounds. Absent ventilation, absent pulse and dilating pupils are cardinal signs; however, it must be remembered that, if there is significant hypothermia, the peripheral circulation may be shut down to such an extent that a peripheral pulse is not palpable. Palpation of the carotid artery and listening over the apex of the heart should be undertaken for 60 seconds in the presence of hypothermia.

> In the presence of significant hypothermia, the peripheral circulation may be shut down to such an extent that a peripheral pulse is not palpable

An ECG will occasionally show slow sinus rhythm, even though no peripheral pulse can be palpated. The danger of assuming death from cardiac arrest in the presence of hypothermia cannot be overestimated. There are many examples in the world literature over the last 30 years of prolonged submersion in cold water being compatible with recovery. Periods of cardiopulmonary resuscitation (CPR) in excess of 2 hours have been compatible with cerebrally normal survivors in some circumstances. The maximum period of cold-water immersion known to be compatible with normal recovery was in a child of 2 years, submerged in water of 5°C for 66 minutes. Most survivors have been children, in whom the high body surface to weight ratio may have led to more rapid cooling than in the adult, but adult survivors have also been recorded. The vital considerations are the length of submersion and the temperature of the water. Before assuming death in an immersion victim rescued from cold water, it is important to ask the following questions.

- What was the period of immersion?
- What was the temperature (or estimated temperature) of the water?
- If the period of submersion was short and in cold water, what does an ECG show?

If there is any doubt, the wisest policy is to commence and maintain CPR during transfer to a major hospital centre. A decision to resuscitate may be difficult but, once made, resuscitation should follow conventional ABC lines and be continued during transfer to hospital.

Hospital management

Initial hospital treatment is really an extension of the immediate care phase. Even those victims who appear to have recovered at the accident site should be taken to a hospital with a well-equipped accident and emergency (A&E) department and an intensive care unit. Near-drowning is a medical emergency and any serious immersion victim should be met on arrival by a resuscitation team with facilities for suction, ECG, endotracheal intubation and ventilation with 100% oxygen. Ideally, initial assessment and treatment should take place in the ambulance or helicopter as soon as it arrives on site. The patient should not be transferred to the intensive care unit until the initial assessment and treatment have been made and instigated. For the purposes of hospital management, it is convenient to divide patients into four categories according to their respiratory distress:

1. Patients with no apparent inhalation
2. Patients with inhalation but adequate ventilation
3. Patients with inadequate ventilation
4. Cardiac arrest group.

Group 1: patients with no apparent inhalation

There will be patients brought to an A&E department who have had to be rescued from the water, and some who may have received expired air resuscitation but who appear to have completely recovered by the time they are first seen in A&E. It is important for the triage nurse to impress upon these patients, or the relatives of children, that they should be assessed in A&E and admitted if there is any suggestion that they may have inhaled water. Late-onset deterioration, often called secondary drowning, occurs in < 3% of these patients but deterioration can be dramatic with potentially fatal sequelae. Evidence of inhalation is usually easy to recognise on auscultation,

and clinical findings are almost always confirmed by radiological examinations. Any relatives should be reassured that a period of observation of pulse, respiratory rate and blood pressure is necessary to avoid the small risk of what is effectively respiratory failure.

Monitoring should continue for at least 6 hours, looking for ominous signs of deterioration, the onset of cough with sticky, frothy sputum, accompanied by a rising pulse rate and respiratory rate. Pulse oximetry is the simplest guide to adequate oxygenation. A falling oxygen saturation level accompanied by a rising respiratory rate and cough should be an urgent indication to transfer from an observation ward to an intensive care ward. The European Resuscitation Council guidelines from 1994 suggest that discharge could be considered at 6 hours, if the patient has a clear chest x-ray, normal observations and a normal oxygen saturation breathing room air.

Group 2: patients with inhalation but adequate ventilation

These patients are frequently extremely distressed with retrosternal pain on inspiration and paroxysmal coughing. They need reassurance in the A&E department, and then a rapid assessment as to whether the depth and rate of their respiratory rate are adequate to maintain normal oxygenation. It is wise to give high-flow oxygen by mask while this assessment is taking place. As well as basic monitoring, it is also wise to confirm that hypoxia is not present by either serial pulse oximetry measuring SaO_2 or, if the peripheral circulation is shut down and oximetry is unreliable, by a single arterial blood sample. If an intravenous line is not already sited, this should be performed, as there will undoubtedly be a degree of hypotension, which will respond to the rapid infusion of warmed crystalloid solution. It is quite safe in all categories of patients to give 10 ml/kg of fluid warmed to 40°C via a giving set, and it seems sensible to use 5% dextrose for salt water accidents and normal saline for fresh water incidents. The effect on circulation can be assessed after the initial infusion.

Any patient who does not respond to the above measures requires urgent transfer to an intensive care unit. Priorities in intensive care are to restore cardiorespiratory normality as rapidly as possible. This will mean in most cases monitoring by pulse oximetry or peripheral arterial line. It is mandatory to make every effort to raise the SaO_2 to > 90% or, if using arterial blood gas monitoring, to maintain partial pressure oxygen (Pa O_2) of > 8 kPa. If high-flow oxygen therapy by mask does not rapidly achieve this, then consideration can be given to continuous positive pressure airway (CPAP) circuits or elective airway intubation. Initial reports of the use of CPAP circuits are encouraging but, if they are not rapidly successful, there should be no delay in opting for intubation and ventilation. Most patients, however, will respond to conservative management but will require a lot of reassurance; the physiotherapist should be called to aid in breathing and coughing control.

Cardiovascular resuscitation has already been mentioned and further aliquots of warm crystalloid fluid may be necessary to restore circulating blood volume. It is important, however, to avoid circulatory overload, although, in this group of patients, it is unlikely that central venous pressure monitoring (CVP) will be necessary.

These patients will by and large be conscious and only mildly hypothermic. It could be expected that a central temperature would be above 34°C, as below this consciousness starts to decline. This mild hypothermia will be accompanied by a degree of metabolic acidosis but, as long as cardiorespiratory normality is restored, then rewarming can be passive; a warm room, warm blankets and warm drinks are appreciated by the patient and help restore temperature. Treatment of mild hypothermia needs to be no more active than this and a mild metabolic acidosis means that the pH is above 7.2, and both temperature and acidosis will be self-correcting as long as the patient is steadily recovering.

Investigations should consist of a portable chest x-ray and venous blood samples for urea, electrolytes, full blood count and film and blood glucose. The chest x-ray frequently shows an alarming amount of diffuse white infiltration. This is due to aspirated water rather than any left ventricular problem and there is no place for diuretic therapy at this stage. Similarly, blood investigations will rarely show any evidence of haemoconcentration

or haemolysis, but it is important to note that blood glucose is normal, as hypoglycaemia has been mentioned as a precipitating factor in causing the drowning process. There is little benefit in nasogastric tube or urinary catheter insertion. There is no evidence that the prophylactic use of steroids improves outcome and their use has largely been abandoned. Similarly, there seems little place for the prophylactic use of antibiotics unless the victim is known to have fallen into heavily polluted water, when a broad-spectrum intravenous antibiotic can be commenced after sputum or tracheal aspirate has been sent to the laboratory for culture. Otherwise, it is wiser to wait for the result of definite bacteriology before commencing therapy. Given careful early management, the vast majority of patients recover completely and major organ dysfunction or the later onset of adult respiratory distress syndrome is surprisingly rare.

Group 3: patients with inadequate ventilation

Care of the immersion victim who is unconscious after rescue remains a medical emergency, as relief of hypoxia and the prevention of cardiac arrest is paramount. Ambulance paramedics should be instructed to give advance notice of the arrival of such a patient to the A&E department. The patient should be met on arrival by the resuscitation team, usually involving A&E and intensive care medical and nursing personnel together with the necessary equipment to suction the airway, intubate and ventilate with 100% oxygen. Such patients are cold and peripherally shut down with gasping diaphragmatic breathing. Exhalation may be accompanied by the production of small amounts of greyish fluid from the mouth or nose. Hypotension may be profound but an ECG will show slow sinus rhythm.

Treatment should be directed at initial airway clearance using suction and, wherever possible, endotracheal intubation and ventilation with 100% oxygen. Damage to the cervical spine must be borne in mind, but care of the airway and early effective ventilation is a priority. Glottic reflexes are severely obtunded and there is little need for depressant or paralysing drugs to achieve endotracheal intubation. Similarly, the patient's own respiratory drive is weak and easily overridden by moderate hyperventilation. It may be that initial inspiration is accompanied by water regurgitating up into the endotracheal tube and endobronchial suction may be required regularly. Venous access should be secured as soon as possible and, if hypotension is profound, then a rapid infusion at 10 ml/kg of a warmed plasma volume expander will lead to a faster improvement in blood pressure and circulating blood volume.

When the airway is secure and venous access has been achieved, the patient should be transferred to the intensive care unit undergoing intermittent positive pressure ventilation (IPPV) with 100% oxygen. Mechanical ventilation can commence in the intensive care unit using an inspired oxygen percentage of 100% and, if necessary, high inflationary pressures, as compliance will initially be poor. If consciousness starts to return, then this is the time when sedative drugs may need to be employed, as it is vital to maintain ventilation during early treatment. An arterial line needs to be inserted and repeated blood gas analysis undertaken to ensure a PaO_2 of 8 kPa is achieved and maintained. Carbon dioxide levels should be maintained at the lower end of the normal range, as deliberate hyperventilation is now not considered to be of any benefit. When fluid resuscitation of the cardiovascular system has taken place, the use of positive end expiratory pressure (PEEP) may be employed, if high inspired oxygen concentrations continue to be necessary. The PEEP can be commenced at 2.5 cm of water and increased stepwise, but this should only be done after adequate restoration of circulating blood volume and with invasive cardiovascular monitoring.

Cardiovascular resuscitation should commence with fluid therapy, but it is important to avoid fluid overload, particularly in the elderly or those with pre-existing cardiac disease. Children will usually respond quickly to initial transfusion and central venous or pulmonary artery catheters are rarely needed. In the middle-aged or elderly, however, further fluid therapy after the initial challenge should be titrated against the central venous pressure and, where facilities exist, either pulmonary capillary wedge pressure or cardiac output studies using a Swan–Ganz catheter or oesophageal Doppler. If high wedge pressures and

low cardiac output persist despite adequate fluid replacement, the use of beta inotropic support should be considered. Appropriate mixtures of dobutamine and dopamine have been reported in the literature, and should be accompanied by regular monitoring of cardiac output and, whenever possible, systemic vascular resistance and oxygen delivery and oxygen consumption.

Supplementary treatment involves insertion of a urinary catheter, which enables hourly urine volumes to be monitored, and a nasogastric tube, which may lead to the aspiration of large amounts of swallowed water. Radiological, biochemical and haematological investigations should be as before. Electrolyte imbalance is rare, but serious abnormalities of sodium, potassium and chloride estimations can be treated by haemofiltration or even peritoneal dialysis.

The initial chest x-ray will usually reveal large whitish areas in one or both lung fields, and limited areas for normal gas exchange. As long as hypoxia is relieved and cardiovascular normality restored as quickly as possible, this picture is rapidly reversible. Positive pressure ventilation should be continued and sedative drugs employed as necessary until the chest x-ray is virtually normal and ventilation is possible at low pressures with a normal arterial oxygen level using an inspired concentration of not more than 40%. Sedatives can then be discontinued and extubation performed when the cough reflex and consciousness return. Spontaneous ventilation should be aided by mask therapy and it may be that CPAP circuits again may be helpful here. Patients should remain in intensive care until they are clinically recovered and have normal blood gas results with no or minimal enhanced oxygen therapy.

Group 4: patients with absent ventilation and cardiac output

The decision of whether to resuscitate or not should have been made at the accident site as already outlined. It is accepted practice that, once resuscitation has been commenced, it must be continued until either spontaneous cardiac output returns or the patient is warmed to above 32°C. This is because the cerebrally protective influence of hypothermia means that a decision should not be made to abandon resuscitation in the presence of significant hypothermia. Providing the heart can be restarted, then treatment can proceed along the lines indicated for the previous group. However, attempts at rewarming should be started at an early stage. In a hospital without extracorporeal rewarming facilities, this can be a difficult and long procedure. It is important to persevere; however, as survivors have been reported after periods of CPR amounting to 2–3 hours. The inspired gases on the ventilator can be warmed to 42°C and all intravenous fluids warmed to 37°C. The use of surface rewarming intragastric or intravesical warm fluid seems to be of little help. Haemofiltration alone seems to afford little additional heat but haemofiltration in line with an efficient blood warmer has been successfully utilised. However, the most efficient and controlled method of rewarming is with right heart bypass and a heating interchanger. This is the preferred method of rewarming in any hospital with such facilities. Once 32°C has been reached, then the use of defibrillation, atropine and adrenaline can follow conventional protocols. It is only after this that a decision can reasonably be made as to whether to continue or abandon resuscitation.

> Once resuscitation has been commenced, it must be continued until either spontaneous cardiac output returns or the patient is warmed to 32°C

Advice to relatives

The supportive role of the nurse to the family of a serious immersion victim cannot be overstated. Relatives are frequently distraught, particularly when children are involved. The most tragic event is probably the accidental drowning of a baby or toddler in a warm bath, but immersion accidents frequently occur during family leisure activities. Knowledge that prognosis can be excellent, if the patient is treated before cardiac arrest occurs, can be very helpful. Overall, cerebrally damaged survivors are fortunately much rarer than many people envisage. A guarded prognosis must, however, be given, if there has been a prolonged period of submersion, delayed immediate care, fixed dilated pupils or asystole on the initial ECG. Prolonged resuscitation with delayed spontaneous

breathing and a Glasgow coma score of < 5 after the initial resuscitation are also bad prognostic factors, as is the onset of fitting after cardiorespiratory normality has been achieved. Fortunately, the prognosis for anyone who has not suffered cardiac arrest is excellent and persistent cerebral damage is rare in the extreme. Indeed, complications after successful resuscitation are rare but include respiratory distress syndrome, chronic pulmonary infection, renal failure, haemodialysis and diffuse intravascular coagulation.

It should be appreciated by any nurse involved in trauma care that drowning and near-drowning accidents need urgent attention from the time of rescue to the time the patient leaves the ward. It is attention to scrupulous care in A&E and intensive care that will see remarkably good results overall.

ACCIDENTAL HYPOTHERMIA

Hypothermia is defined as being clinically significant when a central temperature recording is less than 35°C. Further definitions splitting into mild or moderate hypothermia are artificial, but most recognise hypothermia as being severe below 30°C. These are important figures, as overall survival is approximately 66% between 30°C and 35°C, but only 33% below 30°C. Patients with multiple trauma and hypothermia have a 40% mortality rate, if the initial core temperature is below 34°C (Lloyd, 1999).

Aetiology

Hypothermia can be primary or secondary to a precipitating cause. Primary hypothermia occurs when a patient is exposed to cold for a prolonged time without adequate insulation. This can occur in many social spheres as well as in immersion incidents. People becoming lost or injured when mountain walking or climbing may not be prepared for prolonged exposure. Accidents still occur to workers in cold environments, fishermen in very cold winter waters or essential workers conducting repairs after severe gales or snowstorms. Professional divers are usually adequately insulated but accidents still do occur to recreational scuba divers.

Secondary hypothermia occurs largely as a result of a primary event causing unconsciousness or inability to escape from an abnormally cold environment. Falls leading to head injuries and head injuries of any kind causing a reduced or unconscious state will lead to increasing hypothermia in a cold environment. Unfortunately, the inappropriate use of drugs or alcohol abuse lead to a significant number of deaths from hypothermia. It should be remembered also that normal thermoregulatory mechanisms are not as efficient in elderly people as in the young. The elderly, particularly if malnourished, are vulnerable to even mildly cold environments. If none of the above seem to be precipitating causes, then the following list of medical conditions should be considered: cerebrovascular event, hypothyroidism, hypoglycaemia, myocardial infarction, Addison's disease, hypopituitarism, pancreatitis and hepatic failure. By far the commonest of these is a cerebrovascular event, occurring to a person who is alone at the time of the accident and subsequently not found for several hours.

Effects of hypothermia

The normal physiological response to cold is shivering and there is normal cerebral activity in the conscious individual down to 35°C. Below this critical temperature, there is a period of disorientation, confusion and lack of motor coordination, which is akin to drunkenness or mild cerebral hypoxia. It is important to differentiate between these three causes as the appropriate treatment for each is vital. Below 32°C, there is a steady reduction in conscious level and, below 30°C, most individuals will become unconscious from hypothermia *per se* notwithstanding any other precipitating cause. Below 30°C, there is an increasing risk of ventricular fibrillation but, if the heart remains in sinus rhythm, blood pressure is reduced, the heart rate slows and cardiac output falls steadily. Most individuals will go into asystole below 20°C. The ECG in severe hypothermia may show ventricular fibrillation, asystole or, rarely, a slow broad complex sinus rhythm. The J-wave after the QRS complex is a classic sign but seems to be quite rare in practice. This low-voltage, low cardiac output, slow rhythm

may not be detectable on palpation of the peripheral pulses.

Cardiovascular responses are important and need careful consideration. The initial response is marked peripheral vasoconstriction, which will increase the blood volume of capacitance vessels and may be interpreted by the body as circulatory overload leading to a diuresis. Relative hypovolaemia can occur owing to this and the later movement of fluid from the intravascular space to the extravascular space. These pathophysiological changes are best seen in slow-exposure hypothermia. In immersion hypothermia, the picture always seems to be that of an acute hypovolaemic state, as there is insufficient time for diuresis or significant intracellular or extracellular shifts.

Pathophysiological effects on the respiratory system lead to a reduction in the rate of breathing and tidal volume, resulting in reduced gas transfer in the lung. The oxygen dissociation curve shifts to the left, which means that the red blood cells tend to retain oxygen rather than give it up in the tissues. The net effect of all these changes, if severe, is tissue hypoxia. Changes in renal and acid–base metabolism lead to a reduced glomerular filtration rate with metabolic acidosis and renal failure gradually ensues. There is general reduced metabolic activity with lowering of blood sugar levels but cerebral metabolism itself is reduced quite markedly by hypothermia. It is this reduced requirement of the brain for oxygen and glucose that has been responsible for some remarkable recoveries from profound hypothermia.

Immediate care

The important thing to consider in hypothermia is to be aware that it may exist. Methods of measuring temperature at an accident site may not be available or, indeed, may be inaccurate. An axillary temperature recording can be misleading; therefore, a rectal or mid-oesophageal reading should ideally be used to make the diagnosis. When hypothermia is suspected or confirmed, the victim should be carefully removed from the cold environment and insulated from further heat loss. Unnecessary or excessive handling of the patient should be avoided, although the risk of precipitating ventricular fibrillation (VF) has perhaps been overstated in the past. In conscious individuals, the temperature will normally be above 34°C and warm dry blankets or clothing, warm drinks and a warm environment are all that is required. Warm showers and baths have their advocates but, if this form of treatment is undertaken, the individual should be carefully observed, as vasodilatation with fainting owing to a fall in cardiac output can be dangerous. In the semiconscious or unconscious hypothermic patient, priority should be given to clearing and supporting the airway and administering oxygen therapy by mask, if spontaneous ventilation is present. The patient should be removed from the cold environment, insulated as described and then transported in a horizontal position to a hospital with both Emergency Department and intensive care facilities.

> Unnecessary or excessive handling of the hypothermic patient should be avoided owing to the risk of precipitating ventricular fibrillation

Hospital management

All patients suspected of being hypothermic after rescue should be taken to hospital and any patient who is semiconscious or unconscious should be admitted to an intensive care unit for careful monitoring and treatment. The airway remains the priority, and it must be kept clear and supported as necessary. Oxygen therapy should be employed to reverse any hypoxia as quickly as possible. In the presence of vasoconstriction, pulse oximetry to measure oxygen saturation is unreliable. Although excessive handling and invasive procedures have to be weighed against the risk of precipitating cardiac dysrhythmias, a peripheral arterial line to measure PaO_2 at regular intervals will usually be essential. This should be inserted under local anaesthesia to avoid any potential painful stimulation. There is little value in correcting blood gas samples from a patient to 37°C, as this will rarely affect management. The aim should be to maintain a PaO_2 of > 8 kPa at all times. If this cannot be achieved with mask therapy, then careful laryngoscopy and intubation followed by ventilation with appropriate inspired oxygen concentrations should be carried out.

Fluid shifts and fluid resuscitation are complex matters, and venous lines and CVP monitoring will be needed in the unconscious patient. Each invasive procedure has to have its risks weighed against benefits. In most cases. the passage of a Swan–Ganz catheter through the right side of the heart to enable pulmonary artery and pulmonary capillary wedge pressures to be measured should be avoided. Volume resuscitation of the cardiovascular system aims to restore an adequate circulating blood volume but avoid circulatory overload. There is little risk of this in immersion hypothermia but in slow-onset accidental hypothermia the fluid sequestrated in the extracellular compartment or even in the cells can move back into the circulation during rewarming. This can lead to circulatory overload with respiratory or cerebral oedema. It is important, therefore, that any fluid therapy is carefully and constantly monitored. Fluids should be warmed to 37°C and 5% dextrose is the initial fluid of choice. Lactate containing compounds should be avoided (e.g. Hartmann's solution), as they will exaggerate any metabolic acidosis. The aim should be to restore a normal circulating blood volume and a urine output of at least 30 ml/hour in adult patients.

Rewarming has been the subject of much debate and controversy and, in the past, too much attention has been paid to rewarming in the patient who has not suffered a cardiac arrest. Indeed, there is merit in rewarming these patients slowly while paying attention to restoring cardiac output and oxygenation. The use of a warm environment, warmed intravenous fluids and humidified oxygen may be all that is required to achieve a passive rewarming rate of 0.5°C per hour. In the presence of cardiovascular stability, this is an adequate rewarming rate, which will reduce the risk of violent fluid shifts leading to circulatory overload. However, if these simple methods prove to be inadequate, then peritoneal dialysis or haemofiltration with a Level One blood warmer can be considered, bearing in mind that this is another invasive procedure. In the unconscious patient or the patient being maintained on a ventilator with sedative drugs, a urinary catheter is unavoidable. A nasogastric tube is necessary, if there is marked gastric dilatation, but this can otherwise be avoided in the early stages of resuscitation. The prophylactic use of steroids and antibiotics has largely been abandoned.

Management of hypothermic cardiac arrest

The diagnosis of cardiac arrest in accidental hypothermia can be very difficult. It is recommended that the carotid pulse is palpated for at least 1 minute before a diagnosis of cardiac arrest is made. Wherever possible, this should be supported by ECG evidence. The indications for resuscitation in accidental hypothermia are:

- the cardiac arrest has been witnessed and a previous carotid pulse had been palpated
- no carotid pulse detectable for 1 minute
- there is evidence that the cardiac arrest is of less than 2 hours duration
- rapid transport to hospital with CPR is a practical possibility.

Successful resuscitation in accidental hypothermia involving CPR of 6.5 hours has been reported and success in another case after rescue had been delayed for 20 minutes in a snow avalanche (Gray, 1987). Once the decision has been made to resuscitate, this must be continued until either a pulse is detected or a decision to stop is made after rewarming. The actual resuscitation techniques are the same as standard protocols but chest wall compliance may be reduced. There is controversy regarding the treatment of ventricular fibrillation but most recommendations would now agree that, if VF is shown on the ECG, then three basic shocks can be given but, if not successful, then further direct current (DC) shocks should be withheld until the patient has been rewarmed above 30°C. Rewarming is essential before a decision on death is made. It is probably only in the cardiac arrest situation that active rewarming with cardiopulmonary bypass should be considered a first line of treatment in those hospitals where it is available. The essential components are right heart bypass with a heat interchanger. Hospitals that do not have this facility will have to persevere with the simple methods already outlined but many will have the facility to use a haemofiltration circuit with in-line blood warmer. This can be an effective alternative. It is important that the victim is warmed to above 32°C, when any cerebral protection from hypothermia is going to be minimal, before a decision to abandon resuscitation is taken.

Complications

The results of treatment of accidental hypothermia, particularly severe hypothermia, are disappointing, as indicated previously. It is probable, however, that most deaths in secondary hypothermia are due to a primary precipitating cause rather than the hypothermia itself. Even with successful initial resuscitation, many potentially life-threatening complications may arise and require immediate management. These include cerebral damage, bronchopneumonia, acute renal failure, pancreatitis, peripheral ischaemia, diffuse intravascular coagulation and thrombocytopenia.

Summary

Successful management of accidental hypothermia involves alertness to the diagnosis, meticulous immediate care at the scene, and intensive nursing and monitoring in hospital. Trauma nurses play a key role in the resuscitation of these patients not only by rewarming them, but also in observing and monitoring them closely in order to detect complications early and initiate appropriate treatment.

FROSTBITE

Frostbite is relatively uncommon in the UK, but can occur in conditions of exposure to the elements. It is a primary indication for admission to a high-dependency area, where the patient may be monitored for signs of sepsis and assessment of fluid balance; a central venous cannula may be required in severe cases. Other injuries should be sought according to 'Advanced trauma life support' (ATLS®; American College of Surgeons, 1977) guidelines and the temperature of the patient should be measured as soon as possible. Coexistent hypothermia may frequently be present and should be treated concomitantly.

The extremities are most commonly affected, and patients may present with painful, oedematous and purple discoloration of the affected part of the body. Frostbite can cause local tissue necrosis and mummification.

The affected area should be rewarmed and analgesia provided for the patient. The area may blister; such areas should be left intact to prevent secondary infection and fluid loss. Topical antibiotics may be applied to the area of skin loss and the patients referred for surgical assessment and further management. Immediate management involves immersing the area in warm water and resuscitating the patient whilst performing a secondary survey and treating any other injuries. Intravenous access should be secured early and correction of hypotension with warmed fluids using normal saline or 5% dextrose solution. As part of the initial treatment, analgesia should be provided as soon as possible. This may involve the use of intravenous opiates or more simple analgesics, such as non-steroidal anti-inflammatory agents. Areas where blisters have ruptured should be debrided and topical antibiotics applied. The affected area should be elevated and splinted with a non-adherent dressing *in situ*. After initial management, the mainstay of treatment involves daily dressing changes and surgical intervention when required. Tetanus status should be sought and antitetanus toxoid given, if required.

CHEMICAL INCIDENTS

Chemical incidents can lead to severe morbidity and mortality, occurring more commonly in adults than children and in the industrial work place. No ideal definition exists for a chemical incident, although one definition can be quoted from Hill and O'Sullivan (1992): 'An unforeseen event leading to acute exposure of two or more individuals to any non-radioactive substance resulting in illness or potentially toxic threat to health'.

There are approximately 1000 incidents per year in the UK, and there are a wide variety of causes and treatment requirements. Incidents range from chemical leaks and spills to fire, malicious damage and explosions. Unlike other major incidents arriving in the emergency room, the safety of the rescuers is also of paramount importance and must be included in any major incident plan.

Management

It is vital to ensure the safety of the rescuers at the scene and at the receiving Emergency Department. Resuscitation can continue as long as there is no risk of injury or contamination to the team. Secondary contamination of medical personnel is common and made more difficult, as the potential hazard may not be visible to the naked eye.

As well as the immediate risk to the individual, the site of the accident is enlarged and will lead to an increase in the size of the incident, wasting resources and time. Determination of the type of chemical involved in the incident should be made as soon as practical. Where this may involve a vehicle, symbols may be found on the side of the tanker, thus allowing early identification and planning for the treatment of casualties.

As well as protecting personnel, it is also important to keep the number of rescuers involved to a minimum to decrease the risk of secondary contamination. Triage at the scene is the first aim of clinical management. Casualties can be graded according to the severity of their illness and those most likely to respond to treatment. It is of great importance to remember that there may be other injuries not immediately apparent and, as with other trauma, a full primary and secondary survey should be completed and recorded in the case notes.

There are three broad groups in the triage of chemically injured patients as follows.

> Priority 1 (P1) – resuscitation required during decontamination.
>   Priority 2 (P2) – resuscitation after decontamination.
>   Priority 3 (P3) – minor injuries able to walk to a decontamination area prior to treatment.

Decontamination

In the organisation of the rescue, clean (uncontaminated) and dirty (contaminated) areas should be pre-arranged with different personnel working in the separate areas. The initial decontamination process should consist of a 'rinse–wipe–rinse' routine. This can be repeated as often as required to achieve decontamination and copious amounts of water may be required (Fisher, 1998). The waste can be either contained (collected for later disposal) or non-contained (diluted and let into the drainage system). An obvious result of this process is hypothermia, which should be actively and urgently treated. Areas of obvious importance are the eye, which should be irrigated as soon as possible with care taken not to contaminate the other eye, and open sores or wounds.

Dry decontamination can be used when the chemicals react with water. Special vacuum cleaners or Fuller's earth can adsorb the chemical residues.

Resuscitation

Resuscitation should be performed along the ATLS® guidelines (American College of Surgeons 1997), with particular care taken of the cervical spine if an explosion has occurred.

The patient should be fully exposed and all articles that may be contaminated placed in a dirty area. The removal of clothes itself performs 70–80% of the decontamination process. Primarily, attention is made to the airway and breathing, and supplemental oxygen should be given to all patients as soon as it is practical and safe to do so. Intravenous access should be secured by two large-bore cannulae and warm fluids given appropriately. In the majority of cases, supportive measures are all that are usually required, although there should be a low threshold for seeking more expert advice and antidotes given if appropriate.

Types of chemical injury

The reaction with a chemical injury is similar to that of a burn. There are four common types of chemical injury and the treatment varies according to the substance.

Phosphorus
Phosphorus ignites spontaneously and will continue to burn in the presence of water. Copper sulphate 1% is used to react with the phosphorus and there is a colour change to black. The area can then be cleaned by removing the individual pieces of the phosphorus and a further survey then performed. Care must be taken with large areas, as copper may be toxic in large doses.

Phenol
Phenol can produce systemic toxicity and rarely causes a full-thickness burn. Charcoal should be applied to adsorb the phenol; if the area is soaked with water, absorption is increased and toxic side effects can result.

Hydrofluoric acid
Hydrofluoric acid is used in the manufacture of glass and industrial cleaning. Hypocalcaemia can result secondary to skin colliquation. A large burn may be fatal, and patients should be referred to a burns unit for immediate excision and debridement. Immediate treatment may include calcium gluconate gel and, rarely, intra-arterial calcium to prevent distal limb ischaemia.

Cement
Cement is a weak alkali, which can produce full-thickness burns even in a small area if left applied to the skin.

RADIATION

Radiation injuries are uncommon in the UK, but give rise to a combination of problems including internal and external radiation. They may be associated with traumatic injuries, which should be sought for as a priority and the treatment not delayed whilst the patient is decontaminated.

Radiation has its effect by passing energy from the radiation source to the target. The units of radiation are measured as becquerels from the source. In man, the amount and type of radiation that the subject is exposed to determine the radiation dose. This is measured as the equivalent dose and can be derived by the following equation:

Absorbed dose × radiation weighting factor =
Equivalent dose

The unit of equivalent dose is the sievert.

Over 80% of the radiation dose comes from natural sources in the UK. Cells in the body vary in their sensitivity to radiation with the rapidly dividing cells being the most sensitive. All hospitals should have a major incident plans that include the treatment of radiation victims. It is important that there is no contamination of the staff treating the victims. Measures should also be taken to avoid contamination of the centre where treatment is carried out.

On-scene treatment

In the event of a radiation incident, a health physicist is required in addition to the emergency services to provide suitable monitoring equipment and to advise on the treatment required for the casualties.

Decontamination should be carried out as soon as is practical. In rare cases, the external radiation is life threatening and needs to be carried out urgently, as in the incident at Chernobyl. Usually, the external radiation dose is not sufficient to cause burns or radiation sickness to the victim or the rescuers. A primary survey should be carried out as soon as possible and other life-threatening injuries treated. In the ideal situation, the decontamination is carried out early to prevent the cross-contamination of the staff and the hospital. The extent of contamination (both internal and external) should be determined within a few hours, if possible, in order that further treatment can be proposed. This can, however, be delayed for more urgent treatment.

With the aid of the emergency services, the area should be secured and the risk assessment for the rescuers established. Any airborne contaminants must be sought and appropriate protective gear provided for the rescuers. This may include the use of respiratory protection.

Firstly, simple measures should be taken to protect the staff and the victims. Initial measures include the removal of all external clothing, if contaminated, and the securing of these contaminated clothes in a safe area. At the initial assessment of the site, the degree of contamination can be predicted. If there has not been release of radioactive substances into the atmosphere and the source is known, although the victims may have suffered radiation exposure, there is no risk of them being radioactive; therefore, they pose no threat to the staff or hospital. No special precautions need be taken and transport need not be any different to that of a non-radiation incident.

Radiation dosimeters should be available to all staff and simple precautions taken to decrease any risk of contamination. If dosimeters are not available, time should be monitored in the field so a risk assessment can be made at a later date. By decreasing the time spent in the radiation field and keeping as far away from the source as possible, the risk is decreased for the rescuers. In the hospital setting, staff can be protected behind dense materials, such as lead gowns. Radiation fields are very unlikely to produce a dose sufficient for acute sickness; therefore, although it is important to remove the patient from the area as soon as possible, it is not justified to remove the subject without sufficient care for other injuries and stabilisation of any injuries noticed in the primary survey.

At the scene, simple protective equipment can be given to staff, which may include waterproof clothing and gloves. Surgical gloves should be changed frequently to protect the wearer but also the victim. Ideally, two pairs can be worn with the outer pair replaced between patients and the inner for the protection of the staff. The assessment should also include whether any radioactive iodine has been released, as prophylaxis should be given to all in the form of stable potassium iodate. This will be taken up by the thyroid gland preferentially and saturate the thyroid, thus preventing gland irradiation and subsequent hypothyroidism.

Initial hospital treatment

An initial assessment should be performed at the site of accident and initial treatment commenced. The 'on-scene' team should also have reported back to the receiving hospital and appropriate staff and equipment prepared in advance. If there are many casualties expected, the staff on scene can divide the patients into clean and contaminated (dirty) patients and thus divide the hospitals into the different receiving sites to minimise the contamination of the buildings and the staff.

Intravenous access is not vital at the scene unless there are other injuries. In these situations, access should be sought through a non-contaminated area of skin to prevent further contamination. Opsite dressings can be used in the severely contaminated to protect the surrounding skin, if intravenous access is near to a penetrating wound.

Prior to the arrival of the patients, the hospital should notify the appropriate health physics team and the department should be prepared to decrease the amount of contamination that occurs. This will involve the removal of non-essential personnel and equipment from the receiving area. Carpeted areas should be covered in non-permeable material and securely taped down. All trolleys and waste bins should also be covered in waterproof materials so the casualties do not contaminate them and the coverings can be disposed of safely with all other contaminated clothes and non-reusable equipment. Air conditioning should also be turned off to prevent spread through the duct system in the hospital.

Staff in the dirty team should wear caps, gowns, masks and boots. They should also wear two pairs of gloves and aprons. The clean and dirty areas of the department should be well divided and the clean team should wear caps, masks, gloves and overshoes. In this way, both the department and the staff are well protected against the risk of contamination from the casualties.

Triage

Triage is vital in this situation and should be dictated by the severity of the injury as in standard ATLS® teaching (American College of Surgeons, 1997) and not dependent on the degree of contamination.

All clothing should be bagged and marked appropriately, and the surface of the body should be monitored for the degree of contamination. Areas particularly at risk are the skin folds, wounds and the head. Medical personnel should also be monitored and, as well as standard washing procedures from the neck down, swabs should be taken from the mouth, including nostrils, lips, tongue and teeth. Areas of contamination can be noted on an anatomical diagram for the different areas of radioactivity.

> Patients who present as a result of a chemical incident must be triaged based on the severity of their injury and not on their degree of contamination

Initial management

Skin, if intact, is an effective barrier to radioactive materials. After full assessment and treatment of life-threatening injuries, patients should be washed with a mild detergent and care taken not to break the integrity of the skin by overvigorous scrubbing. Repeated washing may be required to fully decontaminate. Washing from the periphery to the centre of the area is recommended, and sponging and swabbing to prevent spread from water running over non-contaminated areas.

Potassium permanganate can be used to fix the area of contamination. The area should be left to dry for a few minutes and the colouring then removed with 2.5% solution of sodium metasulphite. This process confirms that all the area has been treated and also allows some desquamation of the affected area. Showering should be from the neck downwards and the head dealt with separately. Facial hair should be trimmed and not shaved to avoid the risk of breaking the skin's integrity. All hair and swabs should be sent for monitoring by the physics health laboratory. Any areas that are resistant to decontamination should be covered with a non-porous material and recleaned the following day. Following each cleansing, the area should be monitored for the degree of contamination and recorded.

Any penetrating wounds should be dealt with according to their severity. If there is wound contamination, then the area should be surgically toileted. Any less severe wounds that can be covered with a non-porous dressing should be covered so that the surrounding skin can be cleaned to ensure that the contamination is in the wound and all other areas are clean. Foreign material should be removed and any excised tissue sent for monitoring as well as the surgical instruments used. Areas of wound contamination should be frequently monitored and recorded levels of contamination noted. If there are areas of continuing contamination, then a decision about tissue removal should be discussed with the plastic surgeons and the risk–benefit ratio worked out for that area of contamination.

Radiation effects

Acute radiation affects radiosensitive tissues in the body. These include the bone marrow, gastrointestinal tract, blood vessels and nerves. There is a threshold below which radiation damage will *not* occur and, in the vast majority of incidents, this dose is not exceeded. Therefore, for both treatment schedules and reassurance for the patient, it is important to work out the whole body radiation dosages.

Symptoms occur soon after exposure, some within hours, but the majority within days or weeks. This is the main reason that the more conventional injuries should be treated first. Whole-body absorbed doses exceeding 2 Gy are likely to produce symptoms and those above 4 Gy will produce serious effects and may be life threatening. In these circumstances, it is important to involve haematologists and radiotherapists early. Bone marrow effects, including short-lived neutrophilia followed by neutropenia, are frequent; there is an immediate fall in the lymphocyte count and thrombocytopenia. An early full blood count is advisable. If there is confirmed bone marrow damage, then specialist advice is needed for the long-term management, which may include the use of blood products and antibiotics (owing to the immunocompromisation). Cytokine therapy and transplantation may be required in serious cases. There may be transient erythema (occurring within 2–3 hours) and headache, nausea, vomiting, diarrhoea and hyperpyrexia can ensue. Radiation burns occur within a week of exposure and need care by a dermatologist, which may involve the use of analgesia and antibiotics for ulceration and infection.

Internal radiation

If a patient has suffered internal contamination, then the most important treatment is to administer stable iodine. This will compete for take-up in the thyroid gland and so reduce the dose to the organ. If given within 12 hours of exposure, then there will be reduced uptake by the gland.

Summary

Following a radiation exposure, the casualties should first be assessed at the scene and a report made to the hospital with the provision made for dirty and clean areas. Their basic resuscitation should not alter, the priority being the treatment of life-threatening conditions followed by assessment and treatment of the radiation injury.

The majority of radiation injuries are not severe, the level being lower than the threshold dose. Despite this, there should be early liaison with the local health physicist, and dose meters made available for the staff and hospital. Simple cleaning methods are suitable for the majority of patients and these techniques may need to be repeated for a few days, if contamination is not cleared with the first cleaning.

CONCLUSION

Patients who sustain trauma in unusual or special circumstances must be assessed and treated according to ATLS® guidelines (American College of Surgeons, 1997). It is essential that such patients are also assessed based on the severity of their injury or condition, and not on the basis of the circumstances in which they are found (e.g. radiation incident). Trauma nurses play a vital role in the ongoing assessment and monitoring of these patients; their early identification and treatment of complications have a direct impact on morbidity, and the outcome from trauma and should not be underestimated. An awareness of the roles and expertise of public health and other appropriate agencies will contribute to an effective team approach to managing such trauma patients successfully.

References and further reading

American College of Surgeons. *Advanced trauma life support manual*, 6th edn. Chicago: American College of Surgeons, 1997

Barnet PN. *Arctic Aerospace Laboratory Report*, AA1 – TDR. 1962; 61: 65b

Botte RG, Black PG, Bowers RS, et al. The use of extra corporeal rewarming in a child submerged for 66 minutes. *JAMA* 1933; 260: 377–379

Driscoll P, Skinner D. (eds) *Trauma care*. London: BMJ, 1998

European Resuscitation Council. *ALS manual*. Antwerp: European Resuscitation Council, 1994: BH9, 40

Garrard G, Foex P, Westaby S. (eds) *Principles and practice of critical care*. Oxford: Blackwell Science, 1997

Golden FStC, Harvey GR, Tipton MJ. Circum-rescue collapse: collapse, sometimes fatal, associated with rescue of immersion victims. *Journal of the Royal Naval Medical Service* 1991; 77: 139–149

Gray D. Survival after burial in avalanche. *British Medical Journal* 1987; 611–612

Greaves I, Porter K. (eds) *Pre-hospital medicine*. London: Arnold, 1999

Hill PM, O'Sullivan DG. *A study of arrangements for the identification and investigation of incidents of acute exposure of the public to toxic substances*. London: Department of Health, 1992

Lexoff K. Severe accidental hypothermia: survival after 6 1/2 hours of CPR. *Arctic Medical Research* 1991; 50(Suppl): 112–114

Lloyd EL. Hypothermia. In: Greaves, Porter K (eds) *Pre-hospital medicine*. London: Arnold, 1999

Modell JH. Pathophysiology and treatment of drowning. *Acta Anaesthesiologica Scandinavica* 1968; (Suppl. xxix): 263–279

Orlowski JP. Drowning, near drowning and ice-water submersion. *Pediatric Clinics of North America* 1987; 30: 75–92

Simcock AD. Near drowning and hypothermia. In: Goldhill DR, Withington SP (eds) *Intensive care*. London: Chapman & Hall, 1997: 680

Chapter 38

Sudden death

Rose Ann O'Shea

INTRODUCTION

Few situations engender more emotion and psychological distress among health care providers than that of witnessing a sudden death or caring for the recently bereaved. This is particularly true in traumatic events, where the death is often unexpected and much is left unfinished or unsaid, where the young are involved, and where precautionary or preventative measures may have changed the outcome. The period immediately following this can have a profound effect on the family and friends of the deceased, often with long-lasting consequences or sequelae. Understanding the grieving process, grief reactions and their impact on all those concerned are essential if those affected are to emerge able to continue with their lives in a productive way. The role of emergency and trauma team members, and trauma nurses in particular, is vital to the process of grieving and to ensuring that those left behind are cared for appropriately when they are at their most vulnerable.

SUDDEN DEATH

The death of a loved one, whether family member or friend, is one of the most traumatic events that most people will experience in their lifetime. Where the death is sudden and unexpected, the response invoked will often be one of great intensity, leaving those left behind unprepared and struggling to deal with the consequences of their loss. Numerous studies addressing grief and grief reactions have provided valuable insight into the issues that need to be faced in the immediate period following the death, as well as those which may occur in later phases and which may be associated with long-term difficulties. Their findings have formed the basis of many bereavement and crisis intervention programmes that have been established to help facilitate the grieving process, and in particular the giving and receiving of bad news.

Many individuals emerge from this experience able to continue leading positive and productive lives. Others, however, encounter greater difficulty in returning to a form of normality, the impact of the experience being so overwhelming as to have a negative impact upon them, potentially permeating every aspect of their lives. The nature of the circumstances surrounding the death and the way in which these are handled are key determinants in the process of grieving and are of paramount importance. Whatever the circumstances surrounding the death, the aim of those caring for the bereaved is to make it manageable by decreasing its impact and the potential for damage through addressing its physical, emotional, intellectual, social and spiritual components. Such a framework is designed to instil order into the chaos and disarray that often ensues, in the hope of preventing or minimising the far-reaching consequences and implications, many of which continue to affect those involved for many years.

> The loss of a loved one is one of the most difficult life events that can be experienced

As carers, trauma nurses find themselves in a privileged, yet to many unenviable, position of being with those faced with a life event that cannot be equalled in terms of its ability to impose emotional pain and distress on another person (Wright, 1991). Although ideally placed to provide a special and important dimension of care, and to play an important part in the life of the bereaved, many carers experience great difficulty at this time, leaving them feeling overwhelmed, drained and damaged. This is found to be particularly the case for many who have performed this role for many years and who eventually succumb to the cumulative effects of stress. Management of the sudden death situation needs, therefore, to focus on the needs of both the bereaved and their carers, and must include immediate and long-term support mechanisms.

Interventions at this time are aimed at channelling emotions positively, and enabling them to be experienced and released in a supportive environment and in such a manner to minimise potentially incapacitating effects on both carers and those being cared for. Reactions can vary enormously ranging from quiet acceptance to overt anger and denial. Much depends on the nature of the attachment prior to the death, the relationship between the parties, whether the death was anticipated, the mode of death and the circumstances surrounding it. Where violence, foul play or human factors are involved, this reaction is likely to be intensified, often with an overt need to apportion blame. The trauma situation can also trigger intense responses, which others may find difficult to understand. Whatever the reaction, it is important that those caring for them are non-judgemental and non-confrontational, display sensitivity, and validate their feelings and beliefs, all of which can contribute towards successful re-emergence.

Grieving is a process that begins on the news of a death. Some studies have found that where death is unexpected, feelings of remorse, self-reproach and distress were more marked than in those who anticipated the death (Lundin, 1984). Anticipatory grief (i.e. the grief experienced where the death is expected) occurs prior to the loss. Lindemann (1944) suggests that, where knowledge of this is not suppressed or withheld, a better outcome ensues, and that where it has been withheld, even when the death is expected and anticipated, the actual moment of death may mimic all the hallmarks of a sudden death reaction. Whether anticipated or not, the effect of death may be compounded by other life events occurring at or around the same time (e.g. occupation, relationships, marital problems or status, domestic circumstances and family or financial pressures).

Some circumstances at the time of death are associated with particularly difficult and sensitive issues, and potentially poor outcomes. These include suicide, murder, violence, trauma and deaths involving children, particularly cot death or *sudden infant death syndrome* (SIDS). These present a unique array of problems and difficulties, leaving those affected incapacitated and unable to cope for considerable periods after the event. Indeed, many focus on the need for answers and are unable to focus on anything else without them. Where spiritual or religious values and beliefs are challenged, the grieving process may be further complicated, with feelings of guilt commonly expressed.

Death may occur in a range of settings, such as the home, workplace, hospital or out-of-hospital setting. Where trauma in particular is concerned, events occurring in the out-of-hospital setting can assume even greater significance. Relatives may sometimes be present in the out-of-hospital setting; however, more commonly, they arrive in the emergency department seeking help and looking for their loved ones. Whatever the environment, open and honest communication is vital; where possible, a named or designated person should be allocated this responsibility. Generally speaking, once health care professionals and trauma/emergency teams become involved, particularly in hospital, it is believed that the patient no longer belongs entirely to the family. Families may be reluctant to state their own needs, and often do not know or understand what boundaries have been imposed. This feeling of loss of autonomy and control may be enhanced where there is a prolonged wait for news or an update on their loved one's progress. For example, where serious head injuries have been sustained, and the result of scans, investigations and procedures are awaited, tensions may rise and apparently rigid and hierarchical hospital processes become overwhelming. Giving false hopes or unrealistic expectations at this time does little to help, and instead delays the process of understanding and coming to terms with what has occurred. Where death has been confirmed, seeing the deceased can in many instances go a long way to restoring this autonomy. Even where the body has been mutilated and disfigured, reality is seen to be more acceptable than fantasy and provides an opportunity to say goodbye. Where bystanders and other laypersons have been involved, for example, in performing cardiopulmonary resuscitation (CPR) in the cardiac arrest situation, the effect on them should not be underestimated. It is essential that their needs are attended to, support is provided and their contribution acknowledged.

Some staff handle these situations well and are able to empathise with the bereaved, acting as their advocate and ensuring that as far as possible their wishes are adhered to. Others experience great difficulty and stumble over what to say and do, resulting in them being dissatisfied with their performance, finding difficulty in letting go, and feeling less effective than they should. For carers, it is important to feel useful, provide comfort and have a valuable contribution, making a difference in what is for many people one of the greatest challenges and adjustments they will have to make in their lives. The role of support services and staff, and the involvement of religious and spiritual leaders and chaplains, can be an invaluable source of strength, and should be offered even if not requested. Some people feel embarrassed to request such support, yet are relieved and thankful when it is offered.

Legal, professional and forensic considerations

Issues surrounding the pronouncing and certification of death pose many questions for staff, and are often key stressors for the bereaved and their family and friends. Where the death is anticipated, this is usually relatively straightforward; where the death is sudden, unexpected or involves outside influences, this process can be complicated greatly. The involvement of police or coroner's/Procurator Fiscal's officers is not uncommon and, indeed, is to be expected where trauma or violence is involved, where the death is unexpected, and where there are suspicious circumstances. In such circumstances, the need for a post mortem or autopsy is evident, although the bereaved may require explanation and convincing of this. The preservation of evidence, particularly at accident scenes or scenes of crime, is central to forensic examinations. This can extend to leaving bodies *in situ* until authorisation to move them has been given by the police or accident investigation officers.

Recent developments in nursing roles, both in-hospital and out-of-hospital emergency and trauma care, have expanded to include the pro-nouncing of death. To date, however, legislation has not been passed to permit nurses and other non-medical staff to issue death certificates. Recognition of the increasing role of nurses responding on behalf of UK ambulance services is evidenced, however, in pre-hospital guidelines issued by the Joint Royal Colleges Ambulance Liaison Committee (JRCALC), such as that relating to the Recognition of Life Extinct (ROLE, v2.2 and v3.0). These permit staff trained in their use to pronounce death according to specified criteria, in the absence of suspicious or untoward circumstances, which may enable family and friends to remain with the deceased at home prior to the involvement of undertakers or funeral staff, and thereby avoid the unnecessary and sometimes unwanted input of hospital staff.

Major-incident, multiple-casualty or disaster situations are exceptional events characteristically associated with sudden or unexpected death. In these instances, responsibility for the dead remains with the police and forensic teams. Retrieval and preservation of evidence and identification of the dead are key elements of the investigation process; adherence to instructions and compliance with directives are, therefore, essential.

Issues relating to the requesting of organs for donation may be discussed in these situations and must be treated with extreme sensitivity. For those left behind, such requests can result in additional stress and trauma to what will, undoubtedly, be one of the most traumatic situations they will face. Consent that is valid, unsolicited and freely given is essential. The involvement of transplant team coordinators, specially trained in this area, should be invited at an early stage to ensure that adequate time, information and explanations are given to family and friends, and to ensure that their needs are not only identified, but are met and appropriately addressed. The use of advance directives or living wills is increasingly being adopted, and their use gaining wider accept-ance and understanding by health care teams. Although not legally binding, these written instructions outlining wishes in the event of death must be considered in the clinical decision-making process.

BREAKING BAD NEWS

The role of breaking bad news has in recent years increasingly become the domain of nursing staff. Once associated with performing a supportive role to medical colleagues, many emergency and trauma nurses now assume responsibility for this, and act as advocate for the bereaved and their liaison with the wider trauma team. Preparation for this is sporadic, with input mainly given in the form of lectures and skill stations on advanced life support (ALS) or similar training courses. While helpful, this is considered by most to be inadequate, leaving them with strong feelings of trepidation on entering the room to inform relatives. The need for education, training and preparation for this role is evident.

In the out-of-hospital setting, this can be even more difficult, especially, for example, after traumatic road traffic accidents or other traumatic incidents, particularly where there may be disfigurement or where those present may seek to apportion blame. This uncontrolled setting serves to add an extra dimension to an already difficult situation, where the responses of those involved may be extreme and unpredictable.

It is essential that carers and those breaking bad news are aware of their own feelings, beliefs and prejudices, and confront them before undertaking this role. An awareness of body language, and all forms of verbal and non-verbal communication, including tone of voice and terminology used, is essential, as the bereaved are noted to remember the incident in detail, even down to the colour of eyes of the person breaking the news to them (Wright, 1991). Also, at this time of intense vulnerability, they may misinterpret information, further exacerbating their pain and distress. Clear unambiguous information should be given and repeated as often as required; where possible, information should also be given to friends or family members, as they may be more able to absorb and retain this, maintain a logical and clear focus, and offer practical guidance and support. Written documentation regarding what to do after a death, including registering it and obtaining a death certificate can prove invaluable.

Most sudden deaths are associated with vigorous resuscitation. Very often relatives are absent, arriving later at the scene of the incident or at hospital. Some are not given the opportunity to witness the resuscitation and are instead left waiting in another room, typically the 'relatives room'. While waiting, the need for answers to questions grows, particularly to questions such as 'was s/he conscious?' and 'did s/he suffer?'. Providing honest comprehensive information may help, including that relating to treatment administered.

The types of reactions that can be evoked in response to receiving bad news are varied and complex, ranging from anger, bewilderment, numbness, protest, hostility, aggression, fight and flight, to shock and disbelief. Confusing and sometimes unpredictable, a wide array of emotions, and potentially erratic and disordered behaviour may ensue. Much often depends on culture, race and religious beliefs; accordingly, the reaction to grief may be noisy and emotional, or very quiet with little emotion shown. In many instances, the initial reaction is one of disbelief followed by denial, with anxiety, guilt or anger experienced later. Preoccupation with events and repeated reflections on every part of their relationship with the deceased may engulf some, while others demonstrate the need to make sense of something senseless; a need that often remains unmet. Later, there may be a shift towards having to take control, to get on with things and to depersonalise the loss.

> Initial reaction is usually one of disbelief, then denial

In the event of a sudden death, it is not uncommon for family and friends to arrive at hospital or at the scene with offers of help and support, often seeking confirmation of the event itself. One of the key roles of carers is to advocate for the bereaved, and to prevent the most closely bereaved person from being swamped with care and thus lose their autonomy. This includes preventing others who are trying to help taking over the role of answering questions. This is the only opportunity that the bereaved will have to work through this difficult time in the immediate term and to begin the process of grieving, and will not be afforded to them unless they are given the space and time to do so.

In his extensive review of sudden death and the effects on those bereaved, Wright (1991) cites criticisms of those giving bad news as mainly related to communication. Beating about the bush, preamble, poor non-verbal communication including stance, positioning, standing rather than sitting, and poor eye contact featured as the main culprits. Returning personal property and valuables was also seen as being of great significance, and associated with causing distress and pain for the bereaved. In many instances, clothing was returned unfolded in carrier bags; the type of bag used and the manner in which clothing and other valuables was presented was seen by some to be an indication of how the person was considered in life.

The relatives room

Wright's study (1991) also included perceptions of the bereaved of the hospital facilities provided for them and, in particular, that of the relatives room. Access to a telephone capable of national dialling, washbasins with hot and cold water and a towel, chairs and a coffee table, privacy, drinks and access to toilet facilities were seen as being essential. Criticisms offered related mainly to the size and oppressive nature of rooms, particularly where there were no windows or access to the outside walls, and where lighting was poor, as these could induce feelings of panic, fear or isolation when left alone. Guidance on when and whether the bereaved were able to leave the room was also highlighted.

In the emergency department setting, news of the death will usually be given in the relatives room. Many people experience fear and apprehension on entering this room, the mere act of which starts to prepare them for what is to come. Establishing a rapport with them is an essential responsibility of the nurse or carer tasked with imparting information about the patient. Although many individuals can liaise with families and deliver news effectively, many believe that nurses are ideally placed for this, as they can liaise between the resuscitation room and the relatives more comfortably than most, and will have some understanding about the emergency treatment required. Attributes required for this role include the ability to communicate and answer questions, honesty, and the ability to deal with a range of reactions or emotions.

Identifying and viewing the body

Formal identification of the body in the presence of a police officer is required in most, if not all, cases of sudden death. This is particularly the case in the event of cot deaths, and all trauma or violence-related incidents. After the brief initial contact and the formal identification has been made, it is usual for police officers to withdraw, allowing family members to remain with the deceased and spend time with them. It is essential that the bereaved are advised of this, as some may wish to leave hospital very quickly before this formality has been completed; if they are not so advised, it is possible that they will have to return and repeat the whole procedure again.

Identifying patients or establishing their identity is often an issue for those not present when the emergency initially occurred. This may involve taking them into the resuscitation area at an appropriate moment; this is especially important if the patient is critical and emergency surgery is imminent. This can also help prevent relatives sitting waiting for lengthy periods where there is uncertainty over the patient's identification. Where death has occurred or is imminent, religious, spiritual and cultural issues may become more prominent. Relatives may give instructions on whether or the extent to which the patient's body may be touched. Trauma nurses should comply with these and should, ideally, have a general understanding of customs and rituals.

Viewing the body can be traumatic for relatives and friends. This is particularly so in cases involving mutilation, or where there is a distorted or disfigured body image, such as that which may occur in trauma, road traffic accidents, fires, suicide and assault or murder. Despite the intense trepidation, anxiety and fear that many relatives report at this stage, the vast majority report the reality of the situation as being far less than their imagination had allowed them to believe, particularly where they were informed beforehand of the nature of any discolorations, mutilations or injuries. Indeed, many reported obtaining comfort from being in the place where their loved one died. Conversely, in those who declined to see their relative or loved one or to say goodbye, many report having regretted this for years to come.

Leaving the hospital or place of death

The act of leaving the hospital or place of death can present tremendous difficulties for people, particularly when the nature of the relationship has been close. The initial feeling of flight, and of wanting to turn around and run may now be replaced with the opposite reaction and a reluctance to leave. Coming to terms with the separation and loss may engender renewed feelings of distress; those bereaved need to know that everything possible has been done. Prior to leaving, all valuables and personal property should be returned, including jewellery, and documentation completed according to local policy. Assurances must be given that the procedures to be followed are understood; written documentation outlining these and providing details of names of those to contact in the event of confusion or difficulty once the initial reaction has passed can prove invaluable. As far as possible, it must be ensured that they are accompanied and that help, if needed, is given with transport arrangements. Where relatives insist on leaving the scene or hospital alone, even going so far as to insist on driving, steps should be taken to ensure their safety and every effort made to liaise with their family and/or friends.

Follow-up

In recent years, the need for ongoing support of the bereaved has been identified and, in many places, formalised. The role of bereavement liaison nurses, bereavement counsellors and organisations, such as CRUISE and 'compassionate friends', are a few such examples. Some kinds of sudden death are known to be associated with more pain and long-term difficulties (e.g. suicide and loss of a child). Counselling and support can prove to be invaluable. The use of sedation or medication to help with grieving, more common in the past, should be avoided where possible; indeed, many people regret having turned to chemicals to help them at this time.

GRIEF RESPONSES AND THE GRIEVING PROCESS

The grieving process

Wordon (1991) states that a healthy grieving process involves four key factors: accepting the reality of the loss; working through the pain of grief; adjusting to an environment in which the deceased is missing; and emotionally relocating the deceased and moving on with life. The notable works of Kubler-Ross (1969) in which the stages through which the bereaved may pass, are still quoted today. Awareness of these stages – denial, anger, bargaining, depression and acceptance – is necessary to understand the grief process and the reactions and emotions expressed (Box 38.1). Interestingly, Wordon (1983) makes a distinction between the process that occurs after loss and the personal experience of the loss; the former he terms 'mourning' and the latter 'grief'.

Active and passive components of the grieving process have been identified. Currency is given to the approach which suggests that Kubler-Ross' work relates to the more passive phases and Wordon's to the more active stages, seen as giving some control back and going some way to resolving issues of autonomy. The need to allow feelings to emerge and be explored, and to help the bereaved deal with them is accepted by all. In his studies of grief in adult life, Parkes (1975) supports this, going on to state that the feelings of alarm, searching, mitigation, anger and guilt end with gaining a new identity. This guilt may overwhelm the bereaved with sadness and may incapacitate them for a period or until resolution has been reached, if, indeed, this is ever achieved.

Grief responses

Those who have been affected by a sudden death will often talk about a loss of control over their lives and feelings of powerlessness or helplessness. As their advocate, one of the goals of trauma nurses should be to help them regain control and power, whilst giving them the freedom and space to express their emotions and pain. Some circumstances are associated with particularly strong grief responses and difficulties in coming to terms with the situation. Suicide is one such situation where the need to blame someone may be strong. For many, suicide is a taboo subject and one that creates hostility or relationship breakdown. Negative social reactions towards surviving relatives and spouses have serious adverse and lasting consequences. The need for emotional support at this time is huge, particularly where relationship difficulties prior to death were difficult and stressful, as feelings of guilt or responsibility can be overwhelming.

A number of factors are known to determine some of the difficulties that may be encountered when working with the bereaved, and which may become recurring issues in the counselling process. These determinants identified in Parkes' Harvard study (1975) are of great value in helping support those bereaved, as they enable those counselling to understand where they are at in terms of relationships and grief reactions and the part that these components play in their responses to grief (Box 38.2).

Mode of death

Where death is due to natural causes or occurs subsequent to a long illness, it is usually easier to come to terms with. Traumatic deaths, deaths

---

Box 38.1   Stages of the grieving process

- Denial
- Anger
- Bargaining
- Depression
- Acceptance

Box 38.2   Determinants of grief

1. Mode of death
2. Nature of the attachment
3. Who was the person?
4. Historical antecedents
5. Personality variables
6. Social variables

by injury or violence, or those which damage the body are more likely to be considered as having caused more suffering and pain and are, therefore, more likely to be regarded as being unjust. This is a particularly important issue for the bereaved as well as knowing the extent to which the victims were aware of what was happening to them. Where suffering is involved, a not uncommon reaction is to try to apportion blame – whether blaming themselves or others. Where death is perceived to have been due to a delay of failure in treatment, the National Health Service or health care professionals may be blamed. Where industry, employment or road traffic incidents are involved, an increased sense of anger, injustice and blame may result. In the latter, such feelings may be further exacerbated where human factors are believed to have played a vital part (e.g. hit-and-run or drink-driving situations).

The role of the deceased in their death may also come under scrutiny and may be discussed in the Coroner's or Procurator Fiscal's inquiries. Indeed, organisations or society itself may be blamed, resulting in altered dynamics and potential feelings of isolation. The location in which the death occurred is also important; where death has occurred in familiar territory, this is generally more acceptable, as the role of the deceased in the community or society is perceived to have been better understood, and they are perceived to have been among friends. The location of family and friends at the time of death and thereafter is also important; where families and close networks are expanded over a wider geographical area, the grieving process may be more difficult and prolonged. Where suicide has occurred, the grieving process may become increasingly complicated emotionally, intellectually and psychologically; indeed, physical ill health may also ensue. Questions surrounding what might have been, how else might the victim have emerged from the situation and the parts played by all those concerned are often repeated in the hope of finding answers or explanations.

Nature of the attachment

The type of relationship that the bereaved had with the deceased, its strengths and weaknesses, and what its loss represents may be suggestive of potential or actual vulnerability, and must be understood.

Who was the person?

Family roles, relationships and hierarchies may or may not be significant; assumptions should, therefore, be avoided and time taken instead to learn more about the individual relationship dynamics.

Historical antecedents

Previous life crises and how these were addressed and managed, especially sudden death, may affect the ability to cope after the bereavement. Where positive outcomes have been experienced in the past, there is an increased likelihood that this may again be the case. There is no place for complacency, however, and each situation should be addressed on its own merits. Where negative outcomes have resulted from previous experiences, these may again raise their head, resulting in a resurgence of previous problems. Similarly, previously unresolved loss or previous failure to confront loss may result in its re-emergence, and the potential impact of other coexisting life factors, such as concomitant illness (e.g. depression), compound difficulties in dealing with the loss.

Personality variables

Personality attributes of the bereaved may affect their ability to deal with grief, in both the short and long term. A positive immediate reaction to grief does not always suggest a positive long-term response, and long-term problems themselves may or may not be due to negative factors. Earlier personal experiences of death and grief may also contribute to vulnerability.

Social variables

Bereavement may result in alteration in the role of the bereaved in their community and society in general. Sexism may have existed in relationships, or domination by one party over another; death may alter this, and dictate that new or existing relationships are re-established.

THE LOSS OF A CHILD

While the loss of loved one cannot be imagined, few would disagree that no loss can be more intense than that of a child, particularly one's own child. The emotional and psychological turmoil associated with such an event can be devastating, leaving those concerned drained and incapacitated. Added to this is the attention focused on such situations by police and forensic teams, who may be called upon to investigate. One situation in particular seems to evoke a strong reaction and display of emotion – that of *sudden infant death syndrome* or cot death.

Slightly more common in boys than girls and more frequent in the winter months, SIDS is the name given to the situation where apparently healthy babies are put down to sleep, suffering only from minor ailments, such as upper respiratory tract infections or difficulty in feeding. When next looked on by their carers, they are found to be unresponsive with death confirmed soon thereafter. In the vast majority of cases, the cause of death is difficult, if not impossible, to determine. Recriminations and feelings of guilt can be overwhelming, with each part of the infant or child's life revisited. The need for answers and explanations is often immense and the need to apportion blame voiced. Why infants die in their sleep, or become unconscious and die seems inexplicable, yet the statistics rise year on year. Research into the cause of SIDS suggests that no pain or distress is suffered. Numerous campaigns are launched outlining the preferred sleeping position for children, yet the problem remains. Post-mortem examination in some infants reveals previously undiagnosed or unsuspected problems, possibly congenital, or overwhelming infection. Vomitus may sometimes be found in or around the infant's mouth or on bedclothes, leading to a possible conclusion of aspiration. In most instances, however, this is not the case, as the presence of vomit may occur during or after death, and is not a cause of death in itself.

Very often, the first health care professions to attend such situations are ambulance paramedics or immediate care practitioners. In most, if not all, cases, the infant is immediately transferred to hospital with resuscitation attempted en route, ideally accompanied by the parents or other close relatives/carers. Where circumstances prevent this (e.g. other small children at home who cannot be left), every attempt should be made to enable them to follow to the emergency department as soon as possible. Feelings of intense grief and distress are to be expected, and consideration should be given to religious or cultural beliefs or customs. Time must be given for the parents and family to say goodbye, to hold the baby, and to let go.

As well as exercising great sensitivity in breaking the news of the death, this sensitivity needs to be extended to imparting information on the role of the police and the Coroner's (or Procurator Fiscal's) officer. Such information will include health records and details of the child's history to date, vaccination and immunisation records, and details of the last days or hours prior to death. All clothing should be removed from the body and placed in separate bags for collection by the Coroner's officer, including soiled nappies and clothing, as this will form an important part of any investigation or inquiry. Nothing should be discarded or destroyed. Contact with paediatricians can be helpful and may help explain the rationale behind actions, interventions and the need for a post mortem. It may also be helpful in dealing with feelings of helplessness, confusion and perplexity. Open access to the dead baby prior to post mortem is also hugely important; grandparents and other family members may also wish to say goodbye and should not be forgotten. Although a clean gown may have been placed on the baby, or clothing provided by the emergency department staff, the family should be offered the opportunity to return with the child's own clothes and toys. Taking photographs of the baby can also be helpful, especially at a later date, as can handprints and footprints, which may be presented to the parents in specially handmade cards.

The parents of the infant should not be left alone unless requested by them; even when this request has been made, help should remain close at hand. Every attempt should be made to ensure that opportunities have been given to review the whole of the event prior to their departure. If the mother is breastfeeding, she will need immediate advice and support regarding the suppression of lactation. Written information explaining what SIDS is, and contact details of people and organisations that can provide help should be given (e.g. the Foundation for the Study of Infant Deaths).

WITNESSED RESUSCITATION

The practice of enabling family members to witness the resuscitation of their loved ones has gained increasing acceptance among emergency and trauma teams over recent years. Yet, despite this, little preparation or training is given to equip those performing this role, leaving many feeling vulnerable and reluctant to discuss it with relatives and friends. A range of factors may explain this, including confidence within the resuscitation team, adequacy of explanations, answering difficult questions, taking the decision to stop resuscitation, dealing with reactions and fear of reprisal, or even, in extreme cases, litigation. The dilemma regarding whether or not to admit relatives into the resuscitation room essentially relates to the relative's and the staff's perception of witnessed resuscitation, and the effect of witnessed resuscitation on them.

Those against the concept believe that trauma resuscitations can be visually disturbing, even to the most experienced clinical staff, and that, at an olfactory level, burns, blood and other secretions can result in unpleasant and upsetting smells in the trauma room, and may adversely affect those unfamiliar with the environment. Similarly, some believe that, where patients are conscious and crying out due to pain, hypoxic confusion or anxiety, this would cause disturbance and distress for the relatives. Confidentiality is also a frequent consideration in the debate. Where patients are unconscious, they are unable to give their consent; consequently, patient confidentiality may be broken, if their wishes are not known. Furthermore, Fulbrook (1998) suggests that, not only would the relatives see everything happening to the patient, but they may also hear information of an intensely personal nature.

In the trauma or resuscitation situation, clinical staff are known to use a variety of methods to deal with the resulting stress. Some bleak situations may be peppered with a small degree of humour, which can help to keep the team functioning under stress. Those against witnessed resuscitation believe that where relatives are present, not only may they find this difficult, offensive or distressing, but that their presence may inhibit this coping mechanism and thereby affect team performance. The possibility of unpredictable emotional responses on the part of relatives is also often cited as an argument. Emergency room staff asked about this relay the belief that panic by relatives can disrupt medical efforts, and fear potentially uncontrollable grief which could disrupt the team performance.

With relatives present, the pressure for the trauma team to perform well is increased. Some believe that their clinical performance may be inhibited by a reluctance to discuss the patient's condition in front of relatives, resulting in delayed decision-making and resuscitation attempts potentially continuing for considerably longer than usual. Moreover, many procedures learned by doctors and nurses are undertaken for the first time during trauma calls, for example, the insertion of a chest drain. Senior doctors talking through this procedure with more junior staff may not be viewed positively by grief-stricken relatives. Finally, the fear of complaints or litigation is increasingly cited as a reason for not to have family presence during resuscitation. Some staff fear that, during a witnessed resuscitation, an observed action or remark may offend relatives, leading to a complaint, and allowing the observation of medical procedures may lead to the risk of litigation against the hospital or the practitioner.

Those in favour of witnessed resuscitation cite respect for persons as a central facet of their argument. It is presumed that patients are resuscitated to save their lives and return them to their family and friends. By allowing relatives to see what is happening to their loved one, even for short periods of time, this may help to dispel unhealthy imagery or anxiety, and reassure them that everything possible is being done for their loved one. Permitting them to touch the patients while they are still warm may also be comforting to the general public as, to them, being warm equates to being alive. They may also feel able to say whatever they need to, to the dying person, while there is a remote chance that they may hear them, before saying goodbye.

Media influences can also play a part in the decision to enable or deny witnessed resuscitation. Whilst it is naïve to assume that television medical dramas or documentaries can completely prepare relatives for trauma resuscitation, the public may be more informed than first thought. Whether or not in favour of such influences, media obsession with this type of programme can graphically bring to the home the close up workings of trauma rooms as never seen before.

Some emergency personnel accept and are comfortable with witnessed resuscitation. Studies into the attitude of medical and nursing staff have shown that the more senior and experienced the members of staff, the more likely they were to agree to allow relatives into the emergency room. Establishing some basic ground rules that are understood by family members can be helpful in ensuring that resuscitation is maintained. These may include the following:

- The resuscitation team will determine the best time for the relatives to enter the area
- Relatives may be asked to leave depending on the patient's condition and the interventions being performed
- Family members will be escorted from they area, if they become overwhelmed or disturb the resuscitation efforts of the team
- Family members will never be left alone during resuscitation or a procedure (Royal College of Nursing, 2002).

The acclaimed Foote Hospital study (Jezierski, 1993), which resulted from the insistence of the relatives of two patients on being present during resuscitation, one a trauma victim, has led to the development of guidelines and a support structure for these interactions. Among its published findings demonstrating the success achieved in this area were: no evidence of relatives interfering, some incidence of hysteria where relatives were led away from the resuscitation, the presence of children permitted, the availability of a support system for relatives, and staff regarding patients as part of the community, not merely a clinical challenge.

In their study into whether relatives wished to be present during resuscitation, and their psychological sequelae, Robinson et al. (1998) reviewed the relatives of 25 patients, including trauma victims. Their findings revealed that none commented on any technical procedures or problems (including a difficult intubation), all felt that the experience had been beneficial to be present, there was less of a tendency to intrusive imagery, post-traumatic stress disorder and grief-related symptoms, and that staff viewed the patient as a valued family member. Their conclusion supported the view that there was little evidence to support the exclusion of relatives who wished to be present during resuscitation.

This complex and controversial issue clearly has many implications, not only for the initial stages of trauma care but also for the definitive care setting. It is an area in need of research and review, including the language and cultural barriers that can prove to be problematic when discussing it with relatives. Moreover, considerations of staff availability, support, personnel, training costs and follow-up all need to be addressed.

The enabling considerations and positive outcomes of witnessed resuscitation are shown in Box 38.3 and a checklist for practice outlined in Figure 38.1.

Box 38.3   Prerequisites to enable witnessed resuscitation

Enabling considerations

Organisational policies in place/Familiarity and understanding of policies
- Designated team member to support person in need
- Assessment and preparation of relatives/loved ones
- Resuscitation team in agreement with decision
- Systems in place to audit actions and interventions
- Education and development programmes in place

Positive outcomes

Processes
- Provides opportunity to say goodbye
- Assists with the grieving process
- Bereavement counselling in place
- Formal and informal debriefing systems available for staff

Witnessed resuscitation enabled

Witnessing Resuscitation: A checklist for practice			
	Yes	No	Comments
1. Organisational policies identified and in place			
2. Does guidance exist to cope with stopping resuscitation?			
3. Do bereavement guidelines exist?			
4. Are there accessible educational policies for all team members which cover:			
• Dealing with grieving relatives?			
• Dealing with witnessed resuscitation?			
• Dealing with bereaved relatives and follow-up services?			
• Communication skills?			
5. Is there a system in place that allows access to experienced staff who can support relatives when required?			
6. Is there guidance in place for accessing security staff if required?			
7. Are there mechanisms in place for critical incident debriefing?			
8. Is there any access to stress debriefing in place?			

Figure 38.1 Witnessing resuscitation: a checklist for practice.

THE STRESS ON CARERS

For those who are called upon to care for the bereaved, the emotional and psychological impact can take its toll, and may even leave some feeling burnt out. There is no right or wrong response to sudden death; accordingly, the range of responses that may be expressed is extensive. Teaching and training in this area should be designed to help manage responses effectively, and to provide carers with insight into the responses and difficulties that may be encountered. It can also lessen feelings of chaos and disorder because staff can identify the response early on in the grieving process, and where this occurs in the lifespan. Gaining insight into what can render nurses and other health care professionals feeling ineffective may also be beneficial, as this can help them better manage the sudden death situation.

Caring for the bereaved can be one of the most rewarding yet challenging experiences for nurses. To perform effectively in this role, however, personal reflection and analysis are necessary to identify areas of personal strengths, weaknesses and vulnerabilities, and to recognise areas of prejudice or unfinished business. Of particular importance is the need to develop and harness effective listening and interpersonal skills, and an ability to communicate effectively using unambiguous and jargon-free language.

Identifying stress, stressors and factors that incapacitate carers or cause difficulty should form part of training programmes. The bereaved very quickly pick up on these, thus self-awareness and a strategy for dealing with the issues is essential. Of all the responses encountered, withdrawal and silence typically cause the most difficulty, while acceptance, crying and sobbing cause the least. Difficult responses can make carers feel ineffective and question their communication skills. In his study, Wright (1991) found that non-verbal communication was greatly valued by relatives; indeed, just being there was found to help enormously in allaying fears of being alone. No response should, therefore, not be taken to assume that they wish to be alone; indeed, unless this is clearly verbalised, it may be best to remain with them. Other responses known to induce distress include denial and anger, particularly anger directed at the deceased. Ultimately, the bereaved attempt to regain control of the situation, often having gone through stages of bargaining, self-reproach and guilt. The aim is to help them to accept what has happened, to forgive themselves where this is an issue, and to move on.

Although dealing with individual situations is manageable for many nurses, problems may be encountered when the cumulative effects of stress are experienced. The ability to recognise this in oneself and in others is essential if burnout is to be avoided. Stress itself is not necessarily destructive or negative, but instead is suggestive that internal and external resources have been exceeded by demands, and that some intervention or coping mechanism is required. Burnout, on the other hand, results when coping mechanisms have been exhausted, resulting in carers becoming emotionally and psychologically overwhelmed. Where burnout is present, this can be manifest in a range of ways. Physical manifestations include fatigue, loss of energy and drive, tiredness and exhaustion, general aches and pains, malaise, sleep disturbances or sleeplessness, gastrointestinal disturbances, minor illnesses or hyperventilation, and other breathing difficulties. Emotional indicators include oversensitivity, irritability, tearfulness, distress and anger – often with little warning or stimulus – strong feelings of sadness or hopelessness, avoidance of people and places, and difficulties in concentrating.

The role of support systems and networks – whether formal or informal – should not be underestimated and are often recommended as first-line sources of help. In many cases, these are able to help address and manage problems, and avoid the impact of lasting consequences. Where events are of a particularly sensitive or critical nature, their effect on staff may be considerable. Critical incidents, classed as any situations faced by emergency or trauma personnel that cause them to experience unusually strong emotional reactions which have the potential for incapacitating them or rendering them ineffective, require structured intervention. Structured debriefing sessions, known as *critical incident stress debriefing* (CISD) sessions, soon after these events can facilitate the process of coping, go some way towards resolving feelings of inability to cope, restore normality, and are central to effective management of the cumulative effects of stress and the avoidance of disabling sequelae.

SUMMARY

Death is an inevitable event for everyone, fraught with potential emotional turmoil and unparalleled distress. Where the death is sudden and unexpected, these emotions may become heightened and more intense. At times of such vulnerability, those caring for the bereaved are in the privileged and delicate, yet unenviable, position of advocating for them during one of the most traumatic experiences that they will experience in their lives. The giving and receiving of bad news, personal interactions, interpersonal communication and the manner in which events are conducted may have lasting consequences well beyond the time of the incident, and are central to the grieving process. In ensuring that the bereaved receive the necessarily high standard of care at this time, the needs of those caring for them must not be forgotten.

References

Fullbrook S. Medico legal insights, legal implications of relatives witnessing resuscitation. *British Journal of Theatre Nursing 7* 1998; 10: 33–35

Jezierski M. Foote Hospital Emergency Department: shattering a paradigm. *Journal of Emergency Nursing* 1993; 19: 266–267

Kubler-Ross E. *On death and dying.* New York: Macmillan, 1969

Lindemann F. Symptomatology and management of acute grief. *American Journal of Psychiatry* 1944; 101: 141–149

Lundin T. Morbidity following sudden and unexpected bereavement. *British Journal of Psychiatry* 1984; 144: 84–88

Parkes CM. Bereavement – studies of grief in adult life. Harmondsworth: Penguin, 1975

Raphael B. *When disaster strikes.* London: Hutchinson, 1986

Robinson SM, Mackenzie-Ross S, Campbell-Hewson GL, Egleston CV, Prevost AT. Psychological effect of witnessed resuscitation on bereaved relatives. *Lancet* 1998; 22(352): 614–617

Royal College of Nursing (RCN). *Witnessing resuscitation: guidance for nursing staff.* London: RCN, 2002

Wordon JW. *Grief counselling and grief therapy.* London: Tavistock, 1983

Wordon JW. *Grief counselling and grief therapy: a handbook for the mental health practitioner*, 2nd edn. London: Routledge Publishers, 1991

Wright B. *Sudden death: intervention skills for the caring professions.* Edinburgh: Churchill Livingstone, 1991

Further reading

Adams S, Whitlock M, Higgs R, Bloomfield P, Baskett P. Should relatives be allowed to watch resuscitation? *British Medical Journal* 1994: 308: 1687–1692

Back KJ. Sudden, unexpected padiatric death: caring for the parents. *Pediatric Nursing* 1991; 17: 571–575

Back D, Rooke U. The presence of relatives in the resuscitation room. *Nursing Times* 1994; 90(30): 34–35

British Association for Accident and Emergency Medicine (BAEM) and Royal College of Nursing (RCN). *Bereavement care in A&E Departments. Report of the Working Group.* London: BAEM/RCN, 1995

Blomfield RA. Relatives in the resus room: don't overlook the patient. *Accident and Emergency Nursing* 2000; 8: 52–53

Bloomfield P. Good information and time with the body are more important. *British Medical Journal* 1994; 308, 1688–1689

Burgess K. Supporting bereaved relatives in A&E. *Nursing Standard* 1992, 6(19): 36–39

Chalk A. Should relatives be present in the resuscitation room? *Accident and Emergency Nursing* 1995; 3(2): 58–61

Clark AP, Calvin AO, Meyers TA, Eichhorn DE, Guzzetta CE. Family presence during CPR and invasive procedures: a research-based intervention. *Critical Care Nursing Clinics of North America* 2001; 13: 569–575

Connors P. Should relatives be allowed in the resuscitation room? *Nursing Standard* 1996; 10(44): 42–44

Cooke MW, Cooke HM, Glucksman EE. Management of sudden bereavement in the accident and emergency department. *British Medical Journal* 1992; 304: 1207–1209

Dimond B. Death in accident and emergency. *Accident and Emergency Nursing* 1995; 3: 38–41

Doyle CJ, Post H, Burney RE, Maino J, Keefe M, Rhee KJ. Family participation during resuscitation: an option. *Annals of Emergency Medicine* 1987; 16: 6

Eichhorn DJ, Meyers TA, Mitchell TG, Guzzetta CE. Opening the doors: family presence during resuscitation. *Journal of Cardiovascular Nursing* 1996; 10(4): 59–70

Eckle N, Baker P eds. *Presenting the option for family presence.* Park Ridge, IL: Emergency Nurses Association 1995.

Emergency Nurses Statement. Family presence at the bedside during invasive procedures and/or resuscitation. *Journal of Emergency Nursing* 1994; 21(2)

Fraser S, Atkins J. Survivors' recollections of helpful emergency nurse activities surrounding sudden death of a loved one. *Journal of Emergency Nursing* 1990; 16: 13–16

Gregory CM. I should have been with Lisa as she died. *Accident and Emergency Nursing* 1995; 3: 136–138

Hampe SO. Needs of the grieving spouse in a hospital setting. *Nursing Research* 1975; no 24: 113–120

Hampe SO. Needs of the grieving spouse in the hospital setting. *Nursing Research* 1995; 2: 113–119

Hanson C, Strawser P. Family presence during CPR, Foote Hospital Emergency department 9 year perspective. *Journal of Emergency Nursing* 1992; 18: 104–106

Higgs R. Relatives wishes should be accommodated. *British Medical Journal* 1994; 308: 1688

Kidby J. Family-witnessed cardiopulmonary resuscitation. *Nursing Standard* 2003; 17(5): 33–36

Meyers TM, Eichhorn DJ, Guzzetta CE. Do families want to be present during CPR? A retrospective survey. *Journal of Emergency Nursing* 1998; 24: 400–405

Meyers T, Eichhorn D, Guzzetta C et al. Family presence during invasive procedures and resuscitation. *America Journal of Nursing* 2000; 100: 32–43

Mitchell MH, Lynch MB. Should relatives be allowed in the resuscitation room? *Journal of Accident and Emergency Nursing* 1997; 14: 366–369

Morgan J. Introducing witnessed resuscitation in A&E. *Emergency Nurse* 1997; 5: 13–18

McGuinness S. Sudden death in the emergency department. *Management and practice in emergency nursing.* London: Chapman & Hall, 1988

McGenathan BM, Torrington KG, Uyehara FT. Family member presence during cardiopulmonary resuscitation. *Chest* 2002; 122: 2204–2211

Osuagwu CC. Keeping the family out: rethinking traditional thoughts. *Journal of Emergency Nursing* 1991; 17: 363–364

Osuagwu CC. More on family presence during resuscitation. *Journal of Emergency Nursing* 1993; 19: 276–277

Phillips BM. Supporting relatives following a cot death. *Postgraduate Medical Journal* 1996; 72: 648–652

Raphael B. *The anatomy of bereavement. A handbook for the caring professions.* London: Unwin Hyman, 1984

Read S. Loss and bereavement: a nursing response. *Nursing Standard* 2002; 16: 47–53

Redley B, Hood K. Staff attitudes towards family presence during resuscitation. *Accident and Emergency Nursing* 1996; 4: 145–151

Resuscitation Council (UK). *Should relatives witness resuscitation?* London: Resuscitation Council, 1996

Sacchetti A, Carracio C, Leva E, Hams RH, Lichenstein R. Acceptance of family member presence during pediatric resuscitation in the emergency department: effects of personal experience. *Pediatric Emergency Care* 2000; 16: 85–87

Samford M, Pugh D, Warren NA. Family presence during CPR: new decision in the twenty-first century. *Critical Care Nursing Quarterly* 2002; 25(2): 61–66

Stead CE. Sudden infant death syndrome (SIDS) on the 'other side'. *Accident and Emergency Nursing* 1998; 6: 24–27

Tippett J. Providing comfort in the resuscitation room.

Accident and Emergency Nursing 1993; 2: 155–159

Tucker TL. Family presence during resuscitation. *Critical Care Nursing Clinics of North America* 2002; 14(2): 177–185

Tye C. Qualified nurses' perceptions of the needs of suddenly bereaved family members in the accident and emergency department. *Journal of Advanced Nursing* 1993; 18: 948–956

Van der Woning M. Should relatives be invited to witness a resuscitation attempt? *Accident and Emergency Nursing* 1997; 5: 215–218

Van der Woning M. Relatives in the resuscitation area: a phenomenological study. *Nursing in Critical Care* 1999; 4: 186–192

Wellesley A, Glucksmann EE, Crouch R. Organ donation in the accident and emergency department: a study of relatives' views. *Journal of Accident and Emergency Medicine* 1997; 14: 24–25

Williams JM. Family presence during resuscitation: to see or not to see? *Nursing Clinics of North America* 2002; 37(1): 211–220

Wright B. Sudden death: nurses' reactions and relatives' opinions. *Bereavement Care* 1989; 8: 2–4

Wright B. *Caring in crisis: a handbook of intervention skills.* Edinburgh: Churchill Livingstone, 1993

Yates DW, Ellison G, McGuiness S. Care of the suddenly bereaved. *British Medical Journal* 1990; 301: 29–31

SECTION **6**

Professional dimensions

Chapter **39**

Legal aspects of trauma nursing

Bridgit Dimond

INTRODUCTION

Nurses are increasingly taking on new and advanced roles within a range of health care settings, none more so than those involved in emergency and trauma care. Advances in technology have contributed to these developments as has a political agenda which openly accepts the valuable and growing contribution that nurses can make to the delivery of high-quality patient care. While such nurses are willing to accept these new and increasingly autonomous roles, and understand their professional accountability in relation to them, most express a degree of uncertainty and sometimes confusion when confronted with their legal responsibilities. This chapter aims to address these concerns and ambiguities, and to clarify those areas of the law that particularly relate to nurses involved in caring for trauma patients.

THE LEGAL SYSTEM

In the UK, there are two main sources of law: statute law (Acts of Parliament) and common law (also known as case law or judge-made law). Statute law is also known as primary law and may sometimes give powers for a Minister of the Crown to draw up secondary legislation in the form of statutory instruments. In recent years, the Human Rights Act 1998 has become one of the most important new statutes. Common law develops as judges, in deciding disputes over the interpretation of statutes or filling in gaps not covered by legislation, lay down principles known as precedents, which should be followed by lower courts. The House of Lords' rulings are binding on all other courts. As members of the European Community, directives and regulations of the European Commission are binding upon us. Since devolution of powers to Scotland, Wales and Northern Ireland, these countries have varied and limited law-making powers.

THE LAW AND NEGLIGENCE – GENERAL PRINCIPLES

Four forums of accountability

Where harm occurs to patients or there is a failure to follow approved standards of care, practitioners could face action in four different courts of law or hearings.

Criminal law

The criminal law derives from both statutes and common law, and identifies actions or omissions (offences), which can be pursued by criminal proceedings. Health and safety laws, as laid down by the Health and Safety at Work Act 1974, and the regulations made under that statute are enforced in the criminal courts. Professional misconduct could also be the subject of a criminal prosecution, if it amounts to an offence. For example, in R v Adomako (1994), an anaesthetist was found to be guilty of gross negligence when a patient died on the operating table as a result of a tube bringing gases to him becoming disconnected. Whilst the anaesthetist had accepted that he may have been negligent, he denied that he was guilty of a criminal offence. The House of Lords held that the judge had correctly directed the jury on establishing beyond reasonable doubt gross negligence as a criminal offence. In another case, following the removal of the wrong kidney, a urologist and surgeon were prosecuted for causing the death of the patient. However the judge stopped the trial after it became evident from prosecution evidence that the prosecution could not prove that the removal of the kidney had actually caused the death of the patient.

Civil law

The most frequently brought cause of action in the civil courts in relation to health care is an action

for negligence. This is one of a group of civil wrongs known as 'torts'. To establish grounds for compensation in the law of negligence, a claimant has to show that a duty of care was owed to him or her, that the duty was broken by a failure to follow the reasonable standard of care, and that as a reasonably foreseeable consequence of this breach of duty harm occurred.

> The most frequently brought cause of action in the civil courts in relation to health care is an action for negligence

A duty of care clearly exists towards patients. However, UK law does not recognise any duty to volunteer help and be a 'good Samaritan'. The Code of Professional Conduct of the Nursing and Midwifery Council (2004a) recognises a 24-hour professional duty owed by the registered practitioner inside or outside of the workplace. However, nurses who volunteer help in such circumstances would not be covered by the vicarious liability of their employer should they cause harm, and would, therefore, require to have professional indemnity cover.

The courts have used the Bolam Test to determine the reasonable standard of care (Bolam v. Friern Hospital Management Committee, 1957). In the case from which the test takes its name, the court laid down the following principle to determine the standard of care that should be followed: 'the standard of the ordinary skilled man exercising and professing to have that special skill' (Judge McNair).

> The reasonable standard of care is that of the ordinary skilled man exercising and professing to have that special skill – the Bolam Test

Whilst individual practitioners may have been negligent, it is unlikely that they would be sued personally, unless they were self-employed, since the employer is seen in law as being vicariously liable for the negligence of employees who are acting in the course of employment. This ensures that the complainant is able to recover compensation. Most National Health Service (NHS) trusts are members of the Clinical Negligence Scheme for Trusts (CNST), which operates a pool from which compensation payments over a fixed amount are paid to claimants. The CNST requires the member Trusts to comply with specified standards in relation to such topics as record keeping and risk management, and carries out inspections to ensure that these standards are in place. The NHS Litigation Authority (NHSLA) handles the actual law cases on behalf of NHS Trusts. Failure to follow approved practice, which leads to personal injury or death, could be subject of litigation. Expert evidence would be given to the court regarding the standards that should have been in place.

Professional conduct

All registered practitioners face the possibility of a fitness to practise hearing before the Competence and Conduct Committee or Health Committee of the Nursing and Midwifery Council (NMC) with the ultimate sanction of being struck off the register. New procedures were introduced in August 2004 and their impact has yet to be determined (Statutory Instrument 2004/1761). The main aim of the registration provisions is the protection of the public.

> All registered practitioners face the possibility of a fitness to practise hearing before the Competence and Conduct Committee or Health Committee of the NMC with the ultimate sanction of being struck off the register

Disciplinary action by the employer

A contract of employment contains terms from diverse sources, including express terms agreed between the parties, terms required by statute, terms agreed through collective bargaining and also terms that are implied by law. The latter include the implied terms that an employer will take reasonable care of the health and safety of its employee, and the implied terms that the employee will act with all reasonable care and skill, and obey the reasonable instructions of the employer.

NATIONAL STANDARD SETTING

The government has developed plans as shown in the White Paper, in the document 'Making a

difference' and in 'The NHS plan' (Department of Health, 1997, 1999a, 2000). Legislation implementing these plans is to be found in the Health Act 1999, the Health and Social Care Act 2001, the NHS Reform and Health Care Profession Act 2002, and the Health and Social Care (Community Health and Standards) Act 2003. The National Institute for Clinical Excellence (NICE), Commission for Health Improvement (from April 2004 the Commission for Healthcare Audit and Inspection, known as the Health Commission), National Service Frameworks (NSFs) and the National Patient Safety Agency (NPSA) are to name but a few organisations that have also been established to set and monitor performance against national standards.

Clinical governance

One of the most important recent government initiatives was the introduction of the concept of clinical governance, which derives from the statutory duty under Section 18 of the Health Act 1999 as revised by the Health and Social Care (Community Health and Standards) Act 2004 section 45, as shown below.

> It is the duty of each NHS body to put and keep in place arrangements for the purpose of monitoring and improving the quality of health care provided by and for that body. Health care means the services provided to individuals for or in connection with the prevention, diagnosis or treatment of illness and the promotion and protection of public health

This statutory duty to deliver the standards expected falls primarily upon the chief executive of each health authority, primary care trust and NHS Trust. The result of this duty is that NHS bodies and their chief officers are responsible for the standard of clinical care within their organisations. If they fail to ensure that reasonable standards of care are in place, then the Secretary of State can replace the board, its chairman and its chief officers. As a consequence of this power, greater freedom has been granted to those NHS Trusts whose hospitals have reached high standards in the league tables and the management of 'poor performers' has been taken over (Department of Health, 2002a). In 2002, the poorly rated Trusts were given 3 months to show clear signs of improvement. Those that failed to deliver such improvements had their management taken over by successful managers from other Trusts or from the private sector (Department of Health, 2002b). The successful trusts have since been able to apply for NHS foundation trust status under the watchful eye of the Independent Regulator according to the arrangements set up under the Health and Social Care (Community Health and Standards) Act 2003.

National Institute of Clinical Excellence

This statutory body was established on 1 April 1999 to promote clinical and cost effectiveness. The then Secretary of State stated that its task would be to abolish variation in care across the country, so that there would be national standards for the provision of health care. Some of the functions of NICE are to issue clinical guidelines, clinical audit methodologies and information on good practice. NICE has a major role to play in the setting of standards of practice, by disseminating the results of research of what is proved to be clinically effective research-based practice. It is essential that practitioners are aware of its reports and its recommendations. It does not follow that they will automatically become binding on practitioners, since practitioners will still have to use their professional discretion in deciding whether the guidelines are appropriate for the care and treatment of the individual patient. However, if practitioners fail to follow the guidelines, they would have to give clear reasons why these were not appropriate for the circumstances of that individual patient. Hurwitz (1998) considers the legal position of clinical guidelines and protocols, and shows that, in certain circumstances, there could be liability in failing to follow the guidelines; in other situations, there may be liability because the guidelines were followed slavishly without regard to the individual circumstances of the patient. Comprehensive and clear documentation is also essential to provide evidence for the actions taken by practitioners.

Health Care Commission (Commission for Healthcare Audit and Inspection)

Sections 19–24 of the Health Act 1999 establish the Commission for Health Improvement and sets out its functions and powers. It was replaced by the Commission for Healthcare Audit and Inspection under the provisions of the Health and Social Care (Community Health and Standards) Act 2003; it is a body corporate (i.e. it can sue and be sued on its own account). It undertakes inspections of NHS Trusts, health authorities and primary care trusts over a 5-year cycle and, in addition, will carry out additional inspections at the request of the Secretary of State. Its reports are likely to influence standards of health care provision across the NHS. It also acts as the independent review stage of the new complaints procedure established in July 2004 under the new Regulations (Statutory Instrument 2004/1768).

National Service Frameworks

National Service Frameworks have been set up for several specialties, including mental health, coronary heart disease (CHD), cancer care, older peoples' services and diabetes. An NSF for maternity care and child health care was published in September, 2004. The NSF sets minimum standards to be achieved across the specific specialty and could become a major justification for the redistribution of resources.

Kennedy Report

The report on paediatric heart surgery in Bristol has made significant recommendations for a fundamental change in the relationship between patients and professionals within the NHS (Bristol Royal Infirmary, 2001). Implementation of these recommendations should ensure that there is openness and honesty between professionals and patients and, where concerns are raised, these are dealt with honestly. Patients should also be told of untoward events.

HEALTH AND SAFETY

General principles

Health and safety laws, which protect the health and safety of employees, patients and the general public, derive from many statutory and common law sources. The principal legislation is the Health and Safety at Work Act 1974 (HASWA) and the statutory instruments made under it. Section 2 places a duty on the employer to take reasonable care of the health, safety and welfare of its employees, and Section 3 places a duty on the employer to all those whose health or safety may be affected by its enterprise. Under Section 7, each employee has a duty to take reasonable care of the health and safety of himself (or herself) and others, and to cooperate with the employer in obeying health and safety laws. The Health and Safety Executive and its inspectors enforce these statutory duties by way of criminal proceedings. These statutory duties are paralleled by duties under the contract of employment under which the employer has an implied duty to take reasonable care for the health and safety of the employee, and the employee a duty to obey the reasonable instructions of the employer; and by the laws of negligence, where a duty of care is owed to patients and others. Other statutory provisions cover the liability of the occupier to visitors (Occupier's Liability Act 1957) and to trespassers (Occupier's Liability Act 1984), the regulations relating to substances hazardous to health (COSHH), the reporting of incidents of disease (RIDDOR) and the medical devices regulations (see later).

Manual handling regulations

The manual handling regulations set out the statutory requirements, which are binding on employers in relation to manual handling. The 1992 Regulations are amplified by the Provision and Use of Work Equipment Regulations 1998 (PUWER) and by the Lifting Operations and Lifting Equipment Regulations 1998 (LOLER), which came into force on 5 December 1998, and apply in all premises and work situations subject to the Health and Safety at Work Act 1974.

Medical devices

The Medical Devices Agency (MDA) was established to promote the safe and effective use of devices. In April 2003, together with the Medicines Control Agency, it was brought into a single body known as the Medicines and Health Care Products Regulatory Agency (MHRA). Its role is to ensure that, whenever a medical device is used, it is suitable for its intended purpose, is properly understood by the professional user, and is maintained in a safe and reliable condition.

Clarity is often required regarding what constitutes a medical device. Annex B to safety notice 9801 gives examples of medical devices (Medical Devices Agency, 1998a) and includes the following:

- equipment used in the diagnosis or treatment of disease or monitoring of patients (e.g. syringes, needles, dressings, catheters, beds, mattresses, bedcovers and physiotherapy equipment)
- equipment used in providing life support (e.g. ventilators and defibrillators)
- *in-vitro* diagnostic medical devices and their accessories (e.g. blood gas analysers) – regulations came into force in 2002 in relation to *in-vitro* diagnostic devices
- equipment used in the care of disabled people (e.g. orthotic and prosthetic appliances, wheelchairs, special support seating, patient hoists, walking aids and pressure care prevention equipment)
- aids to daily living (e.g. commodes, hearing aids, urine drainage systems, domiciliary oxygen therapy systems, incontinence pads and prescribed footwear)
- equipment used by ambulance services, but not the vehicles themselves (e.g. stretchers, trolleys and resuscitation equipment).

Other examples of medical devices include condoms, contact lenses and care products, and intrauterine devices.

Regulations (Statutory Instrument 1994/3017) require that from 14 June 1998:

> All medical devices placed on the market (made available for use or distribution even if no charge is made) must conform to "the essential requirements" including safety required by law, and bear a CE marking as a sign of that conformity. Although most of the obligations contained in the Regulations fall on manufacturers, purchasers who are positioned further down the supply chain may also be liable – for example, for supplying equipment which does not bear a CE marking or which carries a marking liable to mislead people. (Medical Devices Agency, 1998b)

This is the requirement of the European Commission (EC) Directive on medical devices (EC, 1993). The manufacturer who can demonstrate conformity with the regulations is entitled to apply the CE marking to a medical device.

Control of infection

The highest standards of sterile practice and cleanliness are required in all areas of health care, and particularly in trauma and orthopaedics, where open wounds and severely ill patients give rise to reasonably foreseeable risks. A recent report by the National Audit Office (2000) has raised major concerns about the level of hospital-acquired infection. The report suggested that hospital-acquired infection could be the main or a contributory cause in 20 000 or 4% of deaths each year in the UK, and that there are at least 100 000 cases of hospital-acquired infection, with an estimated cost to the NHS of one billion pounds. Far-reaching recommendations on the control of hospital-acquired infection have resulted.

PROFESSIONAL PRACTICE

Advanced nursing roles

Increasingly specialist nurses, nurse practitioners and, more recently, nurse consultants have been appointed who have a greatly expanded scope of professional practice. The onus of ensuring that they are competent to perform within this extended role is their personal responsibility. The law does not permit a lower standard of care to be provided to patients because the role has been delegated to another person to be carried out. Nor does the law accept any concept of team liability. Each individual practitioner is personally and professionally accountable for his or her actions and omissions, and for all decisions taken. Where activities normally carried out by a doctor or nurse are delegated to other health care professionals, then it is the responsibility of the practitioner delegating that activity to ensure that the person carrying it out has the requisite experience, training and knowledge to undertake the activity safely.

Independent nurse prescribing

Following publication of the first Crown Report (Department of Health, 1989), the powers of prescribing were extended to nurses and health visitors. The Medicinal Products Act 1992 enables a registered nurse, either health visitor or district nurse, who has the requisite additional training, to prescribe those medicinal products contained in the nurse's formulary as set out in a Schedule to the Prescription Only Medicines Order (Statutory Instrument 1994/3050). Section 58 of the Medicines Act 1968 (as amended by the 1992 Act) enables an appropriate practitioner to provide a prescription to be dispensed by the registered pharmacist. Nurse prescribing in the community, therefore, has a clear statutory basis and can take place within certain clearly defined parameters (Dimond, 1995). In February 2000, an amendment by Statutory Instrument 2000/121 added nurses employed by a doctor whose name is included in a medical list (e.g. practice nurses) and those assisting in the capacity of a nurse in the provision of services in a walk-in centre.

Second Crown Report

Dr Crown was appointed in 1997 to review the prescribing, supply and administration of medicines. Its terms of reference included the development of a consistent policy framework to guide judgements on the circumstances in which health professionals might undertake new responsibilities with regard to the prescribing, supply and administration of medicines. The review group was also asked to advise on the likely impact of any proposed changes: to consider possible implications for legislation, professional training and standards, and to advise on prescriptions under group protocols and related safeguards. An interim report was published in 1998 that was concerned with the prescribing, supply and administration of medicines under group protocols (Department of Health, 1998). It recommended that the majority of patients should continue to receive medicines on an individual basis. However, current safe and effective practice using group protocols, which are consistent with criteria defined in the report, should continue. As a consequence of this interim report, a statutory instrument was published specifying the minimum requirements for a patient group direction, originally known as group protocol. These requirements are shown in Box 39.1.

Box 39.1   Patient group directions (PGDs): minimum requirements

- The period during which the PGD shall have effect
- The description or class of prescription-only medicines to which the PGD relates
- Any restrictions on the quantity of medicine that may be supplied
- The clinical situations in which the PGD may be used to treat
- The clinical criteria under which persons are eligible for treatment
- The class of persons excluded from treatment under the PGD
- The circumstances in which further advice should be sought from a doctor or dentist
- The pharmaceutical form or forms in which the prescription-only medicines may be administered
- The strength, or maximum strength, at which the specified prescription-only medicines may be administered
- The applicable dosage and maximum dosage
- The route of administration
- The frequency of administration
- The minimum or maximum period of administration
- Details of any relevant warnings
- Details of any follow-up actions required
- Referral arrangements
- Details of the clinical records to be kept of the supply or administration of medicines under the PGD

The final Crown Report

The recommendations of the Final Report of the Crown Committee (Department of Health, 1999b) include the following recommendations:

1. The legal authority in the UK to prescribe should be extended beyond currently authorised prescribers.
2. The legal authority to prescribe should be limited to medicines in specific therapeutic areas related to particular competence and expertise of the group.
3. Two types of prescribers should be recognised: the independent prescriber and the dependent prescriber (known as supplementary).
4. A UK-wide advisory body, provisionally entitled the 'New Prescribers Advisory Committee' should be established under

Section 4 of the Medicines Act to assess submissions from professional organisations seeking powers for suitably trained members to become independent or dependent prescribers.
5. Newly authorised groups of prescribers should not normally be allowed to prescribe specified categories of medicines including controlled drugs.
6. Current arrangements for the administration and self-administration of medicines should continue to apply. Newly authorised prescribers should have the power to administer those parenteral prescription-only medicines, which they are authorised to prescribe.

As a consequence of these recommendations, legislation contained in Section 63 of the Health and Social Care Act 2001 amends Section 58 of the Medicines Act 1968 to enable 'other persons who are of such a description and comply with such conditions as may be specified in the order' to be eligible to write prescriptions for medicinal products. Section 63(3) lists those persons who are eligible, including persons who are registered by a board established under the Professions Supplementary to Medicine Act 1960 or by a body set up under the Health Act 1999, for example, the Health Professions Council or the Nursing and Midwifery Council.

Further developments in extending prescribing powers came into force on 1 April 2002. A statutory Instrument (2000/549) laid down arrangements for nurses registered in Parts 1, 3, 5, 8, 10, 11, 12, 13, 14 or 15 of the professional register (The NMC register changed in August 2004 with a reduction in the number of parts), and who are recorded in the register as qualified to order drugs, medicines and appliances from the Extended Formulary, and to prescribe products listed in the Extended Formulary. The Extended Formulary nurse prescribers are able to prescribe all pharmacy and general sales list medicines prescribable by a general practitioner and also those prescription-only medicines that are set out in Schedule 3A of the Order. These cover minor injuries, minor ailments, health promotion and palliative care. In April 2002, the Department of Health (2002c, 2002d) published proposals to give nurses and pharmacists further prescribing powers to cover chronic conditions. These 'supplementary prescribing' proposals were implemented in 2003, and enable appropriately trained nurses and pharmacists to prescribe medications for chronic conditions as asthma, diabetes, hypertension and arthritis. Prescriptions for inhalers, hormone replacement therapy and anticoagulants were included in the proposals.

Revisions to the Nurse Prescribers Extended formulary are ongoing.

Trained nurse practitioners may have a role to play in prescribing as well as the administration of medicines to trauma patients. It is essential, however, that they define the legal basis on which they can lawfully 'prescribe' (i.e. through the use of patient group directions, or as an extended independent or supplementary prescriber). All nurses are responsible for ensuring that they are personally, professionally and legally competent to prescribe.

> Nurses prescribing medicines must understand and be able to define the legal basis on which they can lawfully 'prescribe'

Record keeping

All registered health professionals have a professional duty to ensure that they document all interventions, including their assessment, care and treatment of patients. If clear comprehensive records are kept in the interests of the patient, then they will also provide valuable evidence of the care provided should the practitioner be faced with any legal or disciplinary forums described earlier. Internal audit on a regular basis should assist in ensuring that reasonable standards of documentation are maintained. In addition, the Clinical Negligence Scheme for Trusts examines standards of record keeping in determining the level of membership of the clinical risk pool. New guidance on records and record keeping was published by the NMC in August 2004 (NMC, 2004b).

PATIENTS' RIGHTS

Human rights

The UK was a signatory of the European Convention in 1951 and accepted the articles on human rights. However, the Convention was not incorporated into UK law at that time. If a person considered his or her rights had been infringed, then he or she would need to take the case to the European Court of Human Rights in Strasbourg and argue the case there. The UK parliament has now passed the Human Rights Act 1998, which came into force on 2 October 2000 in England, Wales and Northern Ireland (in Scotland the Act came into force earlier). The Articles of the European Convention on Human Rights are set out in Schedule 1 to the Human Rights Act 1998. The Act requires all public authorities to implement the articles of the European Convention on Human Rights, gives a right to anyone who alleges that a public authority has failed to respect those rights to bring an action in the courts of his country, and enables judges who consider that legislation is incompatible with the Articles of the Convention to refer that legislation back to Parliament.

A right to treatment

The Secretary of State has a statutory duty to provide a reasonable health service. This duty has been interpreted by the courts as not being an absolute duty but one dependent upon the resources that are made available. Several cases where patients have sued because they have been waiting for a long time for operations have failed because the courts have held that there was no breach of the statutory duty (R. v. Secretary of State for Social Services ex parte Hincks and others, 1979; R. v. Central Birmingham Health Authority ex parte Walker, 1987). The health service organisations are, however, obliged to follow the guidelines of the Department of Health in determining whether certain medicines should be made available (R. v. North Derbyshire Health Authority, 1997) and not to have blanket policies prohibiting the provision of services (North West Lancashire Health Authority v. A, D, and G, 1999); each individual patient should be assessed on her or his individual circumstances. The reduction of waiting times for orthopaedic surgery is a political priority as well as a clinical one. However, it is unlikely, in view of the legal precedents, that patients who have waited longer than the time outlined in the national guidelines would have a successful claim in law for breach of statutory duty or negligence, nor are they likely to succeed in a case brought under Article 2 or Article 3 of the European Convention of Human Rights.

CONSENT

The mentally competent adult

Two legal actions can arise in relation to consent. The first is an action for trespass to the person, where there is no consent to the touching of another person or other legal justification, or there has been fraud or duress in obtaining the consent. In this action, harm need not be proved: merely the touching or apprehension of touching. Trespass to the person includes both *battery*, the actual touching of the person and *assault*, the apprehension of the touching. Battery and assault are also criminal offences, but here they are considered as civil wrongs. The other action that can arise in relation to consent is that of *negligence*, where the person has not been informed or given significant information regarding the procedure or intervention in question. In this action, the claimant would have to prove that harm has been suffered, which would not have been suffered if the information had been given. The basic principle of law is that no mentally competent adult person can be treated, whatever the motive, without their consent or statutory justification (e.g. the Mental Health Act 1983). The main defences to an action for trespass to the person are consent by a mentally capacitated person, acting out of necessity in respect of a mentally incapacitated person and statutory justification, such as the Mental Health Act 1983. The consent must have been given by a mentally competent person, voluntarily without duress or fraud, and with the knowledge of what was proposed. Guidance has been provided by the Department of Health on consent (Department of Health, 2001a).

Evidence of consent

Consent can be given in a variety of ways, including non-verbal behaviour that implies agreement with the intended action, such as rolling up a sleeve for an injection or blood pressure reading to be taken; by word of mouth, or in writing. Clearly, if there is a dispute, then written consent is the preferred evidence that consent was given. However, the signature on the consent form should not be seen as the consent itself, but rather evidence, following a process of communication between health professional and patient, with the result that the patient understands the proposed intervention and gives his or her consent to this. Forms were distributed by the Department of Health (2001b) as part of its Good Practice in Consent implementation guide, replacing those issued by the NHS Management Executive in 1990 that were later updated in 1992. The recommended forms can be used by any health professional.

Children

Consent to treatment by 16- and 17-year-olds

These young persons have a statutory right to give consent under the Family Law Reform Act 1969 Section 8. Consent can be given for surgical, medical and dental treatment, the definition of treatment covering any procedure undertaken for the purpose of diagnosis and any ancillary procedures, such as the administration of anaesthesia.

Parents also have the right to give consent on behalf of their 16- and 17-year-old children. This is preserved by Section 8(3) of the Family Law Reform Act 1969. Where there is a clash between parents and minors, the health care professional would normally follow the wishes of the minor. However, much depends upon the circumstances.

Refusal of treatment by 16- and 17-year-olds

In the case of Re W (1992), a 16-year-old, who suffered from anorexia, refused to attend a specialist unit for treatment. The courts decided that she could be compelled to attend against her wishes, since it was in her best interests to receive treatment. The Court of Appeal held that the refusal of a minor should only be overruled in extreme circumstances, in life and death situations. However, this decision was made before the Human Rights Act 1998 became part of English law. It could be argued that failure to recognise the right of a young person to refuse treatment was a breach of Article 3 of the Human Rights Act, and his or her right not to be treated in an inhuman degrading way. If, for example, W had been a Jehovah's Witness and had refused blood in a life-saving situation, then to overrule the refusal could have been seen as a violation of Article 3 and also Article 9 (freedom of thought, religion and practice). The point has yet to be considered by the House of Lords.

Children aged under 16 years

Whilst children under 16 years of age do not have a statutory right to consent to treatment, the right to give consent at common law (i.e. judge-made law) was recognised by the House of Lords in the case of Gillick v. W. Norfolk and Wisbech Area Health Authority (1986). This asserted that, if a child has the maturity to understand the nature, purpose and likely effects of any proposed treatment, then he or she could give valid consent without the involvement of the parents. Whilst the Gillick case itself was concerned with family planning and treatment, the principle applies to other forms of treatment. The principle that the ascertainable wishes and feelings of the child concerned, considered in the light of his or her age and understanding, should also be taken into account is also stated in the Children Act 1989 Section 1(3)(a), as one of the factors that the court will consider when determining what, if any, orders should be made or varied. Parents can also give consent to treatment on behalf of their children up to the age of 18 years; however, such treatment must be in the best interests of the child. Persons who do not have parental responsibilities also have power under the Children Act 1989 Section 3(5), which enables a person who (a) does not have parental responsibility for a particular child but (b) has care of the child, to do what is reasonable in all the circumstances of the case for the purposes of safeguarding or promoting the child's welfare.

Parental refusal to give consent

Should the parent or guardian of a minor under the age of 18 refuse to give consent to treatment that is necessary in the best interests of the minor,

doctors can act out of necessity in the best interests of the minor according to the principle set out in Re F v. West Berkshire Health Authority (1989). Alternatively, the authority of the court could be sought for treatment to proceed against the parents' wishes. Should the parents fail to give consent to essential treatment or arrange for the treatment to take place, they can face prosecution in the event of harm befalling the child. For example, a Rastafarian couple who had refused on religious grounds to allow their diabetic daughter, who was 9 years old, to be given insulin, were convicted of manslaughter. The father was given a sentence of imprisonment and the mother a suspended sentence (*The Times*, 1993).

Mentally incompetent adults

Whilst legislation has been passed in Scotland [The Adult Incapacity (Scotland) Act 2000], in the rest of the UK there is statutory provision covering the making of treatment decisions on behalf of mentally incapacitated adults. The situation is covered by a House of Lords decision, which recognised the duty of the health professional to act in the best interests of the mentally incapacitated adult (Re F v. West Berkshire Health Authority, 1989). Following extensive consultation, the Law Commission in 1995 published its proposals on decision-making on behalf of mentally incapacitated adults, which included a mental incapacity bill. In 1997, a new consultation document was issued by the Lord Chancellor's office, which was followed by a White Paper setting out the government's proposals for decision-making on behalf of mentally incapacitated adults (Lord Chancellor, 1999). At the time of writing, legislation to implement these proposals is being debated in Parliament.

Caring for mentally incapacitated patients places considerable burdens upon health care professionals and, in particular, those dealing with the trauma patient. It would not be correct in law to say that an unconscious patient gives implied consent to be treated. There is no consent from such a patient. However, the practitioner has a duty to take reasonable care of such a person, until such time as they are competent to make their own decisions. The power to act in the person's best interests is recognised by the common law. Reasonable care must be followed in their treatment. The Department of Health's (2001b) guidelines for implementation can be used in the case of mentally incapacitated adults by any health professional who gives treatment in the best interest of the patient, without the patient's consent. It must be emphasised that relatives do not have the right to give consent on behalf of a mentally incapacitated adult, but they should, where reasonably practicable, be involved in the discussions and their involvement and understanding of the necessity to give treatment in the patient's best interest documented according the guidance referred to.

CONFIDENTIALITY – BASIC PRINCIPLES

The Data Protection Act 1998 applies to both manually held and computerised records; the data protection principles as set out in the Data Protection Act should, therefore, be followed (Box 39.2).

The duty of confidentiality derives from the trust that is created between patient and professional, from the professional codes of practice of registered health professionals and from specific statutory provisions. If there is a breach of confidentiality that is not justified in law, then the patient can apply for an injunction to prevent its publication, or, if not, sue for damages for the breach of confidentiality. In the case of X v. Y (1988) doctors working in the NHS who were suffering from acquired immunodeficiency syndrome (AIDS) were granted an injunction against a newspaper preventing it publishing their names. The Court held that the information obtained from hospital records should be kept confidential and the public interest did not require the publication of the names. The Court did not order the disclosure by the press of their informant, as the circumstances did not constitute one of the exceptional grounds on which the disclosure could be ordered against the press. More recently, however, the Court ordered the press to disclose the name of their informant at Ashworth Hospital who had given information about patients. Clearly, in the management of major incidents and mass casualty situations, there should be careful handling of press inquiries to prevent any un-

---

Box 39.2   Data Protection Act principles

1. Personal data shall be processed fairly and lawfully and, in particular, shall not be processed unless:
   a. at least one of the conditions in Schedule 2 is met; and
   b. in the case of sensitive personal data, at least one of the conditions in Schedule 3 is also met.
2. Personal data shall be obtained only for one or more specified and lawful purposes, and shall not be further processed in any manner incompatible with that purpose or those purposes.
3. Personal data shall be adequate, relevant and not excessive in relation to the purpose or purposes for which they are processed.
4. Personal data shall be accurate and, where necessary, kept up to date.
5. Personal data processed for any purpose or purposes shall not be kept for longer than is necessary for that purpose(s).
6. Personal data shall be processed in accordance with the rights of data subjects under this Act.
7. Appropriate technical and organisational measures shall be taken against unauthorised or unlawful processing of personal data and against accidental loss or destruction of, or damage to, personal data.
8. Personal data shall not be transferred to a country or territory outside the European Economic Area unless that country or territory ensures an adequate level of protection for the rights and freedoms of data subjects in relation to the processing of personal data.

---

justified and unlawful disclosure of confidential information. The media's interest in obtaining personal sensational stories must be placed in the context of the duty of confidentiality to the patients.

Exceptions to the duty of confidentiality

The basic presumption is that confidentiality should be respected but there are specific exceptions recognised both in statute and at common law. These include the following recognised exceptions:

- consent of the patient
- information given to other professionals in the interests of the patient

- order from the Court before or during legal proceedings
- statutory justification, for example,
  - notification of registration of births and stillbirths
  - infectious disease regulations
  - Police and Criminal Evidence Act
  - Health and Social Care Act 2001
- public interest.

The latter exception of public interests is recognised as a legitimate justification for disclosure of confidential information by all health registration bodies. The public interest would cover situations where serious harm is feared to the patient or another person, or in a child protection situation. Section 60 of the Health and Social Care Act 2001 enables the Secretary of State to draw up regulations covering the processing of confidential patient information. The Patient Information Advisory Group must be consulted and due regard given to its views, before any such regulations are placed before Parliament. A Statutory Instrument (2002/1438) was published in May 2002, and permits disclosure of confidential information for the purposes of the Cancer Registries and Public Health.

Access to records

Section 7 of the Data Protection Act 1998 enables an individual to be informed of data held about him and to access that data. Special provisions exist in relation to health, education and social work under Section 30. Section 30 enables the Secretary of State to draw up specific provisions setting exemptions from the statutory rights of access in relation to health, education and social work records. Statutory Instruments (2000/413, 2000/414, 2000/415) have been enacted setting out details of the restrictions on access to these records.

Right to withhold access

Access can be withheld under the Data Protection Act 1998 in the following circumstances:

- Where in the opinion of the holder of the record, serious harm would be caused to the mental or physical health or condition of the applicant, or of any other individual.

- Where the identity of a third person would be made known and this person has not consented to access. This does not apply where the other person is the health professional caring for the patient.
- Where the reports are confidential under a statutory provision, such as information supplied in a report or other evidence given to the court by a local authority, Health or Social Services Board, Health and Social Services Trust, or probation officer.

COMPLAINTS

Several years ago, research was commissioned by the Department of Health on the effectiveness of the current complaints system. In the light of the results of that research, the Department of Health (2001c) published a document suggesting a number of ways to improve the current procedure. It also issued a consultation document on which feedback was invited (Department of Health, 2001d). A new complaints procedure was introduced in July 2004, which has made significant changes to the previous complaints system. In particular, the independence of the second stage of the complaints system is ensured by enabling a complainant, who is not satisfied by the response from the health service organisation or primary care practitioner, to take the complaint to the Healthcare Commission and, if dissatisfied with the outcome from that, to take the complaint to the Health Service Commissioner.

SUMMARY

There are many legal issues arising from trauma care. The aim of this chapter has been to provide a basic coverage of the main legal principles that apply, so that trauma nurses can have an understanding of the legal context within which they practise and follow this up with more detailed reading of legal sources. Nurses must understand their legal and professional responsibilities and be aware of their clinical practices, not only to protect themselves but also to protect the patients who place their trust in them, especially when they are at their most vulnerable.

References

Bolam v. Friern Hospital Management Committee (1957) 1 WLR 582

Brian H. *Clinical guidelines and the law.* Abingdon: Radcliffe Medical Press, 1998

Bristol Royal Infirmary. *Learning from Bristol: the report of the public inquiry into children's heart surgery at the Bristol Royal Infirmary 1984–1995.* Command Paper CM 5207 July 2001 (http://www.bristol-inquiry.org.uk/)

Department of Health. Report on nurse prescribing and supply, Advisory Group chaired by Dr June Crown. London: HMSO, 1989

Department of Health. *The new NHS: modern, dependable.* London: HMSO, 1997

Department of Health. *Review of prescribing, supply and administration of medicines: a report on the supply and administration of medicines under group protocols.* London: HMSO, 1998

Department of Health. *Making a difference: the new NHS.* London: HMSO, 1999a

Department of Health. *Final report on the prescribing, supply and administration of medicines, chaired by Dr June Crown.* London: HMSO, 1999b

Department of Health. *Reference guide to consent for examination or treatment.* London: HMSO, 2001a (www.doh.gov.uk/consent)

Department of Health. *Good practice in consent implementation guide: consent to examination or treatment.* London: HMSO, 2001b (www.doh.gov.uk/consent)

Department of Health. *The NHS complaints procedure: national evaluation.* London: HMSO, 2001c

Department of Health. *Reforming the NHS complaints procedure: a listening document.* London: HMSO, 2001d

Department of Health. *Milburn announces radical decentralisation of NHS control.* Press Release 2002/0022, 2002a

Department of Health. *Management of four NHS trusts to be franchised.* Press release 2002/0069, 2002b

Department of Health. *Groundbreaking new consultation aims to extend prescribing powers for pharmacists and nurses.* Press release 2002/0189, 2002c

Department of Health. *Pharmacists to prescribe for the first time. Nurses will prescribe for chronic illness.* Press release 2002/0488, 2002d

Dimond B. *Nurse prescribing.* Merck Dermatology and Scutari Press, 1995

European Commission. *93/42/EEC Directive concerning medical devices,* 1993

Gillick v. W. Norfolk and Wisbech Area Health Authority (1986) 1 AC 112

Law Commission. *Mental incapacity.* Report no. 231. London: HMSO, 1995

Lord Chancellor. *Who decides? Decision making on behalf of the mentally incapacitated adult.* Lord Chancellor's Office. London: HMSO, 1997

Lord Chancellor. *Making decisions: the government's proposals for decision making on behalf of the mentally incapacitated adult.* Lord Chancellor's Office. London: HMSO, 1999

Medical Devices Agency. *Reporting adverse incidents relating to medical devices.* SN 9801, January 1998a

Medical Devices Agency. Medical device and equipment management for hospital and community-based organizations. DB 9801, January 1998b

National Audit Office. The management and control of hospital acquired infection in acute NHS Trusts in England. London: HMSO, 2000

North West Lancashire Health Authority v. A, D, and G (1999) *Lloyds Law Reports Medical,* p. 399 (Refusal to fund transsexual surgery)

Nursing and Midwifery Council (NMC). *Code of professional conduct: standards for conduct, performance and ethics 2002 (renamed 2004).* London: NMC, 2004a

Nursing and Midwifery Council. *Guidelines for records and record keeping.* London: NMC, 2004b

R. v. Adomako House of Lords. *The Times Law Report* 1994; July 4

R. v. Central Birmingham Health Authority ex parte Walker (1987) 3 BMLR 32. *The Times* 1987; 26 November

R. v. North Derbyshire Health Authority (1997) 8 Med L R 327 (Refusal to supply beta interferon to multiple sclerosis patient)

R. v. Secretary of State for Social Services ex parte Hincks and others. 29 June 1979. *Solicitors Journal* 1979; 123: 436

Re F v. West Berkshire Health Authority (1989) 2 All ER 545

Re W (A minor) (Medical treatment) 1992 4 All ER 627

Secretary of State for Health. *The NHS plan.* Cm 4818-1 July. London: HMSO, 2000

Statutory Instrument 1994 no. 3017. *Medical devices regulations 1994.* (Came into force 1 January 1995, mandatory from 14 June 1998)

Statutory Instrument 1994 no. 3050. *Prescription only medicines*

Statutory Instrument 2000 no. 121. *The National Health Service (pharmaceutical services) amendment regulations 2000*

Statutory Instrument 2000 no. 413. *Data protection (subject access modification) (health) order 2000*

Statutory Instrument 2000 no. 414. *Data protection (subject access modification) (education) order 2000*

Statutory Instrument 2000 no. 415. *Data protection (subject access modification) (social work) order 2000*

Statutory Instrument 2002 no. 549. *The prescription only medicines (human use) amendment order*

Statutory Instrument 2002 no. 1438. *The health service (control of patient information) regulations*

Statutory Instrument no 1761. *The Nursing and Midwifery Council (Fitness to Practise) Rules Order of Council 2004*

Statutory Instrument 2004 no 1768. *The National Health Service (Complaints) Regulations 2004*

The Times. Insulin ban parents killed their daughter. 1993; 29 October

X v. Y (1988) 2 All ER 648

Further reading

Dimond B. *Legal aspects of patient confidentiality*. Salisbury: Quay Publications, Mark Allen Press, 2002

Dimond B. *Legal aspects of pain management*. Salisbury: Quay Publications, Mark Allen Press, 2002

Dimond B. *Legal aspects of radiography and radiology*. Oxford: Blackwell Scientific Publications, 2002

Dimond B. *Legal aspects of health and safety*. Salisbury: Quay Publications, Mark Allen Press, 2004

Dimond B. *Legal aspects of nursing*, 4th edn. Harlow: Pearson Education, 2004

Health and Safety Commission. *Manual handling regulations and approved code of practice*. London: HMSO, 1992

Hurwitz B. *Clinical guidelines and the law*. Abingdon: Radcliffe Medical Press, 1998

Kennedy I, Grubb A. *Medical law and ethics*, 3rd edn. London: Butterworth, 2000

McHale J, Tingle J. *Law and nursing*. London: Butterworth Heineman, 2001

Pitt G. *Employment law*, 4th edn. London: Sweet and Maxwell, 2000

Selwyn N. *Selwyn's law of employment*, 11th edn. London: Butterworth, 2000

Wilkinson R, Caulfield H. *The Human Rights Act: a practical guide for nurses*. London: Whurr Publishers, 2000

Chapter 40

The future of trauma care delivery

Rose Ann O'Shea and Lynda Sibson

INTRODUCTION

Recent years have seen the structure and function of the National Health Service (NHS) come under unparalleled scrutiny, resulting in unprecedented change in the direction and delivery of emergency care amid a plethora of government policies and directives. Successive governments have maintained the momentum of change, each enthusiastic to recognise and maximise the individual and collective contribution that all health care professionals can make to improve patient care. At a time when clinical effectiveness, quality measures and the achievement of targets are so vital in the commissioning of services and the delivery of health care, the expanded role and contribution of these individuals within the health care team, particularly nurses, are now paramount.

This chapter will outline recent developments in the delivery of first-line and immediate medical care by nurses to patients with a range of traumatic presentations. Focusing on the development and advancement of the nursing role and that of other pre-hospital workers, it will address changes in levels of autonomy and their impact on patient care, both in terms of quality of care and quality of service. The infrastructure to support these advancements and initiatives will also be discussed from both clinical and political perspectives, and educational frameworks proposed. Finally, advances in telemedicine and the role of electronic health technologies (e-technologies), which are set to influence trauma care delivery for decades to come, will be considered within a context of enabling and supporting care, and potential models for future service delivery explored.

TRAUMA CARE IN CONTEXT

The delivery of health care in the UK has changed over recent decades and the momentum is set to continue. Historically perceived in the hand-maiden role acting to support their medical colleagues while having little scope to practise autonomously, nurses have gradually evolved with their role now recognised as one in which they increasingly accept responsibility and accountability for their practice, and take on roles traditionally associated with medicine. This is most evident in relation to minor injuries and the emergency nurse practitioner role, where suitably trained nurses independently assess selected patients, diagnose their injuries and treat them accordingly, without direct referral to a doctor. The success of such initiatives has greatly enhanced the nursing profile, so much so that there is now growing support for further blurring of the interprofessional boundaries of clinical practice, most notably in the field of minor illnesses, but also in relation to other undiagnosed health care problems. Advances in relation to major trauma have, however, been slower to evolve, perhaps owing to resistance from those unwilling to challenge traditional roles and who perceive this advancement as unacceptable in terms of clinical risk.

The foundation for new roles

Presently, much of the care delivered by nurses acting independently is facilitated through the use of clinical standards and protocols. This paradigm shift towards independent nursing care without referral to a doctor, which has occurred in primary and secondary health care sectors, has a rationale that is both complex and varied. A direct relationship can be seen in the increased shift in the delivery of care from the secondary to the primary care sector, which, in addition to the development of advanced nursing, has been a significant driver

in changing practice, perhaps nowhere more notable than for nurses involved in the delivery of front-line emergency care.

For many years, the only access to treatment for accidents and emergencies resided at one port of call – the local accident and emergency (A&E) department – usually within a district general hospital. This often meant patients travelling some distance, particularly in geographically remote areas. Even in more locally situated A&E departments (now referred to as Emergency Departments), access to care was, and in some cases still is, preceded by a long wait. Many of these A&E departments provided care for a spectrum of patients suffering from complaints ranging from major trauma to minor injuries and illnesses. These groups of patients, often accounting for a substantial minority of patients in A&E departments, were identified as being in need of care that could arguably be delivered in either a more appropriate environment or by a more appropriate health care professional.

Traditionally, the underpinning model of care was one in which care was supervised by junior doctors with variable levels of experience, who invariably had considerably less experience than many of the senior A&E nurses with whom they were working; informally, many of these nurses directed their medical colleagues in the care required. Greater organisational changes also provided a catalyst for change. A number of smaller A&E departments, unable to justify their existence financially, were closed, often in the face of considerable public disquiet. Major trauma centres, staffed with expensive personnel and equipment that were largely underutilised, were unable to provide cost-effective services to local communities and were, therefore, under threat.

Introduced to reduce waiting times in A&E departments, triage resulted in patients being assessed by A&E nurses upon arrival and having a triage priority allocated related to their degree of clinical urgency. This often resulted in patients being moved to different areas to wait for doctors to provide medical consultations and to prescribe care, while those with less urgent clinical conditions continued to wait for long periods of time to be seen.

The evolution of nurse practitioners and specialist nurses

As a response to the situation described above, local communities were provided with a growing number of minor injury units (MIUs). These units, many of which were nurse-led with sessional medical support, provided care for patients with a range of injuries that could be managed outside major trauma centres. Injuries in this category included minor burns, lacerations, bony and soft tissue injuries, foreign bodies and other minor trauma. The role of the emergency nurse practitioner (ENP) was also gathering pace, with skills acquired in a range of techniques, including the management of simple undisplaced fractures, the application of plaster of Paris, suturing of wounds, and trephining of subungual haematomas. As these MIUs were almost entirely nurse-led, ENPs developed skills in patient consultation, history taking and physical examination. This signified the beginning of increased autonomy amongst emergency nurses, support for which was given by professional bodies, including the English National Board (ENB) and the National Board for Scotland (NBS) in various forms, including autonomous practice courses.

> Nurse practitioners diagnose, refer, prescribe and provide complete episodes of care for patients with undifferentiated health care problems

Not exclusive to the emergency setting, this significant role change extended further into the primary care setting with the evolution of the more generic nurse practitioner (NP) role. Initially established in the USA in the 1960s in response to a lack of primary health care provision, this role provided the foundation for further developments within the UK (Jordan, 1993). Pioneering the British cause, Stilwell established the role within an inner-city practice in England, culminating in the inception of the first NP training and education programme at the Royal College of Nursing (RCN) (Drury et al., 1988). Success was subsequently evidenced in its protégés practising in the primary health care arena as practice nurses or emergency nurse practitioners, having developed the role to meet the needs of the local populations.

In the 1990s, posts began to emerge in secondary care with titles such as nurse practitioner, advanced practitioner and advanced nurse practitioner, which frequently involved nurses giving care or performing tasks previously carried out by doctors.

Of necessity, knowledge of clinical examination skills, advanced anatomy and physiology, and applied pharmacology and its application to disease processes, became central curricular components. Having completed such educational programmes, some nurses advanced their practice to include the organisation and management of clinics, such as those focusing on chronic disease management including asthma, diabetes and hypertension, and the management of independent caseloads, including patients with minor self-limiting illnesses. Others embraced not only the management of patients with minor illnesses, such as self-limiting viral infections, but also those with minor injuries, since many patients chose to attend their general practitioner (GP) surgeries with such injuries rather than waiting in A&E departments.

Official recognition of the nurse practitioner role has, however, been less clear. Replaced by the Nursing and Midwifery Council (NMC) in 2002, the United Kingdom Central Council (UKCC), regulator of the nursing profession, did not recognise the title. Retrospectively, this may have been appropriate, given that the range of educational programmes, which evolved to prepare a growing number of nurses for this role, varied in content and duration ranging from 3 months certificate courses to 2-year first-level degree courses. Frustration among nurses became increasingly evident, resulting in a 'higher level of practice' status being awarded to nurses, health visitors and midwives who had completed the requisite educational preparation and who worked in these areas (UKCC, 1999; Box 40.1).

Recognition of a higher level of clinical practice is founded on the attainment of clinical competence with underpinning post-registration education and the need to develop a method of accrediting practitioners who work at this level. Education to underpin practice competence is undoubtedly crucial; the preferred academic level of this education, however, remains controversial.

> **Box 40.1 Higher level of practice standards (UKCC, 1999)**
>
> - Promotion of effective health care
> - Development of clinical judgement and autonomy
> - Developing a questioning approach and exploring alternatives
> - Improvement in quality and health outcomes
> - Evaluation and research
> - Leading and developing practice
> - Innovation and changing practice
> - Staff development
> - Working across professional and organisational boundaries

In recent years, growing recognition has been given to the need for higher-level practitioners to have an appropriate first degree, particularly if they are to be respected by their professional peers. Those in favour of an all-graduate nursing profession support this, indeed, specifying a masters-level degree as a prerequisite for advanced practice. Overall, most favour the development of a generic UK-wide educational standard to enable not only transparency but also cross-boundary and cross-country transferability.

> Education to underpin practice competence is crucial

The advent of nurse prescribing and independent diagnostic rights

The conferring of independent diagnostic rights upon nurses has been slow to evolve, even among those with a proven record of safety and efficacy in their advanced roles. X-ray requesting of upper and lower limbs in patients presenting with minor injuries has, however, increasingly become a recognised part of many advanced roles, most notably the emergency nurse practitioner role (Macleod and Freeland, 1992). Supported by legislation and a growing body of evidence, the requesting and interpretation of such radiographic investigations have been shown to be procedures that may safely and accurately be undertaken by nurses who first see the patients (Lindley-Jones and Finlayson, 2000).

Advances in the independent prescribing of medicines by nurses in their own right have similarly been slow to progress. Galvanised by success from the first prescribing formulary for district nurses and health visitors, the Crown Report, commissioned by the Department of Health (1989), paved the way for further advances in prescribing and medicines management. Published in 2001, proposals to enable nurses to prescribe independently from an extended formulary known as 'Nurse presciber's extended formulary' (Department of Health, 2002c) gave licence to nurses to prescribe a limited range of prescription-only medicines without recourse to their medical colleagues. Further amendments in the form of supplementary prescribing expanded this scope, acknowledging the restrictions that existing legislation placed on the delivery of care (Department of Health, 2003). Aimed at enhancing access to care and improving the patient's experience, these initiatives heralded turning points for the nursing profession. No longer viewed in a subordinate supporting role, nurses were perceived as independent professional practitioners in their own right, with the inherent legal and professional responsibilities.

Despite providing a portal of entry for the independent prescribing of medicines, this avenue has, however, met the needs of only a small proportion of nurses. Requiring a lengthy period of education in higher education institutes (HEIs) and clinical practice consolidation (RCN, 2002) many nurses have not been afforded the opportunity to undertake this course of study, forcing them to continue to practise within traditional boundaries. Initiatives to widen the availability and accessibility of independent prescribing courses continue to grow, including proposals to embed them into postgraduate education programmes and undergraduate curricula. In the intervening period, an alternative solution has been found; the facility to enable nurses to administer and supply a range of prescription-only medicines against agreed criteria, patient group directions (PGDs), has gained increasing momentum and acceptance among staff, serving as a positive interim step towards achieving the ideal (National Prescribing Centre, 2004).

Evolution of consultant nurses

Among the most recent and most significant innovations and advancements in nursing practice has been the evolution of the consultant nurse role (Department of Health, 1997, 1999a, 2001a, 2002a, 2002b). Having the same status within nursing as their medical colleagues in medicine, their role is rooted in clinical practice, providing a focus for developing and supporting other nursing roles and offering an alternative career pathway (Box 40.2).

Designed primarily to retain senior nurses in the clinical arena while empowering them to liberate their clinical talents and realise their full potential, this role has heralded the advent of a vision for nursing that was formerly unheard of. Combining research and clinical practice, it was envisaged that the consultant nurse would officially lead nursing into previously untapped dimensions, incorporating an evidence base to practice as far as possible. In so far as these nurses worked within their scope of practice and carried out only those activities for which they were suitably prepared, and both confident and competent to perform, no restrictions were brought to bear upon their clinical role/activities (NMC, 2002). Now increasingly welcomed as part of the nursing team and striving to move forward leading-edge practice, consultant nurses have provided a new and innovative clinical career pathway for those who may otherwise have sought new challenges in other, less directly patient-focused ways (Manley, 2000a, 2000b).

To date, evaluations of the role have focused on its implementation and acceptance by other health professionals, and its clinical, organisational and professional dimensions (Box 40.3). Associated with inevitable teething problems and interprofessional tensions, the years since their inception have brought both wisdom and clarity: wisdom in terms of the unique contribution and expertise that senior specialist nurses can bring, and clarity regarding their role within the multiprofessional team. Increasing recognition has been given to their involvement in formulating future strategies for the profession at both local and national levels. Providing visionary leadership, and acting as role models and clinical champions of patient care, they should also ideally be involved in ambassadorial roles across the local health economy.

Role expansion and new ways of working

These developments, which have occurred in the past decade, have led to a cohort of highly educated nurses with expert skills and competencies, and many years of experience, who are able to provide rapid access to a complementary health care route previously unavailable to patients. Medical colleagues, often suspicious of these *new* nurses who were undertaking clinical examinations and diagnostic investigations previously the domain of medicine, viewed such nurses as potentially increasing their workload by virtue of feared increases in referral rates from nurse-led units. These fears, however, were not usually borne out; rather the ability to meet previously unmet and unexpressed patient needs was realised.

Emergency care practitioners
In response to government initiatives to reduce waiting times in emergency departments and to

---

Box 40.2   Consultant nurse roles

- Clinical leadership
- Focus on education and clinical development
- Focus on research and evidence-based practice
- Development of clinical guidelines and frameworks
- Consultation and advice
- National and international networking
- Implementation and review of new systems of emergency nursing care

---

Box 40.3   Consultant nurses: dimensions of expertise

- Delivery of expert nursing practice
- Development of a learning culture in the organisation/department
- Implementation and evaluation of evidence-based practice
- Clinical consultancy at all levels within the organisation
- Leadership and management of change

improve the patient's experience, including access to treatment, a number of alternative health care roles have been piloted nationally and a number evaluated. Most notable among these in relation to emergency care, the emergency care practitioner role, has been proposed as a means to provide safe, timely and effective care to patients while avoiding unnecessary hospital attendances and admissions. Aimed at providing a whole-systems approach to care crossing the primary and secondary care interface, the emergency care practitioner (ECP) is an initiative that is focused on expanding the existing knowledge and expertise of a range of qualified health care professionals drawn from a range of clinical backgrounds including nurses, ambulance paramedics, physiotherapists, occupational therapists and pharmacists. Focused on enhancing the patient's experience and providing care that is patient-focused rather than system-focused, it is aimed at enabling ECPs to make autonomous decisions based on sound clinical assessment and judgement, and to complete episodes of care in a range of settings, including the out-of-hospital setting when it is safe and appropriate to do so, and to arrange appropriate referrals when it is not (O'Shea, 2003).

Trauma nurse coordinators

An organised approach to the care of trauma patients should extend beyond the pre-hospital and resuscitation room phases of their care and into the intensive, acute and rehabilitative phases. This coordinated response is essential to maximise the chances of survival and to work towards achieving a positive patient outcome. In many instances, however, this coordinated approach becomes somewhat fragmented, particularly when several disciplines and specialties are involved. It is here that the benefits of a 'trauma nurse coordinator' (TNC) are evident.

As an integral member of the trauma team, the trauma nurse is superbly placed to act as the patient's advocate and to ensure that all team members are working together in the best interests of the patient. Aimed at coordinating all decisions affecting the trauma patients through their admission, the TNC should work towards ensuring that optimal care is provided (Box 40.4). To date, the majority of trauma units and receiving

---

Box 40.4 Role of the trauma nurse coordinator

Provision of optimal care through:
- Coordination of care, clinical activities and teamwork
- Education of staff
- Continuous professional development
- Continuous quality assurance
- Delivery of clinical effectiveness through evidence-based practice

---

emergency departments do not have such a post embedded within their clinical structure or clinical establishment, often as a consequence of financial constraints. Despite a lack of scientific evidence in this country to support such an initiative, the TNC role appears to be gaining increasing favour (Dekeyser et al., 1993; Von Rotz et al., 1994; McInulty, 1998). This is mainly in recognition of the fact that effective links between trauma units, emergency departments and staff caring for trauma patients later in their progress are known to lead to more coordinated care, reduced complication rates, shorter hospital stays and greater satisfaction for patients and their families.

MODELS OF SERVICE DELIVERY

Minor injury units

Minor injury units first came into being in the early 1990s, the first nurse-led units emerging at the Western General Hospital in Edinburgh and Treliske, Cornwall. The former was developed as a consequence of an emergency department closure and the latter due to geographical distance from the local emergency department. Both served the needs of populations with considerable minor injury presentations, relying heavily on the use of clinical protocols and strong clinician input.

The subject of a 2-year independent review of the service conducted by Heaney and Paxton (1997), the Western General Unit emerged as successful, with 98% of patients seen citing their treatment as satisfactory. A total of 18% of patients attending were found to have been referred to the emergency department with cost comparisons favourable for similar London-based services.

Over the years, the Cornish MIU service has since expanded with a number of MIUs adopting a similar model (Wootton et al., 2000). Further models also existed, including the London model, which consisted of minor treatment centres (MTCs) based in four central London sites. These differed in that they had a predominantly primary care focus, although minor injuries accounted for 60% of their attendances (Darkins et al., 1996).

In a review of minor injuries services extending over 300 British units, Cooke et al. (2000) analysed the degree of on-site senior medical presence to support them. Their findings revealed that, of the 67% who responded to a postal questionnaire, 67% reported medical responsibility as lying with a general practitioner, and only 22% with emergency department clinicians. Only 15% had permanent medical presence on site, despite the main service provider being the reported main care provider in nearly half of the responses. This trend in a lack of medical presence has subsequently been addressed though the use of technology, with a number of MIUs adopting the concept of telemedicine and communication technology to support practitioners, to reduce waiting times, and to facilitate safe and effective practice.

Walk–in centres

The Department of Health first announced walk-in centres in April 1999 as an initiative to support patient access to primary care. Designed to offer fast access to health advice and treatment, they are open to anyone on a drop-in basis, providing minor treatments, information about local health services and self-help advice. In its national evaluation of walk-in centres, the Department of Health identified such units as delivering a high quality of care and increased accessibility for some groups who had not previously accessed primary care. In addition to the core services provided, a number of walk-in centres also focus on particular areas of need, for example, work with refugees and those suffering with mental health problems.

Primary care centres

Alternative models for the delivery of care for minor illnesses and injuries can be found in primary care centres organised and run by primary care trusts (PCTs). Here, care is delivered in facilities centred around the primary care domain and out-of-hours organisations rather than being situated within traditional hospital settings. Likely to be staffed by a variety of health care professionals, including emergency nurse practitioners, emergency care practitioners and general practitioners working in concert, they have for the most part been met with enthusiasm and acceptance by practitioners and patients alike.

Emergency departments

Throughout the UK, most large teaching hospitals and district general hospitals (DGHs) that serve a population in excess of 300 000 are required to maintain functional resuscitation facilities ready to receive both trauma patients and those suffering medical or surgical emergencies throughout the 24-hour period. Such facilities include access to advanced diagnostics, such as computerised tomography scanning and magnetic resonance imaging. Such departments are increasingly supported by teams, such as 'critical care outreach' teams, who offer a service to assist in the stabilisation and transfer of critically ill or injured patients, and the identification and management of those identified as being at risk.

Tasked with the responsibility for providing evidence-based care to vulnerable and often critical patients, such units are expected to participate in trauma audits and benchmarking exercises through which comparisons can be made both locally and nationally, looking in particular at the quality of care delivered and clinical outcomes. The Trauma Audit Research Network (TARN), a voluntary national outcomes audit that produces severity-adjusted hospital case fatality rates following admission with severe trauma, is one such initiative involving 50% of trauma hospitals (Box 40.5). Upon participating in the database, they are given their own identifiable data, presented in the context of the performance of anonymised peers. Trauma patients admitted to hospital who meet at least one of the following inclusion criteria – admitted for more than 72 hours, admitted to the intensive care unit or high dependency area, died in hospital, or transferred to another hospital for further emergency care –

> **Box 40.5   The Trauma Audit Research Network: the clinical audit loop**
>
> ● Agreed trauma care standards
> ● Collect an agreed trauma dataset
> ● Analyse
> ● Report to clinicians and managers to improve delivery of trauma
> ● Review trauma standards
> ● Reaudit

may be included in the database. Formerly known as the Major Trauma Outcome Study (MTOS), TARN is the vehicle through which such activities are coordinated, lessons learned and best practice shared (Trunkey, 1983; American College of Surgeons Committee on Trauma, 1986; Yates et al., 1992; Nicholl and Turner, 1997; Royal College of Surgeons of England, 2000; Lecky 2002; Lecky et al., 2002).

Alternative pathways of care

In support of initiatives occurring within emergency departments, many other health care agencies are developing alternative ways of treating patients in the community, thus minimising referrals to the emergency department. Through rapid assessment of patients' health and social care needs, it is intended that appropriate care is supported in the community through the development of multiagency and multidisciplinary 'treat and refer' protocols, as an alternative to hospital admission. In developing such alternatives to admission, account also needs to be taken of the substantial benefits of telemedicine to such initiatives.

Alternative care pathways can deliver more streamlined access to care end points in primary and social care. These include a reduction in referral to emergency departments and subsequent admissions to hospital; a reduction in hospital attendances and, as a result, improved trolley waits and NHS waiting times; a reduction in unnecessary visits for primary and other health/social care workers; and a reduction in unnecessary responses by ambulance services. Such projects take account of a focus on prevention rather than 'future crises', the development

of multiagency approaches to patient assessment and staff development, delivery of the NHS Plan and National Service Frameworks, delivery of 'Information for health' initiatives, including access to electronic health records, patients' services tailored to individual needs that support the 'independence' agenda, development of and integration with NHS Direct, and development of new practitioners in out-of-hospital emergency care.

In any health care encounter, the final outcome is often largely determined by actions taken at the outset. This is obviously important in emergency and trauma situations, and is particularly true in other situations. Alternative care pathways, therefore, support a more modern response, and take advantage of available opportunities incorporating real-time information management and technology systems to deliver suitable, safe and consistent alternatives to hospital admission. In developing these alternatives, account is taken of current referral patterns. There is much to improve in delivering a more modern service designed to reduce the need for admission by identifying the potential for future crises earlier than is possible at the moment.

> Alternative care pathways deliver safe and consistent alternatives to hospital admission

Using information held on electronic clinical records (ECRs), it is intended that decisions regarding the most appropriate time, location, type and source of care for patients will be made through real-time consultation with appropriate involved care providers, either in person or via 'virtual care centres'. These care packages may include admission, health care advice, medical or social care at home, mental health referral or other appropriate dispositions. In turn, when required, these could be supported by remote monitoring systems using telemedicine in the home. The process may be analysed under the headings of initiation, triage, action plan and disposition as shown below.

Initiation and triage
Anyone attending a call for help should be able to initiate a process that will, with appropriate

support, lead to appropriate and consistent triage processes. It is expected that the triage process could be delivered by a number of different carers, including: individuals alone (e.g. GPs, district nurses); individuals using decision support software (e.g. nurses, health care providers); those working with others through the virtual care centre (virtual case conference); or groups of people working together with or without the virtual care centre.

Action plan and virtual care centre

Virtual care centres (VCCs) could provide the core of the service. Those initiating the process of contact, triage and action plan development may contact the VCC, which would be responsible for either giving the appropriate advice, accessing the electronic clinical record if remote access is not available, and for setting up virtual case conferences with appropriate agencies. It is possible that the VCCs could utilise on-call practitioners from agencies to contribute to any care conference, if those who have personal knowledge of patients are unavailable in the required time frame.

Using current technologies, those involved will, if required, be able to communicate using telephone, multiparty telephone conferencing and telemetry of ECRs. In addition, existing systems could support case conferences through video links and remote vital sign monitoring with telemetry, for example, 12-lead electrocardiograms (ECGs).

Disposition

It is anticipated that, by utilising the decision pathways outlined above, a significant number of patients will be empowered to remain at home, given an appropriate package of care delivered in a timely fashion. Any agencies may be involved; it is important that, for the concept to succeed, all those involved understand, accept and acknowledge the roles of the other agencies concerned. Thus, for example, a mental health team might be required to act on an action plan initiated by another health care provider and where the GP may not have been directly involved, rather than accepting direct referrals from GPs only. Another example is patients requiring admission to hospital being directed straight to a ward rather than spending time in assessment units or emergency departments before a bed is found.

It can be seen, therefore, that new ways of working, alternative care pathways and new style practitioners can significantly impact upon care delivered out of hospital in emergency situations, including minor trauma, with a resultant reduction in pressure on emergency departments and hospital beds.

PROFESSIONAL DEVELOPMENT OF THE TRAUMA NURSE – THE WAY AHEAD

The educational dimension: a toolkit for change

Over the last decade, many factors have accelerated nursing role developments in a number of health care environments and across numerous specialities. These include an increasing evidence base in relation to effective care delivery, government commitment to interprofessional working and new role development, advances in medical and other technologies, a heightened emphasis on improving service quality, developments in primary care, and changes in the medical and paramedical workforce. It is also evident that, when new roles are developed jointly with medical and other colleagues, and where competence is acquired and maintained through appropriate practice experience and supportive education programmes, significant benefits accrue to patients, practitioners and the service as a whole (Dowling et al., 1996; Hopkins, 1996; Read et al., 1998).

> Autonomous practice involves having the power to make decisions, to act upon them and to take responsibility for them

Many nurses who reshape their practice and expand their sphere of authority increasingly share a skill base with medical and other clinical colleagues. At first, many embarking on new roles at the edge of their traditional boundaries cite a range of emotions and concerns with which they must come to terms. These include uncertainty, unknown and unexpected challenges, the potential for confrontation, lack of understanding of their role by others, and confusion and role ambiguity.

> **Box 40.6   Toolkit for autonomous practice**
>
> - Advanced clinical assessment skills
> - Ability to prescribe or administer medicines without recourse to medical staff, e.g. independent prescribing rights or patient group directions
> - Ability to request diagnostic tests and investigations, e.g. pathology and radiology
> - Autonomous clinical decision-making skills
> - Knowledge of boundaries of own practice and when to refer to other agencies

> **Box 40.7   Benefits of competency standards and professional accreditation**
>
> - Patients receive the same explicit standards of care across the UK
> - There is an explicit, identifiable career structure within nursing
> - The impact of nursing care can be demonstrated
> - Transferability of skills across the UK is facilitated
> - A model for lifelong learning, and practice and professional development is provided
> - Organisations are provided with prerequisites for effective patient-centred, evidence-based services

> The authority, and consequent autonomy, of 'advanced nurses' is derived from a sound educational base to practice and the ability to apply theoretical concepts to the provision of high-quality care

To overcome such concerns, it is essential that those undertaking new roles or expanding their practice into as yet uncharted territory are adequately prepared, having received the necessary education and competence to be both safe and effective practitioners (Box 40.6). In support of a competency-based approach to care, a number of frameworks are starting to evolve across the various disciplines, including those devised by the Royal College of Nursing Faculty of Emergency Nursing, and Skills for Health. Not without its critics, proponents of the competency-based approach cite the development of national, transferable standards, a national education framework, public protection and securing the confidence of consumers among its major benefits (Box 40.7). The adoption of individual clinical competence rather than titular frameworks as the basis for practice is also seen as an important benefit, and as a structured and meaningful step towards true, multidisciplinary, multiprofessional working.

Emergency and trauma nurses are increasingly expanding their practice and their nursing role to incorporate some of the skills of their medical colleagues. This has the benefit of offering patients wider access to services through making clinical diagnoses, and referring patients for care and treatment based on their own decisions as practi-

tioners. These attributes, combined with a generally heightened interest in their role, have caused many 'advanced' nurses to consider their vulnerability. Such nurses may consider themselves vulnerable and exposed because they constantly manage clinical uncertainty and undertake innovative practice. Legally, this vulnerability may be associated with fear of litigation; however, this must be considered in the light of vicarious liability, whereby employers are, generally speaking, the persons sued if things go wrong. Emergency and trauma nurses, similar to nurse practitioners, therefore, are no more exposed to claims of negligence than other nurses, 'particularly if their practice is underpinned by a comprehensive educational programme which enhances self-awareness and the ability to acknowledge and remedy their limitations' (RCN, 2002: 5).

Clinical governance

Since the Department of Health (1997) introduced clinical governance to the NHS through 'The new NHS: modern, dependable', a lot has changed. The emphasis on clinical care delivery has shifted away from quantity to quality, with the balance of power shifting from the clinical professions to patients. Patients now rightly expect and demand best clinical practice in a setting that is appropriate for that care and in a time frame that gives them the best chance of recovery.

Providing safe and high-quality health care is no longer optional but a statutory obligation, recognised under the Health Act of 1999. Health

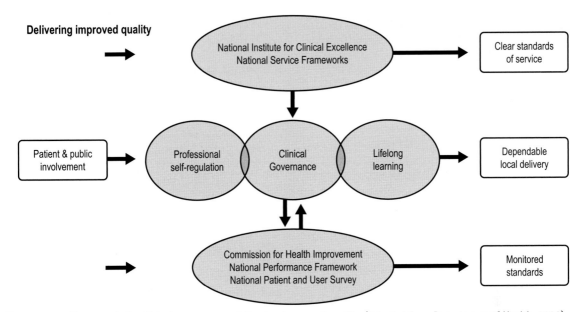

Figure 40.1   Framework for clinical governance: delivering improved quality. (Adapted from Department of Health, 1998).

care organisations and their chief executives are now held accountable for ensuring that clinical governance arrangements are in place, supported within their organisation and make a real difference to patient care. Lack of resources as an excuse to delay progress towards improved care no longer carries the weight it once did, with extra money being passed down through national improvement programmes. Ongoing initiatives to recruit and educate more staff, to break down the demarcation between professional roles and to strengthen patient advocacy are all geared towards ensuring that effective clinical governance becomes a reality.

The documents 'A first class service: quality in the new NHS' (Department of Health, 1998) and 'Clinical governance: quality in the new NHS' (Department of Health, 1999b) both spell out the quality strategy for the NHS for the next 10 years. At the heart of these initiatives is a framework for clinical governance as depicted in Figure 40.1.

Clinical governance affects all NHS Trusts and all departments within them, including the trust board and directorates, and every member of staff concerned with providing patient care including support services. As a consequence, they should implement the guidance published within the above documents. Clinical governance consists of

> **Box 40.8   Components of clinical governance**
>
> - Staffing and management
> - Information management
> - Education and continuing professional development
> - Risk management
> - Patient satisfaction
> - Clinical audit
> - Research

seven main components, namely: staffing and staff management, information management, education and continuing professional development, risk management, patient satisfaction, clinical audit and research (Box 40.8).

With the patient as an equal partner in the process, and using the key components of governance as a foundation, a model known as the 'seven pillars' has been devised to demonstrate the technical and process tools required to deliver effective change. These elements are summarised as clinical effectiveness, risk management effectiveness, patient experience effectiveness, communications effectiveness, resource effectiveness, strategic effectiveness and learning effectiveness (Box 40.9).

> **Box 40.9   The seven pillars of clinical governance**
>
> - Clinical effectiveness
> - Risk management effectiveness
> - Patient experience effectiveness
> - Communications effectiveness
> - Resource effectiveness
> - Strategic effectiveness
> - Learning effectiveness

Clinical governance ensures that both the organisation as a whole and its people are accountable for the clinical quality of the service they provide. Ultimately, accountability for implementing and achieving clinical governance in an organisation lies with the chief executive; however, through professional self-regulation, each member of staff is also accountable for the quality of the service they provide. In support of this, many initiatives have had a significant impact on the delivery of care. Through these, the clinical governance processes that must be put in place to ensure that best practice is delivered can be supported. These initiatives include the following:

- *The Commission for Health Improvement,* which has recently become *The Commission for Healthcare Audit and Inspection,* or the *Healthcare Commission,* as it is commonly called, is tasked with reviewing performance and clinical governance processes across the whole NHS.
- *The NHS Plan,* which sets out clear targets of improvement and service development.
- *Reforming Emergency Care,* a programme of work that will result in great changes in working practice for all those involved in the delivery of emergency care.
- The *National Institute for Clinical Excellence* (NICE), which sets out best practice care pathways for the NHS.
- *Clinical Negligence Scheme for Trusts* (CNST), which ensures that basic risk management processes are in place to ensure that best clinical practice is delivered.
- The *National Patient Safety Agency,* which will

monitor progress and collate adverse clinical events at a national level.

- The *Risk Pooling Scheme for Trust* (RPST) and *Controls Assurance* – structured approaches to both corporate and clinical risks within the NHS.
- The establishment of new ways of governing the activities of health care professions through the Nursing and Midwifery Council (NMC), the General Medical Council (GMC) and the Health Professions Council (HPC).

> Each member of staff is responsible for the clinical quality of the service they provide

The work required to back up the principles and supporting initiatives for clinical governance can be challenging in all areas of care and at all levels of an organisation. It is easy to argue that it is impossible to get more out of people without huge investments in staff and resources. Most people in the NHS are already highly committed, work extremely hard and do the best possible job within the time available to them. Recent high-profile cases, such as that of Bristol (Department of Health, 2001d) have demonstrated, however, that the absence of reflective practice, effective communication and teamwork result in dysfunctional ways of working. In many cases, errors occur as a consequence of organisational systems and processes. Changes in organisational culture and the adoption of an open and supportive reporting system to enable everyone to learn from errors are, therefore, fundamental to the development of robust clinical governance in any NHS organisation.

Electronic clinical records

Nationally and locally, the hardest challenge in health care is the provision of patient-centred integrated services within constrained capacity. This is particularly real in unscheduled care, where each of several organisations separately provide highly intensive, expert and often highly expensive services, but without effective coordination. Information is repeatedly sought but not shared, assessments are made from different standpoints and often the most important decisions about individuals' needs are overcentralised in hospital emergency departments, even when many decisions could be far more speedily and appropriately taken elsewhere: at the scene of an accident, at the patient's home, in a minor injuries or walk-in unit, or at the end of a telephone.

Until now, it has not been possible to obtain clinical information that supports reliable data analysis, benchmarking or continuous clinical improvement, nor can Trusts readily monitor the day-to-day quality of care delivered by their staff. This represents a considerable risk to both patients and Trusts; a discrepancy that needs to be addressed urgently.

Further problems arise when emergency departments receive patients from multiple ambulance services, each of which use different reporting formats. This poses considerable risks with hospital staff becoming confused and not utilising the ambulance clinical records. Major clinical errors can then ensue, as the full picture of the patients' journey is not available. It is recognised by the NHS Litigation Authority (NHSLA) that much of the financial loss incurred as a result of claims against the NHS arises from failures of communication at the point of care 'handover'. The current system, therefore, poses both a clinical threat to patients, and both fiscal and financial ones to the NHS.

In some areas, a number of important but as yet disparate initiatives aim to bring a more coordinated and more appropriate response to unscheduled care in local areas. These include investment in intermediate care teams and walk-in centres, development of integrated care pathways for older people, designated acute medical assessment unit beds and equalising emergency workloads through automated emergency capacity management systems (ECMS). Ambulance services have developed working systems over the past few years, including the use of mobile computers to support the acquisition of clinical records, 12-lead ECGs, increased diagnostic capability with telemedicine links for remote clinician support and, importantly, the potential integration of such systems with other patient records and other health care systems.

What is needed is to bring the learning from these initiatives together to support the rollout of a national system that will see such systems implemented in all emergency care environments including ambulance services. This will, in turn, support the systematic integration of unscheduled care services across the relevant agencies and professions (Box 40.10). This need has recently been recognised by the Department of Health, which in 2003 launched one of the most ambitious information technology programmes ever seen in health care; the programme 'The National Programme for Information Technology' (NPfIT) is run by the NHS Information Authority and will provide the framework and infrastructure for integrated electronic care records for all patients in every sector of health care.

E-HEALTH – THE ADVENT OF TECHNOLOGY ENABLED CARE

The NHS of the future will be driven by technologies that will make geographical history

Revolutions within the computer and technology industry have had a profound effect on the way nursing is practised and health care delivered. One area where this is apparent is that of telemedicine. From a clinical perspective telemedicine, defined as 'medicine at a distance' (Wootton, 1996), combines computer and communications technology with medical expertise. From a technological perspective, it is simply a multimedia extension of the telephone advice that has been part of clinical practice for many years.

Telemedicine is not a new concept. In existence for decades, it can best be described as combining computer and telecommunications technology with medical expertise from locations remote to patients and their nurses. Indeed, it has existed for such a length of time that the terminology has changed, and is now often referred to as e-health. Neither the name nor the technology of e-health/telemedicine is important; what is important, however, is the way in which e-health as a tool can be applied to support, enable and advance nursing practice, whilst preserving autonomy with appropriate and timely clinical support.

Box 40.10 Benefits of electronic care records

- More seamless response, delivery of treatment and improved outcomes in unscheduled care, leading to shorter waits at the key points in the patient's journey
- Consistent assessment and consequent treatment, irrespective of point of entry into the system
- Improved patient choice regarding speed, type and location of care
- Optimisation of treatments by access to a clinical decision support system
- Intermediate care, social care and other community-based services are able to respond to urgent needs, providing practical alternatives to dispatch to emergency departments for ambulance crews or general practitioners
- Faster diagnostic responses to patients using a growing range of telemedicine and teleconferencing facilities to apply expert advice at the point of need
- Reduced clinical risk from electronically supported evidence-based medicine in the home and at accident sites
- Reduction in avoidable deaths from coronary heart disease and other acute life-threatening illnesses
- Reduction in avoidable deaths from accidents

- Reduced pressure on emergency departments and on general practitioners
- Better and safer support mechanisms for front-line staff, including:
  - early warning to emergency departments and coronary care/stroke units from ambulance services
  - pre-hospital thrombolysis
  - evidence-based medicine at the bedside helping to deliver consistent, safe and effective care
  - online decision/pathway support, particularly for acute and complex medical histories
  - online advice (virtual case conferences)
- Modernised and improved training for front-line staff, such as the development of emergency care practitioners, building major bridges of coworking between nurses in emergency departments, walk-in centres, minor injuries units and ambulance staff
- Early local evidence of improved emergency care to illustrate national policy, from bringing together acute services, ambulance services, NHS Direct, intermediate care, and primary and social care services
- The provision of comparable data for use in benchmark audits, research and risk management

Telemedicine can be defined as the combination of computer and telecommunications technology with remote medical expertise

Perednia (1997) identified five essential requirements for effective e-health, the absence of which can limit its effectiveness. These are distance, data, telecommunications, an expert to interpret the data and the ability to effect care (Box 40.11). Distance may be social, such as reduced access to health care facilities, as well as geographic, although the majority of e-health systems that have been implemented have occurred as a direct consequence of travelling distances for both patient and clinician. To be effective, the data needs to be of adequate quality and quantity for an expert to provide an opinion. Telecommunications could be as simple as a functional facsimile machine; however, as technology continues to advance rapidly, for example, increasing broadband availability, larger quantities of data can be

Box 40.11 Essential prerequisites for effective e-health

- Location affecting access to health care
- Quality and quantity of data provided
- Functional telecommunication system
- Clinical expert to interpret data
- The ability to effect delivery of care

transmitted quickly, thereby reducing telecommunication charges. Finally, for e-health to be effective, an identified and available expert is essential and, of equal importance, an individual to deliver the suggested management plan. If either the expert or teleconsultant is unavailable, or the nurse is unable to deliver the prescribed care, then e-health may be seriously compromised.

A sixth requirement could also be added, namely, the need to look at the way in which e-health can impact upon health care delivery at a macro level. In its early inception, telemedicine, as it was then referred to, was implemented for the sake of technology rather than in response to clinical need. This quickly limited the efficacy of the service, with technology rapidly changing and soon becoming obsolete.

In considering the merits of using and investing in telemedicine, for example, installing a videoconferencing system to support a minor injuries unit, clear justification of the clinical need, both financially and strategically, is required. The long-term future of the technology system in question needs also to be addressed. In the videoconferencing scenario, for example, the potential for the technology to provide links for 'virtual tutorials' to facilitate teaching sessions between emergency nurse practitioners and A&E consultants would need to be explored. The potential for professional isolation to ensue rapidly, particularly in remote units, is all too real, particularly where links are ill maintained. Integration of the system with existing technology, including maintenance and upgrading facilities is, therefore, vital in determining success. Scalability of the service itself is similarly important. Image capturing devices may be useful in managing wounds, for example, in dermatology, as they can support nursing workload, a large percentage of which is due to wound care, particularly in minor injury units.

> Integration of telemedicine systems with existing technology is essential

E-health in practice

E-health essentially consists of two components: 'videoconferencing' and 'store-and-forward'. *Videoconferencing* permits a two-way sound and vision teleconsultation, enabling nurses to seek immediate access to clinicians for expert advice, while *store-and-forward* enables them to capture, store and refer a range of images electronically to an identified expert on a routine basis.

Videoconferencing
Essentially combining telephone and video technology, videoconferencing enables voice and vision links between two or more parties. This real-time access is particularly beneficial when urgent clinical opinions are required. Not only the patient and referrer, but also the specialist must be available simultaneously. Practical examples in the use of the videoconferencing option include management of acute clinical episodes, such as bony injuries, acute wound management and skin rashes. Real-time access to emergency specialist opinion can, therefore, be particularly useful in the management of a range of minor injuries. Tele-radiological links using relatively low technology, such as document-scanning equipment for the first-line management of bony injuries, can be achieved with high levels of diagnostic agreement (Tachakra et al., 1996). Tele-radiological systems that facilitate nurse requesting of radiological tests, which are in turn interpreted by emergency department or orthopaedic clinicians, offer efficient and rapid services for radiology reporting. Although this has been shown to be the primary use of e-health/telemedicine in minor injury units today, the potential use of videoconferencing provides a valuable medium for group clinical supervision within a network of ENPs, including links for training and education.

Store-and-forward
Store-and-forward involves the capture and storage of clinical data for later review by specialists. This deferred technique, which has been used in a variety of specialities when non-urgent clinical opinions are sought, eliminates the need for both the referrer and expert to be available simultaneously, which may be an advantage over videoconferencing. The clinical data may consist of multimedia electronic files, such as text, digital stills and moving images, audio clips or radiology images stored on storage devices such as servers. These files can then be accessed at a later date for review and consultation before being transmitted back to the referrer.

Practical examples of the capabilities offered by the store-and-forward option include digital image capture of acute and chronic wounds, enabling nurses to communicate electronically with emergency department clinicians or dermatologists for wound management treatment and advice. This can be particularly useful for patients being followed up in the minor injury unit or fracture clinic setting. Digital images of almost any anatomical areas, for example, the retina in diabetic patients, could be used to support the work of nurse practitioners in the primary care setting.

The concept of using telemedicine to support nurses is relatively new in the UK (Darkins et al., 1996; Tachakra et al., 1996). Yet to be formally evaluated in terms of its benefits to nurses, both videoconferencing and store-and-forward offer nurses a network of expertise within their present referral environment, and enable access to clinical expertise beyond their geographical boundaries (MacLean, 1996). In essence, it offers the notion of a natural community moving towards a virtual health care system where medical services are 'traded' in a broader and more efficient health care environment. Consultations could involve nurses accessing specialist opinions from distant experts by transmitting the patient's medical history (either in voice or text), medical images (e.g. rash or mole), laboratory test results and other clinical information. Specialists could then conduct 'virtual clinics' with several 'stored' cases, review these cases on their computers, and send opinions and management plans electronically to the nurses' computers.

Despite this, the adoption of such technology has been slow to evolve. For example, within 25 minor injury units and minor treatment centres in the Greater London region in 2001 seeing between 150 and 1950 attendances each month, few utilised telemedicine support. Of these, five replaced emergency departments, nine were stand-alone units/centres, 11 were coterminus with emergency departments and six were integral to the general emergency service provision.

Current and future developments

Health care in the future will undoubtedly continue to evolve at a remarkable rate. Indeed, the electronic era has already begun to exert its influence, and is integral to all but a few developments and advances. A number of successful nurse-led innovations have already been established, with the proposed expansion in the number of walk-in centres and primary care centres providing scope for further innovation and expanded access to health care. Staffed by

nurse practitioners, such units have a wide remit, managing patients with primary care issues as well as those with chronic diseases. Frequently nurse-led with little if any on-site medical support and geographically located within the community to improve access, they provide a range of health care services designed to meet the needs of the local community. It is anticipated that, as the scope of nursing practice expands further, the absence of permanent medical support may increasingly lead some walk-in centres and primary care centres to adopt e-health to support clinical practice.

> The absence of medical support is inversely proportional to the uptake of e-health technology

NHS Direct, the national nurse-led helpline, designed to provide support and advice for those telephoning a local rate number, has experienced a meteoric rise. Not without its critics, it has developed to provide UK-wide coverage in less than 4 years. Now with an interactive website and associated healthcare guide, its aim is to provide information and advice to individuals on a wide variety of health problems, the premise being that a proportion may be managed with self or home care. Nurses undertaking this role utilise national, evidence-based clinical decision support guidelines and associated software to guide their consultations, with a view to providing safe and effective care and positive outcomes. Viewed by some as the largest telemedicine project in the world, NHS Direct (and NHS24, its Scottish equivalent) continues to evolve amid studies investigating its use and the use of interactive television to add visual images and interactivity to this 'remote consultation' for greater clinical effectiveness (Box 40.12).

Allied health professionals

A range of health care professionals other than nurses have delivered out-of-hospital care for years. The role of the paramedic has changed rapidly over the years with academic qualifications now underpinning advanced clinical practice and life support skills. Ambulance paramedics provide mobile intensive therapy units, providing vital care to those seriously ill or injured, as well

Box 40.12   Benefits of equipping nurses with e-health support

- Increased autonomy and skill base
- Integration of nurse and clinician electronic patient records
- Development of clinical governance, including quality assurance and audit
- Patients receiving care from within a holistic nursing paradigm
- Reduced patient anxiety and travelling time
- Reduced waiting times for secondary care consultations
- Reduced clinician travelling time
- Appropriate use made of clinician time
- Utilisation of standards/proformas
- Development of evidence-based nursing/health care practice

as immediate medical treatment, such as the delivery of thrombolytic therapy to those who have suffered myocardial infarction (Roth et al., 1990; GREAT Group, 1992; Weaver et al., 1993; Foster et al., 1994; Grijseels et al., 1995; Department of Health 2000a, 2000b). Clinical decision support systems (CDSS), combined with ECG transmission technology, aim to reduce 'door to needle' and more recently 'pain to needle times' to within recommended time frames for such patients, improving clinical outcomes and overall prognosis (Freeman, 1999; Cox, 2002). Additionally, videoconferencing has been utilised by some ambulance trusts to provide real-time access to emergency department clinicians supervising life-saving procedures at the scene of accidents (Curry and Harrop, 1998).

Recommendations from the Joint Royal Colleges Ambulance Liaison Committee (JRCALC, 2000) suggested a role for a practitioner in emergency care (PEC), the aim of which was to provide a generic health care worker able to engage in cross-boundary working to improve and facilitate access to patient care, while enhancing the role and future career progression of paramedics. The need for a 'seamless' transition between the out-of-hospital and in-hospital settings was also seen as being fundamental to this role. The JRCALC recommendations also proposed that health care

professionals undertaking this role underwent an intensive university-based educational programme extending over 3 years, encompassing core elements, with a number of pre-hospital care components focusing on clinical skill acquisition. Intended for nurses as well as ambulance paramedics and technicians, the growing trend towards a recognised academic basis for paramedic training and recognition of the paramedic as a professional in their own right gave substance to this diversion from traditional pre-hospital practice, and paved the way for a new education platform and career pathway. This new breed of health care professional was also seen as being able to provide holistic and thorough assessment of patients on scene, supported by clinical decision support systems and/or e-health technologies where possible, and to make appropriate referral decisions. This PEC model has since evolved and has in fact become the cornerstone of development for emergency care practitioners.

CONCLUSION

The unprecedented pace of change seen in the NHS makes it reasonable to assume that the role developments already seen in nursing are likely to continue, including changes that have increased the skills and decision-making capacity required of its practitioners. There is also little doubt that e-health technologies can work harmoniously with present practice policies and procedures, and that they are ideally placed to support the increasing array of initiatives embraced by the NHS in recent years. Providing a seamless extension to support and complement existing health care delivery systems, including new ways of working and the development of new professional roles, e-health technologies must be congruent with existing technologies and modalities.

Facilities should be established to enable nurses to refer patients directly to minor injury units and walk in centres, and to wards and departments within acute hospital settings, a practice that is not yet commonplace. Telecommunication technologies provide an avenue designed to enable nurses and allied healthcare professionals to provide improved health care services for their patients, ensuring that, as far as possible, the right care is delivered to patients in the right place at the right time and by the right person.

Most nurses have no wish to practise medicine, but to practise nursing in the fullest sense and aim to work in collaboration, rather than competition, with their medical colleagues. To further develop the philosophy of nurse-led care and autonomous practice, the implementation and development of an e-health facility is required. Linking expert nurses and health care professionals to geographically distant clinicians can deliver high-quality health care to patients, when and where it is required.

References

Ambulance Service Association. *National electronic care records project.* Ambulance Service Association, 2004

American College of Surgeons Committee on Trauma. Hospital and prehospital resources for optimal care of the injured patient. *American College of Surgeons Bulletin* 1986; 77: 4–12

Cooke M, Higgins J, Bridge P. Minor injury services – the present state. *Emergency Nurse* 2001; 9: 12–16

Cox H. Transmission of a 12-lead electrocardiograph via telemedicine: a pilot study. *Nursing in Critical Care* 2002; 7: 7–14

Curry CR, Harrop N. The Lancashire telemedicine ambulance. *Journal of Telemedicine and Telecare* 1998; 4: 231–238

Darkins A, Dearden CH, Rocke LG, Martin JB, Sibson L, Wootton R. An evaluation of a telemedical support for a Minor Treatment Centre. *Journal of Telemedicine and Telecare* 1996; 2: 93–99.

Department of Health. *Report of the Advisory Group on Nurse Prescribing: the Crown Report.* London: HMSO, 1989

Department of Health. *NHS and Community Care Act.* London: HMSO, 1990

Department of Health. *The new NHS: modern, dependable.* 1997

Department of Health. *A first class service: quality in the new NHS.* London: HMSO, 1998

Department of Health. *Making a difference: strengthening the nursing, midwifery and health visiting contribution to health and health care.* London: HMSO, 1999a

Department of Health. *Clinical governance: quality in the new NHS.* London: HMSO, 1999b

Department of Health. *Coronary heart disease. National service framework.* London: HMSO, 2000a

Department of Health. *The NHS Plan. A plan for investment, a plan for reform.* London: HMSO, 2000b

Department of Health. *Reforming emergency care.* London: HMSO, 2001a

Department of Health. *Shifting the balance of power.* London: HMSO, 2001b

Department of Health. *Liberating the talents.* London: HMSO, 2002a

Department of Health. *Making a difference: reducing burdens in hospitals.* London: HMSO, 2002b

Department of Health. *Items prescribable by nurses through the Nurse Prescriber's Extended Formulary.* London: HMSO, 2002c

Department of Health. *Learning from Bristol: The Department of Health's response to the Report of the Public Inquiry into children's heart surgery at the Bristol Royal Infirmary 1984–1995.* London: HMSO, 2002d

Department of Health. *National programme for information technology.* London: HMSO, 2003

Dekeyser FG, Paratore A, Camp L. Trauma nurse co-ordinator: three unique roles. *Nursing Management* 1993; 24(12): 56A, 56D, 56H.

Dowling S, Martin R, Skidmore P, Doyal L, Cameron A, Lloyd S. Nurses taking on junior doctors' work: a confusion of accountability. *British Medical Journal* 1996; 312: 1211–1214

Drury M, Greenfield S, Stilwell B, Hull FM. A nurse practitioner in general practice: patient perspectives and expectations. *Journal of the Royal College of General Practitioners* 1988; November: 503–505

Endacott, et al. *RCN Faculty Project*, 1999.

Foster B, Dufendach J, Barkoll C, Mitchell B. Pre-hospital recognition of AMI nurse/paramedic 12-lead ECG evaluation impact on in-hospital times to thrombolysis in a rural community hospital. *American Journal of Emergency Medicine* 1994; 12: 25–31

Freeman S. Direct transmission of electrocardiograms to a mobile phone for management of a patient with acute myocardial infarction. *Journal of Telemedicine and Telecare* 1999; 5: 67–69

GREAT Group. Feasibility, safety and efficacy of domiciliary thrombolysis by general practitioners: Grampian Region EArly Thrombolysis (GREAT) trial. *British Medical Journal* 1992; 305: 548–553

Grijseels E, Bouten M, Lenderink T, et al. Pre-hospital thrombolytic therapy with either alteplase or streptokinase. Practical applications, complications and long term results in 529 patients. *European Heart Journal* 1995; 16: 1833–1838

Hadfield-Law L, Kent A, McInulty L. Role of the trauma nurse. In: *ABC of major trauma.* London: BMJ, 2000: 93–98

Heaney D, Paxton F. Evaluation of nurse-led minor injuries units. *Nursing Standard* 1997; 12: 35–38

Hopkins A, Solomon J, Abelson J. Shifting boundaries in professional care. *Journal of the Royal Society of Medicine* 1996; 89: 364–371

Joint Royal Colleges Ambulance Liaison Committee. *The future role and education of paramedic ambulance service personnel (emerging concepts)*. Joint Royal Colleges Ambulance Liaison Committee, 2000

Jordan S. Nurse practitioners, learning from the USA experience: a review of the literature. *Health & Social Care* 1993; 2: 173–185

Lecky FE. Trauma care in England and Wales: Is this as good as it gets? *Emergency Medical Journal* 2002; 19: 488–489

Lecky FE, Woodford M, Bouamra O, Yates DW. Lack of change in trauma care in England and Wales since 1994. *Emergency Medical Journal* 2002; 19: 1–3

Lindley-Jones M, Finlayson BJ. Triage nurse requested X-rays – are they worthwhile? *Journal of Accident and Emergency Medicine* 2000; 17(2): 103–107

Macduff C, West B, Harvey S. Telemedicine in rural care part 1: developing and evaluating a nurse-led initiative. *Nursing Standard* 2001a; 15(32):33–38

Macduff C, West B, Harvey S. Telemedicine in rural care part 2: assessing the wider issues. *Nursing Standard* 2001b; 15(33): 33–37

MacLean JR. Telemedicine and the nurse: the benefit of burden of new technology? *Journal of Telemedicine & Telecare* 1996; 2(1): 54–55

Macleod AJ, Freeland P. Should nurses be allowed to request X-rays in an accident and emergency department? *Archives of Emergency Medicine* 1992; 9(1): 19–22

Manley K. A conceptual framework for advanced practice: an action research project operationalising an advanced practitioner/consultant nurse role. *Journal of Clinical Nursing* 1997; 6: 179–190

Manley K. Organisational culture and consultant nurse outcomes: part 1 organisational culture. *Nursing Standard* 2000a; 14(36): 34–38

Manley K. Organisational culture and consultant nurse outcomes: part 2 nurse outcomes. *Nursing Standard* 2000b; 14(37): 34–38

McInulty L. Trauma nurse co-ordinator – the way forward in trauma care? *A & E Focus* 1998; 8: 3–4

National Prescribing Centre. *Patient Group Directions – a practical guide and framework of competencies for all professionals using PGDs*. National Prescribing Centre, 2004

Nicholl J, Turner J. The effectiveness of a regional trauma system in reducing mortality from major trauma: before and after study. *British Medical Journal* 1997; 315: 1349–1354

Nursing and Midwifery Council. *Code of professional conduct*. London: Nursing and Midwifery Council, 2002

O'Shea RA. National documentation to support development of the Emergency Care Practitioner role. London: NHS Modernisation Agency, Department of Health, 2003

O'Shea RA, McNeil ID. *Consistent integrated response – alternative care pathways*. National Electronic Library for Health, 2002

Perednia DA. Fear, loathing, dermatology and telemedicine. *Archives in Dermatology* 1997; 133: 151–155

Read S, Collins K, McDonnell A, et al. *Exploring new roles in clinical practice*. Sheffield: Sheffield Centre for Health and Related Research, 1998

Roth A, Barbash B, Hod H, et al. Should thrombolytic therapy be administered in the mobile intensive care unit in patients with evolving myocardial infarction? A pilot study. *Journal of the American College of Cardiology* 1990; 15: 932–936

Royal College of Nursing. *Nurse practitioners – an RCN guide to the nurse practitioner role, competencies and programme accreditation*. London: RCN, 2002

Royal College of Surgeons of England. *Report of the working party on the management of patients with major injuries*. London: Royal College of Surgeons of England, 1988

Royal College of Surgeons of England. *Better care for the severely injured*. London: Royal College of Surgeons of England, 2000

Tachakra S, Freij R, Mullett S, Sivakumar A. Teleradiology or teleconsultation for emergency nurse practitioners. *Journal of Telemedicine & Telecare* 1996; 2(1): 56–58

Trunkey DD. Trimodal distribution of death. Trauma. *Scientific American* 1983; 249(2): 20–27

United Kingdom Central Council. *A higher level of practice*. London: UKCC 1999

Von Rotz NP, Yates JR, Schare BL. Application of the case management model to a trauma patient. *Clinical Nurse Specialist* 1994; 8(4) 180–186

Weaver W, Cerqueira M, Haalstrom A, et al. Pre-hospital initiated vs hospital initiated thrombolytic therapy. *Journal of the American Medical Association* 1993; 270: 1211–1216

Wootton R. Telemedicine: cautious welcome? *British Medical Journal* 1996; 313: 1375–1377

Wootton R, McKelvey A, McNicholl B, et al. Transfer of telemedical support to Cornwall from a national telemedicine network during a solar eclipse. *Journal of Telemedicine and Telecare* 2000; 6(1+): 182–186

Yates DW, Woodford M, Hollis S. Preliminary analysis of the care of injured patients in 33 British hospitals: first report of the United Kingdom major trauma outcome study. *British Medical Journal* 1992; 305: 737–740

Further reading

Bullock I, Pottle A. The Nurse Consultant: rhetoric and reality! Personal reflections from one NHS Trust. *Care of the Critically Ill* 2003; 19(1): 18–22

Chiarella M. *The legal and professional status of nursing*. Edinburgh: Churchill Livingstone, 2002

Coopers & Lybrand Health Practice. *Nurse Practitioner Evaluation Project. Final Report: Solutions for Business*. London: NHS Executive, 1996

Cross M. Towards the 'Virtual NHS' – technology brought to heal. *British Journal of Health Care Management* 1998; 4(2): 3–5

Gerrard L, Grant AM, Maclean JR. Factors that may influence the implementation of nurse-centred telemedicine services. *Journal of Telemedicine and Telecare* 1999; 5(4): 231–236

Gerrard L, Grant AM, Maclean JR. *The human resource implications for the nursing profession in developing telemedicine within the NHS*. Unit report number 11. Aberdeen: Health Services Research Unit, University of Aberdeen, 1999

Horrocks S, Anderson E, Salisbury C. Systematic review of whether nurse practitioners working in primary care can provide equivalent care to doctors. *British Medical Journal* 2002; 324: 819–823

Humphris D, Masterson A. *Developing new clinical roles: a guide for health professionals*. London: Churchill Livingstone, 2000

Hunt G, Wainwright P. Expanding the role of the nurse: the scope of professional practice. Oxford: Blackwell Scientific Publications, 1994

Institute of Health Services Management. *Telemedicine and telecare: impact on healthcare*. Oxford, Institute of Health Services Management, 1998

Macduff C, Harvey S. An evaluation of the impact of developing nurse-led treatments for minor injuries in community hospital casualty units. *Nursing Times Research* 2000; 5(4):276–284

Maclaine K. Clarifying higher level roles in nursing practice. *Professional Nurse* 1998; 1(14): 159–163

Nelson R, Schlachta L. Nursing and telemedicine: merging the expertise into 'telenursing'. *Healthcare Information Management* 1995; 9(3):17–22

Royal College of Nursing. *Faculty of Emergency Nursing competence framework*. London: RCN, 1995

Schum C, Humphreys A, Wheeler D, Cochrane MA, Skoda S, Clement S. Nurse management of patients with minor illnesses in general practice: multicentre, randomised controlled trial. *British Medical Journal* 2000; 320: 1038–1043

Skills for Health. *Emergency care national workforce competence framework guide*. Bristol: Skills for Health, 2004

Tripp C, Screaton M, Sharples LD, Kearsley N, Caine N. Development and evaluation of the critical care practitioner role. *Nursing in Critical Care* 2002; 7(5): 227–234

Walsh M. *Nursing frontiers: accountability and the boundaries of care*. Oxford: Butterworth-Heineman, 2000

Watt I. Access to care. In: Cox J, Mungall I (eds) *Rural healthcare*. Oxford: Radcliffe Medical Press, 1999

Woods LP. *The enigma of advanced nursing practice*. Salisbury: Quay Books, Mark Allen Publishing, 2000

Wootton R, Loane M, Mair F, et al. A joint US–UK study of home telenursing. *Journal of Telemedicine and Telecare* 1998; 4(1):83–85

Appendix

APPENDIX CONTENTS

Disease	Organism	Morphology and reservoir	Mode of transmission	Prevention
Acquired immunodeficiency syndrome (AIDS)	Human immunodeficiency virus (HIV)	Humans	By blood, sexual transmission and mother to baby (vertical transmission)	Health education, needle-exchange schemes, safe disposal of sharps, blood and body fluid precautions, safe sex
Anthrax	Bacillus anthracis	Gram-positive spore forming encapsulated rods, which are formed after the organism is shed from the body. Survives in soil for many years and is a significant pathogen in domestic and wild animals	Infection occurs in humans when spores enter abrasions on the skin or are inhaled by the lungs (woolsorters' disease)	Formalin decontamination of animal hides. Strict control of domestic animals and immunisation of veterinary laboratory workers at risk
Argentinian haemorrhagic fever	Junin virus (member of the arenaviruses)	Wild rodents (bush mice) in cornfields	Airborne transmission by dust contaminated with infective excreta from rodents. Also laboratory infections occur and the virus can enter through breaks and abrasions on the skin	Control of rodents and isolation of infected cases. No vaccine available
Aspergillosis	Aspergillus fumigantus, A. flavus and A. niger	Filamentous fungi, which cause opportunistic infections in immunocompromised patients. It occurs widely in the environment, especially in the soil	Inhalation of airborne stages, not person-to-person transmission	None known
Athlete's foot (see ringworm)				
Blastomycosis	Blastomyces dermatitidis	Diamorphic fungus thought to be found in the soil in America and parts of Africa	Inhalation of airborne spores, which causes lung infections sometimes mistaken for tuberculosis. Not person to person transmission	Unknown
Chlamydia	Chlamydia trachomatis	Obligate intracellular parasite found in humans. Causes trachoma, urethritis and other genital tract infections	Sexual transmission, newborns may acquire conjunctival and pneumonic strains during birth from infected mothers	Health and sex education with emphasis on use of condoms during sexual intercourse
Cholera	Vibrio cholerae	Curved Gram-negative rods. Human pathogen with no animal reservoir. Possibility of environmental reservoirs in coastal estuary waters	Ingestion of contaminated water or food	Provision of clean water supply and adequate sewerage disposal. Whole-cell vaccine is available but of limited used. New vaccines are now being developed
CJD (see Spongiform encephalopathies)				
Cold sores	Herpes simplex virus (HSV1)	Humans	Contact with saliva, vesicle fluid	Health education and personal hygiene directed towards the minimising of transfer of infectious material

Disease	Organism	Morphology and reservoir	Mode of transmission	Prevention
Common cold	Coronaviruses	Humans	Respiratory droplets, airborne and direct contact	Improved personal hygiene and use of disposable tissues. Reducing overcrowding in living conditions
	Rhino viruses	Humans, more than 100 serotypes are responsible for the common cold	Respiratory droplet spread	As above
Cryptosporidiosis	Cryptosporidium spp.	Protozoa found in humans, cattle and other domestic animals	Via the faecal–oral route, person-to-person spread. Transmission from infected animals and contaminated water is also important	Water treatment, education in personal hygiene, especially hand hygiene practices. Safe disposal of faeces. Especially from domestic pets. Guidelines required for educational farm visits by groups
Cytomegalovirus (CMV)	Herpes virus 5	Humans, rarely causes symptomatic disease, although infection is nearly universal throughout the world. The presence of antibodies varies in populations from 30–40% in developed countries to 100% in developing countries	Intimate contact with infectious tissues. Found in saliva, urine, semen, cervical secretions, milk, transplacental tissues and across the placenta	Strict hand hygiene after changing nappies of babies and toileting of infants. Screening of blood donations for the immunosuppressed and organ donations
Diarrhoea (antibiotic related)	Clostridium difficile	Gram-positive spore-forming rods found as part of the normal gut flora in humans	Flourishes under selective pressure of antibiotics, can cause pseudomembranous colitis. It may be spread from person to person by the faecal–oral route and contamination of their surrounding environment	Stopping of antibiotics, if possible, and attention to personal hygiene and cleaning of the environment
Diarrhoea (bacterial); other bacteria are also responsible for causing diarrhoeal illness	Escherichia coli	Gram-negative rods found in the gut of humans and animals (cattle)	Spread is by contact and ingestion via the faecal–oral route. It may be food associated and also endogenous spread. Enterotoxigenic E. coli is a common cause of traveller's diarrhoea	Strict attention to personal and environmental hygiene
Diarrhoea (viral)	Rotavirus	Humans	Faecal–oral route and possibly airborne	Improved hygiene and sanitation
	Small, round, structured viruses	Humans	Probably faecal–oral route with possibility of airborne spread	Improved hygiene and sanitation

Disease	Organism	Morphology and reservoir	Mode of transmission	Prevention
Diphtheria	*Corynebacterium diphtheriae*	Gram-positive organism found in the nasopharynx and occasionally on the skin of humans	Spread is by aerosol route	Immunization is effective in areas where herd immunity becomes sufficient to protect whole populations (85% or more). Babies acquire their immunity from their mothers for a few months after birth
Dysentery	*Shigella* sp.	Gram-negative rods whose normal reservoir is humans	Direct or indirect faecal–oral route. By contaminated food and milk	Good food hygiene and personal hygiene. No vaccine is available
Ebola and Marburg disease	Ebola and Marburg viruses (members of the Filoviridae family)	Unknown	Person-to-person spread by direct contact with infected blood and body fluids, including organs and semen	Isolation of individual cases and villages; restrict sexual intercourse until semen is free from the virus
Food poisoning	*Bacillus cereus*	Gram-positive spore-forming rods; a soil organism found in low levels in raw, dried and processed foods	Spores are found on many foods, surviving cooking and improper food storage, which encourages multiplication of vegetative organisms. Infection is acquired by ingestion of the organisms or toxin	Majority of illnesses are short lived and self-limited. Hygenic preparation of food is essential, cooked food should be stored in a fridge and reheated thoroughly before serving
Gas gangrene	*Clostridium perfringens* and other species	Anaerobic Gram-positive spore-forming rods. Part of the normal intestinal flora of humans and animals. The spores and vegetative organisms survive in soil	Infection is by contact either when wounds become contaminated with the patients own faecal flora or with contaminated soil. Food poisoning is caused by ingestion of contaminated food	Gangrene requires rapid intervention with extensive debridement of the wound. Prevention of food poisoning is by hygienic preparation and thorough cooking
Genital herpes	Herpes simplex virus (HSV 2)	Humans	Sexual transmission	Health education and use of condoms during sexual intercourse
Glandular fever (mononucleosis)	Epstein–Barr virus	Humans	Person-to-person spread via saliva	Education on personal hygiene (intimate contact)
Gonorrhoea	*Neisseria gonorrhoea*	Gram-negative organism; human pathogen that may be carried in the genital tract, nasopharynx and anus	Infection is spread by sexual or intimate contact causing pelvic inflammatory disease and salpingitis in women and ophthalmia neonatorum in infants born to infected mothers	Prevention requires education and contact tracing. There is no vaccine available
Hand, foot and mouth disease	Coxsackie virus	Humans	Direct contact with nose and throat discharges, and faeces	Reduce person-to-person contact and promote hand hygiene.

Disease	Organism	Morphology and reservoir	Mode of transmission	Prevention
Hepatitis A	Hepatitus A virus	Humans and rarely other primates, e.g. captive chimpanzees	Person-to-person spread by the faecal–oral route and common source outbreaks related to contaminated food and water	Education in public hygiene, good sanitation and catering practices. Immunoglobulin and immunisation are available
Hepatitis B	Hepatitis B virus (HBV)	Humans	Sexual transmission, via infected blood and vertical transmission from mother to baby across the placenta	Vaccination of health care workers and babies born to mothers who are carriers of the virus. Safe disposal of needles
Hepatitis C	Hepatitis C virus	Humans (the cause of most cases of non-A and non-B hepatitis)	Via blood through contaminated needles, blood transfusion, drug users. Transmission from mother to baby is uncertain	Health education and use of needle-exchange schemes. Screening of blood donations
Hepatitis D (delta hepatitis)	Hepatitis delta virus	Humans, requires HBV to cause infection and either causes a co-infection or may be superimposed upon someone who is a carrier of HBV	Similar to hepatitis B	As for hepatitis B
Hepatitis E	Hepatitis E virus	Humans and primates	Contaminated water and person-to-person spread by the faecal–oral route	Education in personal hygiene and improved sanitation
Impetigo	*Staphylococcus aureus* and *Streptococcus pyogenes*	Gram-positive cocci found in humans and animals associated with them	Self-infection and by direct contact	By attention to hand hygiene and the treatment of carriers in high-risk areas in hospitals
Influenza	Influenza types A and B	Humans, though animals have been thought to act as sources of new subtypes of influenza A	By respiratory droplet spread	Education in public hygiene, especially related to unprotected coughing and sneezing. Immunisation should be offered to those considered to be at particular risk
Lassa fever	Lassa virus (Arenavirus)	Widely distributed over West Africa by wild rodents (bush rat)	By contact with excreta of rodent. Person-to-person spread and laboratory infections occur by contact with infected body secretions	Control of specific rodents. No vaccine is available. Source isolation of infected person
Legionnaires' disease	*Legionella pneumophila*	Gram-negative rods, which are an environmental saprophyte found in water supplies, streams and ponds	Infection is caused by inhalation of contaminated water from showers, air-conditioning, cooling towers, jacuzzis, etc. There is no person-to-person spread	Prevention by maintenance of hot water and air-conditioning systems, particularly in buildings, such as offices, hospitals and hotels. No vaccine is available

Disease	Organism	Morphology and reservoir	Mode of transmission	Prevention
Leprosy (Hansen's disease)	*Mycobacterium leprae*	Aerobic rods found in humans	Droplet spread is aided by the ability of the organism to survive in the environment. Infection requires close prolonged contact through the upper respiratory tract and possibly through broken skin	Education on the availability of drug therapy and detection of cases. Prophylactic BCG vaccination reduces the incidence among contacts of cases
Leptospirosis (Weil's disease)	*Leptospira interrogans*	Finely coiled spirochaetes with hooked ends. A zoonosis: its usual hosts are rodents, bats, cattle, sheep, goats and other domestic animals	Leptospires are excreted in urine and contaminate food and water. Infection occurs either through occupation (sewage workers, farmers, abattoir workers) or by recreation activities on inland waters, e.g. canoeing, windsurfing, etc. on canals, rivers and reservoirs. Organisms may penetrate intact skin and conjunctiva	By early treatment of symptoms with penicillin
Listeriosis	*Listeria monocytogenes*	Gram-positive rods. Enteric organism widely found in nature and survives well in the cold. It enters the food chain when silage is used as manure directly on to vegetables. Also through contamination of soft cheeses, paté, etc. Humans may carry the organism in their gut as part of the normal flora	Infection may be acquired by ingestion and via the placenta to the fetus	Widespread distribution of the organism in nature makes prevention of acquiring the organism difficult. Pregnant women have been advised against eating uncooked food, which is thought to be of particular risk, e.g. coleslaw, paté, soft cheeses and unpasteurised milk
Lyme disease	*Borrelia burgdorgeri*	Finely coiled spirochaetes. A zoonosis transmitted to humans by hard ticks associated with deer	Ticks are found on bracken and in undergrowth and attach to exposed skin. Lyme disease is slowly progressive with 50% of cases having a characteristic skin lesion. Joint pains and fatigue are common	Avoid contact with vectors by using protective clothing for walkers and forestry workers
Marburg disease (see Ebola)				
Measles	Measles virus	Humans	Respiratory droplets	Immunisation

Disease	Organism	Morphology and reservoir	Mode of transmission	Prevention
Meningitis: bacterial	Haemophilus influenzae	Gram-negative rods found in the upper respiratory tract of humans	Person-to-person by the airborne route	Hib vaccine is give to children in the UK and USA
	Neisseria meningitidis	Gram-negative diplococci found in the pharynx of humans. Carriage rates are higher in populations during epidemics	Droplet spread with several immunologically distinct capsular types (A, B, C)	A vaccine is available for types A and C, but ineffective with type B strains. Rifampicin is used for prophylaxis of close contacts
	Streptococcus pneumoniae	Gram-positive diplococci found in the respiratory tract of humans with up to 4% of the population carrying it in small numbers	Droplet spread	A vaccine is available
MOTT (mycobacteria other than tuberculosis)		Aerobic rods ubiquitous in nature. Of the numerous species identified approximately 15 are recognised as being pathogenic to humans	With the exception of skin lesions there is no evidence of person-to-person spread. Host tissue damage and immunodeficiency may predispose to infection	
Mumps	Mumps virus	Humans	Respiratory droplet spread	Immunisation
Necrotising fasciitis	Streptococcus pyogenes (group A Strep.)	Gram-positive cocci found in the upper respiratory tract and on the skin of humans	By airborne droplets and contact spread. Survival in dust may be important	No available vaccine. Education about the method of transmission
Pneumonia	Mycoplasma pneumonia	Found in humans, an important cause of atypical pneumonia	Person-to-person spread by the airborne route	Avoidance of crowded living conditions, especially in institutions
	Streptococcus pneumoniae	Gram-positive coccus organisms found in the respiratory tract of humans, with up to 4% of the population carrying it in small numbers	Transmission is by droplet spread	A vaccine is available (pneumovax) composed of antigens of the most common serotypes
Polio	Poliovirus types 1, 2 an 3	Humans. Genus Enterovirus	Direct contact via the faecal-oral route, contamination of drinking water by sewage	Immunisation; education on the importance of hand hygiene
Prion diseases (see Spongiform encephalopathies)				
Pseudomonas infection	Pseudomonas aeruginosa	Gram-negative rods; opportunistic pathogen widespread in moist environments. A small percentage of people carry the organism as part of their normal gut flora	By direct or indirect contact; endogenous infection may occur in compromised patients	Prevention depends on good aseptic techniques when undertaking invasive procedures, e.g. urinary catheterisation

Disease	Organism	Morphology and reservoir	Mode of transmission	Prevention
Rabies	Rabies virus	Wild and domestic biting mammals, including dogs, foxes, coyotes, wolves, jackals and bats	By the bite or scratch of an infected animal. The virus is found in the saliva of the infected animal	Vaccination of pets, especially dogs and cats, education of the public and immunisation of those whose profession is considered to be in a high-risk group
Respiratory syncytial virus (RSV)	Respiratory syncytial virus	Humans	Respiratory droplet spread	Isolation of children in hospitals is desirable
Ringworm	Dermatophytes	A filamentous fungus invading the surface of keratinised structures of skin, hair and nails. Found in humans rarely in soil or animals	By direct or indirect contact with infected skin scales	Improved skin care, hygiene and frequent cleaning of communal areas, e.g. showers and changing areas in public swimming baths, etc.
Rubella (German measles)	Rubella virus	Humans	By respiratory droplet spread	Immunisation and screening for immunity
Salmonellosis	Salmonella sp.	Gram-negative, non-sporing rods. Widespread in animals in the food chain, affecting especially poultry, eggs, meat, milk and cream	Acquired by ingestion of contaminated food or person-to-person spread by the faecal–oral route	Prevention by education of the need for cooking and handling of food properly. Strict hygiene and sanitation systems
Scabies	Sarcoptes scabiei	Human parasite	By direct skin-to-skin contact; can be sexually acquired. Norwegian scabies is highly transmissible because of the large numbers of mites. Infection occurs 2–6 weeks before itching starts	Education of mode of transmission, need for early diagnosis and proper treatment of patients and contacts. Investigation of contacts and index case
Scarlet fever	Streptococcus pyogenes (group A strep.)	Gram-positive cocci found in the human respiratory tract and skin	Airborne droplet spread and by direct contact	Exclusion of infected people from handling and preparing food
Septicaemia	Streptococcus agalactiae (group B strep.)	Gram-positive cocci; causes neonatal septicaemia and meningitis. Found in the human gut and vagina; carriage rate in pregnant women is 10–30%	Babies acquire the organism from colonised mothers at birth or by contact spread between babies in the nursery after birth	Screening of pregnant women is not reliable but prophylactic antibiotics may be given to babies of carriers
Shingles	Herpes zoster (chickenpox virus)	Humans	Direct contact with vesicle fluid may cause chickenpox	Checking of immune status for pregnant women who do not know if they have previously had chickenpox

Disease	Organism	Morphology and reservoir	Mode of transmission	Prevention
Spongiform encephalopathies (prion diseases)	Scrapie-type agents (slow viruses)	Probably not viruses; their structure and mode of replication is unknown. They contain little or no nucleic acid. A host-coded prion protein is associated with infectivity. Highly resistant to heat, chemical agents and irradiation. Very slow replication with a very long incubation period. These agents infect a variety of mammals, and can be transmitted to cows, mink, cats, mice, etc. When food contains infected material	*Kuru:* from infected human brain by contact during burial rites. *Creutzfeldt–Jakob disease (CJD):* in most cases, unknown. Occasionally transmission is from infected human nerve tissue (brain) by medical or surgical procedures. Familial cases have a possible genetic transmission	Prevention of iatrogenic CJD when genetically engineered growth hormone was introduced. Discarding of surgical instruments used on cases
Staphylococcal diseases:				
- Boils, skin sepsis, post-operative wound infections	*Staphylococcus aureus*	Gram-positive cocci found in humans and animals associated with them. Skin, especially the nose and perineum, with carriage rates higher in hospital patients and staff	Contact spread	Attention to hand hygiene, isolation techniques and treatment of carriers in high-risk areas in hospital
- Methicillin-resistant *Staphylococcus aureus* (MRSA)	As above	As above	As above	Multiple resistance to antibiotics is of concern and antibiotic policies have been developed to address this issue
- Toxic shock syndrome	*Staphylococcus aureus*	Syndrome caused by infection or colonisation with toxin-producing strains	Increased risk in high users of tampons and contraception devices, e.g. diaphragms and vaginal sponges	Education that objects (tampons, sponges, etc.) inserted into the vagina should not be left in place longer than 30 hours. Education of women that, if symptoms of fever, vomiting or diarrhoea occur during menstruation, they should discontinue tampon use immediately and consult a doctor
- Urinary tract infections (UTIs)	*Staphylococcus saprophyticus*	Gram-positive cocci on humans, skin and genitourinary mucosa	UTIs in previously healthy women associated with sexual intercourse, endogenous spread to the urinary tract in colonised women	Urination after intercourse helps to wash the organisms out of the bladder and so prevent infection

Disease	Organism	Morphology and reservoir	Mode of transmission	Prevention
Syphilis	*Treponema pallidum*	Humans	Sexually transmitted, requiring very close contact. It may also be transmitted vertically *in utero* to the unborn child and by blood transfusion	Prevention relies on detection and treatment of cases, contact tracing and serological testing of pregnant women
Tapeworms	Beef and pork tapeworms	Intestinal infection due to adult stage of the tapeworm. Humans are the definitive hosts, with cattle and pigs acting as intermediate hosts	Transmission is by eating raw or undercooked meat from animals infected with larval stages of worms	Adequate cooking of meat. Prevention of human faeces contaminating grazing/feeding areas of cattle and pigs
	Dwarf tapeworm	Small tapeworms. Humans are the main host; insects may act as intermediate hosts	Ingestion of eggs in contaminated food or water	Education in personal hygiene and improved sanitation
	Fish tapeworm	Large tapeworms in fish; humans are the main host; intermediate hosts are snails and fish	Eggs excreted in the faeces mature in water to larval stage in snails and fish. Infection occurs when raw or undercooked fish are eaten by humans	Cooking of fish and improved sanitation
Tetanus (lockjaw)	*Clostridium tetani*	Anaerobic Gram-positive spore-forming rods with the organisms widespread in the soil	Acquired by humans when contaminated soil enters wounds. There is no person-to-person spread	Prevention is readily available and effective in the form of immunisation with toxoid. It is usually given in childhood but, if immunization status of the patient is unknown, toxoid is given in addition to antitoxin
Toxocariasis	*Toxocara canis*	Larvae of roundworm; the eggs are excreted in dog faeces	Ingestion of infective eggs by direct or indirect contact	Improved hygiene and sanitation. Importance of adequate cooking of meat
Tuberculosis	*Mycobacterium tuberculosis*	Aerobic rods, primarily found in humans but in some areas diseased cattle, badgers or other animals	Droplet spread is aided by the ability of the organism to survive in the environment	BCG vaccination is valuable to those who are not exposed to heavy loads of mycobacteria early in life. Contact tracing of close contacts and public health measures. Pasteurisation of milk, and improved living conditions and diet has played a major role in prevention. Testing and slaughter of cattle

Disease	Organism	Morphology and reservoir	Mode of transmission	Prevention
Typhoid and paratyphoid (enteric fevers)	*Salmonella typhi* and *Salmonella paratyphi*	Gram-negative non-sporing rods found in humans. A carrier state may follow acute illness, mild or subclinical infections	Ingestion of contaminated food and water, and by the faecal-oral route	Prevention by education of the need for strict hygiene, sanitation systems and cooking of food adequately
Typhus	*Rickettsia prowazekii*	Parasite of which humans are the reservoir. Associated with unhygienic living conditions in times of war and famine	Not directly person-to-person spread. Infection occurs when lice become infected after feeding on the blood of an infected person with acute typhus fever and excreting the infection in their faeces. In louse-infected communities, humans become infected when they rub the faeces or crushed lice into bites and superficial abrasions of the skin	Improved living conditions with bathing and washing facilities. Insecticides can be used on both clothes and people. Immunisation is possible for susceptible people or groups, e.g. military personnel
Viral haemorrhagic fever (see Argentinian and Bolivian haemorrhagic fevers, Ebola and Marburg disease, and Lassa fever)				
Weil's disease (see Leptospirosis)				
Whooping cough	*Bordetella pertussis*	Gram-negative rods; human pathogen; carriage by healthy individuals is not documented.	Spread is by the airborne route from those already infected with the disease.	Vaccine is administered to young children in three doses with diphtheria and tetanus toxoid.

Index

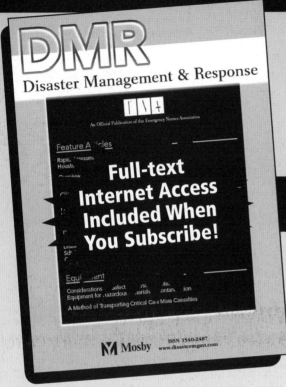
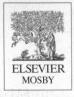
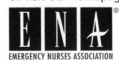